Immunology and Parasitology

Immunology and Parasitology

Editor: Arron Henderson

AMERICAN
MEDICAL PUBLISHERS
www.americanmedicalpublishers.com

AMERICAN
MEDICAL PUBLISHERS
www.americanmedicalpublishers.com

Cataloging-in-Publication Data

Immunology and parasitology / edited by Arron Henderson.
p. cm.
Includes bibliographical references and index.
ISBN 979-8-88740-204-8
1. Immunology. 2. Parasitology. 3. Clinical immunology.
4. Medical parasitology. I. Henderson, Arron.
QR181 .I46 2023
616.079--dc23

American Medical Publishers,
41 Flatbush Avenue,
1st Floor, New York,
NY 11217, USA

ISBN 979-8-88740-204-8 (Hardback)

Contents

Preface

Immunology is a sub field of biology and medicine which studies the immune system. Parasites are the organisms which reside in or on their host and obtain food by harming their hosts. Parasitology, refers to the study of parasites and their hosts, along with the interactions that take place between them. Immunoparasitology is the combination of immunology and parasitology, which studies the immunological interactions that take place between the parasite and the host, along with the immune responses generated by hosts to fight against parasitic infections. One of the primary motivations for investigating parasite resistance is the requirement to comprehend, reduce and eradicate the harm caused by parasites. The host responses to parasites are more than just passive reactions after infection. Different host immune responses indicate different defense methods used by the host for creating protective immunity. Parasites have developed several ways to evade host immune surveillance, such as molecular mimicry and decoys that helps in parasite's survival. This book contains some path-breaking studies in immunology and parasitology. It covers in detail some existent theories and innovative concepts revolving around this domain. This book aims to serve as a resource guide for students and experts alike and contribute to the growth of the disciplines.

This book is a comprehensive compilation of works of different researchers from varied parts of the world. It includes valuable experiences of the researchers with the sole objective of providing the readers (learners) with a proper knowledge of the concerned field. This book will be beneficial in evoking inspiration and enhancing the knowledge of the interested readers.

In the end, I would like to extend my heartiest thanks to the authors who worked with great determination on their chapters. I also appreciate the publisher's support in the course of the book. I would also like to deeply acknowledge my family who stood by me as a source of inspiration during the project.

Editor

1

Protective Efficacy Against Acute and Chronic *Toxoplasma gondii* Infection Induced by Immunization with the DNA Vaccine TgDOC2C

Nian-Zhang Zhang[1]*, Qi Gao[1,2], Meng Wang[1], Jun-Ling Hou[1], Fu-Kai Zhang[1], Ling-Ying Hu[3] and Xing-Quan Zhu[1,4]*

[1] State Key Laboratory of Veterinary Etiological Biology, Key Laboratory of Veterinary Parasitology of Gansu Province, Lanzhou Veterinary Research Institute, Chinese Academy of Agricultural Sciences, Lanzhou, China, [2] Hunan Entry-Exit Inspection and Quarantine Bureau, Changsha, China, [3] Fujian Yongcheng Agricultural and Animal Husbandry Sci-Tech Group, Fuzhou, China, [4] Jiangsu Co-innovation Center for the Prevention and Control of Important Animal Infectious Diseases and Zoonoses, College of Veterinary Medicine, Yangzhou University, Yangzhou, China

***Correspondence:**
Nian-Zhang Zhang
nianzhang919@163.com
Xing-Quan Zhu
xingquanzhu1@hotmail.com

Toxoplasma gondii is a ubiquitous intracellular apicomplexan parasite that can cause zoonotic toxoplasmosis. Effective vaccines against *T. gondii* infection are necessary to prevent and control the spread of toxoplasmosis. The present study analyzed the B-linear epitopes of *T. gondii* DOC2 (TgDOC2) protein and then cloned the C-terminus of the TgDOC2 gene (TgDOC2C) to construct the pVAX-TgDOC2C eukaryotic vector. After intramuscular injection of pVAX-TgDOC2C, immune responses were monitored. Two weeks after the last immunization, the protective effects of pVAX-TgDOC2C against acute and chronic toxoplasmosis were evaluated by challenges with *T. gondii* RH tachyzoites (genotype I) and PRU cysts (genotype II). The DNA vaccine elicited strong humoral and cellular immune responses with high levels of IgG antibody, IL-2 and IFN-γ production compared to those of the controls. The percentage of CD4+ and CD8+ T cells in mice immunized with pVAX-TgDOC2C was significantly increased compared to that of mice injected with empty pVAX I or PBS. After acute infection with 10^3 lethal tachyzoites, mice immunized with pVAX-TgDOC2C survived longer (12.5 days) than mice treated with pVAX I (8 days) and PBS (7.5 days). Mice immunized with pVAX-TgDOC2C had significantly less brain cysts (1600.83 $\pm$ 284.61) compared to mice immunized with pVAX I (3016.67 $\pm$ 153.84) or PBS (3100 $\pm$ 246.98). Together, these results demonstrated that TgDOC2C confers protective immunity against *T. gondii* infection and may be a promising candidate antigen for further development of an effective multicomponent vaccine for veterinary use against toxoplasmosis in livestock animals.

Keywords: *Toxoplasma gondii*, toxoplasmosis, TgDOC2C, DNA vaccine, protective efficacy

INTRODUCTION

Infections by the intracellular parasite *Toxoplasma gondii* are common in all warm-blooded animals, including birds and humans (Dubey, 2008; Innes, 2010; Zhou et al., 2011). If women acquire primary infection with the parasite during gestation, the fetus is at high risk of developing congenital toxoplasmosis that would manifest clinical signs of chorioretinitis, cerebral calcifications, mental retardation and hydrocephalus (Gao et al., 2012; Robert-Gangneux and Dardé, 2012; Aleixo et al., 2016). For immunocompromised individuals, reactivation of latent *Toxoplasma* infection may lead to encephalitis, ophthalmopathy and focal neurological lesions or even fatal damage (Holland, 1989; Pereira-Chioccola et al., 2009; Robert-Gangneux and Dardé, 2012; Wang et al., 2017). Toxoplasmosis in animals can cause heavy economic losses, especially in sheep and goats, arising from miscarriage, stillbirth, and neonatal death (Innes et al., 2009; Gebremedhin et al., 2014). Of more serious concern is the fact that the infected meat-producing animal is considered an important source of infection for humans (Dubey, 2009; Belluco et al., 2017; Pan et al., 2017).

Development of a safe and effective vaccine against *T. gondii* is an attractive option to prevent tissue cyst formation that can improve food safety in meat production (Zhang et al., 2013; Hiszczyńska-Sawicka et al., 2014). A DNA vaccine has elicited strong Th1-bias humoral and cellular immune responses in a mouse model to prolong the survival time after *Toxoplasma* acute infection and reduce brain cyst formation after chronic infection, which is considered a promising strategy to prevent toxoplasmosis (Gurunathan et al., 2000; Zhang et al., 2015a; Li and Zhou, 2018). Because no evaluated antigen can completely protect hosts against *T. gondii* infection, the identification of new potential vaccine candidates is a crucial step toward the development of an effective vaccine against *T. gondii* infection (Zhang et al., 2013; Li and Zhou, 2018).

Ca^{2+} is a crucial secondary messenger in the regulation of intracellular parasite attachment, invasion and egress of eukaryotic cells (Nagamune et al., 2008; Billker et al., 2009; Stewart et al., 2017). Calcium-dependent protein kinases (CDPKs) have been shown to participate in the downstream calcium-related signaling cascades as signaling mediators involved in distinct developmental processes of *T. gondii* (Billker et al., 2009; McCoy et al., 2012). TgDOC2 is another identified calcium signaling mediator that constitutes a second level of the pathway, operating downstream of CDPKs (Farrell et al., 2012; Jean et al., 2014). The DOC2 protein facilitates the membrane fusion of *T. gondii* secretory vesicles with the plasma membrane during the process of egress through regulating the Ca^{2+} signal pathway (Farrell et al., 2012). A previous study has shown that a TgDOC2-deficient strain has a disability in microneme secretion (Farrell et al., 2012). Together, these findings suggested that TgDOC2 may be a novel drug target or a vaccine candidate (Lourido and Moreno, 2015). However, there are no reports about the immunogenicity of TgDOC2 and its potential application as a vaccine candidate.

Thus, the aims of this study were to predict the potential epitopes of TgDOC2 and to evaluate its immunogenicity in the Kunming mouse model through a DNA strategy. Furthermore, the present study aimed to analyze the ability of the DNA vaccine against the infection with the highly virulent RH strain and the less virulent PRU strain.

MATERIALS AND METHODS

Animals

Specific pathogen-free (SPF) female Kunming mice aged 6–8 weeks were obtained from the Center of Laboratory Animals, Lanzhou Institute of Biological Products (Lanzhou, China). The present study was approved by the Animal Administration and Ethics Committee of Lanzhou Veterinary Research Institute, Chinese Academy of Agricultural Sciences (Approval No. LVRIAEC2012-011). All mice used for the experiments were raised and handled in strict accordance with the Good Animal Practice requirements of the Animal Ethics Procedures and Guidelines of the People's Republic of China.

Parasites

Tachyzoites of the *T. gondii* RH strain (genotype I) were maintained in the State Key Laboratory of Veterinary Etiological Biology through serial passage in Kunming mice *via* intraperitoneal injection. Tachyzoites were harvested from the peritoneal exudates. The obtained tachyzoites were also used for the preparation of *Toxoplasma* lysate antigen (TLA). The PRU cysts (genotype II) were maintained monthly through oral passage in Kunming mice, and they were purified from infected brains.

Amplification and Bioinformatics Analysis of the TgDOC2 Gene

Total RNA of *T. gondii* was extracted from the tachyzoites of the RH strain using the Trizol reagent (Invitrogen) according to the manufacturer's protocol. The TgDOC2 gene was amplified by reverse transcription-polymerase chain reaction (RT-PCR) using the following pair of primers: C2F (5′-ATGATGAAACTAAAGGAAATGG-3′) and C2R (5′-TCAGGTGCGCCCAGCCAGATCCAGTTG-3′). The PCR product was sequenced by Sangon Biotech Co., Ltd. (China). The potential epitopes of TgDOC2 were predicted using DNAStar 8.0 (DNAStar, United States) software with the Jameson-Wolf index.

Construction of Recombinant Plasmids

The C-terminus of the TgDOC2 gene (TgDOC2C) was amplified by PCR from the TgDOC2 gene using a pair of primers, namely, C2CF (5′-CGGGGTACCACGGAGAGAGAACGGAGAC-3′) and C2CR (5′-CCGGAATTCTCAGGTGCGCCCAGCCAGATCCAGT-3′), in which *Kpn* I and *Eco*R I restriction sites were introduced and underlined. PCR products were ligated into the pVAX I eukaryotic vector (Invitrogen, United States) through *Kpn* I/*Eco*R I sites to construct the recombinant pVAX-TgDOC2C plasmid. The concentration of extracted recombinant plasmids was determined by spectrophotometry at OD260 and OD280. The pVAX-TgDOC2C vector was diluted in sterile phosphate buffered saline (PBS) at a concentration of 1 μg/μl.

Expression of pVAX-TgDOC2C *in vitro*

The pVAX-TgDOC2C recombinant plasmid was transfected into HEK293 cells using Lipofectamine™ 2000 reagent

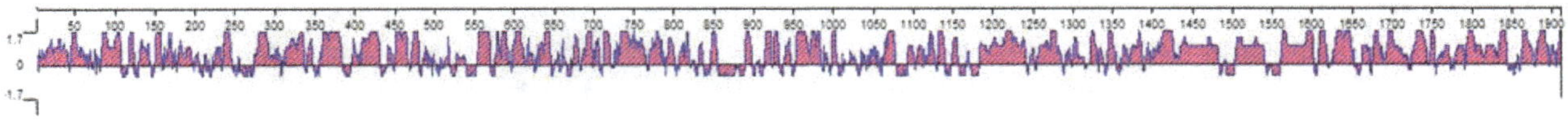

FIGURE 1 | Analysis of the antigenic index of TgDOC2 protein by DNAStar 8.0 software with the Jameson-Wolf index. Linear B-cell epitopes were predicted to widely distribute in the whole TgDOC2 protein but were mainly clustered in the C-terminal.

(Invitrogen, United States) following the manufacturer's instructions. Forty-eight hours posttransfection, the expression of pVAX-TgDOC2C *in vitro* was assayed by indirect immunofluorescence assay (IFA). In brief, pVAX-TgDOC2C-transfected cells were fixed with absolute acetone and washed with PBSTr (0.1% Triton-X-100 in PBS). Cells were then incubated with goat anti-*T. gondii* tachyzoites polyclonal antibody (in PBSTr at 1:50) for 1 h. After washing with PBSTr, cells were stained by fluorescein isothiocyanate (FITC)-labeled rabbit anti-goat IgG antibody (1:2000, Sigma, United States) for 1 h. HEK293 cells transfected with the empty pVAX I vector were treated as the negative control.

The expression of pVAX-TgDOC2C in HEK293 cells was detected by Western blot analysis. Briefly, transfected HEK293 cells (approximately 10^6) were lysed by freezing and thawing five times, and the lysates were then subjected to SDS-PAGE. After electrotransfer, the nitrocellulose (NC) membrane (Pall, United States) was incubated with 5% bovine serum albumin (BSA) in PBST (PBS with 0.05% Tween-20) at room temperature (RT) for 1 h to block the non-specific binding sites. The membrane was washed 3 times with PBST and then was cultured with pVAX-TgDOC2C-vaccinated mouse sera (diluted in 1:500; collected at 2 weeks after the third immunization) at RT for 1 h. After washing 3 times with PBST, the membrane was incubated with goat anti-mouse IgG-HRP antibody (diluted at 1:3000, Sigma, United States) for 1 h at RT. The specific band was visualized with Clarity™ Western ECL Blotting Substrates (Bio-Rad, United States) according to the manufacturer's protocol. Mouse sera from PBS-treated mice were used as the negative control.

Immunization and Challenge

Sixty-six female Kunming mice were randomly divided equally into three groups. Mice were intramuscularly immunized with 100 μl of pVAX-TgDOC2C and boosted with a 2-week interval. Mice treated with pVAX I vector alone or PBS served as controls. Blood samples were collected prior to each vaccination from the mouse tail vein and were centrifuged at 3,000 × *g* for 10 min to separate blood samples. Preimmune serum samples were used as negative controls.

For evaluation of the protective effect against acute *T. gondii* infection, 10 mice from each group were intraperitoneally infected with 10^3 tachyzoites of the virulent RH strain 2 weeks after the final immunization. The challenged mice were monitored daily until total death. In addition, another six mice from each group were orally infected with 10 brain cysts of the PRU strain as the chronic infection model. Five weeks after the challenge, the numbers of brain cysts were determined under microscopic examination.

IgG Antibody Assay

The levels of IgG antibodies in sera from mice in each group were determined by ELISA using the SBA Clonotyping System-HRP Kit (Southern Biotech Co., Ltd., Birmingham, AL, United States) following the manufacturer's protocol. In brief, 96-well microtiter plates were coated with 5 μg/ml TLA at 4°C overnight. After washing with PBST, plates were then treated with 1% skim milk in PBST for 1 h while shaking at RT to block non-specific binding sites. Serum (100 μl; 1:10 diluted with PBS) from each mouse was pipetted into a well and incubated for 1 h at 37°C. Each well was then incubated with 100 μl of anti-mouse IgG (HRP, 1:250 dilution, Sigma, United States) for 1 h at 37°C. Peroxidase activity was revealed by incubating with 100 μl of substrate solution (pH 4.0; 1.5% ABST, 0.03% H_2O_2 and 1.05% citrate substrate buffer). The reaction was stopped after the addition of 1 M H_2SO_4, and the absorbance was measured at 450 nm. All samples were performed in triplicate.

Purified Splenocyte Collection

Two weeks after the last immunization, six mice per group were sacrificed to aseptically harvest the spleen. Splenocytes were obtained by filtering spleens through a nylon membrane and were purified using erythrocyte lysis buffer (Solarbio, Shanghai, China). Harvested splenocytes were resuspended in DMEM medium supplemented with penicillin/streptomycin (p/s) and 10% fetal bovine serum (FBS).

Lymphocyte Proliferation Assay by MTS Assay

The density of purified splenocytes was adjusted into 2 × 10^5/well in 96-well microtiter plates. Cells were cultured in DMEM medium supplemented with 10% FBS and 100 U/ml p/s. Splenocytes were then incubated with 10 μg/ml TLA or 5 μg/ml concanavalin A (ConA; Sigma, St. Louis, MO, United States) at 37°C in 5% CO_2. Splenocytes cultured with medium alone (M) served as the blank control. The levels of proliferative responses *in vitro* were estimated using the MTS assay (Promega, Madison, WI, United States) after 92 h. The stimulation index (SI) was calculated using the following equation: OD_{570TLA}/OD_{570M} or $OD_{570ConA}/OD_{570M}$.

Flow Cytometry

CD4+ and CD8+ T lymphocytes were examined according to previous methods (Li et al., 2014). Splenocytes were first adjusted into a concentration of 10^6 cells/ml in PBS containing 2% FBS. Staining with phycoerythrin (PE)-labeled anti-CD3 (eBioscience, San Diego, CA, United States), allophycocyanin (APC)-labeled anti-CD4 (eBioscience) and fluorescein isothiocyanate (FITC)-labeled anti-CD8 (eBioscience) was performed at 4°C for 30 min in the dark. After rinsing twice with PBS, cells were fixed in FACScan solution (1% BSA and 0.1% sodium azide diluted in PBS) and 2% paraformaldehyde. The fluorescence profiles of stained samples were analyzed using a FACScan flow cytometer (BD Biosciences) using SYSTEM II software (Coulter).

Cytokine Assays

Purified splenocytes from mice in each group were stimulated with TLA (10 μg/ml) in 96-well flat-bottom microtiter plates. Supernatants in each well were harvested to determinate IL-4 and IL-2 levels at 24 h and IFN-γ levels at 96 h using ELISA kits according to the manufacturer's instructions (BioLegend, United States). Briefly, the supernatants and assay buffer A were pipetted into the same well, and plates were then incubated while shaking at 200 rpm for 2 h at RT. After washing the plates four times with 1× wash buffer, 100 μl of IL-4, IL-2 or IFN-γ detection solution was added into each well and incubated at RT. After 1 h, the contents of the plates were discarded, and the avidin-HRP solution was added after washing four times and incubated while shaking for 30 min at RT. The substrate solution E was then added and incubated for 20 min in the dark. To stop the reaction, 100 μl of stop solution was added. Absorbance was read by a Model 680 microplate reader (Bio-Rad, Hercules, CA, United States) at 450 nm. Sensitivity limits for the assays were 50 pg/ml for IL-2, 20 pg/ml for IFN-γ and 10 pg/ml for IL-4. Three independent experiments were performed for analysis of the data.

Statistical Analysis

The differences in IgG levels, CD4+ T cells and CD8+ T cells as well as the reduction in brain cysts were calculated by one-way ANOVA among at least three groups and by the *t*-test between two groups. The difference in survival time was calculated by the *Chi*-square test. All figures regarding the statistical analysis were prepared by GraphPad Prism version 5.0 (San Diego, CA, United States). A value of $P < 0.05$ was considered significant.

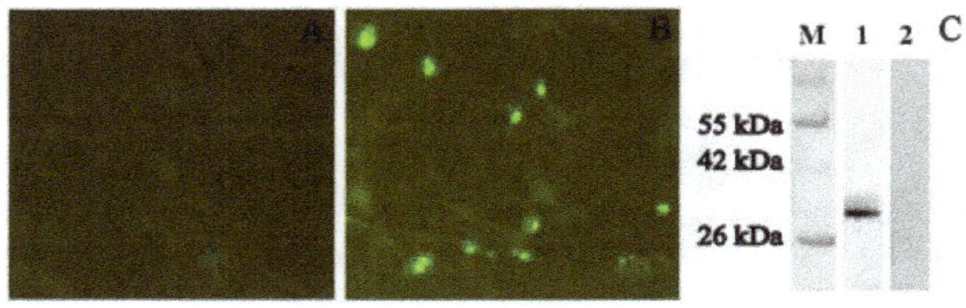

FIGURE 2 | Analysis of pVAX-TgDOC2C expression *in vitro*. Expression of the pVAX I empty vector **(A)** and pVAX-TgDOC2C **(B)** in HEK293 cells was detected by indirect immunofluorescence (IFA). **(C)** The pVAX-TgDOC2C product in HEK293 cell lysate was detected by Western blot analysis. M: protein molecular weight; lane 1: membrane incubated with mouse sera from the pVAX-TgDOC2C-vaccinated group at 2 weeks after the last immunization; lane 2: membrane incubated with mouse sera from the PBS group.

RESULTS

Analysis of the Amplified TgDOC2 Gene

The amplified TgDOC2 gene was identified through alignment with the corresponding sequence from the http://toxodb.org/ website. The cloned TgDOC2 gene showed 100% identity to the reference sequence (Gene ID: TGGT1_240910).

The potential B-linear epitopes of the TgDOC2 protein was predicted using DNAStar 8.0 software. The results showed that potential B-linear epitopes of the TgDOC2 protein were mainly gathered in the C-terminal end (**Figure 1**). Thus, the nucleotide positions distributed between 3550 (position at 1183 aa) and the end were selected for further amplification to construct the DNA vaccine.

Detection of pVAX-TgDOC2C Plasmid Expression in HEK293 Cells

The expression of pVAX-TgDOC2C *in vitro* was first examined by IFA. Green fluorescence was identified in HEK293 cells transfected with pVAX-TgDOC2C plasmids, but no fluorescence was observed in cells transfected with pVAX I alone (**Figures 2A,B**). These results indicated that pVAX-TgDOC2C was successfully expressed in HEK293 cells. As shown in **Figure 2C**, the specific band was detected in the membrane incubated with pVAX-TgDOC2C-vaccinated mouse sera but not in the membrane incubated with sera from the PBS-treated group. The size of the band was approximately 30 kDa, which was the expected size.

TABLE 1 | Splenocyte proliferative responses and the percentages of T cell subsets in immunized mice 2 weeks after the last immunization.

Groups	SI (Mean ± SD)		CD3 + CD4 + CD8 - (%)	CD3 + CD8 + CD4 - (%)
	TLA	ConA		
pVAX-TgDOC2C	1.51 ± 0.08***	1.80 ± 0.04*	13.33 ± 2.86***	8.45 ± 1.27*
pVAX I	1.32 ± 0.04	1.44 ± 0.09	3.28 ± 1.18	5.13 ± 1.84
PBS	1.30 ± 0.05	1.56 ± 0.1	3.27 ± 0.94	5.61 ± 1.11

*SI, stimulation index; TLA, Toxoplasma lysate antigen; ConA, concanavalin A. n = 6, *P < 0.05, **P < 0.001, ***P < 0.0001.*

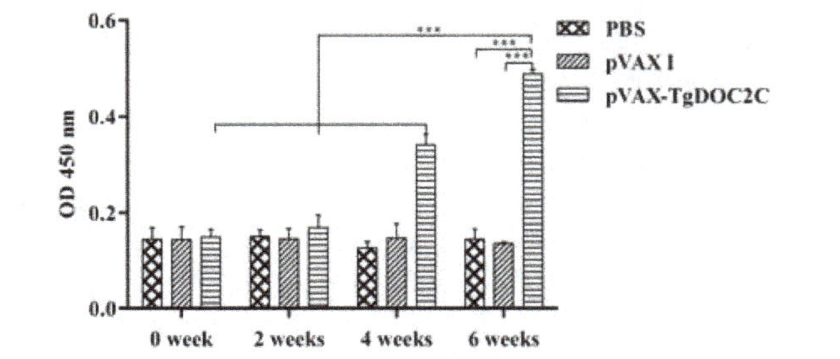

FIGURE 3 | Determination of IgG antibodies in the sera of Kunming mice at 0, 2, 4, and 6 weeks. Each bar represents the mean OD (±SE, $n = 3$). $^{***}P < 0.0001$.

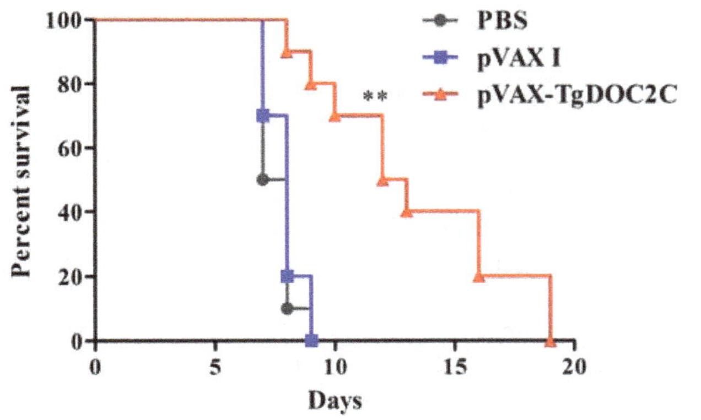

FIGURE 4 | Survival rate of mice immunized with pVAX-TgDOC2C, pVAX I and PBS followed by challenge with 10^3 tachyzoites 2 weeks after the last immunization. The mice immunized with pVAX-TgDOC2C died from day 9 to 19, which resulted in an increased survival time (12.5 days) compared to mice in the pVAX I (8 days) and PBS (7.5 days) groups ($n = 10$). $^{**}P < 0.001$.

Humoral Responses Induced by DNA Immunization of pVAX-TgDOC2C

The antibody levels in the sera of mice injected with pVAX-TgDOC2C increased with successive immunization and were reached the highest levels at 2 weeks after the last vaccination [$F(3,8) = 66.21$, $P < 0.0001$]. However, no differences were detected in serum samples of mice from pVAX I [$F(3,8) = 0.04$, $P = 0.99$] and PBS [$F(3,8) = 0.27$, $P = 0.84$] groups following immunization. After the third immunization, a significantly higher level of IgG antibody was examined in the sera of mice inoculated with pVAX-TgDOC2C compared to those receiving pVAX I [$t(4) = 29.20$, $P < 0.0001$] and PBS [$t(4) = 10.78$, $P < 0.0001$] (**Figure 3**).

Analysis of Cellular Immune Response

As shown in **Table 1**, an enhanced proliferative response was detected in the splenocytes of mice immunized with pVAX-TgDOC2C after incubation with TLA [$F(2,15) = 23.95$, $P < 0.0001$] and ConA [$F(2,15) = 4.131$, $P = 0.04$] compared to those from the pVAX I and PBS groups.

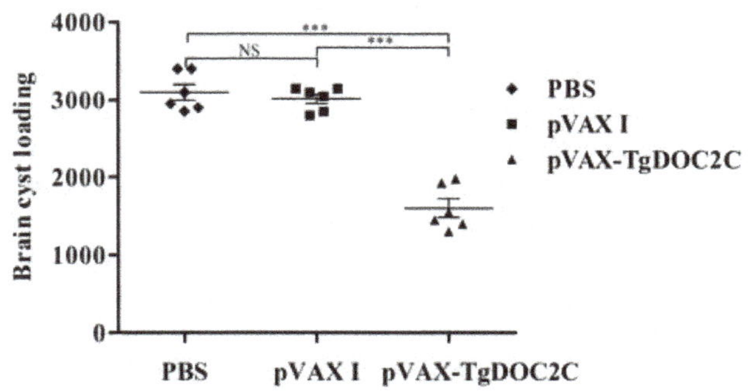

FIGURE 5 | Protection against chronic toxoplasmosis in mice injected with pVAX-TgDOC2C, pVAX I and PBS 2 weeks after the last immunization. Each bar represents the mean number of brain cysts (±SE, $n = 6$). $^{***}P < 0.0001$. NS, not significant.

Percentages of CD4+ and CD8+ T cells were determined in spleens of mice from each group by flow cytometry analysis. The CD3+ CD4+ T lymphocytes in mice injected with pVAX-TgDOC2C were significantly higher than those in mice from the pVAX I and PBS groups [$F(2,15) = 57.53$, $P < 0.0001$] (**Table 1**). The ratio of CD3+ CD8+ T cells in mice of the pVAX-TgDOC2C group was higher than that in controls [$F(2,15) = 9.3$, $P = 0.002$] (**Table 1**).

Cytokine Assays

Splenocytes from mice injected with pVAX-TgDOC2C had significantly higher levels of IFN-γ [$F(2,15) = 52.66$, $P < 0.0001$] and IL-2 [$F(2,15) = 15.87$, $P = 0.0002$] than those in mice in the pVAX I and PBS groups (**Table 2**). However, the level of IL-4 production was not significantly difference among the three groups ($P > 0.05$).

Protective Efficacy Elicited by pVAX-TgDOC2C Vaccination

To evaluate the protective activity of the pVAX-TgDOC2C recombinant plasmid against acute *T. gondii* infection, 10 mice in each group were intraperitoneally administered with 10^3 lethal tachyzoites 2 weeks after the last vaccination. The average survival time of mice inoculated with pVAX-TgDOC2C (12.5 days) was significantly longer than those injected with pVAX I (8 days) and PBS (7.5 days) ($P = 0.0004$) (**Figure 4**). Moreover, the

TABLE 2 | Cytokine production by splenocytes of immunized Kunming mice after stimulation by toxoplasma lysate antigen[a].

Groups	Cytokine production (pg/ml)		
	IFN-γ	IL-2	IL-4
pVAX-TgDOC2C	1584.8 ± 474.4***	178.03 ± 58.55**	< 10
pVAX I	172.21 ± 11.5	< 50	< 10
PBS	182.12 ± 24.03	< 50	< 10

[a]*Splenocytes from mice were harvested 2 weeks after the last immunization.* $n = 6$, $^{**}P < 0.001$, $^{***}P < 0.0001$.

survival times of mice in the control groups were not significantly different ($P > 0.05$).

The protective effect of the pVAX-TgDOC2C vaccine against *T. gondii* chronic infection was assessed through examination of brain cyst number per mouse from each group 35 days after infection of 10 cysts of the PRU strain. As depicted in **Figure 5**, mice immunized with pVAX-TgDOC2C (1600.83 ± 284.61) had significantly decreased brain cyst loadings compared to those injected with pVAX I (3016.67 ± 153.84) [$t(10) = 10.72$, $P < 0.0001$] and PBS (3100 ± 246.98) [$t(10) = 9.75$, $P < 0.0001$]. Immunization of mice with pVAX-TgDOC2C resulted in a cyst reduction rate of 48.36% compared to that of PBS-injected mice.

DISCUSSION

The present study showed that a DNA vaccination encoding the TgDOC2C gene in a mouse model promoted humoral and cellular immune responses, which contributed to a prolonged survival time (12.5 days, $P = 0.0004$) during acute infection and a decrease in brain cysts (1600.83 ± 284.61, $P < 0.0001$) during chronic infection. Significant progress has been made in recent years in the investigation of immune effects of various *T. gondii* antigens, such as ASP3 (Zhao et al., 2017), GRA2 (Ching et al., 2016), ROM5 (Zhang et al., 2015b), ROP18 (Yuan et al., 2011), ROP1 (Hiszczyńska-Sawicka et al., 2011), MIC6 (Peng et al., 2009), and SAG1 (Couper et al., 2003), and most of these antigens provide partial protection against *T. gondii* infection. The present results first demonstrated the potentiality of TgDOC2C as a vaccine candidate against acute and chronic toxoplasmosis.

DOC2, a calcium-binding protein, acts on membrane fusion and spontaneous neurotransmission in a murine model (Pinheiro et al., 2016; Ramirez et al., 2017). In intracellular parasites, the DOC2 protein impairs microneme secretion and is an essential component for exocytosis (Farrell et al., 2012; Jean et al., 2014). In the present study, the TgDOC2 protein was used to predict potential B-linear epitopes using DNASTAR software. The C-terminal end of the protein had more epitopes, suggesting that this sequence had potential to become an effective DNA vaccine against *T. gondii*. Analyses of epitopes, functions, or gene structures by emerging bioinformatics programs are widely used to design new vaccine candidates using an experimental methodology that discards non-functional sequences (Bai et al., 2012; Bastos et al., 2016; Zhou et al., 2016; Zhou and Wang, 2017). As expected, TgDOC2C is an effective vaccine candidate to improve the protective immunity against *T. gondii* challenges. Further study should design an epitope-based vaccine using calcium-dependent antigens in view of the ability of several TgCDPKs to protect mice from toxoplasmosis (Zhang et al., 2015a).

T cell-mediated immune defense is relevant to the control of toxoplasmosis (El Bissati et al., 2017), and CD8+ and CD4+ lymphocytes play a critical role during the adaptive immune response against *T. gondii* infection and reactivation (Gazzinelli et al., 1992). CD4+ T cells perform important roles in adaptive immune responses and limit intracellular pathogens in the early stage of infection (Kemball et al., 2007), while CD8+ T cells participate in the resistance in the later stage of intracellular infection through cytolytic activity (Ely et al., 1999). Enhanced CD8+ and CD4+ T cells contribute to the increasing protective immunity against *T. gondii* acute and chronic infection after DNA immunization with TgSOD (Liu et al., 2017), TgROM5 (Zhang et al., 2015b), TgeIF4A (Chen et al., 2013a) and other cocktail vaccines (Cao et al., 2015; Zhang et al., 2018). In the present study, the increased CD8+ and CD4+ T cells in mice immunized with TgDOC2C prolonged the survival time against acute infection and decreased brain cysts against chronic infection.

During the course of CD8+ and CD4+ T cell proliferation, polarization and activation, IFN-γ and IL-2 participate in certain stages and drive the immune response into Th1 type (Suzuki et al., 2011). IFN-γ is not only crucial to restrict tachyzoite growth in the early stage of infection but also important to inhibit the reactivation of dormant *T. gondii* cysts (MacMicking, 2012). Several previous studies have shown the correlation between the Th1 type immune response, characterized by the increase in IFN-γ and IL-2 production, and the enhanced resistance against toxoplasmosis in mice (Li et al., 2014; Zhao et al., 2017; Zheng et al., 2017). In the present study, significantly higher levels of IFN-γ and IL-2 production were detected in mice immunized with pVAX-TgDOC2C compared to those that received empty pVAX I and PBS, which conferred the extent of survival time after acute infection and the decrease in brain cysts after chronic infection. However, IL-4, which is associated with the Th2 immune response, was not significantly changed among the three groups. A promoted protective immunity against *T. gondii* infection along with a low secretion of IL-4 production has also been indicated in mice immunized with TgROP8 (Parthasarathy et al., 2013) and TgIF2α (Chen et al., 2013b).

The IgG antibodies against toxoplasmosis control *T. gondii* infection through inhibiting *T. gondii* duplication, facilitating the parasite attachment to immune cells and promoting macrophages to kill intracellular parasites *via* the process of antibody-dependent cell-mediated cytotoxicity (ADCC). In the present study, the increasing humoral immune response was associated with the enhanced protection against *T. gondii* infection, which was similar to the results from DNA immunization with TgROM5, TgeIF4A, TgROP18, and other antigens (Peng et al., 2009; Yuan et al., 2011; Cui et al., 2012; Chen et al., 2013a; Zhang et al., 2015b).

CONCLUSION

The present study demonstrated that immunization of mice with pVAX-TgDOC2C induces a strong humoral and cellular Th1-type immune response, resulting in reduced brain cyst numbers and the extent of survival time. The vaccine potential of pVAX-TgDOC2C indicates the possibility of inclusion in further development of a multicomponent or an epitope-based vaccine against toxoplasmosis in food-producing animals.

AUTHOR CONTRIBUTIONS

X-QZ and N-ZZ conceived and designed the experiments. QG, MW, F-KZ, and L-YH performed the experiments. N-ZZ and J-LH analyzed the data and wrote the paper. N-ZZ, QG, and X-QZ critically revised the manuscript. All authors read and approved the final version of the manuscript.

REFERENCES

1. Aleixo, A. L., Curi, A. L., Benchimol, E. I., and Amendoeira, M. R. (2016). *Toxoplasmic retinochoroiditis*: clinical characteristics and visual outcome in a prospective study. *PLoS Negl. Trop. Dis.* 10:e0004685. doi: 10.1371/journal.pntd. 0004685
2. Bai, Y., He, S. Y., Zhao, G. H., Chen, L., Shi, N., Zhou, H., et al. (2012). *Toxoplasma gondii*: bioinformatics analysis, cloning and expression of a novel protein TgIMP1. *Exp. Parasitol.* 132, 458–464. doi: 10.1016/j.exppara.2012.09.015
3. Bastos, L. M., Macêdo, A. G. Jr., Silva, M. V., Santiago, F. M., Ramos, E. L., Santos, F. A., et al. (2016). *Toxoplasma gondii*-derived synthetic peptides containing B- and T-cell epitopes from GRA2 protein are able to enhance mice survival in a model of experimental toxoplasmosis. *Front. Cell Infect. Microbiol.* 6:59. doi: 10.3389/fcimb.2016.00059
4. Belluco, S., Simonato, G., Mancin, M., Pietrobelli, M., and Ricci, A. (2017). *Toxoplasma gondii* infection and food consumption: a systematic review and meta-analysis of case-controlled studies. *Crit. Rev. Food Sci. Nutr.* 11, 1–12. doi: 10.1080/10408398.2017.1352563
5. Billker, O., Lourido, S., and Sibley, L. D. (2009). Calcium-dependent signaling and kinases in apicomplexan parasites. *Cell Host Microbe* 5, 612–622. doi: 10.1016/ j.chom.2009.05.017
6. Cao, A., Liu, Y., Wang, J., Li, X., Wang, S., Zhao, Q., et al. (2015). *Toxoplasma gondii*: vaccination with a DNA vaccine encoding T- and B-cell epitopes of SAG1, GRA2, GRA7 and ROP16 elicits protection against acute toxoplasmosis in mice. *Vaccine* 33, 6757–6762. doi: 10.1016/j.vaccine.2015.10.077
7. Chen, J., Huang, S. Y., Li, Z. Y., Yuan, Z. G., Zhou, D. H., Petersen, E., et al. (2013a). Protective immunity induced by a DNA vaccine expressing eIF4A of *Toxoplasma gondii* against acute toxoplasmosis in mice. *Vaccine* 31, 1734–1739. doi: 10.1016/j.vaccine.2013.01.027
8. Chen, J., Huang, S. Y., Zhou, D. H., Li, Z. Y., Petersen, E., Song, H. Q., et al. (2013b). DNA immunization with eukaryotic initiation factor-2α of *Toxoplasma gondii* induces protective immunity against acute and chronic toxoplasmosis in mice. *Vaccine* 31, 6225–6231. doi: 10.1016/j.vaccine.2013.10.034
9. Ching, X. T., Fong, M. Y., and Lau, Y. L. (2016). Evaluation ofimmunoprotection conferred by the subunit vaccines of GRA2 and GRA5 against acute toxoplasmosis in BALB/c mice. *Front. Microbiol.* 7:609. doi: 10.3389/fmicb.2016.00609
10. Couper, K. N., Nielsen, H. V., Petersen, E., Roberts, F., Roberts, C. W., and Alexander, J. (2003). DNA vaccination with the immunodominant tachyzoite surface antigen (SAG-1) protects against adult acquired *Toxoplasma gondii* infection but does not prevent maternofoetal transmission. *Vaccine* 21, 2813–2820. doi: 10.1016/S0264-410X(03)00163-4
11. Cui, X., Lei, T., Yang, D., Hao, P., Li, B., and Liu, Q. (2012). *Toxoplasma gondii* immune mapped protein-1 (TgIMP1) is a novel vaccine candidate against toxoplasmosis. *Vaccine* 30, 2282–2287. doi: 10.1016/j.vaccine.2012.01.073
12. Dubey, J. P. (2008). The history of *Toxoplasma gondii*-the first 100 years. *J. Eukaryot. Microbiol.* 55, 467–475. doi: 10.1111/j.1550-7408.2008.00345.x Dubey, J. P. (2009). Toxoplasmosis in pigs–the last 20 years. *Vet. Parasitol.* 164,89–103. doi: 10.1016/j.vetpar.2009.05.018
13. El Bissati, K., Zhou, Y., Paulillo, S. M., Raman, S. K., Karch, C. P., Roberts, C. W., et al. (2017). Protein nanovaccine confers robust immunity against *Toxoplasma*. *NPJ Vaccines* 2:24. doi: 10.1038/s41541-017-0024-6
14. Ely, K. H., Kasper, L. H., and Khan, I. A. (1999). Augmentation of the CD8+ T cell response by IFN-gamma in IL-12-deficient mice during *Toxoplasma gondii* infection. *J. Immunol.* 162, 5449–5454.
15. Farrell, A., Thirugnanam, S., Lorestani, A., Dvorin, J. D., Eidell, K. P., Ferguson, D. J., et al. (2012). A DOC2 protein identified by mutational profiling is essential for apicomplexan parasite exocytosis. *Science* 335, 218–221. doi: 10. 1126/science.1210829
16. Gao, X. J., Zhao, Z. J., He, Z. H., Wang, T., Yang, T. B., Chen, X. G., et al. (2012). *Toxoplasma gondii* infection in pregnant women in China. *Parasitology* 139, 139–147. doi: 10.1017/S0031182011001880
17. Gazzinelli, R., Xu, Y., Hieny, S., Cheever, A., and Sher, A. (1992). Simultaneous depletion of CD4+ and CD8+ T lymphocytes is required to reactivate chronic infection with *Toxoplasma gondii*. *J. Immunol.* 149, 175–180.
18. Gebremedhin, E. Z., Abdurahaman, M., Hadush, T., and Tessema, T. S. (2014). Seroprevalence and risk factors of *Toxoplasma gondii* infection in sheep and goats slaughtered for human consumption in Central Ethiopia. *BMC Res. Notes* 7:696. doi: 10.1186/1756-0500-7-696
19. Gurunathan, S., Wu, C. Y., Freidag, B. L., and Seder, R. A. (2000). DNA vaccines: a key for inducing long-term cellular immunity. *Curr. Opin. Immunol.* 12, 442–447. doi: 10.1016/S0952-7915(00)00118-7
20. Hiszczyn´ska-Sawicka, E., Gatkowska, J. M., Grzybowski, M. M., and Długon´ska, H. (2014). Veterinary vaccines against toxoplasmosis. *Parasitology* 141, 1365–1378. doi: 10.1017/S0031182014000481
21. Hiszczyn´ska-Sawicka, E., Li, H., Xu, J. B., Holec-Ga̧sior, L., Kur, J., Sedcole, R., et al. (2011). Modulation of immune response to *Toxoplasma gondii* in sheep by immunization with a DNA vaccine encoding ROP1 antigen as a fusion protein with ovine CD154. *Vet. Parasitol.* 183, 72–78. doi: 10.1016/j.vetpar.2011. 06.010
22. Holland, G. N. (1989). Ocular toxoplasmosis in the immunocompromised host. *Int. Ophthalmol.* 13, 399–402. doi: 10.1007/BF02306488
23. Innes, E. A. (2010). A brief history and overview of *Toxoplasma gondii*. *Zoonoses Public Health* 57, 1–7. doi: 10.1111/j.1863-2378.2009.01276.x
24. Innes, E. A., Bartley, P. M., Buxton, D., and Katzer, F. (2009). Ovine toxoplasmosis. *Parasitology* 136, 1887–1894. doi: 10.1017/S003118200999 1636
25. Jean, S., Zapata-Jenks, M. A., Farley, J. M., Tracy, E., and Mayer, D. C. (2014). *Plasmodium falciparum* double C2 domain protein, PfDOC2, binds to calcium when associated with membranes. *Exp. Parasitol.* 144, 91–95. doi: 10.1016/j. exppara.2014.06.015
26. Kemball, C. C., Pack, C. D., Guay, H. M., Li, Z. N., Steinhauer, D. A., Szomolanyi- Tsuda, E., et al. (2007). The antiviral CD8+ T cell response is differentially dependent on CD4+ T cell help over the course of persistent infection. *J. Immunol.* 179, 1113–1121. doi: 10.4049/jimmunol.179.2.1113
27. Li, Y., and Zhou, H. (2018). Moving towards improved vaccines for *Toxoplasma gondii*. *Expert Opin. Biol. Ther.* 18, 273–280. doi: 10.1080/14712598.2018. 1413086
28. Li, Z. Y., Chen, J., Petersen, E., Zhou, D. H., Huang, S. Y., Song, H. Q., et al. (2014). Synergy of mIL-21 and mIL-15 in enhancing DNA vaccine efficacy against acute and chronic *Toxoplasma gondii* infection in mice. *Vaccine* 32, 3058–3065. doi: 10.1016/j.vaccine.2014.03.042
29. Liu, Y., Cao, A., Li, Y., Li, X., Cong, H., He, S., et al. (2017). Immunization with a DNA vaccine encoding *Toxoplasma gondii* Superoxide dismutase (TgSOD) induces partial immune protection against acute toxoplasmosis in BALB/c mice. *BMC Infect. Dis.* 17:403. doi: 10.1186/s12879-017-2507-5
30. Lourido, S., and Moreno, S. N. (2015). The calcium signaling toolkit of the *Apicomplexan parasites Toxoplasma gondii* and Plasmodium spp. *Cell Calcium* 57, 186–193. doi: 10.1016/j.ceca.2014.12.010
31. MacMicking, J. D. (2012). Interferon-inducible effector mechanisms in cell- autonomous immunity. *Nat. Rev. Immunol.* 12, 367–382. doi: 10.1038/nri3210 McCoy, J. M., Whitehead, L., van Dooren, G. G., and Tonkin, C. J. (2012).
32. TgCDPK3 regulates calcium-dependent egress of *Toxoplasma gondii* from host cells. *PLoS Pathog.* 8:e1003066. doi: 10.1371/journal.ppat.1003066
33. Nagamune, K., Moreno, S. N., Chini, E. N., and Sibley, L. D. (2008). Calcium regulation and signaling in apicomplexan parasites. *Subcell Biochem.* 47, 70–81. doi: 10.1007/978-0-387-78267-6_5
34. Pan, M., Lyu, C., Zhao, J., and Shen, B. (2017). Sixty Years (1957-2017) of

research on toxoplasmosis in China-an overview. *Front. Microbiol.* 8:1825. doi: 10.3389/ fmicb.2017.01825

35. Parthasarathy, S., Fong, M. Y., Ramaswamy, K., and Lau, Y. L. (2013). Protective immune response in BALB/c mice induced by DNA vaccine of the ROP8 gene of *Toxoplasma gondii. Am. J. Trop. Med. Hyg.* 88, 883–887. doi: 10.4269/ajtmh. 12-0727
36. Peng, G. H., Yuan, Z. G., Zhou, D. H., He, X. H., Liu, M. M., Yan, C., et al. (2009). *Toxoplasma gondii* microneme protein 6 (MIC6) is a potential vaccine candidate against toxoplasmosis in mice. *Vaccine* 27, 6570–6574. doi: 10.1016/j. vaccine.2009.08.043
37. Pereira-Chioccola, V. L., Vidal, J. E., and Su, C. (2009). *Toxoplasma gondii* infection and cerebral toxoplasmosis in HIV-infected patients. *Future Microbiol.* 4, 1363– 1379. doi: 10.2217/fmb.09.89
38. Pinheiro, P. S., Houy, S., and Sørensen, J. B. (2016). C2-domain containing calcium sensors in neuroendocrine secretion. *J. Neurochem.* 139, 943–958. doi: 10.1111/ jnc.13865
39. Ramirez, D. M. O., Crawford, D. C., Chanaday, N. L., Trauterman, B., Monteggia, M., and Kavalali, E. T. (2017). Loss of Doc2-dependent spontaneous neurotransmission augments glutamatergic synaptic strength. *J. Neurosci.* 37, 6224–6230. doi: 10.1523/JNEUROSCI.0418-17.2017
40. Robert-Gangneux, F., and Dardé, M. L. (2012). Epidemiology of and diagnostic strategies for toxoplasmosis. *Clin. Microbiol. Rev.* 25, 264–296. doi: 10.1128/ CMR.05013-11
41. Stewart, R. J., Whitehead, L., Nijagal, B., Sleebs, B. E., Lessene, G., McConville, J., et al. (2017). Analysis of Ca2+ mediated signaling regulating *Toxoplasma* infectivity reveals complex relationships between key molecules. *Cell Microbiol.* 19:e12685. doi: 10.1111/cmi.12685
42. Suzuki, Y., Sa, Q., Gehman, M., and Ochiai, E. (2011). Interferon-gamma- and perforin-mediated immune responses for resistance against *Toxoplasma gondii* in the brain. *Expert Rev. Mol. Med.* 13:e31. doi: 10.1017/S1462399411002018
43. Wang, Z. D., Liu, H. H., Ma, Z. X., Ma, H. Y., Li, Z. Y., Yang, Z. B., et al. (2017).
44. *Toxoplasma gondii* infection in immunocompromised patients: a systematic review and meta-analysis. *Front. Microbiol.* 8:389. doi: 10.3389/fmicb.2017. 00389
45. Yuan, Z. G., Zhang, X. X., Lin, R. Q., Petersen, E., He, S., Yu, M., et al. (2011). Protective effect against toxoplasmosis in mice induced by DNA immunization with gene encoding *Toxoplasma gondii* ROP18. *Vaccine* 29, 6614–6619. doi: 10.1016/j.vaccine.2011.06.110
46. Zhang, N. Z., Chen, J., Wang, M., Petersen, E., and Zhu, X. Q. (2013). Vaccines against *Toxoplasma gondii*: new developments and perspectives. *Expert Rev. Vaccines* 12, 1287–1299. doi: 10.1586/14760584.2013.844652
47. Zhang, N. Z., Gao, Q., Wang, M., Elsheikha, H. M., Wang, B., Wang, J. L., et al. (2018). Immunization with a DNA vaccine cocktail encoding TgPF, TgROP16, TgROP18, TgMIC6, and TgCDPK3 genes protects mice against chronic toxoplasmosis. *Front. Immunol.* 9:1505. doi: 10.3389/fimmu.2018. 01505
48. Zhang, N. Z., Wang, M., Xu, Y., Petersen, E., and Zhu, X. Q. (2015a). Recent advances in developing vaccines against *Toxoplasma gondii*: an update. *Expert Rev. Vaccines* 14, 1609–1621. doi: 10.1586/14760584.2015.109 8539
49. Zhang, N. Z., Xu, Y., Wang, M., Petersen, E., Chen, J., Huang, S. Y., et al. (2015b). Protective efficacy of two novel DNA vaccines expressing *Toxoplasma gondii* rhomboid 4 and rhomboid 5 proteins against acute and chronic toxoplasmosis in mice. *Expert Rev. Vaccines* 14, 1289–1297. doi: 10.1586/14760584.2015. 1061938
50. Zhao, G., Song, X., Kong, X., Zhang, N., Qu, S., Zhu, W., et al. (2017). Immunization with *Toxoplasma gondii* aspartic protease 3 increases survival time of infected mice. *Acta Trop.* 171, 17–23. doi: 10.1016/j. actatropica
51. Zheng, B., Ding, J., Chen, X., Yu, H., Lou, D., Tong, Q., et al. (2017). Immuno- efficacy of a *T. gondii* secreted protein with an altered thrombospondin repeat (TgSPATR) as a novel DNA vaccine candidate against acute toxoplasmosis in BALB/c mice. *Front Microbiol.* 8:216. doi: 10.3389/fmicb.2017. 00216
52. Zhou, J., and Wang, L. (2017). SAG4 DNA and peptide vaccination provides partial protection against *T. gondii* infection in BALB/c mice. *Front. Microbiol.* 8:1733. doi: 10.3389/fmicb.2017.01733
53. Zhou, J., Wang, L., Lu, G., Zhou, A., Zhu, M., Li, Q., et al. (2016). Epitope analysis and protection by a ROP19 DNA vaccine against *Toxoplasma gondii. Parasite* 23:17. doi: 10.1051/parasite/2016017
54. Zhou, P., Chen, Z., Li, H. L., Zheng, H., He, S., Lin, R. Q., et al. (2011). *Toxoplasma gondii* infection in humans in China. *Parasit. Vectors* 4:165. doi: 10.1186/1756- 3305-4-165

2

Immunization with a DNA Vaccine Cocktail Encoding TgPF, TgROP16, TgROP18, TgMIC6 and TgCDPK3 Genes Protects Mice Against Chionic Toxoplasmosis

Nian-Zhang Zhang[1]*, Qi Gao[1,2], Meng Wang[1], Hany M. Elsheikha[3], Bo Wang[4], Jin-Lei Wang[1], Fu-Kai Zhang[1], Ling-Ying Hu[1] and Xing-Quan Zhu[1,5]*

[1]State Key Laboratory of Veterinary Etiological Biology, Key Laboratory of Veterinary Parasitology of Gansu Province, Lanzhou Veterinary Research Institute, Chinese Academy of Agricultural Sciences, Lanzhou, China, [2]Hunan Entry-Exit Inspection and Quarantine Bureau, Changsha, China, [3]Faculty of Medicine and Health Sciences, School of Veterinary Medicine and Science, University of Nottingham, Loughborough, United Kingdom, [4]Department of Mathematics, University of Leicester, Leicester, United Kingdom, [5]Jiangsu Co-Innovation Center for the Prevention and Control of Important Animal Infectious Diseases and Zoonoses, Yangzhou University College of Veterinary Medicine, Yangzhou, China

***Correspondence:**
Nian-Zhang Zhang
zhangnianzhang@caas.cn;
Xing-Quan Zhu
xingquanzhu1@hotmail.com

Toxoplasmosis is a zoonotic disease caused by the intracellular protozoan *Toxoplasma gondii*; and a major source of infection in humans is *via* ingestion of *T. gondii* tissue cysts. Ultimately, the goal of anti-toxoplasmosis vaccines is to elicit a sustainable immune response, capable of preventing formation of the parasite tissue cysts—or, at least, to restrain its growth. In this study, we formulated a cocktail DNA vaccine and investigated its immunologic efficacy as a protection against the establishment of *T. gondii* cysts in the mouse brain. This multicomponent DNA vaccine, encoded the TgPF, TgROP16, TgROP18, TgMIC6, and TgCDPK3 genes, which play key roles in the pathogenesis of *T. gondii* infection. Results showed that mice immunized *via* intramuscular injection three times, at 2-week intervals with this multicomponent DNA vaccine, mounted a strong humoral and cellular immune response, indicated by significantly high levels of total IgG, $CD4^+$ and $CD8^+$ T lymphocytes, and antigen-specific lymphocyte proliferation when compared with non-immunized mice. Immunization also induced a mixed Th1/Th2 response, with a slightly elevated IgG2a to IgG1 ratio. The increased production of proinflammatory cytokines gamma-interferon, interleukin-2, and interleukin-12 ($p < 0.0001$) correlated with increased expression of p65/RelA and T-bet genes of the NF-κB pathway. However, no significant difference was detected in level of interleukin-4 ($p > 0.05$). The number of brain cysts in immunized mice was significantly less than those in non-immunized mice (643.33 ± 89.63 versus 3,244.33 ± 96.42, $p < 0.0001$), resulting in an 80.22% reduction in the parasite cyst burden. These findings indicate that a multicomponent DNA vaccine, encoding TgPF, TgROP16, TgROP18, TgMIC6, and TgCDPK3 genes, shows promise as an immunization strategy against chronic toxoplasmosis in mice, and calls for a further evaluation in food-producing animals.

Keywords: *Toxoplasma gondii*, chronic toxoplasmosis, cocktail DNA vaccine, multistage antigens, mixed Th1/Th2 immune response

INTRODUCTION

Toxoplasma gondii, the causative agent of toxoplasmosis, infects nearly all warm-blooded vertebrates, including birds and humans (1, 2). Toxoplasmosis in immunocompetent people usually manifests as a flu-like, self-limiting infection; however, in immunocompromised patients (cancer, AIDS, and organ transplant recipients), reactivation of chronic toxoplasmosis can cause fatal complications, such as toxoplasmic encephalitis (3, 4). The reactivation of tissue cysts is manifested by their rupture, followed by the conversion of released bradyzoites to tachyzoites, and a proliferation of tachyzoites. Therefore, the removal of *T. gondii* tissue cysts from infected individuals would prevent such reactivation. Tissue cysts of *T. gondii* in animals also present a potential threat to human health if they are consumed in raw or undercooked meat (5, 6). Currently, there are no available drugs to eliminate *T. gondii* tissue cysts (7, 8). It is therefore imperative that new approaches are developed for immunotherapy against this infection.

Development of vaccines to prevent *T. gondii* tissue cyst formation can be an effective approach to ensure the safety of meat products, originating from food-producing animals under backyard and free-ranging conditions (9, 10). Over the last two decades, various anti-*T. gondii* vaccine approaches have been evaluated in animal models. Previous studies have shown that DNA vaccine can induce, through enhanced humoral and cellular immune responses, immune protection against acute and chronic toxoplasmosis in animal models (11–15). Additional advantages of the DNA vaccination, when compared with using live-type vaccines, are their thermal stability, safety, and the low cost of production (12, 14). To date, no single DNA vaccine has provided full protection against *T. gondii* cyst formation (9, 16, 17).

Toxoplasma gondii-specific cytotoxic T lymphocytes (CTLs) induced by immunization can improve the protective immunity against parasite infection (9, 14). Previous studies have shown that a multicomponent vaccine may offer better protection than a single antigen (16–19) due to the elevated numbers of *T. gondii*-specific CTLs, and the subsequent increase in the production of antigen-specific cytokine gamma-interferon (IFN-γ) (19, 20). A combination of different antigens, in theory, contain more CTL epitopes and are considered superior to a single antigen for protecting the host against *T. gondii* infection (14, 21).

This study aimed to examine the protective efficacy of a DNA multicomponent vaccine against chronic *T. gondii* infection. Five well-characterized antigens play key roles in host–parasite interaction including host cell attachment (MIC6) (22), gliding motility and invasion (profilin) (23, 24), signal transduction and egress (calcium-dependent protein kinase 3; CDPK3) (25), intracellular proliferation (ROP18) (26), and modulation of host gene expression (ROP16) (27). These antigens were selected to formulate a cocktail DNA vaccine. We investigated the immunologic efficacy of this vaccine, in protecting Kunming mice against chronic *T. gondii* infection. In addition, we conducted a longitudinal immune analysis and evaluated several immunization strategies, in order to provide some guidance for optimal schedules of vaccine administration in future clinical trials. Utilization of the DNA vaccine with multi-antigens is a step forward in the development of commercial vaccine formulations against chronic toxoplasmosis for use in humans and food-producing animals.

MATERIALS AND METHODS

Ethics Statement

Animal experiments were reviewed and approved by the Animal Administration and Ethics Committee of Lanzhou Veterinary Research Institute, Chinese Academy of Agricultural Sciences. The study was performed in strict compliance with the recommendations set forth in the Animal Ethics Procedures and Guidelines of the People's Republic of China. All efforts were made to minimize animal suffering and to reduce the numbers of animals used in the experiments.

Mice and Parasite Strain

Specific pathogen-free female Kunming mice, aged 6–8 weeks, were purchased from the Center of Laboratory Animals, Lanzhou Institute of Biological Products, Lanzhou, China. They were housed, in pathogen-free conditions, at Lanzhou Veterinary Research Institute in controlled room under stable conditions (12-h/12-h dark/light cycle, 50–60% humidity, and ~22°C temperature). Mice had access to sterilized food and water *ad libitum* and were acclimated for 1 week before use. The avirulent *T. gondii* type II Prugniuad (Pru) was propagated in our laboratory, by oral passage of infected brain homogenates in Kunming mice (28). Bradyzoites of *T. gondii* Pru strain were used to prepare the *T. gondii* lysate antigen (TLA) as described previously (29, 30).

Preparation of Multicomponent DNA Vaccine

The pVAX1 plasmids encoding *T. gondii* profilin (pVAX1-PF), rhoptry protein 16 (pVAX1-ROP16), rhoptry protein ROP18 (pVAX1-ROP18), microneme protein 6 (pVAX1-MIC6), and calcium-dependent protein kinase 3 (pVAX1-CDPK3) were constructed as previously reported (31–35), with the fidelity of all plasmids confirmed by sequencing (Sangon, China). The five eukaryotic plasmids were each transformed into *E. coli* DH5α for propagation and were isolated by anion exchange chromatography (EndoFree Plasmid Giga Kit, Qiagen Sciences, MD, USA) following the manufacturer's instruction. Plasmid concentration and purity was determined by measuring the optical density ratio A_{260}/A_{280}. The purified plasmids were stored at −20°C until used in the mouse immunization protocols.

Immunization and Challenge

Mice ($n = 120$) were randomly allocated to six groups of 20 mice. Mice in groups G1, G2, and G3 were immunized using plasmids encoding either five genes, four genes, or one gene, respectively. Further details of the various vaccination regimens are listed in **Table 1**. Mice received intramuscular (i.m.) injections of 100 μg of plasmids in 100 μl phosphate-buffered saline (PBS), into the tibialis anterior muscles using a 1-ml insulin syringe with a 28-G needle. Three vaccinations at 2-week intervals were

TABLE 1 | Vaccination regimens used in this study.

Group	Immunization protocol	Content	Volume	Administration
G1	pVAX1 plasmids expressing ROP16 + ROP18 + MIC6 + CDPK3 + PF	20 μg/plasmid	100 μl	Intramuscular
G2	pVAX1 plasmids expressing ROP16 + ROP18 + MIC6 + CDPK3	25 μg/plasmid	100 μl	Intramuscular
G3	pVAX1-PF	100 μg	100 μl	Intramuscular
G4	pVAX1	100 μg	100 μl	Intramuscular
G5	Phosphate-buffered saline	–	100 μl	Intramuscular
G6	Healthy control	–	–	–

performed. Mice in G4 and G5 received empty pVAX1 vector and PBS, respectively. Mice in G6 were healthy untreated controls (non-immunized and uninfected). Following the primary immunization, mice in G1–G5 were provided with two booster immunizations at weeks 2 and 4. For the challenge, 2 weeks after the final immunization (6 weeks post initial immunization), 6 mice from each group were inoculated orally with 200 μl of PBS containing 10 tissue cysts of the avirulent *T. gondii* Pru strain. Control mice received 200 μl of PBS without cysts. Six weeks post challenge, the mouse brains were removed, homogenized in 1 ml of PBS and cysts were morphologically identified and counted under a microscope (40× objective) on three aliquots of 20 μl, without staining.

Multicomponent DNA Vaccine Induced a Systemic Humoral Immune Response

The blood samples from three mice in each group were collected from the tail vein pre-immunization, and 2 weeks after each of the three sequential immunizations (i.e., at 2, 4, and 6 weeks post immunization). The sera were separated by centrifugation of blood samples at 3,000 × *g* for 10 min. Levels of anti-*T. gondii*, total IgG, and IgG isotypes (IgG2a and IgG1 antibodies, as markers for Th1 and Th2 responses) were examined in mice in each group using the SBA Clonotyping System-HRP Kit according to the manufacture's instruction (Southern Biotech Co., Ltd., Birmingham, AL, USA). Wells of 96-well microtiter plates were coated with 100 μl (10 μg/ml) TLA diluted in PBS at 4°C overnight, and then washed with PBST (PBS with 0.05% Tween-20). Plates were then treated with PBS-T plus 1% low fat milk for 1 h at ambient temperature, in order to block non-specific binding sites. After washing the wells three times with PBS, mouse serum samples (1:10 diluted with PBS) were added to the wells, and incubated at 37°C for 1 h followed by washing three times with PBST. The serum from non-immunized mice was used as a negative control. Horse radish peroxidase (HRP) conjugated anti-mouse IgG (1:500 diluted with PBS) and anti-mouse IgG1 or IgG2a (1:1,000 diluted with PBS) were added to the wells and incubated for 1 h at 37°C. Wells were then washed five times with PBST, and streptavidin–horseradish peroxidase was added for 1 h at ambient temperature. TMB (3,3′,5,5′-tetramethyl benzidine) in 200 μl citrate-phosphate buffer (0.05 M Na_2HPO_4, 0.025 M citric acid, pH 4.0) and 2 mM H_2O_2 were added to monitor the peroxidase activity. The reaction was stopped after 30 min by adding 2 M H_2SO_4. Analysis of antibody responses was based on absorbance, measured at 450 nm using an ELISA plate reader (iMark microplate absorbance reader; Bio-Rad, Hercules, CA, USA). All measurements were performed in triplicate.

Lymphocyte Proliferation Assay

Spleens from five mice in each group were aseptically collected, 2 weeks after the final/third booster immunization and were pushed through a fine nylon mesh. After removal of red blood cells, using erythrocyte lysis buffer (Sangon, China), the purified splenocytes were re-suspended in RPMI medium, supplemented with 10% fetal calf serum and 100 U/ml penicillin/streptomycin. The number of purified splenic lymphocytes was determined, and cells were cultured at a concentration of 2×10^5 cells/well in 96-well flat-bottom microwell plates, in complete RPMI medium. Cell cultures were stimulated with TLA (10 or 5 μg/ml) in three wells. RPMI media only (no antigen) and Concanavalin A (ConA; 5 μg/ml; Sigma, St. Louis, MO, USA) were used as nonstimulated and positive controls, respectively. After 4 days at 37°C in a humidified 5% CO_2 incubator, the level of *in vitro* proliferative response was determined using the 3-(4,5-dimethylthiazol-2-yl)-5-(3-carboxymethoxyphenyl)-2-(4-sulfophenyl)-*2H*-tetrazolium, inner salt (MTS) assay (Promega, USA). The OD values were measured using a microplate reader (iMark microplate absorbance reader; Bio-Rad, Hercules, CA, USA) at 490 nm. Data were expressed as stimulation index (SI), which was calculated as the ratio of mean OD_{590} values in immunized and control groups.

Antigen-Specific T-Cell Proliferation

The percentages of $CD4^+$ and $CD8^+$ T lymphocytes in the purified splenocytes were determined by flow cytometry. The specific antigen epitope of each T subclass was stained with phycoerythrin-labeled anti-mouse CD3 (eBioscience), allophycocyanin-labeled anti-mouse CD4 (eBioscience), and fluorescein isothiocyanate-labeled anti-mouse CD8 (eBioscience) antibodies. The cell suspension was then fixed with FACScan buffer (PBS containing 1% BSA and 0.1% sodium azide) and 2% paraformaldehyde. All samples were analyzed for their fluorescence profiles on a FACScan flow cytometer (BD Biosciences) using System II software (Coulter).

Cytokines

Splenocytes at a density of 2×10^5 cells/well were co-cultured with TLA and medium only (negative control). Culture supernatants were harvested at 24 h for quantification of interleukin-2 (IL-2) and IL-4 and at 96 h for IFN-γ and interleukin-12 (IL-12). The level of each cytokine was determined using commercial ELISA kits, according to the manufacturer's instructions (BioLegend, USA). The supernatants from each cell culture were pipetted into microplate wells followed by assay buffer A. Then, 100 μl of the detection solution was added into each well. After washing the plate four times, avidin-HRP A solution and the substrate solution E were added sequentially. The reaction was stopped by adding 100 μl of stop solution. The sensitivity limits for the assays were 4 pg/ml for IL-12 (p70), 20 pg/ml for IFN-γ, 10 pg/ml for IL-4, and 50 pg/ml for IL-2. Optical absorbance was read at 450 nm. This experiment was performed in triplicate.

We studied the expression of the two transcription factors, p65/RelA and T-bet of the NF-κB pathway, in an effort to establish their roles in mediating the increased production of T cell cytokine (e.g., IFN-γ and IL-12). Total RNA from 10^7 purified splenocytes of mice from G1 to G6 were extracted using Trizol reagent (Invitrogen, USA), as per the manufacturer's instructions. RNAs were dissolved in RNase-free ddH_2O (TaKaRa, China) and reverse transcribed first-strand cDNAs were used as templates for real-time (RT)-PCR. The primers for amplification of RelA/p65 and T-bet genes are listed in **Table 2**. β-Actin was used as a housekeeping reference gene. The SYBR Green qPCR SuperMix was purchased from Invitrogen (USA). RT-PCR was performed on ABI PRISM® 7500 Sequence Detection System (Applied Biosystems). The amplification reactions were performed under the following conditions: 50°C 2 min, 95°C 2 min, 40 cycles of 95°C for 15 s, and 60°C for 32 s. Melting curve analysis was carried out under the following conditions: 1 min at 95°C, 65°C for 2 min, and progressive increase from 65 to 95°C to ensure that a single product was amplified in each reaction. All measurements were run in triplicate.

Statistical Analysis

Two-way ANOVA with matched data at different weeks was used to compare the total IgG antibody responses between the mouse groups. Tukey's multiple comparisons test was then employed to test the differences between each of the three vaccination groups, and each of the three control groups at each week. One-way ANOVA and Tukey's multiple comparisons test were used for comparison in regards to the levels of IgG1 and IgG2a, and IgG2a/IgG1 ratio, proliferation of splenocytes, the numbers of $CD3^+$ $CD4^+$ $CD8^+$ and $CD3^+$ $CD8^+$ $CD4^+$ T cells, cytokine production, and the numbers of brain cysts. Welch's *t* test was used to compare the qPCR in the three genes (p65/RelA, T-bet, and β-actin) between the blank control group and mice in group 1. Data are presented as mean ± SD. All analyses and graphs were performed using GraphPad Prism version 7.04 (San Diego, CA, USA). The level of significance was defined as $*p \le 0.05$, $**p \le 0.01$, $***p \le 0.001$, and $****p \le 0.0001$.

TABLE 2 | Sequences of primers used for amplification of p65/RelA, T-bet, and β-actin genes.

Primer name	Sequence
T-bet-F	5′-GCCAGGGAACCGCTTATATG-3′
T-bet-R	5′-TGGAGAGACTGCAGGACGAT-3′
RelA-F	5′-GAACCAGGGTGTGTCCATGT-3′
RelA-R	5′-TCCGCAATGGAGGAGAAGTC-3′
β-Actin-F	5′-GCTTCTAGGCGGACTGTTAC-3′
β-Actin-R	5′-CCATGCCAATGTTGTCTCTT-3′

RESULTS

Identification of Plasmids

Five purified plasmids pVAX1-PF, pVAX1-ROP16, pVAX1-ROP18, pVAX1-MIC6, and pVAX1-CDPK3 were confirmed by sequencing prior to use in the immunization experiment. Sequence alignment analysis showed that no base deletion or change was detected after alignment with the corresponding sequences in GenBank: accession numbers AY937257.1, DQ116422, AM075204, EF102772, and AJ488146.2.

Kinetics of Humoral Immune Responses

We characterized temporal changes in the humoral immune responses following immunization. Sera were available pretreatment, and at weeks 2, 4, and 6 post sequential immunizations from mice in all groups. Levels of total IgG and its subclasses (IgG2a and IgG1) from these time points were determined using ELISA. As shown in **Figure 1**, the IgG responses tended to increase with the increased number of immunizations, and with the increased number of plasmids used in immunization. Levels of IgG in mice in G1, G2, and G3 increased proportionally with time following immunization, and peaked at 2 weeks after the third/final booster immunization. Statistical analyses of the results (for weeks 0, 2, 4, and 6 post immunization) were performed using a two-way ANOVA for matched data. Both time and group variables had significant effects ($p < 0.0001$ for time and $p = 0.0140$ for group). Tukey's multiple comparisons test showed no significant differences in all groups at week 0, 2, and 4 after immunization. At week 6 post immunization, the levels of IgG production in mice from G1 were significantly higher than those in the control groups G4, G5, and G6 ($p < 0.0001$, $p < 0.0001$, and $p < 0.0001$, respectively). The levels of IgG in G2 mice were significantly elevated compared with the control groups G4, G5, and G6 ($p = 0.0004$, $p = 0.0004$, and $p = 0.0003$, respectively). The levels of IgG in G3 mice were significantly high compared with the control groups G4, G5, and G6 ($p = 0.6142$, $p = 0.5803$, and $p = 0.5576$, respectively). The levels of IgG antibodies in mice from control groups (G4, G5, and G6) were not significantly different when compared with each other. Within G1, G2, and G3 groups, levels of IgG antibodies were not significantly different in G1 versus G2 ($p = 0.8977$), but were significantly different in G1 versus G3 ($p = 0.0023$) and in G2 versus G3 ($p = 0.0447$).

The levels of IgG1 and IgG2a were determined 2 weeks after the final immunization. One-way ANOVA and Tukey's multiple comparisons test were used for statistical analysis of IgG1 and IgG2a data. The results of IgG1 analysis showed that G1 versus G4, G5, and G6 were all significantly different; G2 versus G4 ($p = 0.0626$), G2 versus G5 ($p = 0.0504$), G2 versus G6 ($p = 0.0335$), whereas G3 versus G4, G5, and G6 were not significant (**Figure 2**). The levels of IgG2a showed that G1 versus G4, G5, and G6 were all significant; G2 versus G4, G5, and G6 were all significant; and G3 versus G4 ($p = 0.0765$), G3 versus G5 ($p = 0.0053$), and G3 versus G6 ($p = 0.0049$). These results suggest that both IgG1 and

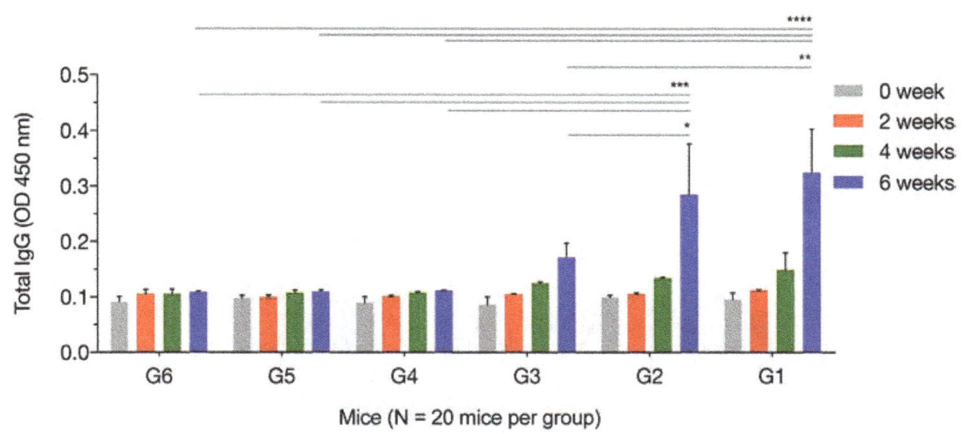

FIGURE 1 | Antigen-specific antibody response in immunized mice. Total IgG antibodies were determined in the sera of mice pre-immunization (0 week) and at 2, 4, and 6 weeks post three consecutive booster immunizations. Experimental groups include G1 mice received pVAX1 plasmids containing five antigens (ROP16, ROP18, MIC6, CDPK3, and PF); G2 mice received pVAX1 plasmids containing four antigens (ROP16, ROP18, MIC6, and CDPK3); G3 mice received pVAX1-PF; G4 mice received an empty pVAX1; G5 mice received phosphate-buffered saline alone; G6 healthy control mice. Data are mean ± SDs for three wells (representative of three independent experiments). $^*p < 0.05$, $^{**}p < 0.01$, $^{***}p < 0.001$, and $^{****}p < 0.0001$, compared with the control groups.

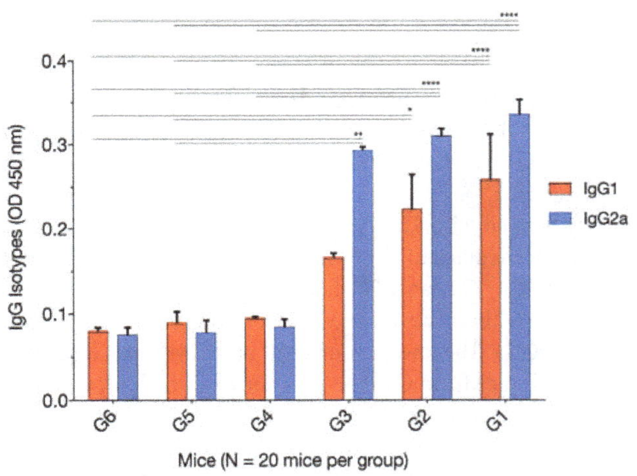

FIGURE 2 | Levels of IgG subclasses (IgG1 and IgG2a) in the sera of mice 2 weeks after the final booster immunization. The patterns of IgG2a to IgG1 post immunization using various immunization regimens suggest the induction of a mixed Th1/Th2 immune response. Experimental groups include G1: mice received pVAX1 plasmids containing five antigens (ROP16, ROP18, MIC6, CDPK3, and PF); G2: mice received pVAX1 plasmids containing four antigens (ROP16, ROP18, MIC6, and CDPK3); G3: mice received pVAX1-PF; G4: mice received an empty pVAX1; G5: mice received phosphate-buffered saline alone; G6: healthy control mice. Each bar represents the group OD_{450} ± SDs for three wells (representative of three experiments). $^*p < 0.05$, $^{**}p < 0.01$, and $^{****}p < 0.0001$, compared with the control groups.

IgG2a antibodies were higher in mice in G1, G2, and G3 than those in control groups at 2 weeks after the third immunization, suggesting a mixed Th1/Th2 immune response. To provide information on the dominant cellular immune type (Th1 or Th2) induced by immunization, ELISA was used to determine the ratio of IgG2a to IgG1 in the sera of all mouse groups. Results showed that immunized mouse groups, in particular, mice immunized with pVAX1-PF, had a slightly Th1-biased immune response as indicated by the higher IgG2a/IgG1 ratio (G1: 1.29; G2: 1.38; G3: 1.75) when compared with that of the control mouse groups (G4: 0.88; G5: 0.87; G6: 0.94; $p = 0.0877$).

Cellular Immune Responses

The MTS assay was used to assess the T lymphocyte's proliferative response following stimulation with TLA or ConA. As expected, there was no difference for the SIs between the immunized groups (G1, G2, and G3). However, *in vitro* lymphocyte proliferation assay revealed that splenic lymphocytes from immunized mice had a significantly higher SI than their counterparts from non-immunized controls, either in the presence of ConA or TLA extract. Exposure to 10 μg/ml TLA increased T-cell proliferation in G1, G2, and G3 compared with that obtained from control mice (**Figure 3**): G1 versus G6 ($p = 0.0010$), G2 versus G6 ($p = 0.0012$), and G3 versus G6 ($p = 0.0001$). Similar results for T lymphocyte proliferation were obtained from splenocytes sensitized with 5 μg/ml TLA in mice from G1, G2, and G3 (**Figure 3**). The results of this *ex vivo* splenic lymphocyte proliferation assay suggested that immunization has induced antigen-specific lymphocyte proliferation.

We further characterized the cellular immune response, using flow cytometry analysis, and found that the numbers of $CD3^+$ $CD4^+$ $CD8^-$ T cells in spleens of mice from G1, G2, and G3 were significantly higher than those from the controls (**Figure 4**). One-way ANOVA and Tukey's multiple comparisons test of the absolute numbers of $CD3^+$ $CD4^+$ $CD8^-$ T cells in spleens, showed that G1 versus G4 ($p = 0.0010$), G1 versus G5 ($p = 0.0003$), G1 versus G6 ($p = 0.0005$); G2 versus G4 ($p = 0.0359$), G2 versus G5 ($p = 0.0130$), G2 versus G6 ($p = 0.0187$); G3 versus G4 ($p = 0.0752$), G3 versus G5 ($p = 0.0287$), G3 versus G6 ($p = 0.0407$). After the third vaccination, mice immunized with various vaccines produced significantly higher $CD3^+$ $CD8^+$ $CD4^-$ T cells in splenic

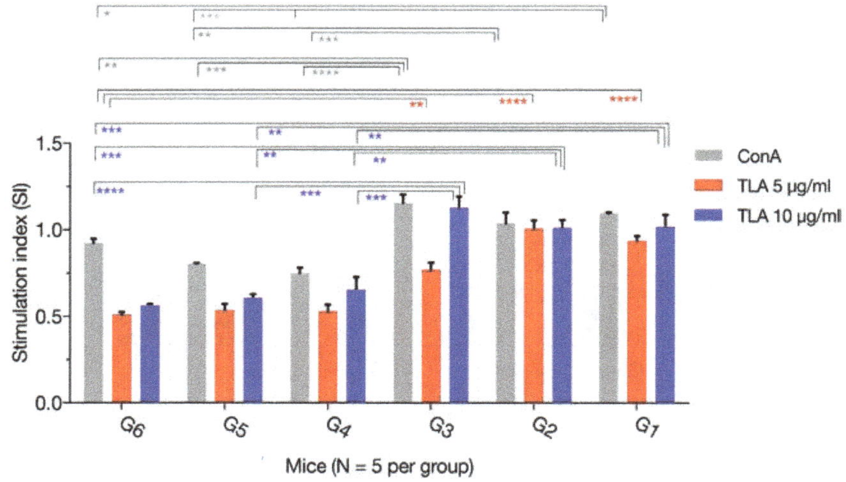

FIGURE 3 | *In vitro* lymphocyte proliferation induced by immunization. Splenocyte proliferation was assessed in mice 2 weeks after the final booster immunization. Exposure of splenocytes to 10 or 5 μg/ml *T. gondii* lysate antigen (TLA) significantly increased T cell proliferation in splenocytes obtained from mice in G1, G2, and G3, compared with proliferation in the control using antigen alone suggesting the induction of antigen-specific T-cell immune response after DNA immunization. Experimental groups include G1: mice received pVAX1 plasmids containing five antigens (ROP16, ROP18, MIC6, CDPK3, and PF); G2: mice received pVAX1 plasmids containing four antigens (ROP16, ROP18, MIC6, and CDPK3); G3: mice received pVAX1-PF; G4: mice received an empty pVAX1; G5: mice received phosphate-buffered saline alone; G6: healthy control mice. Each sample was assayed at least in triplicate. Data represent the mean ± SD (error bars) from the five mice. *$p < 0.05$, **$p < 0.01$, ***$p < 0.001$, and ****$p < 0.0001$, compared with the control groups.

lymphocytes as did the controls. The numbers of $CD3^+$ $CD8^+$ $CD4^-$ T cells in mice from G1, G2, and G3 were significantly increased compared with those from control mice (**Figure 4**). One-way ANOVA and Tukey's multiple comparisons test of the absolute numbers of $CD3^+$ $CD8^+$ $CD4^-$ showed that G1 versus G4 ($p = 0.0026$), G1 versus G5 ($p = 0.0038$), G1 versus G6 ($p = 0.0007$); G2 versus G4 ($p = 0.0381$), G2 versus G5 ($p = 0.0527$), G2 versus G6 ($p = 0.0111$); G3 versus G4 ($p = 0.0590$), G3 versus G5 ($p = 0.0804$), G3 versus G6 ($p = 0.0178$). These findings suggest that the frequency of $CD4^+$ $CD8^+$ T cells were augmented after DNA immunization.

Cytokine Production by Spleen Cells

Following stimulation with TLA, significantly high levels of IFN-γ, IL-2, and IL-12 were observed in splenocyte cultures from mice in G1, G2, and G3 when compared with those from control mouse groups (**Table 3**). In regard to IL-2, G1, G2, and G3 were all significantly higher than G4, G5, and G6 (all $p < 0.0001$). For IL-12, G1, G2, and G3 were all significantly higher than G4, G5, and G6 (all $p < 0.0001$), and for IFN-γ, G1, G2, and G3 are all significantly higher than G4, G5, and G6 (all $p < 0.001$). Levels of IL-4 in mice immunized with various DNA vaccines were not significantly different than those in mice from control groups ($p = 0.5028$). We analyzed the expression level of the transcription factors p65/RelA and T-bet using RT-PCR. We examined the difference between the expression of these two genes between control mice and mice in G1. Results showed that the expression of both p65/RelA and T-bet genes was significantly higher in G1 mice than in the control group ($p < 0.0001$ and $p = 0.0010$) (**Figure 5**). This result indicates that p65/RelA and T-bet are induced by immunization and are likely to increase the production of IFN-γ and IL-12 cytokines.

Assessment of Protective Activity

We evaluated which immunization regimen generated an immune response that was strong enough to protect against the formation of *T. gondii* brain cysts. Six mice from each group were challenged with 10 cysts of *T. gondii* Pru strain; and brain cyst loads were determined 6 weeks later. As shown in **Figure 6**, mice from G1, G2, and G3 had significantly lower numbers of brain cysts than those from control groups G4, G5, and G6 (all $p < 0.0001$). The lowest number of brain cysts was detected in immunized mice from G1 (643.33 ± 89.63), which represented a significant reduction (80.22%, $p < 0.0001$) when compared with the number of cysts found in control non-immunized + challenged mice (3,244.33 ± 96.42). The number of brain cysts in G1 mice was significantly lower than in G2 or G3 mice ($p < 0.0001$).

DISCUSSION

Despite significant research to develop and evaluate anti-*T. gondii* vaccines, there is little consensus on the "best" antigens to target and the optimal means of targeting them. The development of vaccines to prevent cerebral toxoplasmosis disease in high risk populations could reduce the enormous tragedy associated with brain infection with cystogenic (brain cyst-forming) strains of *T. gondii*. A substantially reduced parasite cyst load in the brains of immunized mice in our study, together with enhanced humoral and cell-mediated immune responses—compared with non-immunized infected mice demonstrate that immunization with a DNA cocktail vaccine of five antigens, provides considerable protection in mice against a primary oral challenge with the avirulent cystogenic *T. gondii* Pru strain. These elements are believed to be important in developing an effective therapeutic vaccine. Our results showed that immunization using

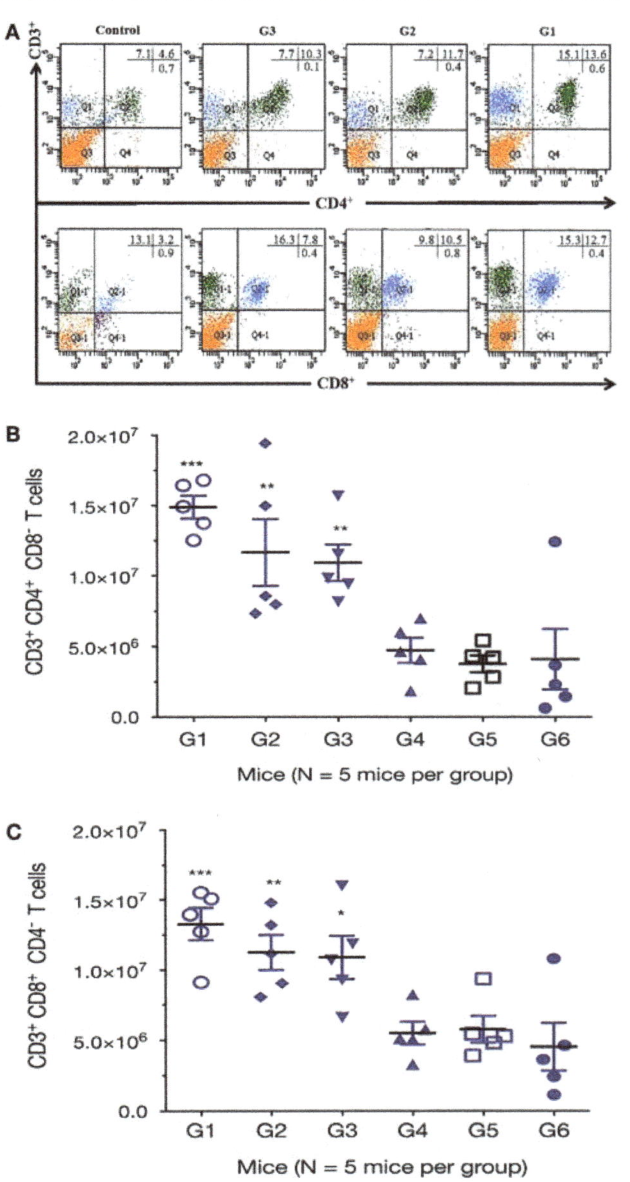

FIGURE 4 | DNA immunization augmented the frequency of antigen-specific T cells. Percentages of $CD4^+$ and $CD8^+$ T cells subsets were determined in the spleen of mice 2 weeks after the final immunization by flow cytometry analysis. **(A)** Representative dot plots showing the percentages of $CD3^+$ $CD4^+$ $CD8^-$ and $CD3^+$ $CD8^+$ $CD4^-$ T lymphocytes. **(B)** Total numbers of $CD3^+$ $CD4^+$ $CD8^-$ T lymphocytes per spleen. **(C)** Total numbers of $CD3^+$ $CD8^+$ $CD4^-$ T lymphocytes per spleen. Experimental groups include G1: mice received pVAX1 plasmids containing five antigens (ROP16, ROP18, MIC6, CDPK3, and PF); G2: mice received pVAX1 plasmids containing four antigens (ROP16, ROP18, MIC6, and CDPK3); G3: mice received pVAX1-PF; G4: mice received an empty pVAX1; G5: mice received phosphate-buffered saline alone; G6: healthy control mice. Data are mean ± SDs (representative of three experiments). $^*p < 0.05$, $^{**}p < 0.01$, and $^{***}p < 0.001$, compared with the control groups.

the cocktail DNA vaccine is a promising approach to control chronic toxoplasmosis, when compared with vaccination based on single antigens (31–35). In this study, cocktail DNA vaccine achieved an 80.22% reduction in the parasite cyst burden, compared with 50% obtained by DNA vaccine expressing *T. gondii* CDPK3 (34) and 39.08% by DNA vaccine (pVAX1-PF) encoding TgPF gene (35). Reduction in the brain cysts' load achieved in our study, was also greater than the 57.8% reduction achieved by vaccination using multiple antigenic peptides encapsulated by chitosan microspheres (36).

The cytokine Th1 immune response is crucial for the control of infection with this obligate intracellular pathogen (14, 37). In our study, immunized mice developed a high level of anti-*T. gondii* IgG antibodies, particularly after the third booster immunization. It is arguable that a high level of antibodies plays an important role in protection against subsequent infection with *T. gondii* tachyzoites, and in controlling *T. gondii* during chronic infection, by preventing cysts' reactivation. A requirement for B cells, in addition to cell-mediated immunity, has been reported for mice challenged with virulent *T. gondii* parasites after vaccination with attenuated tachyzoites—suggesting that antibody-mediated immunity is also critical for *T. gondii*-induced protection (38). Our previous studies have demonstrated that the individual protective immunity offered by pVAX1-PF, pVAX1-ROP16, pVAX1-ROP18, pVAX1-MIC6, or pVAX1-CDPK3 against *T. gondii* infection, elicited a mixed Th1/Th2 or Th1-biased immunity *via* the induction of lymphocyte proliferation, activation of $CD8^+$ T cells and increased IFN-γ production (31–35). In this study, a mixed Th1/Th2 immune response, with a slight bias toward the Th1-type response, was detected in mice in groups G1, G2, and G3, as indicated by a slightly increased lgG2a/IgG1 ratio (i.e., a higher level of IgG2a than IgG1). Vaccination using five antigens evoked an increase in $CD8^+$ T lymphocytes and IFN-γ production along with low levels of IL-4 in G1 mice compared with controls; all are characteristic features of a Th1-type cellular immune response. These findings indicate that a mixed Th1/Th2 protective immune response was elicited following immunization with the cocktail vaccine—consistent with the results of previous studies (14, 39).

A cellular immune response, including high levels of IFN-γ, $CD4^+$, and $CD8^+$ T lymphocytes, is required for protection against chronic *T. gondii* infection (39–43). Both cell types act synergistically to control *T. gondii* infection, and effective control of *T. gondii* infection requires $CD4^+$ for the generation of proficient $CD8^+$-mediated immunity (44). $CD8^+$ T cells possess anti-cyst activity, mediated by a perforin-dependent mechanism (45, 46) and high levels of $CD8^+$ T lymphocytes can contribute to a decrease of brain cyst loads (39, 43, 47–50). In our study, the significantly increased numbers of $CD8^+$ T cells in mice immunized with our cocktail vaccine may have contributed toward reducing the brain cyst burden.

Gamma-interferon, a crucial mediator of immune resistance to *T. gondii* infection, was detected in elevated levels in mice from G1, G2, and G3. IFN-γ can activate macrophages and the CTL response during infection (51). Significantly higher expression of the transcription factor T-bet ($p = 0.0010$) was observed in mice in G1, compared with mice from the control group. This finding indicates that increased IFN-γ production may have resulted from T-bet-mediated activation of $CD4^+$ T cells and natural killer (NK) cells (36). In marked contrast with IFN-γ, the level

TABLE 3 | Cytokine production by splenocytes of immunized Kunming mice after stimulation by *T. gondii* lysate antigen.

Group[b]	Cytokine production (pg/ml)[a]			
	Gamma-interferon	**Interleukin-2 (IL-2)**	**IL-4**	**Interleukin-12 (IL-12)**
G1	1,003.66 ± 311.02	294.24 ± 11.1	<10	411.96 ± 57.94
G2	644.94 ± 190	269.35 ± 19.17	11.1 ± 17.4	184.75 ± 39.95
G3	1,930.26 ± 5.46	277.14 ± 2.24	<10	400.14 ± 54.43
G4	169.29 ± 1.66	<50	<10	15.42 ± 2.01
G5	182.94 ± 33.64	<50	<10	<10
G6	177.75 ± 22.32	<50	<10	<10

[a]*No significant difference ($p > 0.05$) in the level of the four cytokines was observed between the immunized groups (G1, G2, and G3) nor between the control groups (G4, G5, and G6). Differences between immunized groups and control groups were significant for INF-γ ($p < 0.001$), and for IL-2 and IL-12 ($p < 0.0001$). Levels of IL-4 did not show any significant differences between the different mouse groups ($p > 0.05$).*

[b]*Experimental groups included G1: mice received pVAX1 plasmids containing five antigens (ROP16, ROP18, MIC6, CDPK3, and PF); G2: mice received pVAX1 plasmids containing four antigens (ROP16, ROP18, MIC6, and CDPK3); G3: mice received pVAX1-PF; G4: mice received an empty pVAX1; G5: mice received phosphate-buffered saline alone; G6: healthy control mice. Data are mean ± SDs for three wells (representative of three independent experiments).*

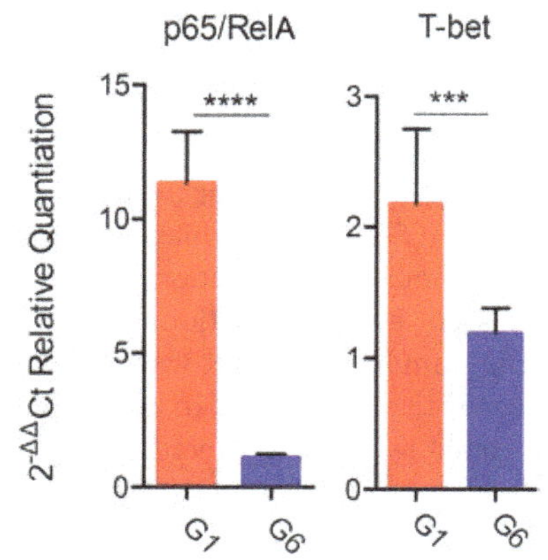

FIGURE 5 | Real-time-PCR expression analysis of the transcription factors p65/RelA and T-bet. β-Actin was used as a housekeeping reference gene. Experimental groups include G1: mice received pVAX1 plasmids containing five antigens (ROP16, ROP18, MIC6, CDPK3, and PF); G6: healthy control mice. Each sample was analyzed in triplicate. Data are mean ± SDs (error bars) from the two mice. ***$p < 0.001$ and ****$p < 0.0001$.

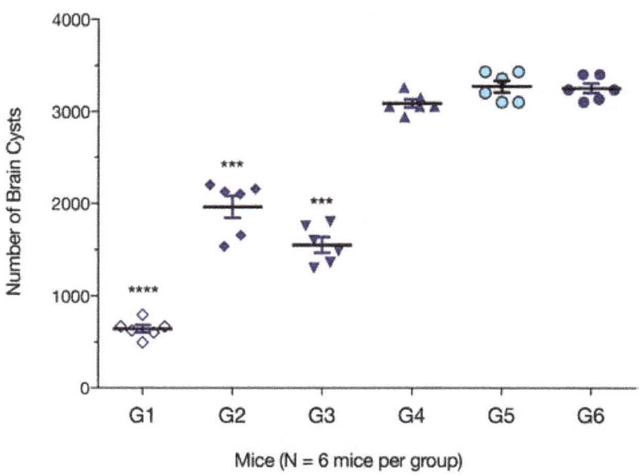

FIGURE 6 | Protection against chronic toxoplasmosis in immunized mice 2 weeks after the final booster immunization. Six mice per group were challenged orally with a dose of 10 cysts of the Pru strain (type II). Cyst load was counted from whole brain homogenates of mice 6 weeks after challenge. Experimental groups include G1: mice received pVAX1 plasmids containing five antigens (ROP16, ROP18, MIC6, CDPK3, and PF); G2: mice received pVAX1 plasmids containing four antigens (ROP16, ROP18, MIC6, and CDPK3); G3: mice received pVAX1-PF; G4: mice received an empty pVAX1; G5: mice received phosphate-buffered saline alone; G6: healthy control mice. Data are mean ± SDs (representative of three experiments). ***$p < 0.001$ and ****$p < 0.0001$, compared with the control groups.

of IL-4 was not statistically different between any mouse groups. IL-4 is a Th2-type cytokine, produced in response to receptor activation by Th2-type $CD4^+$ T cells, basophils, and mast cells, and possesses B-cell stimulatory and Th2-promoting properties (52). IL-4 functions are generally antagonistic to those of IFN-γ, in line with the increased IFN-γ and decreased IL-4 levels seen in our study. Elevated IFN-γ production, together with a low level of IL-4, was also detected in mice immunized with DNA vaccines encoding TgROP1 (15), TgROM5 (39), TgCDPK2 (53), TgSAG1 (54), or multi-antigens (17, 19). IL-4 also promotes isotype-switching in murine B cells to IgG1 and IgE, but inhibits switching to IgG2a, IgG2b, and IgG3. This is in agreement with the reduced IL-4 and a high IgG2a to IgG1 ratio, observed in our study—providing more evidence of a biased Th1 type immune response.

Previous studies have shown that high levels of $CD4^+$ and IL-2 production, increased mouse resistance to chronic toxoplasmosis (30, 41, 42, 55). We also found an increased production of $CD4^+$, IL-2, and IL-12, along with a reduction in the brain cyst load in mice vaccinated with various DNA vaccines. A major role of NF-κB in resistance to *T. gondii* is the induction of IL-12 secretion (56). IL-12, putatively *via* STAT4, is important for the optimal production of INF-γ, which in turn induces differentiation of Th1 T lymphocytes, and possibly $CD8^+$ and NK cells, to control *T. gondii* infection. Significantly increased expression of the transcription factor p65/RelA (a transcription factor of the NF-κB pathway) was observed in mice in G1, when compared with mice in the control group ($p < 0.0001$). This result, in addition to the increased level of IFN-γ, presents activation of NF-κB pathway as an additional mechanism for increased IFN-γ production to limit *T. gondii* infection. Suppressed expression of IL-12 resulted in 100% mortality in mice infected with *T. gondii* (57). High levels of IL-12 contributed to brain cyst reduction in mice (54, 58). Toll-like receptor 11 (TLR11) signaling is an important pathway involved in the production of IL-12 (23, 59). *T. gondii* profilin (TgPF) can act as a ligand for TLR11 to mediate cytokine production (60–62) and has been exploited as a TLR-based vaccine adjuvant to enhance immune responses generated by vaccination (62–65). TgPF also plays an essential role in *T. gondii* gliding motility, invasion and egress from host cells (23, 24) and is an immunodominant antigen (35, 66). These key characteristics of TgPF prompted us to separately evaluate the protective efficacy of immunization with this gene against chronic toxoplasmosis. The specific finding that DNA vaccine encoding TgPF alone induced the production of high level of IL-12 is consistent with previous data (60) and, together with a higher IgG2a/IgG1 ratio and reduced brain cyst numbers may be of particular relevance. The enhanced protective immunity seen in mice from G1, compared with mice from group G2, suggests that TgPF may be necessary to augment the immune response induced by the multicomponent *T. gondii* DNA vaccine used in our study.

CONCLUSION

We have demonstrated that a strong humoral and cellular immune response, conferring significant protection against chronic *T. gondii* infection in mice—after immunization three times at 2-week intervals with a DNA vaccine encoding multiple antigens (TgPF, TgROP16, TgROP18, TgMIC6, and TgCDPK3). Several DNA immunizations were necessary to elicit the specific IgG antibody response. Immunization with several plasmids expressing more antigens produced a greater antibody response when compared with immunization using fewer plasmids expressing less number of antigens. These data support a call for further evaluation of multivalent synthetic plasmids as potential therapeutic *T. gondii* vaccines. Our findings are significant as they open up the possibility that chronic toxoplasmosis can be controlled by the combined action of multiple parasite-derived antigens. Although further studies and clinical evaluations are required, this study puts into place a "proof of concept" that tests the efficacy of the combination of a range of *T. gondii* antigens in preventing a chronic brain infection that is incurable with current therapeutics.

ETHICS STATEMENT

All animal protocols were reviewed and approved by the Animal Administration and Ethics Committee of Lanzhou Veterinary Research Institute, Chinese Academy of Agricultural Sciences. The study was performed in strict compliance with the recommendations set forth in the Animal Ethics Procedures and Guidelines of the People's Republic of China. All efforts were made to minimize animal suffering and to reduce the numbers of animals used in the experiments.

AUTHOR CONTRIBUTIONS

X-QZ, N-ZZ, and HE designed the experiments, interpreted the data, and critically revised the manuscript. N-ZZ, QG, MW, BW, and J-LW performed the experiments and analyzed the data. N-ZZ drafted the manuscript. F-KZ, MW, and L-YH helped in the implementation of the study. All the authors reviewed and approved the final version of the manuscript.

REFERENCES

1. Montoya JG, Liesenfeld O. Toxoplasmosis. *Lancet* (2004) 363:1965–76. doi:10.1016/S0140-6736(04)16412-X
2. Robert-Gangneux F, Darde ML. Epidemiology of and diagnostic strategies for toxoplasmosis. *Clin Microbiol Rev* (2012) 25:264–96. doi:10.1128/CMR.05013-11
3. Wohlfert EA, Blader IJ, Wilson EH. Brains and brawn: *Toxoplasma* infections of the central nervous system and skeletal muscle. *Trends Parasitol* (2017) 33:519–31. doi:10.1016/j.pt.2017.04.001
4. Wang ZD, Liu HH, Ma ZX, Ma HY, Li ZY, Yang ZB, et al. *Toxoplasma gondii* infection in immunocompromised patients: a systematic review and meta-analysis. *Front Microbiol* (2017) 8:389. doi:10.3389/fmicb.2017.00389
5. Hill DE, Dubey JP. *Toxoplasma gondii* as a parasite in food: analysis and control. *Microbiol Spectr* (2016) 4:PFS-0011-2015. doi:10.1128/microbiolspec.PFS-0011-2015
6. Belluco S, Simonato G, Mancin M, Pietrobelli M, Ricci A. *Toxoplasma gondii* infection and food consumption: a systematic review and meta-analysis of case-controlled studies. *Crit Rev Food Sci Nutr* (2017) 11:1–12. doi:10.1080/10408398.2017.1352563
7. Pan M, Lyu C, Zhao J, Shen B. Sixty years (1957-2017) of research on toxoplasmosis in China-an overview. *Front Microbiol* (2017) 8:1825. doi:10.3389/fmicb.2017.01825
8. Alday PH, Doggett JS. Drugs in development for toxoplasmosis: advances, challenges, and current status. *Drug Des Devel Ther* (2017) 11:273–93. doi:10.2147/DDDT.S60973
9. Zhang NZ, Chen J, Wang M, Petersen E, Zhu XQ. Vaccines against *Toxoplasma gondii*: new developments and perspectives. *Expert Rev Vaccines* (2013) 12:1287–99. doi:10.1586/14760584.2013.844652
10. Vercruysse J, Knox DP, Schetters TP, Willadsen P. Veterinary parasitic vaccines: pitfalls and future directions. *Trends Parasitol* (2004) 20:488–92. doi:10.1016/j.pt.2004.07.009
11. Robinson HL. DNA vaccines: basic mechanism and immune responses (review). *Int J Mol Med* (1999) 4:549–55.
12. Gurunathan S, Wu CY, Freidag BL, Seder RA. DNA vaccines: a key for inducing long-term cellular immunity. *Curr Opin Immunol* (2000) 12:442–7. doi:10.1016/S0952-7915(00)00118-7
13. Chen J, Huang SY, Li ZY, Yuan ZG, Zhou DH, Petersen E, et al. Protective immunity induced by a DNA vaccine expressing eIF4A of *Toxoplasma gondii* against acute toxoplasmosis in mice. *Vaccine* (2013) 31:1734–9. doi:10.1016/j.vaccine.2013.01.027
14. Zhang NZ, Wang M, Xu Y, Petersen E, Zhu XQ. Recent advances in developing vaccines against *Toxoplasma gondii*: an update. *Expert Rev Vaccines* (2015) 14:1609–21. doi:10.1586/14760584.2015.1098539
15. Sonaimuthu P, Ching XT, Fong MY, Kalyanasundaram R, Lau YL. Induction of protective immunity against toxoplasmosis in BALB/c mice vaccinated with *Toxoplasma gondii* rhoptry-1. *Front Microbiol* (2016) 7:808. doi:10.3389/fmicb.2016.00808
16. Jongert E, Melkebeekd V, De Craeyeb S, Dewitc J, Verhelst D, Coxd E. An enhanced GRA1-GRA7 cocktail DNA vaccine primes anti-*Toxoplasma* immune responses in pigs. *Vaccine* (2008) 26:1025–31. doi:10.1016/j.vaccine.2007.11.058
17. Fang R, Feng H, Hu M, Khan MK, Wang L, Zhou Y, et al. Evaluation of immune responses induced by SAG1 and MIC3 vaccine cocktails against *Toxoplasma gondii*. *Vet Parasitol* (2012) 187:140–6. doi:10.1016/j.vetpar.2011.12.007
18. Mévélec MN, Bout D, Desolme B, Marchand H, Magné R, Bruneel O, et al. Evaluation of protective effect of DNA vaccination with genes encoding

antigens GRA4 and SAG1 associated with GM-CSF plasmid, against acute, chronical and congenital toxoplasmosis in mice. *Vaccine* (2005) 23:4489–99. doi:10.1016/j.vaccine.2005.04.025
19. Hoseinian Khosroshahi K, Ghaffarifar F, D'Souza S, Sharifi Z, Dalimi A. Evaluation of the immune response induced by DNA vaccine cocktail expressing complete SAG1 and ROP2 genes against toxoplasmosis. *Vaccine* (2011) 29:778–83. doi:10.1016/j.vaccine.2010.11.012
20. Beghetto E, Nielsen HV, Del Porto P, Buffolano W, Guglietta S, Felici F, et al. A combination of antigenic regions of *Toxoplasma gondii* microneme proteins induces protective immunity against oral infection with parasite cysts. *J Infect Dis* (2005) 191:637–45. doi:10.1086/427660
21. Picchio MS, Sánchez VR, Arcon N, Soto AS, Perrone Sibilia M, Aldirico MLA, et al. Vaccine potential of antigen cocktails composed of recombinant *Toxoplasma gondii* TgPI-1, ROP2 and GRA4 proteins against chronic toxoplasmosis in C3H mice. *Exp Parasitol* (2018) 185:62–70. doi:10.1016/j.exppara.2018.01.006
22. Zheng B, He A, Gan M, Li Z, He H, Zhan X. MIC6 associates with aldolase in host cell invasion by *Toxoplasma gondii*. *Parasitol Res* (2009) 105:441–5. doi:10.1007/s00436-009-1401-5
23. Plattner F, Yarovinsky F, Romero S, Didry D, Carlier MF, Sher A, et al. *Toxoplasma* profilin is essential for host cell invasion and TLR11-dependent induction of an Interleukin-12 response. *Cell Host Microbe* (2008) 3:77–87. doi:10.1016/j.chom.2008.01.001
24. Koblansky AA, Jankovic D, Oh H, Hieny S, Sungnak W, Mathur R, et al. Recognition of profilin by toll-like receptor 12 is critical for host resistance to *Toxoplasma gondii*. *Immunity* (2013) 38:119–30. doi:10.1016/j.immuni.2012.09.016
25. McCoy JM, Whitehead L, van Dooren GG, Tonkin CJ. TgCDPK3 regulates calcium-dependent egress of *Toxoplasma gondii* from host cells. *PLoS Pathog* (2012) 8:1003066. doi:10.1371/journal.ppat.1003066
26. El Hajj H, Lebrun M, Arold ST, Vial H, Labesse G, Dubremetz JF. ROP18 is a rhoptry kinase controlling the intracellular proliferation of *Toxoplasma gondii*. *PLoS Pathog* (2007) 3:e14. doi:10.1371/journal.ppat.0030014
27. Jensen KD, Hu K, Whitmarsh RJ, Hassan MA, Julien L, Lu D, et al. *Toxoplasma gondii* rhoptry 16 kinase promotes host resistance to oral infection and intestinal inflammation only in the context of the dense granule protein GRA15. *Infect Immun* (2013) 81:2156–67. doi:10.1128/IAI.01185-12
28. Zhou CX, Zhou DH, Elsheikha HM, Zhao Y, Suo X, Zhu XQ. Metabolomic profiling of mice serum during toxoplasmosis progression using liquid chromatography-mass spectrometry. *Sci Rep* (2016) 6:19557. doi:10.1038/srep19557
29. Bastos LM, Macêdo AG Jr, Silva MV, Santiago FM, Ramos EL, Santos FA, et al. *Toxoplasma gondii*-derived synthetic peptides containing B- and T-cell epitopes from GRA2 protein are able to enhance mice survival in a model of experimental toxoplasmosis. *Front Cell Infect Microbiol* (2016) 6:59. doi:10.3389/fcimb.2016.00059
30. Wang JL, Elsheikha HM, Zhu WN, Chen K, Li TT, Yue DM, et al. Immunization with *Toxoplasma gondii* GRA17 deletion mutant induces partial protection and survival in challenged mice. *Front Immunol* (2017) 8:730. doi:10.3389/fimmu.2017.00730
31. Peng GH, Yuan ZG, Zhou DH, He XH, Liu MM, Yan C, et al. *Toxoplasma gondii* microneme protein 6 (MIC6) is a potential vaccine candidate against toxoplasmosis in mice. *Vaccine* (2009) 27:6570–4. doi:10.1016/j.vaccine.2009.08.043
32. Yuan ZG, Zhang XX, Lin RQ, Petersen E, He S, Yu M, et al. Protective effect against toxoplasmosis in mice induced by DNA immunization with gene encoding *Toxoplasma gondii* ROP18. *Vaccine* (2011) 29:6614–9. doi:10.1016/j.vaccine.2011.06.110
33. Yuan ZG, Zhang XX, He XH, Petersen E, Zhou DH, He Y, et al. Protective immunity induced by *Toxoplasma gondii* rhoptry protein 16 against toxoplasmosis in mice. *Clin Vaccine Immunol* (2011) 18:119–24. doi:10.1128/CVI.00312-10
34. Zhang NZ, Huang SY, Zhou DH, Chen J, Xu Y, Tian WP, et al. Protective immunity against *Toxoplasma gondii* induced by DNA immunization with the gene encoding a novel vaccine candidate: calcium-dependent protein kinase 3. *BMC Infect Dis* (2013) 13:512. doi:10.1186/1471-2334-13-512
35. Gao Q, Zhang NZ, Zhang FK, Wang M, Hu LY, Zhu XQ. Immune response and protective effect against chronic *Toxoplasma gondii* infection induced by vaccination with a DNA vaccine encoding profilin. *BMC Infect Dis* (2017) 18:117. doi:10.1186/s12879-018-3022-z
36. Guo J, Sun X, Yin H, Wang T, Li Y, Zhou C, et al. Chitosan microsphere used as an effective system to deliver a linked antigenic peptides vaccine protect mice against acute and chronic toxoplasmosis. *Front Cell Infect Microbiol* (2018) 8:163. doi:10.3389/fcimb.2018.00163
37. Ismael AB, Sekkai D, Collin C, Bout D, Mévélec MN. The MIC3 gene of *Toxoplasma gondii* is a novel potent vaccine candidate against toxoplasmosis. *Infect Immun* (2003) 71:6222–8. doi:10.1128/IAI.71.11.6222-6228.2003
38. Sayles PC, Gibson GW, Johnson LL. B cells are essential for vaccination-induced resistance to virulent *Toxoplasma gondii*. *Infect Immun* (2000) 68(3):1026–33. doi:10.1128/IAI.68.3.1026-1033.2000
39. Zhang NZ, Xu Y, Wang M, Petersen E, Chen J, Huang SY, et al. Protective efficacy of two novel DNA vaccines expressing *Toxoplasma gondii* rhomboid 4 and rhomboid 5 proteins against acute and chronic toxoplasmosis in mice. *Expert Rev Vaccines* (2015) 14:1289–97. doi:10.1586/14760584.2015.1061938
40. Gazzinelli RT, Hakim FT, Hieny S, Shearer GM, Sher A. Synergistic role of CD4+ and CD8+ T lymphocytes in IFN-gamma production and protective immunity induced by an attenuated *Toxoplasma gondii* vaccine. *J Immunol* (1991) 146:286–92.
41. Jordan KA, Hunter CA. Regulation of CD8+ T cell responses to infection with parasitic protozoa. *Exp Parasitol* (2010) 126:318–25. doi:10.1016/j.exppara.2010.05.008
42. Gazzinelli R, Xu Y, Hieny S, Cheever A, Sher A. Simultaneous depletion of CD4+ and CD8+ T lymphocytes is required to reactivate chronic infection with *Toxoplasma gondii*. *J Immunol* (1992) 149:175–80.
43. El Bissati K, Zhou Y, Paulillo SM, Raman SK, Karch CP, Roberts CW, et al. Protein nanovaccine confers robust immunity against *Toxoplasma*. *NPJ Vaccines* (2017) 2:24. doi:10.1038/s41541-017-0024-6
44. Casciotti C, Ely K, Williams M, Khan I. CD8+-T-cell immunity against *Toxoplasma gondii* can be induced but not maintained in mice lacking conventional CD4+ T cells. *Infect Immun* (2002) 70:434–43. doi:10.1128/IAI.70.2.434-443.2002
45. Hakim FT, Gazzinelli RT, Denkers E, Hieny S, Shearer GM, Sher A. CD8+ T cells from mice vaccinated against *Toxoplasma gondii* are cytotoxic for parasite-infected or antigen-pulsed host cells. *J Immunol* (1991) 147:2310–6.
46. Suzuki Y, Sa Q, Gehman M, Ochiai E. Interferon-gamma- and perforin-mediated immune responses for resistance against *Toxoplasma gondii* in the brain. *Expert Rev Mol Med* (2011) 13:e31. doi:10.1017/S1462399411002018
47. Xu Y, Zhang NZ, Tan QD, Chen J, Lu J, Xu QM, et al. Evaluation of immuno-efficacy of a novel DNA vaccine encoding *Toxoplasma gondii* rhoptry protein 38 (TgROP38) against chronic toxoplasmosis in a murine model. *BMC Infect Dis* (2014) 14:525. doi:10.1186/1471-2334-14-525
48. Scorza T, D'Souza S, Laloup M, Dewit J, De Braekeleer J, Verschueren H, et al. A GRA1 DNA vaccine primes cytolytic CD8(+) T cells to control acute *Toxoplasma gondii* infection. *Infect Immun* (2003) 71:309–16. doi:10.1128/IAI.71.1.309-316.2003
49. Zhou J, Wang L. SAG4 DNA and peptide vaccination provides partial protection against *T. gondii* infection in BALB/c mice. *Front Microbiol* (2017) 8:1733. doi:10.3389/fmicb.2017.01733
50. Landrith TA, Sureshchandra S, Rivera A, Jang JC, Rais M, Nair MG, et al. CD103+ CD8 T cells in the *Toxoplasma*-infected brain exhibit a tissue-resident memory transcriptional profile. *Front Immunol* (2017) 8:335. doi:10.3389/fimmu.2017.00335
51. Bessieres MH, Swierczynski B, Cassaing S, Miedouge M, Olle P, Sequela JP, et al. Role of IFN-gamma, TNF-alpha, IL4 and IL10 in the regulation of experimental *Toxoplasma gondii* infection. *J Eukaryot Microbiol* (1997) 44:87S. doi:10.1111/j.1550-7408.1997.tb05800.x
52. Bao Y, Cao X. The immune potential and immunopathology of cytokine-producing B cell subsets: a comprehensive review. *J Autoimmun* (2014) 55:10–23. doi:10.1016/j.jaut.2014.04.001
53. Chen K, Wang JL, Huang SY, Yang WB, Zhu WN, Zhu XQ. Immune responses and protection after DNA vaccination against *Toxoplasma gondii* calcium-dependent protein kinase 2 (TgCDPK2). *Parasite* (2017) 24:41. doi:10.1051/parasite/2017045
54. Meng M, He S, Zhao G, Bai Y, Zhou H, Cong H, et al. Evaluation of protective immune responses induced by DNA vaccines encoding *Toxoplasma gondii* surface antigen 1 (SAG1) and 14-3-3 protein in BALB/c mice. *Parasit Vectors* (2012) 5:273. doi:10.1186/1756-3305-5-273
55. Hwang S, Cobb DA, Bhadra R, Youngblood B, Khan IA. Blimp-1-mediated

CD4 T cell exhaustion causes CD8 T cell dysfunction during chronic toxoplasmosis. *J Exp Med* (2016) 213:1799–818. doi:10.1084/jem.20151995

56. Mason NJ, Artis D, Hunter CA. New lessons from old pathogens: what parasitic infections have taught us about the role of nuclear factor-kappaB in the regulation of immunity. *Immunol Rev* (2004) 201:48–56. doi:10.1111/j.0105-2896.2004.00189.x
57. Gazzinelli RT, Wysocka M, Hayashi S, Denkers EY, Hieny S, Caspar P, et al. Parasite-induced IL-12 stimulates early IFN-gamma synthesis and resistance during acute infection with *Toxoplasma gondii*. *J Immunol* (1994) 153:2533–43.
58. Yang WB, Zhou DH, Zou Y, Chen K, Liu Q, Wang JL, et al. Vaccination with a DNA vaccine encoding *Toxoplasma gondii* ROP54 induces protective immunity against toxoplasmosis in mice. *Acta Trop* (2017) 176:427–42. doi:10.1016/j.actatropica.2017.09.007
59. Pifer R, Yarovinsky F. Innate responses to *Toxoplasma gondii* in mice and humans. *Trends Parasitol* (2011) 27:388–93. doi:10.1016/j.pt.2011.03.009
60. Yarovinsky F, Zhang D, Andersen JF, Bannenberg GL, Serhan CN, Hayden MS, et al. TLR11 activation of dendritic cells by a protozoan profilin-like protein. *Science* (2005) 308:1626–9. doi:10.1126/science.1109893
61. Denkers EY, Striepen B. Deploying parasite profilin on a mission of invasion and danger. *Cell Host Microbe* (2008) 3:61–3. doi:10.1016/j.chom.2008.01.003
62. Yarovinsky F, Hieny S, Sher A. Recognition of *Toxoplasma gondii* by TLR11 prevents parasite-induced immunopathology. *J Immunol* (2008) 181:8478–84. doi:10.4049/jimmunol.181.12.8478
63. Pyo KH, Lee YW, Lim SM, Shin EH. Immune adjuvant effect of a *Toxoplasma gondii* profilin-like protein in autologous whole-tumor-cell vaccination in mice. *Oncotarget* (2016) 7:74107–19. doi:10.18632/oncotarget.12316
64. Neal LM, Knoll LJ. *Toxoplasma gondii* profilin promotes recruitment of Ly6Chi CCR2+ inflammatory monocytes that can confer resistance to bacterial infection. *PLoS Pathog* (2014) 10:e1004203. doi:10.1371/journal.ppat.1004203
65. Hedhli D, Moiré N, Akbar H, Laurent F, Héraut B, Dimier-Poisson I, et al. The antigen-specific response to *Toxoplasma gondii* profilin, a TLR11/12 ligand, depends on its intrinsic adjuvant properties. *Med Microbiol Immunol* (2016) 205:345–52. doi:10.1007/s00430-016-0452-3
66. Tanaka S, Kuroda Y, Ihara F, Nishimura M, Hiasa J, Kojima N, et al. Vaccination with profilin encapsulated in oligomannose-coated liposomes induces significant protective immunity against *Toxoplasma gondii*. *Vaccine* (2014) 32:1781–5. doi:10.1016/j.vaccine.2014.01.095

3

Galectin-3 and Galectin-9 May Differently Regulate the Expressions of Microglial M1/M2 Markers and T Helper 1/Th2 Cytokines in the Brains of Genetically Susceptible C57BL/6 and Resistant BALB/c Mice Following Peroral Infection with *Toxoplasma gondii*

Jinfeng Liu[1,2], *Shiguang Huang*[3]* *and Fangli Lu*[1,2]*

[1] *Department of Parasitology, Zhongshan School of Medicine, Sun Yat-sen University, Guangzhou, China,* [2] *Key Laboratory of Tropical Disease Control of Ministry of Education, Sun Yat-sen University, Guangzhou, China,* [3] *School of Stomatology, Jinan University, Guangzhou, China*

***Correspondence:**
Shiguang Huang
thshg@126.com;
Fangli Lu
fanglilu@yahoo.com

Toxoplasmic encephalitis (TE), an opportunistic infection, is a severe health problem in immunocompromised patients. Previous studies have revealed that C57BL/6 mice are susceptible and BALB/c mice are resistant to TE. To investigate the mechanisms involved in the immunopathogenesis of TE in susceptible C57BL/6 and resistant BALB/c mice, both strains of mice were perorally infected with the Prugniuad (Pru) strain of *Toxoplasma gondii*. Our results showed that compared with BALB/c mice, C57BL/6 mice infected with *T. gondii* Pru strain had more severe brain histopathological damage, and higher mRNA expression levels of tachyzoite-specific surface antigen 1, bradyzoite-specific antigen 1, interferon gamma (IFNγ), interleukin (IL)-10, arginase1 (Arg1) (M2 marker), galectin (Gal)-3, Gal-9, *T. gondii* microneme protein 1 (TgMIC1), TgMIC4, and TgMIC6 during the course of infection by using quantitative real-time reverse transcription-polymerase chain reaction. Further analysis displayed that BALB/c mice showed higher numbers of microglial cells and higher levels of IL-1β, inducible nitric oxide synthase (iNOS) (M1 marker), and chitinase-3-like protein 3 (Ym1) (M2 marker) in the early infective stage [at day 14 or 35 post infection (p.i.)] compared with C57BL/6 mice, whereas C57BL/6 mice showed higher numbers of microglial cells and higher levels of IL-10, iNOS (M1 marker), and Ym1 (M2 marker) at days 35, 50, or 70 p.i. compared with BALB/c mice. Correlation analysis showed that significant positive correlations existed between Gal-3 and IL-4/IL-10/iNOS/Ym1 and between Gal-9 and IL-4/Ym1 in C57BL/6 mice; between Gal-3 and IFNγ/Arg1 and between Gal-9 and IFNγ/Arg1 in BALB/c mice. Together, our data demonstrated that different Gal-3 and Gal-9 expressions as well as different positive correlations were found between Gal-3 and T helper 1 (Th1)/Th2/M1/M2 cytokines or between Gal-9 and Th1/Th2/M2 cytokines in the brains of *T. gondii* Pru strain-infected C57BL/6 and BALB/c mice.

Keywords: toxoplasmic encephalitis, galectins, microglial M1/M2 markers, *T. gondii* microneme proteins, mice

INTRODUCTION

Toxoplasma gondii, a pathogen of medical and veterinary importance, is an obligate intracellular protozoan parasite that has a global distribution and can infect almost any warm-blooded vertebrate (1). *T. gondii* infection in the immunocompetent individual is effectively controlled by a vigorous immune response (2); however, the infection can cause toxoplasmic encephalitis (TE), a life-threatening disease in immunocompromised patients (3). Although all mice lineages develop a strong T helper 1 (Th1) immune response to *T. gondii* infection (4), the immune response to the parasite infection in the brains can be drastically different between genetically resistant mice (e.g., BALB/c mice) and that of susceptible mice (e.g., C57BL/6 mice) (5). During the late stage of infection, resistant mouse strain establishes a latent chronic infection, while susceptible strain spontaneously develops necrotizing TE (6). So far, the mechanisms behind the differences between the two strains of mice during the development of TE are not fully understood.

It has been proposed that *T. gondii* utilizes innate immune cells such as macrophages to migrate to immunoprivileged sites such as the central nervous system (CNS) to establish chronic infection (7). Macrophages are generally categorized into two distinct subsets as either classically activated (M1) or alternatively activated (M2). M1 type macrophages, characterized by CD86 expression, can release high levels of pro-inflammatory markers such as monocyte chemotactic protein-1β, inducible nitric oxide synthase (iNOS), interleukin (IL)-6, and tumor necrosis factor alpha (TNFα) (8). M2 macrophages can produce a large amount of IL-10, chitinase-3-like protein 3 (Ym1), macrophage and granulocyte inducer-form 1, and arginase1 (Arg1) and play important roles in the protection of the host by decreasing inflammation and promoting tissue repair (9, 10). During *T. gondii* infection, Th1 cells produce cytokines such as interferon gamma (IFNγ) to activate macrophages and cytotoxic T lymphocytes, while Th2 cells secrete cytokines such as IL-4 to induce humoral type immune responses (11, 12). IFNγ-activated microglial cells significantly upregulate iNOS and produce nitric oxide (NO), which can inhibit intracellular *T. gondii* replication (13).

Galectins belong to the family of β-galactoside-binding lectins, which are known to regulate a number of pathways that involve in apoptosis (14), immune tolerance, inflammation (15), and cell adhesion (16). Currently, 15 members of the galectin family have been identified in mammals; some members are widely distributed in different cells and tissue types, while others are more selectively expressed (17). The major galectins expressed in the CNS are galectin (Gal)-1, Gal-3, Gal-4, Gal-8, and Gal-9 (18). Under normal physiological conditions, galectins maintain CNS homeostasis, while in neuronal diseases and experimental neuroinflammatory disease models, galectins may serve as extracellular mediators or intracellular regulators in controlling the inflammatory response or conferring the remodeling capacity in damaged CNS tissues (18). So far, the roles of galectins in TE remains poorly understood.

Apicomplexan parasites such as *T. gondii* and *Plasmodium* spp. utilize apical complex organelles consisting of dense granules, rhoptries, and micronemes to deploy for the release (egress), attachment, and invasion of host cells, as well as the establishment of the parasitophorous vacuole (19). *T. gondii* microneme proteins (TgMICs) are secreted by micronemes upon contact with host cells and play important roles in *T. gondii* motility, invasion, intracellular survival, and egress from host cells (20). TgMIC6 and TgMIC8 genes are expressed in the rapidly dividing tachyzoites, whereas TgMIC7 and TgMIC9 genes are predominantly expressed in the slowly dividing encysted bradyzoites (21). TgMIC1 and TgMIC4 can bind to host cells, while TgMIC6 serves as an escorter for two soluble adhesins TgMIC1 and TgMIC4 and along with adhesins can establish a molecular bridge between the host and parasites (22). So far, limited data are available about the role of TgMICs in the immune response to *T. gondii* infection.

Based on the relationship between galectins and brain diseases, this study was designed to compare the expressions of galectins, microglial activation markers (M1 and M2 phenotypes), TgMICs, and Th1 and Th2 cytokines between C57BL/6 and BALB/c mice infected with *T. gondii* Pru strain. We found that significant positive correlations existed between Gal-3 and Th1/Th2/M1/M2 cytokines as well as between Gal-9 and Th1/Th2/M2 cytokines in C57BL/6 or BALB/c mice after *T. gondii* Pru strain infection.

MATERIALS AND METHODS

Mice, Parasites, and Experimental Infections

This experimental study and all administrations were reviewed and approved by the Ethical Committee of Animal Experiments at Sun Yat-sen University.

Female 6- to 8-week-old C57BL/6 and BALB/c mice were purchased from the Experimental Animal Center at Sun Yat-sen University (Guangzhou, China), and 20 mice were used per each group. All animals were housed under specific-pathogen-free conditions in the animal facility at Sun Yat-sen University. Mice were infected *via* oral route with eight cysts of *T. gondii* Pru strain prepared from the brain of chronically infected mice. To establish a chronic infection by controlling the proliferation of tachyzoites during acute stage, mice were treated with sulfadiazine (Sigma-Aldrich, Shanghai, China) in the drinking water as described previously (23).

Histopathology

Mice infected with *T. gondii* Pru strain were euthanized by CO_2 asphyxiation at 14, 35, 50, and 70 days post infection (p.i.), and their brains were harvested and immediately fixed in 10% buffered natural formaldehyde (Guangzhou Chemical Reagent Factory, China) for over 48 h. The paraffin-embedded tissues from each mouse were sectioned at 5 μm and prepared for hematoxylin and eosin (Sigma-Aldrich, Shanghai, China) staining. The histopathological changes of brains from each group were determined under 200× magnification in three noncontiguous sections from four mice, and histopathological scores were given based on previously described criteria (23) with some modifications. In brief, the histological changes were scored semi-quantitatively as 1, 2, 3, and 4 (e.g., normal, mild inflammation, moderate inflammation and necrosis, and severe inflammation and necrosis, respectively).

Immunohistochemical Staining

The paraffin-embedded brain sections (6-μm) were deparaffinized and rehydrated in distilled water. Heat-induced antigen retrieval was carried out in an 800-W microwave oven for 30 min. Sections were treated with 3% hydrogen peroxide in methanol for 10 min at 37°C, and then incubated in 10% normal goat serum with 1% bovine serum albumin (Sigma-Aldrich, Shanghai, China) in PBS (pH 7.4) for 10 min at room temperature to block nonspecific binding. After washing with PBS, sections were incubated with rabbit anti-Iba1 (1:200 dilutions) (Wako Pure Chemical Industries, Osaka, Japan), rabbit anti-Gal-9 (1:200 dilutions) (Boster Biological Technology, Wuhan, China), and mouse anti-Gal-3 (1:200 dilutions) (R&D Systems, Minneapolis, MN, USA) overnight at 4°C. Those sections incubated with secondary antibodies alone were used as isotype controls. Immunohistochemical staining was then performed with a streptavidin–biotin–peroxidase complex kit and developed with diaminobenzidine tetrahydrochloride (Zhongshan Golden Bridge Technology, Beijing, China). The sections were counterstained with hematoxylin and positive cells were identified by dark-brown staining under light microscopy.

Morphometric Analysis

Serial sections from the brains were immunostained with anti-Iba1. A total of three mice were analyzed in each time point, and four sections per animal were selected for counting of positive cells. In every brain section, the microglial cells expressing Iba1 markers were captured with a digital microscopy under 400× magnification and the numbers of Iba1-positive cells in the brains (0.015066 mm^2 tissue section) were determined by Image-Pro Plus (Image Z1 software, Media Cybernetics, MD, USA), and the density of positive cells was expressed as the number of cells per square millimeter.

Selection of Galectins

Gal-1, Gal-3, Gal-7, Gal-8, and Gal-9 are known to be relevant to brain diseases (18). Therefore, in this study, the specific expression pattern of these five galectins was examined.

Determination of mRNA Expression Using Quantitative Real-Time Reverse Transcription-Polymerase Chain Reaction (qRT-PCR)

Total RNA was extracted from about 100 mg of mouse brain tissues from each group using a RNA Extraction Kit (TaKaRa, Shiga, Japan) as per the manufacturer's protocol. RNA amount was determined by measuring the ratio of absorbance at 260 and 280 nm using a NanoDrop ND-1000 spectrophotometer (NanoDrop Technologies). First-strand cDNA was constructed from 1.0 μg of total RNA with oligo (dT) as primers using a PrimeScript 1st Strand cDNA Synthesis Kit (TaKaRa, Shiga, Japan). To determine tissue mRNA levels of cytokines (IL-1β, IFNγ, IL-4, IL-10, iNOS, Arg1, and Ym-1), galectins (Gal-1, Gal-3, Gal-4, Gal-8, and Gal-9), TgMICs (TgMIC1, TgMIC4, TgMIC6, TgMIC3, and TgMIC8), β-actin, actin of the ME49 strain of *T. gondii*, *T. gondii* tachyzoite-specific surface antigen 1 (SAG1), and *T. gondii* bradyzoite-specific antigen 1 (BAG1), qRT-PCR measurements were performed using SYBR Green QPCR Master Mix (TaKaRa, Shiga, Japan). Primers are listed in **Table 1**. Briefly, a total of 10 μl reaction mixture contained 5.0 μl of SYBR® Premix Ex TaqTM (2×), 0.5 μl of each primer (10 pM), 3.0 μl of dH_2O, and 1.0 μl of cDNA (0.2 μg/μl). Amplification was pre-denaturized for 30 s at 95°C, followed by 43 cycles of 5 s at 95°C and 20 s at 60°C with a LightCycler® 480 instrument (Roche Diagnostics, USA). The mRNA expression levels of cytokines, SAG1, and BAG1 were normalized to that of mouse housekeeping gene, β-actin, and the mRNA levels of TgMICs were normalized to that of *T. gondii* housekeeping gene (actin of *T. gondii* ME49 strain). The results were expressed as fold change compared with uninfected controls.

Statistical Analysis

Results of experimental studies were reported as mean ± SD. Statistical analysis of the data was performed by the Wilcoxon

TABLE 1 | Primer sequences of genes used for quantitative real-time reverse transcription-polymerase chain reaction assays.

Genes	Forward primer (5′→3′)	Reverse primer (5′→3′)	Reference/accession
IL-1β	AATGACCTGTTCTTTGAAGTTGA	TGATGTGCTGCTGCGAGATTTGAAG	(24)
IFNγ	GGAACTGGCAAAAGGATGGTGAC	GCTGGACCTGTGGGTTGTTGAC	(25)
IL-4	ACAGGAGAAGGGACGCCAT	GAAGCCCTACAGACGAGCTCA	(26)
IL-10	AGCCGGGAAGACAATAACTG	CATTTCCGATAAGGCTTGG	(25)
iNOS	GTTCTCAGCCCAACAATACAAGA	GTGGACGGGTCGATGTCAC	(27)
Arg1	CTCCAAGCCAAAGTCCTTAGAG	AGGAGCTATCATTAGGGACATC	(27)
Ym1	AGAAGGGAGTTTCAA ACCTGGT	GTCTTGCTCATGTGTGTAAGTGA	(27)
Gal-1	CGCCAGCAACCTGAATC	GTCCCATCTTCCTTGGTGTTA	(28)
Gal-3	GCTACTGGCCCCTTTGGT	CCAGGCAAGGGCATATCGTA	(29)
Gal-4	CAACCCTCCACAGATGAACACCTT	TCCAGCGTGTCTACCATTTGGAAT	(30)
Gal-8	GGGTGGTGGGTGGAACTG	GCCTTTGAGCCCCCAATATC	(31)
Gal-9	GAGCTTTGCTTCCTGGTACAGA	CGGTGTGAGTACTGTACAAAGAAGT	(29)
β-actin	TGGAATCCTGTGGCATCCATGAAAC	TAAAACGCAGCTCAGTAACAGTCCG	(25)
TgMIC1	GCGAATTTCCTTGATGGATT	GTAGTCGAGGACAACAGCGA	XM_002368490.1
TgMIC3	AGCCATCACACACACACCTT	ATGCACAGAAACGCACTCTC	XM_002369792.1
TgMIC4	CCTGCAAGGCTTCACTGATA	CTATTGTGGGAGCCCTTGAT	XM_002369565.1
TgMIC6	CGCCAGATGCAGTACAGAGT	GCGTCGATTGTCGCTATAAA	XM_002370595.1
TgMIC8	GTAAAGGCGAGGTCGAAGAC	GTACTGCGGGAAAGGATGAT	XM_002366938.1
T. gondii ME49 actin	ATTATGAAGTGCGACGTGGA	TGATCTTCATGGTGGAAGGA	XM_002369622.1

rank sum test and one-way ANOVA followed by Bonferroni's multiple comparison tests using SPSS software for windows (version 19.0; SPSS, Inc., IL, USA). Pearson's correlation coefficient was used to analyze correlations between the levels of cytokines and galectins. All graphs were performed using GraphPad Prism software (version 5.0). A value of $P < 0.01$ was considered significant for correlation analysis, while a value of $P < 0.05$ was considered significant for other statistical analysis.

RESULTS

Comparison of Histopathology and Parasite Burdens in the Brains of *T. gondii*-Susceptible C57BL/6 and *T. gondii*-Resistant BALB/c Mice

Histological observation showed that control sections of the brains from uninfected C57BL/6 and BALB/c mice had no obvious inflammations or structural abnormalities. The brains of *T. gondii* Pru strain-infected C57BL/6 mice showed moderate-to-severe inflammation, diffuse inflammatory cellular infiltration, necrotic focus, and tissue structural damages at days 14, 35, 50, and 70 p.i., while the brains of infected BALB/c mice showed limited infiltration of inflammatory cells at the aforementioned times (**Figure 1A**). Semi-quantitative analysis of the severity of inflammation and necrosis in the brain sections of the two strains of mice were performed. Compared with uninfected controls, the pathological severity scores of brains were significantly increased in both C57BL/6 and BALB/c mice at days 14, 35, 50, and 70 p.i. Compared with BALB/c mice, the histopathological scores in the brains of C57BL/6 mice were significantly higher at days 35 ($P < 0.05$), 50 ($P < 0.01$), and 70 ($P < 0.01$) p.i. (**Figure 1B**).

Stage conversion between tachyzoite and bradyzoite forms is associated with stage specific antigen expression. In this study, the mRNA expression levels of tachyzoite-specific SAG1 and bradyzoite-specific BAG1 in the brains of C57BL/6 and BALB/c mice infected with *T. gondii* Pru strain were detected by using qRT-PCR and the transcript. Levels of SAG1 and BAG1 were relative to day 14 p.i. (e.g., the relative transcript level at day 14 p.i. = 1.0). Compared with day 14 p.i., the SAG1 levels in the brains of both C57BL/6 and BALB/c mice were significantly decreased at days 35, 50, and 70 p.i. The BAG1 levels in the brains of C57BL/6 mice were significantly elevated at days 35 and 70 p.i., while the BAG1 level in BALB/c mice was significantly reduced at day 70 p.i. Compared with BALB/c mice, both SAG1 and BAG1 levels were significantly higher in the brains of C57BL/6 mice at days 35, 50, and 70 p.i. ($P < 0.01$ and $P < 0.05$, respectively) (**Figure 1C**).

Comparison of Microglial Cells in the Brains of *T. gondii*-Susceptible C57BL/6 and *T. gondii*-Resistant BALB/c Mice

A few Iba1-positive microglial cells were observed in the sections of brains of uninfected C57BL/6 and BALB/c mice. However, a large number of activated microglial cells were observed in the brains of both *T. gondii* Pru strain-infected C57BL/6 and BALB/c mice; the majority of activated microglial cells were ameboid shape with thickened and retracted branches (**Figure 2A**). Quantitative analysis of Iba1 staining showed that, compared with uninfected controls, the numbers of Iba1-positive microglial cells in the brains of both C57BL/6 and BALB/c mice were significantly increased at days 14, 35, 50, and 70 p.i. However, compared with BALB/c mice, the microglial cell numbers in the brains of C57BL/6 mice were significantly higher at days 35 ($P < 0.001$), 50 ($P < 0.001$), and 70 ($P < 0.01$) p.i. (**Figure 2B**).

Comparison of mRNA Levels of M1/M2 Markers in the Brains of *T. gondii*-Susceptible C57BL/6 and *T. gondii*-Resistant BALB/c Mice

The mRNA levels of M1 marker (iNOS) and M2 marker (Arg1 and Ym1) in the brains of *T. gondii* Pru strain-infected C57BL/6 and BALB/c mice were examined. Compared with uninfected controls, iNOS levels were significantly increased in the brains of both C57BL/6 and BALB/c mice at days 14, 35, 50, and 70 p.i.; Arg1 and Ym1 levels were significantly increased in C57BL/6 mice at days 14, 35, 50, and 70 p.i., and significantly increased in BALB/c mice at days 14 and 35 p.i. (**Figure 3A**). Compared with BALB/c mice, there were significantly lower iNOS levels at days 14 and 35 p.i. ($P < 0.01$); while there were significantly higher iNOS levels at days 50 and 70 p.i. ($P < 0.001$), significantly higher Arg1 levels at days 14 ($P < 0.05$), 35 ($P < 0.01$), 50 ($P < 0.001$), and 70 ($P < 0.01$) p.i., and significantly lower Ym1 level at day 14 p.i. ($P < 0.001$) and significantly higher Ym1 levels at days 35 ($P < 0.01$), 50 ($P < 0.001$), and 70 ($P < 0.001$) p.i. in the brains of C57BL/6 mice (**Figure 3B**).

Comparison of mRNA Levels of Th1/Th2 Cytokines in the Brains of *T. gondii*-Susceptible C57BL/6 and *T. gondii*-Resistant BALB/c Mice

Compared with uninfected controls, the levels of IL-1β, IFNγ, and IL-10 were significantly increased in the brains of both C57BL/6 and BALB/c mice at days 14, 35, 50, and 70 p.i.; IL-4 levels were significantly increased in both *T. gondii* Pru strain-infected C57BL/6 and BALB/c mice at days 35, 50, and 70 p.i. (**Figure 4A**). Compared with BALB/c mice, significantly lower IL-1β level at day 35 p.i. ($P < 0.05$), significantly higher IL-10 level at day 50 p.i. ($P < 0.01$), and significantly higher IFNγ levels at days 14 ($P < 0.05$), 35 ($P < 0.05$), 50 ($P < 0.01$), and 70 ($P < 0.01$) p.i. were detected in the brains of C57BL/6 mice (**Figure 4B**).

Comparison of mRNA Levels of Galectins in the Brains of *T. gondii*-Susceptible C57BL/6 and *T. gondii*-Resistant BALB/c Mice

Compared with uninfected controls, Gal-3 expression levels were significantly increased in the brains of both *T. gondii* Pru strain-infected C57BL/6 and BALB/c mice at days 14, 35, 50, and 70 p.i.; Gal-9 levels were significantly increased in both C57BL/6 and BALB/c mice at days 14, 35, and 50 p.i., and significantly increased in C57BL/6 mice at day 70 p.i. (**Figure 5A**). Compared

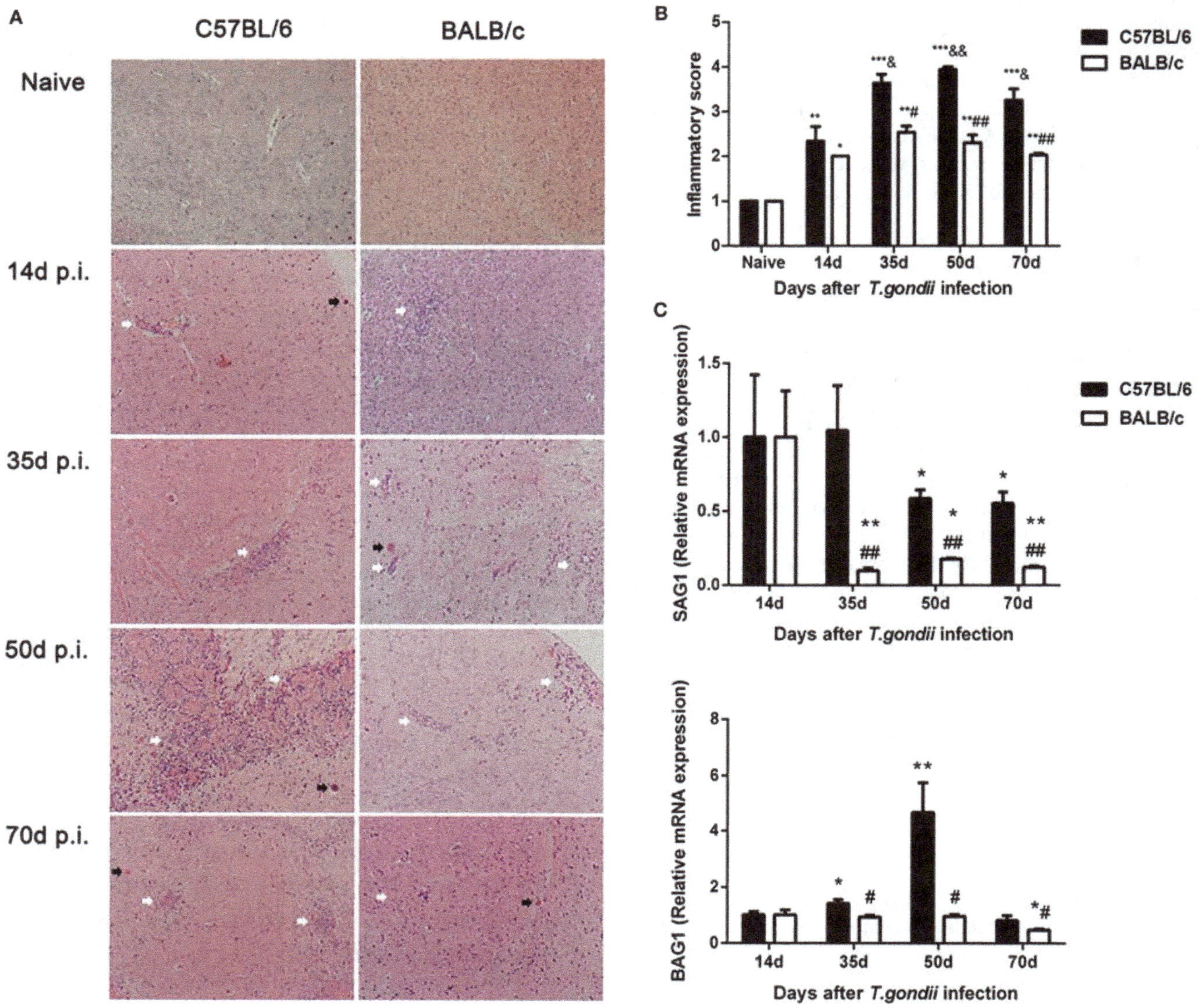

FIGURE 1 | Histopathological changes and parasite burdens in the brains of *Toxoplasma gondii* Pru strain-infected C57BL/6 and BALB/c mice. **(A)** Histopathological changes in the brains at days 14, 35, 50, and 70 post infection (p.i.). Cysts were indicated with black arrow heads and inflammatory cell infiltrates were indicated with white arrow heads. Original magnification 200x; hematoxylin and eosin stain. **(B)** Histopathological score analysis at days 14, 35, 50, and 70 p.i. Data are represented as mean ± SEM. Significant differences between groups are analyzed by the Wilcoxon rank sum test. *$P < 0.05$, **$P < 0.01$, and ***$P < 0.001$ vs naive; &$P < 0.05$ and &&$P < 0.01$ vs 14 days p.i.; #$P < 0.05$ and ##$P < 0.01$ vs C57BL/6 mice. **(C)** Parasite burdens in the brains at days 14, 35, 50, and 70 p.i. Relative mRNA expressions of surface antigen 1 (SAG1) and bradyzoite-specific antigen 1 (BAG1) were detected by using quantitative real-time reverse transcription-polymerase chain reaction. Transcript level at day 14 p.i. was taken as 1. Values are means from triplicate measurements, and data are presented as mean ± SD. *$P < 0.05$ and **$P < 0.01$ vs naive; #$P < 0.05$ and ##$P < 0.01$ vs C57BL/6 mice. There were four mice per group. The data shown are representative of those from two different experiments.

with BALB/c mice, there were significantly higher levels of Gal-3 and Gal-9 in the brains of C57BL/6 mice at days 35 ($P < 0.05$), 50 ($P < 0.01$ and $P < 0.05$, respectively), and 70 ($P < 0.01$) p.i. (**Figure 5B**).

Comparison of mRNA Levels of TgMICs in the Brains of *T. gondii*-Susceptible C57BL/6 and *T. gondii*-Resistant BALB/c Mice

Compared with day 14 p.i., TgMIC1 levels were significantly decreased in the brains of both *T. gondii* Pru strain-infected C57BL/6 and BALB/c mice at days 35, 50, and 70 p.i.; TgMIC3 levels were significantly increased in C57BL/6 mice at days 35, 50, and 70 p.i.; TgMIC4 levels were significantly increased in C57BL/6 mice at days 50 and 70 p.i. and significantly increased in BALB/c mice at day 70 p.i. TgMIC6 levels were significantly decreased in BALB/c mice at days 35, 50, and 70 p.i., and TgMIC8 levels were significantly decreased in both C57BL/6 and BALB/c mice at days 35, 50, and 70 p.i. (**Figure 6A**). Compared with BALB/c mice, there were significantly higher levels of TgMIC1 at days 35 and 70 p.i. ($P < 0.05$) and significantly higher levels of TgMIC4 and TgMIC6 at days

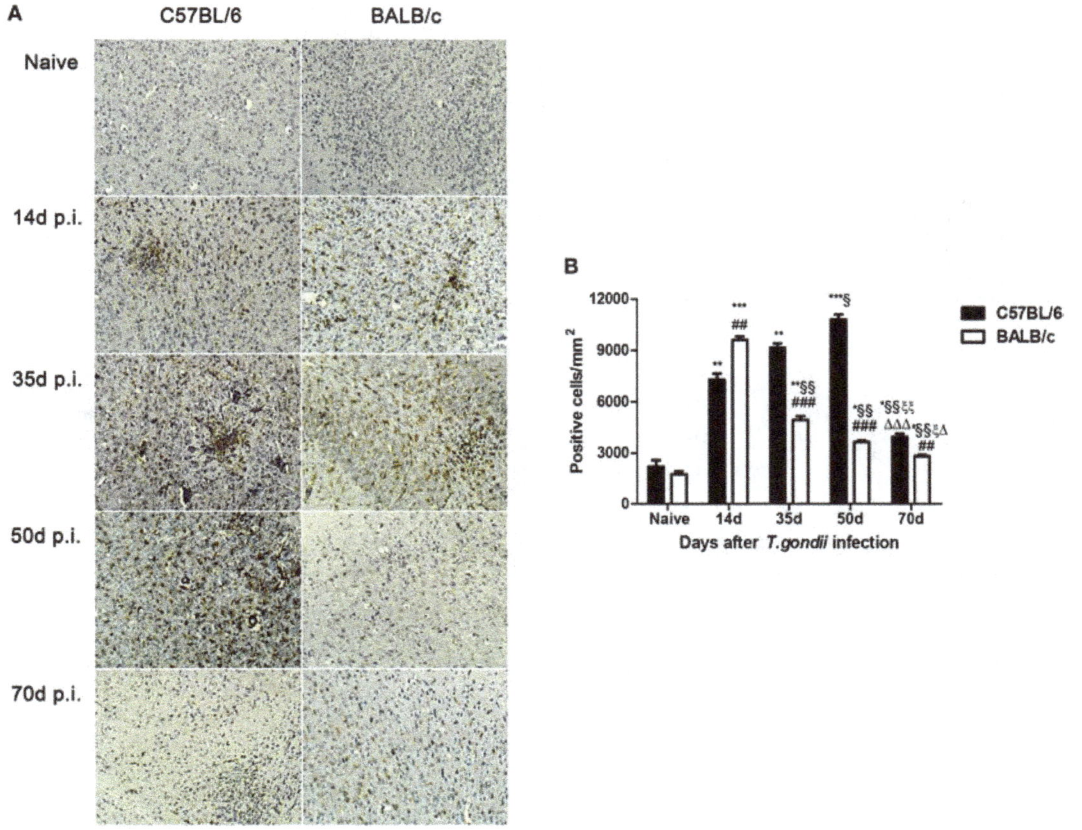

FIGURE 2 | Expression of activated microglial marker Iba1 in the brains of *Toxoplasma gondii* Pru strain-infected C57BL/6 and BALB/c mice. **(A)** Immunohistochemistry for Iba1 in the brains of uninfected mice, and mice infected with *T. gondii* Pru strain at days 14, 35, 50, and 70 post infection (p.i.). Original magnification 200×. **(B)** Quantitative analysis of Iba1-positive microglia. The density of positive cells was expressed as the number of cells per square millimeter. Data are presented as means ± SD; experiments were performed with three mice per group. $^{*}P < 0.05$, $^{**}P < 0.01$, and $^{***}P < 0.001$ vs Naive; $^{§}P < 0.05$ and $^{§§}P < 0.01$ vs 14 days p.i.; $^{ξ}P < 0.05$ and $^{ξξ}P < 0.01$ vs 35 days p.i.; $^{Δ}P < 0.05$ and $^{ΔΔΔ}P < 0.001$ vs 50 days p.i.; $^{\#\#}P < 0.01$ and $^{\#\#\#}P < 0.001$ vs C57BL/6 mice.

35, 50, and 70 p.i. in the brains of C57BL/6 mice ($P < 0.05$) (**Figure 6B**).

Correlations Between Gal-3/Ga-9 and Th1/Th2/M1/M2 Cytokines in the Brains of *T. gondii*-Resistant BALB/c and *T. gondii*-Susceptible C57BL/6 Mice

The correlations between mRNA levels of Gal-3/Gal-9 and Th1/Th2/M1/M2 in the brains of *T. gondii* Pru strain-infected C57BL/6 and BALB/c mice were evaluated, herein only significant correlations were shown. There were significant correlations between the mRNA levels of Gal-3 and IL-4 ($r = 0.8424$, $P = 0.0002$), Gal-3 and IL-10 ($r = 0.6996$, $P = 0.0037$), Gal-3 and iNOS ($r = 0.7344$, $P = 0.0018$), Gal-3 and Ym1 ($r = 0.6866$, $P = 0.0047$), Gal-9 and IL-4 ($r = 0.8293$, $P = 0.0002$), and Gal-9 and Ym1 ($r = 0.6714$, $P = 0.0061$) in *T. gondii* Pru strain-infected C57BL/6 mice (**Figure 7A**). However, there were significant correlations between the mRNA levels of Gal-3 and IFNγ ($r = 0.6993$, $P = 0.0078$), Gal-3 and Arg1 ($r = 0.8099$, $P = 0.0004$), Gal-9 and IFNγ ($r = 0.7378$, $P = 0.0040$), and Gal-9 and Arg1 ($r = 0.7963$, $P = 0.0007$) in *T. gondii* Pru strain-infected BALB/c mice (**Figure 7B**). Taken together, in C57BL/6 mice, significant positive correlations existed between Gal-3 and IL-4/IL-10/iNOS/Ym1 as well as between Gal-9 and IL-4/Ym1; whereas in BALB/c mice, significant positive correlations existed between Gal-3 and IFNγ/Arg1 as well as between Gal-9 and IFNγ/Arg1.

DISCUSSION

When *T. gondii* parasites infect the host, the cysts can exist predominantly in the brain tissue for lifetime, and an immunocompetent host will establish a strong and persistent Th1-biased cell-mediated immunity to resist cyst reactivation and the consequences of TE (4). However, there is a remarkable difference in susceptibility to the infection of *T. gondii* among inbred strains of mice. After peroral infection with *T. gondii* ME49 strain, C57BL/6 mice all died whereas BALB/c mice all survived (32). So far, the immune responses differing between TE-resistant and TE-susceptible hosts are not fully understood. In this study, genetically susceptible C57BL/6 and resistant BALB/c mice were perorally infected with *T. gondii* Pru strain, and significantly more severe histopathological damage (inflammation and necrosis) were found in the brains of C57BL/6 mice

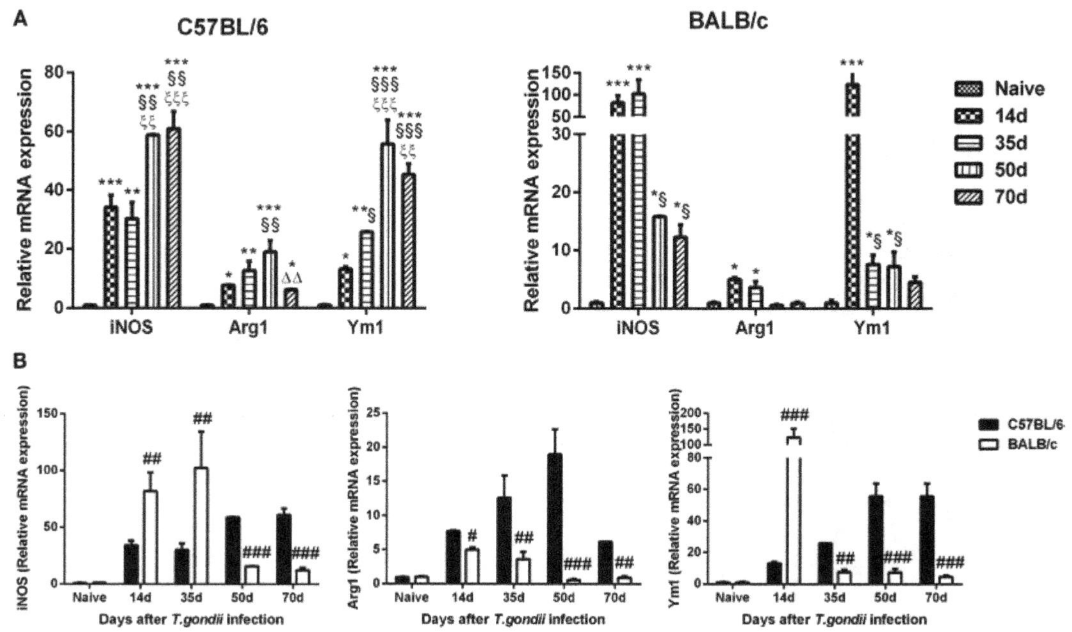

FIGURE 3 | Relative mRNA expressions of inducible nitric oxide synthase (iNOS), arginase1 (Arg1), and Ym1 in the brain tissues of *Toxoplasma gondii* Pru strain-infected C57BL/6 and BALB/c mice were detected by using quantitative real-time reverse transcription-polymerase chain reaction. **(A)** iNOS, Arg1, and Ym1 expressions in the brains of C57BL/6 and BALB/c mice. **(B)** Comparison of iNOS, Arg1, and Ym1 levels in the brains of C57BL/6 and BALB/c mice. Values are means from triplicate measurements, and data are presented as mean ± SD. There were four mice per group. The data shown are representative of those from two different experiments. $^{*}P < 0.05$, $^{**}P < 0.01$, and $^{***}P < 0.001$ vs naive; $^{§}P < 0.05$; $^{§§}P < 0.01$, and $^{§§§}P < 0.001$ vs 14 days post infection (p.i.); $^{ξξ}P < 0.01$ and $^{ξξξ}P < 0.001$ vs 35 days p.i.; $^{ΔΔ}P < 0.01$ vs 50 days p.i.; $^{\#}P < 0.05$, $^{\#\#}P < 0.01$, and $^{\#\#\#}P < 0.001$ vs C57BL/6 mice.

in comparison of those of BALB/c mice at all the times during the observations (e.g., at days 14, 35, 50, and 70 p.i.). The levels of mRNA transcripts of both tachyzoite-specific SAG1 and bradyzoite-specific BAG1 genes were significantly higher in the brains of C57BL/6 mice than those of BALB/c mice at days 35, 50, and 70 p.i. It has been reported that following *T. gondii* ME49 strain infection, C57BL/6 mice showed an intense and progressive inflammatory alteration in the CNS, while BALB/c mice showed slight inflammatory reaction in the CNS (33). After infection with low virulent *T. gondii* DX strain, C57BL/6 mice presented higher tachyzoite and bradyzoite loads than those of BALB/c mice (34). Our data were in accordance with the previous studies.

Microglia activation is recognized as the hallmark of neuroinflammation. Microglial cells are the primary source for inflammatory mediators. Resident microglial cells play a critical role in TE, producing essential pro- and anti-inflammatory cytokines such as IL-1β, IL-10, TNFα, IL-12, and IL-15 (35–37). In this study, we found that microglial cell numbers in the brains of C57BL/6 mice were significantly higher than those of BALB/c mice at days 35, 50, and 70 p.i.; however, the number of microglial cells was significantly higher in BALB/c mice than that of C57BL/6 mice at day 14 p.i. Our data suggest that resident microglia are activated earlier in BALB/c mice, which may be essential for control of the parasite in the early infective stage in *T. gondii*-resistant BALB/c mice; whereas increased microglial activation remains longer in C57BL/6 mice, which may be required for establishing chronic TE in *T. gondii*-susceptible C57BL/6 mice.

It has been reported that activated microglial cells range from the pro-inflammatory M1 phenotype to the alternative/M2 phenotype and play neuroprotective or neurodetrimental roles (38). Therefore, identifying microglia phenotypes is critical for understanding the role of microglia in the pathogenesis of TE. In this study, we found that alterations in M1 and M2 phenotypes differed between the two models. In *T. gondii* Pru strain-infected BALB/c mice, both M1 (iNOS) and M2 (Ym1) phenotypic markers were significantly increased in the early infective stage (at day 14 or 35 p.i.); while in C57BL/6 mice, both M1 (iNOS) and M2 (Ym1) phenotypic markers were significantly increased in the late infective stage (at days 50 and 70 p.i.) and M2 marker (Arg1) was significantly increased at all the times during the study. M1 macrophages are critical for host defense against intracellular pathogens and have roles in antitumor immunity and autoimmune inflammation, whereas M2 macrophages are protective against helminth parasites and are important regulators of the wound healing response, tissue homeostasis, and adiposity (39). Inhibition of iNOS exacerbates chronic TE in *T. gondii*-susceptible C57BL/6 mice but does not lead to reactivation of latent TE in *T. gondii*-resistant BALB/c mice (34). CBA/Ca mice are susceptible to the development of TE. An *in vitro* study demonstrated that microglia from CBA/Ca mice show decreased production of NO and decreased inhibition of *T. gondii* replication after stimulation with lipopolysaccharide or IFNγ plus TNFα compared with microglia from BALB/c mice (40). Our data demonstrated that both M1 (iNOS) and M2 (Ym1 and Arg1) responses may play a role during chronic TE in *T. gondii*-susceptible C57BL/6 mice.

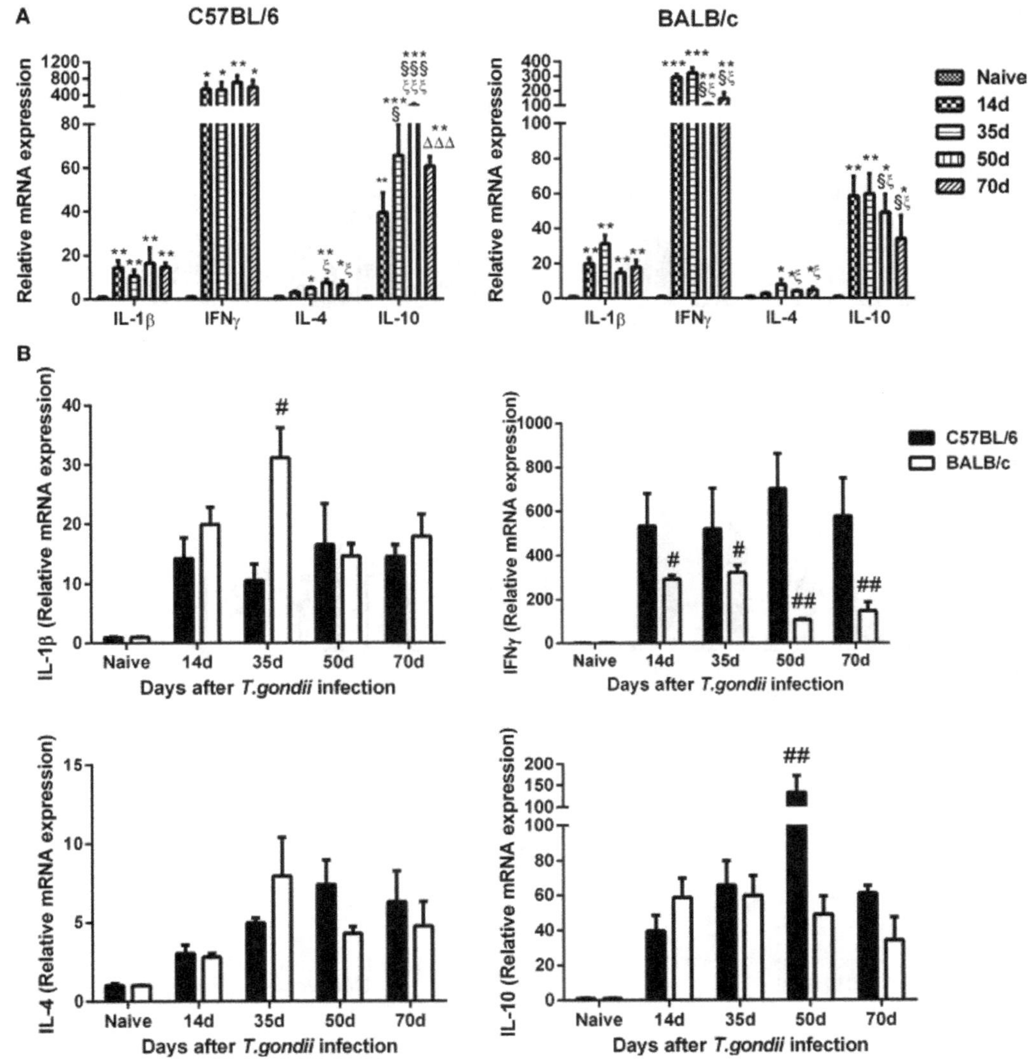

FIGURE 4 | Relative mRNA expressions of interleukin (IL)-1β, interferon gamma (IFNγ), IL-4, and IL-10 in the brain tissues of *Toxoplasma gondii* Pru strain-infected C57BL/6 and BALB/c mice were detected by using quantitative real-time reverse transcription-polymerase chain reaction. **(A)** IL-1β, IFNγ, IL-4, and IL-10 expressions in the brains of C57BL/6 and BALB/c mice. **(B)** Comparison of IL-1β, IFNγ, IL-4, and IL-10 levels in the brains of C57BL/6 and BALB/c mice. Values are means from triplicate measurements, and data are presented as mean ± SD. There were four mice per group. The data shown are representative of those from two different experiments. $^{*}P < 0.05$, $^{**}P < 0.01$, and $^{***}P < 0.001$ vs naive; $^{\S}P < 0.05$ and $^{\S\S\S}P < 0.001$ vs 14 days post infection (p.i.); $^{\xi}P < 0.05$ and $^{\xi\xi\xi}P < 0.001$ vs 35 days p.i.; $^{\Delta\Delta\Delta}P < 0.001$ vs 50 days p.i.; $^{\#}P < 0.05$ and $^{\#\#}P < 0.01$ vs C57BL/6 mice.

Toxoplasma gondii infection induces Th1-biased immune response, which is critical for the prevention of reactivation of TE (41). In this study, although the mRNA levels of Th1-associated cytokines (IFNγ and IL-1β) and Th2-associated cytokines (IL-4 and IL-10) were increased in the brain tissues of both C57BL/6 and BALB/c mice infected with *T. gondii* Pru strain, susceptible C57BL/6 mice presented a dominant Th1 response characterized by high expression of IFNγ at all the times after infection, accompanied by stronger neuroinflammatory outcomes. Our data suggested that the delayed M1 and M2 microglial activation and increased IFNγ expression in C57BL/6 mice after *T. gondii* Pru strain infection may be a part of the reason that C57BL/6 mice are more susceptible than BALB/c mice during TE.

Galectins have recently been demonstrated to play vital roles in host–pathogen interaction (42). Galectins are important modulators participating in homeostasis of the CNS and neuroinflammation; the major galectins expressed in the CNS are Gal-1, Gal-3, Gal-4, Gal-8, and Gal-9 (18). In this study, we compared the dynamic gene expressions of Gal-1, Gal-3, Gal-4, Gal-8, and Gal-9 in the brains between C57BL/6 and BALB/c mice infected with *T. gondii* Pru strain, only Gal-3 and Gal-9 were highly expressed in the brains of both C57BL/6 and BALB/c mice. C57BL/6 mice presented significantly higher mRNA expressions of Gal-3 and Gal-9 than those of BALB/c mice at days 35, 50, and 70 p.i. Gal-3 and Gal-9 are known pro-inflammatory mediators and regulators of apoptosis (29). Gal-9 is produced by activated

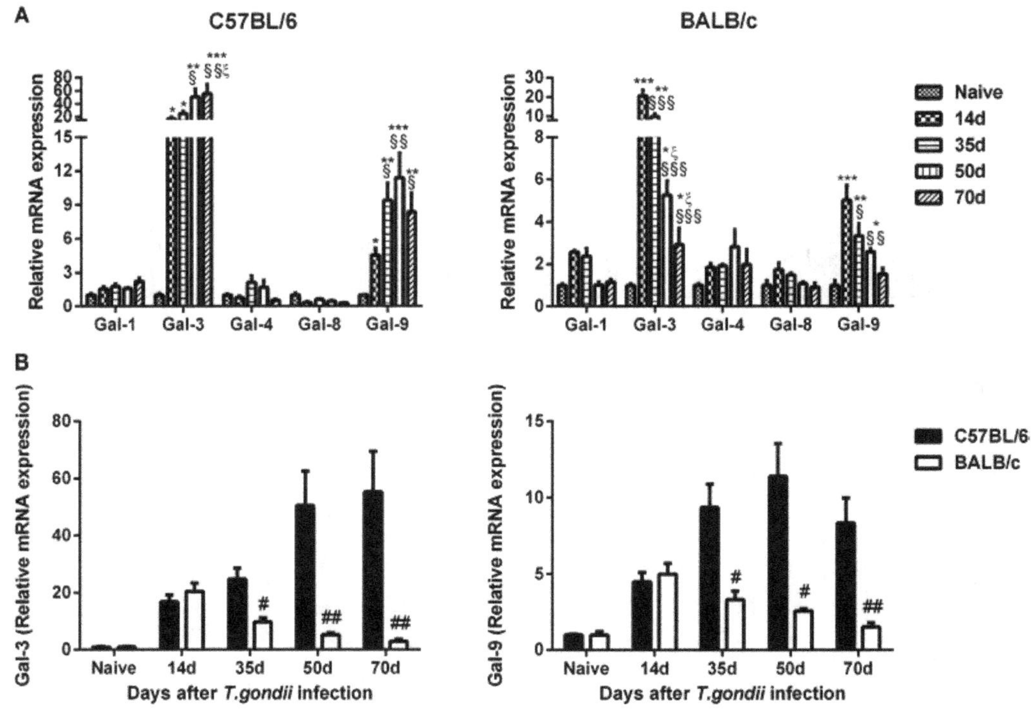

FIGURE 5 | Relative mRNA expressions of Gal-1, Gal-3, Gal-4, Gal-8, and Gal-9 in the brain tissues of *Toxoplasma gondii* Pru strain-infected C57BL/6 and BALB/c mice were detected by using quantitative real-time reverse transcription-polymerase chain reaction. **(A)** Galectin expressions in the brains of C57BL/6 and BALB/c mice. **(B)** Comparison of Gal-3 and Gal-9 levels in the brains of C57BL/6 and BALB/c mice. Values are means from triplicate measurements, and data are presented as mean ± SD. There were four mice per group. The data shown are representative of those from two different experiments. $^{*}P < 0.05$, $^{**}P < 0.01$, and $^{***}P < 0.001$ vs naive; $^{§}P < 0.05$, $^{§§}P < 0.01$, and $^{§§§}P < 0.001$ vs 14 days post infection (p.i.); $^{ξ}P < 0.05$ vs 35 days p.i.; $^{\#}P < 0.05$ and $^{\#\#}P < 0.01$ vs C57BL/6 mice.

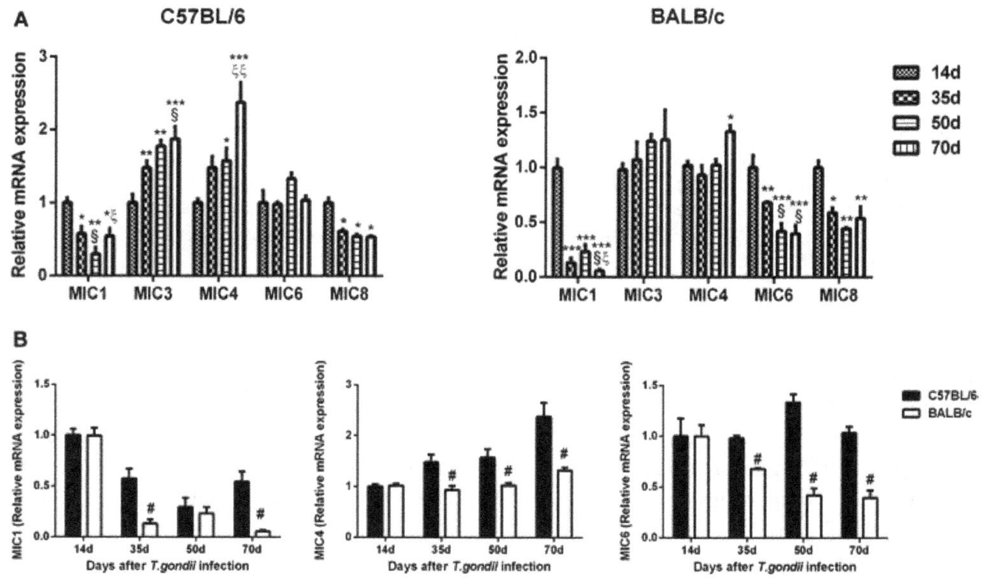

FIGURE 6 | Relative mRNA expressions of TgMIC1, TgMIC4, TgMIC6, TgMIC3, and TgMIC8 in the brain tissues of *Toxoplasma gondii* Pru strain-infected C57BL/6 and BALB/c mice were detected by using quantitative real-time reverse transcription-polymerase chain reaction. **(A)** TgMICs expressions in the brains of C57BL/6 and BALB/c mice. **(B)** Comparison of TgMIC1, TgMIC4, and TgMIC6 levels in the brains of C57BL/6 and BALB/c mice. Transcript level at day 14 post infection (p.i.) was taken as 1. Values are means from triplicate measurements, and data are presented as mean ± SD. There were four mice per group, and data are representative of those from two different experiments. $^{*}P < 0.05$, $^{**}P < 0.01$, and $^{***}P < 0.001$ vs 14 days p.i.; $^{§}P < 0.05$ vs 35 days p.i.; $^{ξ}P < 0.05$ and $^{ξξ}P < 0.05$ vs 50 days p.i.; $^{\#}P < 0.05$ vs C57BL/6 mice.

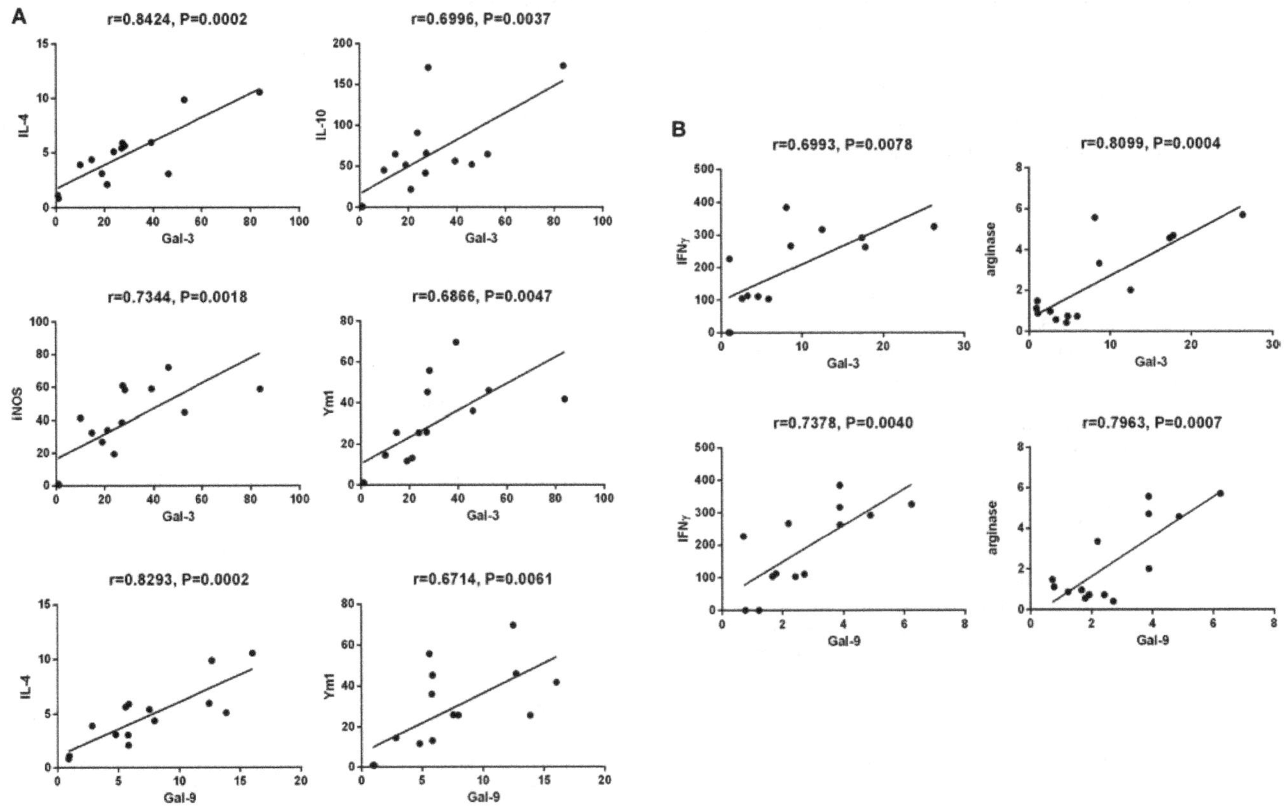

FIGURE 7 | Correlation analysis between Gal-3 and T helper 1 (Th1)/Th2/M1/M2 cytokines as well as between Gal-9 and Th1/Th2/M2 cytokines in the brain tissues of *Toxoplasma gondii* Pru strain-infected C57BL/6 and BALB/c mice ($n = 16$). **(A)** Significant correlations between Gal-3 and IL-4/IL-10/iNOS/Ym1 as well as between Gal-9 and IL-4/Ym1 existed in the brains of *T. gondii*-infected C57BL/6 mice. **(B)** Significant correlations between Gal-3 and IFNγ/Arg1 as well as between Gal-9 and IFNγ/Arg1 existed in the brains of *T. gondii*-infected BALB/c mice. The *r* value generates for the theoretical line of best fit, and the *P* value indicates the significance of the correlation.

astrocytes (43), functions as an astrocyte–microglia communication signal and promotes cytokine production, such as TNF, from microglia (44). After infection with ME49 strain of *T. gondii*, gal3$^{-/-}$ mice exhibits a higher parasite burden, delayed inflammatory response in the CNS, and significantly higher concentrations of IL-12p40 and IFNγ in the sera compared with those of gal3$^{+/+}$ mice (45). Gal-3 is required for resident microglia activation and proliferation in response to ischemic injury in a mouse model (46). Our data demonstrated that both Gal-3 and Gal-9 are important factors in TE-susceptible C57BL/6 and TE-resistant BALB/c mice infected with *T. gondii* Pru strain. In addition, the inflammatory response is more pronounced in the brains of C57BL/6 mice, which are corresponded well with the increased numbers of Iba1-positive resident microglia as well as increased Gal-3 and Gal-9 expressions in C57BL/6 mice. Furthermore, we evaluated the correlations between the gene expressions of Gal-3/Gal-9 and the levels of Th1 and Th2 cytokines, and M1- and M2-associated cytokines in the brains after *T. gondii* Pru strain infection. Positive correlations were found in the mRNA levels between Gal-3 and IL-4/IL-10/iNOS/Ym1 as well as between Gal-9 and IL-4/Ym1 in C57BL/6 mice; whereas positive correlations were found between Gal-3 and IFNγ/Arg1 as well as between Gal-9 and IFNγ/Arg1 in BALB/c mice. These data suggest that Gal-3 is related to Th2 and M1/M2 immune responses while Gal-9 is related to Th2 and M2 immune responses in *T. gondii*-infected C57BL/6 mice. Indeed, both Gal-3 and Gal-9 are related to Th1 and M2 immunity in BALB/c mice with chronic *T. gondii* infection. Our data suggested that Gal-3 and Gal-9 may involve in different immune responses to *T. gondii* Pru strain infection in the two lineages of mice.

Proteins secreted from apicomplexan MICs play important roles in the parasite adhesion and invasion of the host cells (47). MICs, which have been identified with lectin domains, support several key cellular processes including gliding motility, active cell invasion and migration through cells, biological barriers, and tissues (47). Our data showed that C57BL/6 mice expressed significantly higher levels of TgMIC1, TgMIC4, and TgMIC6 at days 35, 50, or 70 p.i. than those of BALB/c mice after *T. gondii* Pru strain infection. Therefore, TgMICs may be expressed differently in the two strains of mice with different genetic background. TgMIC1-4-6 complex contributes to host cell recognition and attachment *via* the action of TgMIC1 as well as contributes to the virulence of *T. gondii* in mice (48). Our data indicate that the different expression levels of TgMIC1, TgMIC4, and TgMIC6 in the two strains of mice may be associated with the different outcomes in *T. gondii* Pru strain-infected C57BL/6 and BALB/c mice.

In conclusion, this study has provided evidences that Gal-3 and Gal-9 may play a critical role in the regulation of M1, M2, Th1, and Th2 cytokines in the hosts with TE. Our data demonstrated that significant different mRNA expressions of Gal-3 and Gal-9 as well as microglial activation markers, cytokines, and TgMICs were found between C57BL/6 and BALB/c mice after *T. gondii* Pru strain infection. Whether these differences are related to the phenomenon that C57BL/6 mice are susceptible while BALB/c mice are resistant to the development of TE needs to be further investigated.

AUTHOR CONTRIBUTIONS

FL designed experiments, wrote, and edited the manuscript. JL conducted experiments, analyzed data, and wrote the manuscript draft. SH revised and edited the manuscript.

REFERENCES

1. Dubey JP. The history of *Toxoplasma gondii* – the first 100 years. *J Eukaryot Microbiol* (2008) 55(6):467–75. doi:10.1111/j.1550-7408.2008.00345.x
2. Weiss LM, Dubey JP. Toxoplasmosis: a history of clinical observations. *Int J Parasitol* (2009) 39(8):895–901. doi:10.1016/j.ijpara.2009.02.004
3. Connolly MP, Goodwin E, Schey C, Zummo J. Toxoplasmic encephalitis relapse rates with pyrimethamine-based therapy: systematic review and meta-analysis. *Pathog Glob Health* (2017) 111(1):31–44. doi:10.1080/20477724.2016.1273597
4. Denkers EY, Gazzinelli RT. Regulation and function of T-cell-mediated immunity during *Toxoplasma gondii* infection. *Clin Microbiol Rev* (1998) 11(4):569–88.
5. Suzuki Y, Kang H, Parmley S, Lim S, Park D. Induction of tumor necrosis factor-alpha and inducible nitric oxide synthase fails to prevent toxoplasmic encephalitis in the absence of interferon-gamma in genetically resistant BALB/c mice. *Microbes Infect* (2000) 2(5):455–62. doi:10.1016/S1286-4579(00)00318-X
6. Suzuki Y. Immunopathogenesis of cerebral toxoplasmosis. *J Infect Dis* (2002) 186(Suppl 2):S234–40. doi:10.1086/344276
7. Da Gama LM, Ribeiro-Gomes FL, Guimaraes U Jr, Arnholdt AC. Reduction in adhesiveness to extracellular matrix components, modulation of adhesion molecules and in vivo migration of murine macrophages infected with *Toxoplasma gondii. Microbes Infect* (2004) 6(14):1287–96. doi:10.1016/j.micinf.2004.07.008
8. Sica A, Mantovani A. Macrophage plasticity and polarization: in vivo veritas. *J Clin Invest* (2012) 122(3):787–95. doi:10.1172/JCI59643
9. Galvan-Pena S, O'Neill LA. Metabolic reprograming in macrophage polarization. *Front Immunol* (2014) 5:420. doi:10.3389/fimmu.2014.00420
10. Martinez FO, Helming L, Gordon S. Alternative activation of macrophages: an immunologic functional perspective. *Annu Rev Immunol* (2009) 27:451–83. doi:10.1146/annurev.immunol.021908.132532
11. Constant SL, Bottomly K. Induction of Th1 and Th2 CD4+ T cell responses: the alternative approaches. *Annu Rev Immunol* (1997) 15:297–322. doi:10.1146/annurev.immunol.15.1.297
12. Kalinski P, Moser M. Consensual immunity: success-driven development of T-helper-1 and T-helper-2 responses. *Nat Rev Immunol* (2005) 5(3):251–60. doi:10.1038/nri1569
13. Chao CC, Anderson WR, Hu S, Gekker G, Martella A, Peterson PK. Activated microglia inhibit multiplication of *Toxoplasma gondii* via a nitric oxide mechanism. *Clin Immunol Immunopathol* (1993) 67(2):178–83. doi:10.1006/clin.1993.1062
14. Hernandez JD, Baum LG. Ah, sweet mystery of death! Galectins and control of cell fate. *Glycobiology* (2002) 12(10):127r–36r. doi:10.1093/glycob/cwf081
15. Rabinovich GA, Toscano MA. Turning "sweet" on immunity: galectin-glycan interactions in immune tolerance and inflammation. *Nat Rev Immunol* (2009) 9(5):338–52. doi:10.1038/nri2536
16. Perillo NL, Marcus ME, Baum LG. Galectins: versatile modulators of cell adhesion, cell proliferation, and cell death. *J Mol Med (Berl)* (1998) 76(6):402–12. doi:10.1007/s001090050232
17. Liu FT, Rabinovich GA. Galectins: regulators of acute and chronic inflammation. *Ann N Y Acad Sci* (2010) 1183:158–82. doi:10.1111/j.1749-6632.2009.05131.x
18. Chen HL, Liao F, Lin TN, Liu FT. Galectins and neuroinflammation. *Adv Neurobiol* (2014) 9:517–42. doi:10.1007/978-1-4939-1154-7_24
19. Child MA, Garland M, Foe I, Madzelan P, Treeck M, van der Linden WA, et al. *Toxoplasma* DJ-1 regulates organelle secretion by a direct interaction with calcium-dependent protein kinase 1. *MBio* (2017) 8(1):e02189-16. doi:10.1128/mBio.02189-16
20. Liu Q, Li FC, Zhou CX, Zhu XQ. Research advances in interactions related to *Toxoplasma gondii* microneme proteins. *Exp Parasitol* (2017) 176:89–98. doi:10.1016/j.exppara.2017.03.001
21. Meissner M, Reiss M, Viebig N, Carruthers VB, Toursel C, Tomavo S, et al. A family of transmembrane microneme proteins of *Toxoplasma gondii* contain EGF-like domains and function as escorters. *J Cell Sci* (2002) 115(Pt 3):563–74.
22. Reiss M, Viebig N, Brecht S, Fourmaux MN, Soete M, Di Cristina M, et al. Identification and characterization of an escorter for two secretory adhesins in *Toxoplasma gondii. J Cell Biol* (2001) 152(3):563–78. doi:10.1083/jcb.152.3.563
23. Dunay IR, Heimesaat MM, Bushrab FN, Muller RH, Stocker H, Arasteh K, et al. Atovaquone maintenance therapy prevents reactivation of toxoplasmic encephalitis in a murine model of reactivated toxoplasmosis. *Antimicrob Agents Chemother* (2004) 48(12):4848–54. doi:10.1128/AAC.48.12.4848-4854.2004
24. Dang Y, Xu Y, Wu W, Li W, Sun Y, Yang J, et al. Tetrandrine suppresses lipopolysaccharide-induced microglial activation by inhibiting NF-kappaB and ERK signaling pathways in BV2 cells. *PLoS One* (2014) 9(8):e102522. doi:10.1371/journal.pone.0102522
25. Jones LA, Roberts F, Nickdel MB, Brombacher F, McKenzie AN, Henriquez FL, et al. IL-33 receptor (T1/ST2) signalling is necessary to prevent the development of encephalitis in mice infected with *Toxoplasma gondii. Eur J Immunol* (2010) 40(2):426–36. doi:10.1002/eji.200939705
26. Jash A, Kwon HK, Sahoo A, Lee CG, So JS, Kim J, et al. Topical application of porcine placenta extract inhibits the progression of experimental contact hypersensitivity. *J Ethnopharmacol* (2011) 133(2):654–62. doi:10.1016/j.jep.2010.10.054
27. Zhang AM, Shen Q, Li M, Xu XC, Chen H, Cai YH, et al. Comparative studies of macrophage-biased responses in mice to infection with *Toxoplasma gondii* ToxoDB #9 strains of different virulence isolated from China. *Parasit Vectors* (2013) 6(1):308. doi:10.1186/1756-3305-6-308
28. Zhou X, Xu Y, Yang G, Li F. Increased galectin-1 expression in muscle of *Astragalus* polysaccharide-treated type 1 diabetic mice. *J Nat Med* (2011) 65(3–4):500–7. doi:10.1007/s11418-011-0527-9
29. Bellac CL, Coimbra RS, Simon F, Imboden H, Leib SL. Gene and protein expression of galectin-3 and galectin-9 in experimental pneumococcal meningitis. *Neurobiol Dis* (2007) 28(2):175–83. doi:10.1016/j.nbd.2007.07.005
30. Markova V, Smetana K Jr, Jenikova G, Lachova J, Krejcirikova V, Poplstein M, et al. Role of the carbohydrate recognition domains of mouse galectin-4 in oligosaccharide binding and epitope recognition and expression of galectin-4 and galectin-6 in mouse cells and tissues. *Int J Mol Med* (2006) 18(1):65–76. doi:10.3892/ijmm.18.1.65
31. Tribulatti MV, Mucci J, Cattaneo V, Aguero F, Gilmartin T, Head SR, et al. Galectin-8 induces apoptosis in the $CD4^{high}CD8^{high}$ thymocyte subpopulation. *Glycobiology* (2007) 17(12):1404–12. doi:10.1093/glycob/cwm104
32. Liesenfeld O, Kosek J, Remington JS, Suzuki Y. Association of CD4+ T cell-dependent, interferon-gamma-mediated necrosis of the small intestine with genetic susceptibility of mice to peroral infection with *Toxoplasma gondii. J Exp Med* (1996) 184(2):597–607. doi:10.1084/jem.184.2.597
33. Silva NM, Manzan RM, Carneiro WP, Milanezi CM, Silva JS, Ferro EA, et al. *Toxoplasma gondii*: the severity of toxoplasmic encephalitis in C57BL/6 mice is associated with increased ALCAM and VCAM-1 expression in the central

nervous system and higher blood-brain barrier permeability. *Exp Parasitol* (2010) 126(2):167–77. doi:10.1016/j.exppara.2010.04.019

34. Schluter D, Deckert-Schluter M, Lorenz E, Meyer T, Rollinghoff M, Bogdan C. Inhibition of inducible nitric oxide synthase exacerbates chronic cerebral toxoplasmosis in *Toxoplasma gondii*-susceptible C57BL/6 mice but does not reactivate the latent disease in *T. gondii*-resistant BALB/c mice. *J Immunol* (1999) 162(6):3512–8.
35. Schluter D, Kaefer N, Hof H, Wiestler OD, Deckert-Schluter M. Expression pattern and cellular origin of cytokines in the normal and *Toxoplasma gondii*-infected murine brain. *Am J Pathol* (1997) 150(3):1021–35.
36. Schluter D, Meyer T, Strack A, Reiter S, Kretschmar M, Wiestler OD, et al. Regulation of microglia by $CD4^+$ and $CD8^+$ T cells: selective analysis in CD45-congenic normal and *Toxoplasma gondii*-infected bone marrow chimeras. *Brain Pathol* (2001) 11(1):44–55. doi:10.1111/j.1750-3639.2001.tb00380.x
37. Fischer HG, Nitzgen B, Reichmann G, Hadding U. Cytokine responses induced by *Toxoplasma gondii* in astrocytes and microglial cells. *Eur J Immunol* (1997) 27(6):1539–48. doi:10.1002/eji.1830270633
38. Jones RS, Lynch MA. How dependent is synaptic plasticity on microglial phenotype? *Neuropharmacology* (2015) 96(Pt A):3–10. doi:10.1016/j.neuropharm.2014.08.012
39. Murray PJ, Wynn TA. Protective and pathogenic functions of macrophage subsets. *Nat Rev Immunol* (2011) 11(11):723–37. doi:10.1038/nri3073
40. Freund YR, Zaveri NT, Javitz HS. In vitro investigation of host resistance to *Toxoplasma gondii* infection in microglia of BALB/c and CBA/Ca mice. *Infect Immun* (2001) 69(2):765–72. doi:10.1128/IAI.69.2.765-772.2001
41. Suzuki Y, Remington JS. The effect of anti-IFN-gamma antibody on the protective effect of Lyt-2^+ immune T cells against toxoplasmosis in mice. *J Immunol* (1990) 144(5):1954–6.
42. Shi W, Xue C, Su XZ, Lu F. The roles of galectins in parasitic infections. *Acta Trop* (2018) 177:97–104. doi:10.1016/j.actatropica.2017.09.027
43. Burman J, Svenningsson A. Cerebrospinal fluid concentration of galectin-9 is increased in secondary progressive multiple sclerosis. *J Neuroimmunol* (2016) 292:40–4. doi:10.1016/j.jneuroim.2016.01.008
44. Steelman AJ, Li J. Astrocyte galectin-9 potentiates microglial TNF secretion. *J Neuroinflammation* (2014) 11:144. doi:10.1186/s12974-014-0144-0
45. Bernardes ES, Silva NM, Ruas LP, Mineo JR, Loyola AM, Hsu DK, et al. *Toxoplasma gondii* infection reveals a novel regulatory role for galectin-3 in the interface of innate and adaptive immunity. *Am J Pathol* (2006) 168(6):1910–20. doi:10.2353/ajpath.2006.050636
46. Lalancette-Hebert M, Swarup V, Beaulieu JM, Bohacek I, Abdelhamid E, Weng YC, et al. Galectin-3 is required for resident microglia activation and proliferation in response to ischemic injury. *J Neurosci* (2012) 32(30):10383–95. doi:10.1523/JNEUROSCI.1498-12.2012
47. Carruthers VB, Tomley FM. Microneme proteins in apicomplexans. *Subcell Biochem* (2008) 47:33–45. doi:10.1007/978-0-387-78267-6_2
48. Cerede O, Dubremetz JF, Soete M, Deslee D, Vial H, Bout D, et al. Synergistic role of micronemal proteins in *Toxoplasma gondii* virulence. *J Exp Med* (2005) 201(3):453–63. doi:10.1084/jem.20041672

4

Characteristics of Infection Immunity Regulated by *Toxoplasma gondii* to Maintain Chronic Infection in the Brain

Young Sang Hwang[1†], Ji-Hun Shin[1†], Jung-Pyo Yang[1], Bong-Kwang Jung[1,2], Sang Hyung Lee[3] and Eun-Hee Shin[1,4*]

[1] Department of Parasitology and Tropical Medicine, Seoul National University College of Medicine, and Institute of Endemic Diseases, Seoul National University, Seoul, South Korea, [2] Institute of Parasitic Diseases, Korea Association of Health Promotion, Seoul, South Korea, [3] Department of Neurosurgery, Seoul National University College of Medicine, SMG-SNU Boramae Medical Center, Seoul, South Korea, [4] Seoul National University Bundang Hospital, Seongnam, South Korea

***Correspondence:**
Eun-Hee Shin
ehshin@snu.ac.kr

[†]These authors have contributed equally to this work.

To examine the immune environment of chronic *Toxoplasma gondii* infection in the brain, the characteristics of infection-immunity (premunition) in infection with *T. gondii* strain ME49 were investigated for 12 weeks postinfection (PI). The results showed that neuronal cell death, microglia infiltration and activation, inflammatory and anti-inflammatory cytokine expression, Stat1 phosphorylation, and microglia activation and inflammatory gene transcripts related to M1 polarization in the brain were increased during the acute infection (AI) stage (within 6 weeks PI), suggesting that innate and cellular inflammatory response activation and neurodegeneration contributed to excessive inflammatory responses. However, these immune responses decreased during the chronic infection (CI) stage (over 6 weeks PI) with reductions in phosphorylated STAT1 (pSTAT1) and eosinophilic neurons. Notably, increases were observed in transcripts of T-cell exhaustion markers (TIM3, LAG3, KLRG1, etc.), suppressor of cytokines signaling 1 protein (SOCS1), inhibitory checkpoint molecules (PD-1 and PD-L1), and Arg1 from the AI stage (3 weeks PI), implying active immune intervention under the immune environment of M1 polarization of microglia and increases in inflammatory cytokine levels. However, when BV-2 microglia were stimulated with *T. gondii* lysate antigens (strain RH or ME49) *in vitro*, nitrite production increased and urea production decreased. Furthermore, when BV-2 cells were infected by *T. gondii* tachyzoites (strain RH or ME49) *in vitro*, nitric oxide synthase and COX-2 levels decreased, whereas Arg1 levels significantly increased. Moreover, Arg1 expression was higher in ME49 infection than in RH infection, whereas nitrite production was lower in ME49 infection than in RH infection. Accordingly, these results strongly suggest that immune triggering of *T. gondii* antigens induces M1 polarization and activation of microglia as well as increase NO production, whereas *T. gondii* infection induces the inhibition of harmful inflammatory responses, even with M1 polarization and activation of microglia and Th1 inflammatory responses, suggesting a host–parasite relationship through immune regulation during CI. This is a characteristic of infection immunity in infection with *T. gondii* in the central nervous system, and SOCS1, a negative regulator of toxoplasmic encephalitis, may play a role in the increase in Arg1 levels to suppress NO production.

Keywords: *Toxoplasma gondii*, brain, chronic infection, microglial polarization, infection immunity

INTRODUCTION

Toxoplasma gondii is an Apicomplexan pathogen of the central nervous system (CNS) (1). Human *T. gondii* infection generally occurs *via* ingestion of oocysts (an environmentally resistant form) released in cat feces or undercooked meat containing tissue cysts (1). Following ingestion, bradyzoites and sporozoites released from cysts and oocysts invade intestinal cells, where they are converted to tachyzoites, which can then be disseminated *via* the blood or lymphatic system to remote organs and can induce an acute infection (AI) or chronic infection (CI) (1). In general, the brain is the most commonly affected site *via* congenital transmission and subsequent CI, which elicits lifelong immunity against toxoplasmosis (1). Immune responses to *T. gondii* infection differ during the proliferative (acute) and dormant (chronic and latent) stages and are dependent on differences in phenotype, virulence, and clinical sequelae of the strains of the clonal lineages, such as the highly virulent strain RH (type I) and the avirulent strain ME49 (type II) (1–3). CI of a type II parasite is maintained by the conversion of tachyzoites into bradyzoites, which produce intracellular tissue cysts. The onset and progression of *T. gondii* encystation result from both intrinsic preprogramming within the parasite and the immune response of the host, which eventually help to maintain a CI (1).

The AI stage of the RH strain is characterized by marked elevations in serum Th1 cytokine levels, such as interferon (IFN)-γ, tumor necrosis factor (TNF)-α, interleukin (IL)-12, and IL-18, and is followed by a lethal outcome in mice at 8 days postinfection (PI) (2). In contrast, non-lethal infection (ME49 strain) is characterized by modest elevations in Th1 cytokines that lead to control of *T. gondii* infection and minimal damage to the host (2). More specifically, in the CNS, IFN-γ plays a critical role in the prevention of toxoplasmic encephalitis (TE) during the late stage of infection in mice *via* inhibition of tachyzoite proliferation. However, simultaneous IFN-γ activation of microglia may cause tissue injury *via* the production of toxic metabolites, such as nitric oxide (NO) (4, 5). However, neurodegeneration does not commonly occur during CI of *T. gondii*, despite potential NO toxicity (4), possibly to control parasitic proliferation and avoid tissue damage in the infected brain *via* regulation of the appropriate induction between the cytokines IFN-γ, IL-10, and transforming growth factor beta (TGF-β), and the toxic mediator NO (4, 6–8).

Microglia, which are a type of glial cell and account for 10–15% of all cells within the brain parenchyma, are macrophages that reside in the brain and spinal cord, and have plasticity due to the CNS immune environment and consequently play a key role the regulation of CNS inflammatory reactions, tissue injury, and tissue homeostasis (9). During *T. gondii* infection, microglia are major effector cells that prevent NO-mediated pathogen proliferation (5). During the immune response of the host, *T. gondii* infection progresses from an acute stage, where tachyzoites replicates for 2 months PI, to the chronic stage, which is characterized by the formation of dormant cysts after 2 months PI (4, 10, 11). Simultaneously, life-threatening toxoplasmosis characterized by encephalitis is gradually decreased in the latent stage of *T. gondii* infection (7). However, the underlying switching mechanisms from the prevention of pathogen proliferation to the inhibition of cellular toxic immune response in the CNS remain unclear, although previous *in vitro* studies have reported a fractional infection period (1–8, 12–15). For example, the cytokines IL-2, IL-12, IFN-γ, and TNF-α, which inhibit the growth of *T. gondii*, and IL-4, IL-10, and TGF-β, which are involved in the downregulation of the intracerebral immune response, favor the growth of *T. gondii* and have been implicated in TE (7). Besides, several reports insisted that the decrease in the expression levels of the effector molecules IFN-γ and NO is important for latent infection of *T. gondii* (4, 5, 8, 15, 16). Hence, active intervention may be a good strategy for prolonged parasitic survival and establishment of a host–parasite relationship without expulsion of the parasites by the host cells.

Our previous study found that a decrease in NO in Tg2576 mice caused Alzheimer's disease even with inflammation of the brain due to TE (8). In particular, because brain tissue is susceptible to the noxious effects of NO, such as wide-spread neurodegeneration, NO production in *T. gondii* infection has been widely studied as an important regulator and indicator of both protective effects and tissue damage (4, 5, 8, 15, 16). In the CNS, microglial cells lead to broad range of immunoregulatory functions with regulation of NO production to prevent further *T. gondii* proliferation (1, 5, 8, 15). However, despite numerous investigations, the time-specific kinetics of microglia activation in chronically infected normal mice have not been defined. Hence, further studies are needed because *T. gondii* infection is very chronic in immunocompetent hosts and can recur with time. Unfortunately, no previous study has investigated the immunomodulation in the brain during long-term CI of *T. gondii* and the key events in the regulation of CI, immunity, and parasite proliferation must be addressed to reduce the harmful effects of CI to brain tissues. As previously revealed, IFN-γ, TNF-α, and IL-12 were found to inhibit parasitic growth both *in vivo* and *in vitro*, and IL-10 and TGF-β are important to reduce the excessive inflammatory response of the brain to CI of *T. gondii* (2–7, 12, 15). The interactions of these cytokines inhibit NO production and promote the conversion of M1-type microglial cells to the M2-type *via* alternative activation accompanying arginase 1 (Argl) activity and expression of the mannose receptor type C (CD206) (3, 5, 7, 12, 15, 16). The effector molecules of *T. gondii* that induce the polarization of macrophages include *Toxoplasma* rhoptry kinase ROP16 in the alternative activation pathway and *Toxoplasma* dense granule protein GRA15 in the classical activation pathway, which activate STAT6 and NF-κB, respectively (3). However, immune modulation may not be limited by the molecular actions

---

Abbreviations: *T. gondii*, *Toxoplasma gondii*; PI, postinfection; CI, chronic infection; (), acute infection; NO, nitric oxide; TGF-β, transforming growth factor-β; GM-CSF, granulocyte-macrophage colony-stimulating factor; IL-12, interleukin-12; STAT1, signal transducer and activator of transcription1; SOCS1, suppressor of cytokines signaling 1 protein; MHCII, major histocompatibility complex II; TLA, *T. gondii* lysate antigen; CNS, central nervous system; TE, toxoplasmic encephalitis; iNOS, nitric oxide synthase; PAMPs, pathogen-associated molecular pattern molecules; DG, hippocampal dentate gyrus; MFI, mean fluorescence intensity; IHC, immunohistochemistry; ME-TLA, lysate antigen of *T. gondii* ME49 strain tachyzoites; (RH-TLA), (COX-2) (Argl), lysate antigen of *T. gondii* RH strain tachyzoites.

of *T. gondii*, but rather may be the result of interactions between the host and parasite to continually change the overall immune response during the latent infection stage due to changes in the immune characteristics and the course of infection. For example, several studies have investigated immune characteristics *via* genetic manipulation, such as the dense granule protein GRA15-KO-T of transgenic *T. gondii* (*Toxoplasma*-Cre) in IL-$10^{-/-}$ mice, but neglected to specify the time-varying infectious immunity during CI in regard to the host–parasite interactions (14, 17–19).

The characteristics of infectious immunity in the *T. gondii*-infected brain have been mainly investigated in TE with a focus on the AI stage (20). The most important effector molecules of TE and protection against *T. gondii* include the IL-12/IFN-γ axis, as well as IFN-γ through signal transducer and activator of transcription 1 (STAT1) and inducible nitric oxide synthase (iNOS) (5, 12, 17). Nevertheless, prolonged *T. gondii* infection results in decreased neurodegeneration and inflammatory immune responses, thus we previously identified components of basic and integrative infection immunity (8). In this respect, we aimed to investigate the processes underlying changes in infection immunity from the AI stage to the CI stage, and identified key responses in the immune regulation between a harmful inflammatory response and restoring neurodegeneration in the brain. To this end, we investigated the changes underlying neurodegeneration during *T. gondii* infection, as well as the activation and polarization of microglial cells as effector cells against *T. gondii* infection. Also, inflammatory and anti-inflammatory responses, changes in transcript expression patterns during the infection period, induction of NO and Arg1, an arginine hydrolytic enzyme, and finally *in vitro* infection of *T. gondii* tachyzoites (RH− or ME49 strain) as well as *in vitro* stimulation of *T. gondii* lysate antigen (TLA) (RH− or ME-TLA) were investigated to reveal the differences in immune-triggering events between *T. gondii* infection in the host–parasite relationship and immune characteristics of TLA as pathogen-associated molecular pattern molecules (PAMPs). The results of the present study are very important and interesting in regard to characterizing the infection immunity processes regulated by the host–parasite relationship through proper control of the protective inflammatory immune response, while reducing the harmful effects of neurodegeneration.

MATERIALS AND METHODS

Experimental Animals

Male, 7-week-old, C57BL/6 mice were purchased from the ORIENT BIO Animal Center (Seongnam, South Korea) and housed at room temperature (20–23°C) on a 12-h light/dark cycle with *ad libitum* access to sterilized (irradiated and autoclaved) food and water. All animal experiments were conducted in accordance with the ethical standards of the Institutional Animal Care and Use Committee of Seoul National University (SNU-110315-5).

Ethics Statement

This study protocol was approved by the Ethics Committee of Seoul National University and conducted in strict accordance with the Guidelines for Animal Experiments (SNUIBC-R110302-1). All surgeries were performed under anesthesia and all efforts were made to ensure minimal animal suffering.

T. gondii Infection

C57BL/6 mice (Orient Bio) at the age of 7 weeks were intraperitoneally injected with *T. gondii* strain ME49 (infection dose of 10 cysts) isolated from *T. gondii*-infected brains harvested at 3 months PI and housed in the animal facility of Seoul National University College of Medicine. Most experiments were conducted at 3 months PI. Six mice were randomly sacrificed at 0, 3, 6, 9, and 12 weeks PI, and brain tissues were collected for histological examinations, cytokine analysis, and microarray analysis.

Neuronal Degeneration in the Hippocampal Dentate Gyrus (DG) Detected by Hematoxylin and Eosin (H&E) Staining

Brain tissues were embedded in paraffin and coronal-sectioned at thickness of 10 μm through the hippocampus, mounted, and stained with H&E. Then, the tissue specimens were dehydrated with a graded alcohol series, cleared in xylene, fixed with Canadian balsam (Caedax; Merck, Darmstadt, Germany), and mounted on cover slips. Neuronal degeneration in the hippocampal DG was determined by the detection of eosinophilic neurons under a light microscope (Olympus PM-20; Olympus Corporation, Tokyo, Japan). The number of degenerative cells were counted in photomicrographs obtained with a digital camera (Leica DFC 280, Leica Microsystems, Wetzlar, Germany) attached to a microscope (BX-51; Olympus Corporation) using Image J software ver. 1.46.[1]

Detection of *T. gondii* Cyst in the Brain by Reverse Transcription Polymerase Chain Reaction (RT-PCR)

Total RNA was isolated from *T. gondii*-infected mouse brain tissue using the RNeasy Mini kit (Qiagen, Hilden, Germany) according to the manufacturer's protocol. All samples were subjected to RT-PCR using the RT premix reverse transcription kit (Elpis Biotech Inc., Daejeon, South Korea) and MG Taq DNA polymerase (Macrogen, Seoul, South Korea) with the following primer pairs: GAPDH (Primer Bank ID 6679937a1): forward 5′-AGG TCG GTG TGA ACG GAT TTG-3′ and reverse 5′-TGT AGA CCA TGT AGT TGA GGT CA-3′ (123 bp); *T. gondii* B1 gene: forward 5′-TCC CCT CTG CTG GCG AAA AGT-3′ and reverse 5′-AGC GTT CGT GGT CAA CTA TCG ATT G-3′ (98 bp). RT-PCR was performed for 35 cycles with an annealing temperature of 54–55°C and the products were analyzed by 1% agarose gel electrophoresis.

Real-time PCR

Total RNA was isolated from Total RNA was isolated from T. gondii-infected mouse brain tissue using the RNeasy Mini kit (Qiagen, Hilden, Germany) according to the manufacturer's protocol. All samples were reverse transcribed using RT premix

[1]http://pga.mgh.harvard.edu/primerbank/.

(Elpis Biotech Inc.). Real-time PCR was performed using the CFX96 (Bio-Rad) and SYBR green (Enzynomics™, Daejeon, Korea) was used to detect amplification products. The reaction conditions used were; initial denaturation at 95°C for 15 min, 40 amplification cycles [denaturation at 95°C for 10 s, annealing at 60°C for 20 s, and extension at 72°C for 30 s], followed by melting curve analysis. Data analysis was performed using CFX96 software (Bio-Rad). The following primer sequences were used for real-time PCR: GAPDH: forward 5′-GGT GAA GGT CGG TGT GAA CG-3′ and reverse 5′-CTC GCT CCT GGA AGA TGG TG-3′ (578 bp); and Socs1: forward 5′-CTG CGG CTT CTA TTG GGG AC-3′ and reverse 5′-AAA AGG CAG TCG AAG GTC TCG-3′ (217 bp); and Nos2 (iNOS): forward 5′-CAG CAC AGA ATG TTC CAG AAT CC-3′ and reverse 5′-TGT CAT GCA AAA TCT CTC CAC TGC-3′ (105 bp); and Arg1: forward 5′-CTT TAA CCT TGG CTT GCT TCG GAA-3′ and reverse 5′-CTT AGT TCT GTC TGC TTT GCT GTG-3′ (140 bp).

Immunostaining of *T. gondii*-Infected Mouse Brain Tissues

Mice were sacrificed by CO_2 asphyxiation at the pre-determined times and brain tissues were collected, then fixed in formalin and embedded in paraffin using the Leica TP1020 Tissue Processor (Leica Microsystems GmbH, Wetzlar, Germany). For specific immunostaining, samples were immunostained using the ChromoMap Kit and the Discovery XT automated staining instrument (Ventana Medical Systems, Inc., Tucson, AZ, USA). Briefly, 4 μm-thick tissue sections were fixed on Probe-On-Plus Slides (Thermo Fisher Scientific, Swedesboro, NJ, USA), deparaffinized in xylene, rehydrated in a graded series of alcohol (100, 95, 80, and 70), and finally rinsed with distilled water. After antigen retrieval, the endogenous peroxidase activity of the samples was blocked by treatment of H_2O_2 with blocking buffer [1% fetal bovine serum in phosphate-buffered saline (PBS)] for 30 min. Then, the samples were incubated for 60 min at room temperature with either rabbit anti-mouse Iba-1 (1:2000, Wako Chemicals, Richmond, VA, USA) or anti-phospho-STAT1 (Tyr701) (58D6, rabbit mAb) (1:500, Cell Signaling Technology, Beverly, MA, USA) primary antibodies, washed thrice with Tris-buffered saline, and incubated with secondary antibodies in UltraMap anti-Rb horseradish peroxidase (HRP) (Ventana Medical Systems, Inc.). Streptavidin-biotin-HRP complex (sABC/HRP) was detected with the ChromoMap DAB detection kit (Ventana Medical System, Inc.). The immunostained sections were then counterstained with hematoxylin (Ventana Medical System, Inc.) and plated on cover slips using Canadian balsam solution (Polysciences Inc., Warrington, PA, USA). Reactions were observed using a light microscope (PM-20; Olympus Corporation) and photomicrographs were acquired with a BX-51 microscope (Olympus Corporation) equipped with a color digital camera (DFC280; Leica Microsystems).

Levels of Inflammatory and Anti-inflammatory Cytokines in *T. gondii*-Infected Brain Tissue

Cytokine levels of IL-6, IL-12 (p70), IFN-γ, TNF-α, granulocyte-macrophage colony-stimulating factor (GM-CSF), IL-10, IL-4, and TGF-β in *T. gondii*-infected mouse brains were examined using the Bio-Plex mouse cytokine assay kit (Bio-Rad Laboratories, Hercules, CA, USA) and enzyme-linked immunosorbent assay (ELISA) kits (R&D Systems, Inc., Minneapolis, MN, USA). Brain tissues of C57BL/6 mice were obtained at 0, 3, 6, 9, and 12 weeks PI, and lysed using the MicroRotofor Cell Lysis Kit (Bio-Rad Laboratories) ($n = 3$). The soluble homogenate proteins were quantified using a bicinchoninic acid (BCA) assay kit (Pierce Biotechnology, Inc., Rockford, IL, USA). The Bio-Plex assay was performed according to the manufacturer's instructions and the raw data [mean fluorescent intensities (MFI)] were analyzed with Bio-Plex Manager Software (Bio-Rad Laboratories) to obtain concentration values. The one-way analysis of variance (ANOVA) was used for statistical analysis, and the results were analyzed using Bio-Plex Data Pro™ software. Cytokine analysis was performed using ELISA kits (R&D Systems, Inc.) according to the manufacturer's protocol. The reaction was measured at 450 nm using an Epoch microplate reader (BioTek Instruments, Inc., Winooski, VT, USA) and cytokine concentrations were calculated using a standard curve of the corresponding cytokine provided with the ELISA kit.

Microarray Analysis of *T. gondii*-Infected Brain

Total RNA of *T. gondii*-infected brain tissues was separately extracted at 0, 3, 6, 9, and 12 weeks PI, and pooled for microarray analysis ($n = 3$), which was performed by Macrogen Inc. (Seoul, South Korea) using an Illumina MouseRef-8 v2 Expression BeadChip array (Illumina, Inc., San Diego, CA, USA). Briefly, 0.55 μg of total RNA was amplified using the Illumina TotalPrep RNA Amplification Kit (Ambion, Austin, TX, USA) and purified using the Ambion Illumina RNA amplification kit (Ambion) to yield biotinylated cRNA. Following fragmentation, 0.75 μg of cRNA were hybridized to the Mouse Expression BeadChip (Illumina, Inc.) according to the manufacturer's protocol. Arrays were scanned with the Illumina Bead Array Reader Confocal Scanner. Array data export processing and analysis was performed using Illumina GenomeStudio v2011.1 (Gene Expression Module v1.9.0), and the data were analyzed with R v. 2.15.1 statistical software. Hierarchical cluster analysis was performed using Permute Matrix EN software. All heat maps were generated using Excel Spreadsheet Software (Microsoft Corporation, Redmond, WA, USA) with conditional formatting. The expression rates of each gene at 3, 6, 9 and 12 weeks PI were compared to baseline (week 0 PI). Positive correlations are depicted in yellow (increased expression) and negative correlations (decreased expression) are depicted in blue. Heat maps of inflammatory and anti-inflammatory cytokines, microglia phenotype markers, and immune regulatory markers are represented by color scales. Each row represents cytokines and immune markers, and each column represents infection times from 0 to 12 weeks PI. The color scale of the heat map corresponds the relative minimum (−3) and maximum (+3) values of each cytokine.

TLAs Prepared from Tachyzoites of *T. gondii* Strains RH and ME49

Toxoplasma gondii lysate antigens of strain RH or ME49 were prepared as previously described with slight modifications (8, 11).

Briefly, peritoneal exudates of infected mice at day 4 PI were passed twice through a 25-gauge needle and then through a 5-µm Millex filter membrane (Merck Millipore, Tullagreen, Ireland) to remove debris and host cells. Then, tachyzoites of *T. gondii* strain RH were recovered and washed with sterilized PBS (pH 7.2). Parasites were then washed and suspended in PBS (pH 7.2) for further antigen preparation. To prepare ME49 tachyzoite antigens, 20 cysts of strain ME49 were intraperitoneally injected to BALB/c mice to obtain ME49 tachyzoites converted from cysts. At 6 to 8 days PI, the tachyzoites were harvested by washing the peritoneal cavity with PBS. Tachyzoites of both *T. gondii* strains RH and ME49 were cultured in Vero cells (monkey kidney cells, KCLB cell line; no. 10081) grown in complete Roswell Park Memorial Institute 1640 media (WelGENE Inc., Daegu, Korea) supplemented with 100 µg/mL of penicillin (Gibco/BRL, Grand Island, NY, USA), 100 µg/mL of streptomycin (Gibco/BRL), and 5% fetal calf serum (Lonza, Walkersville, MD, USA) at 37°C under an atmosphere of 5% CO_2. After culturing in Vero cells, tachyzoites of strains ME49 and RH were passed through a 25-gauge needle twice, and then debris and cells were removed by passing through 5-µm filter membranes. After washing, the tachyzoites were re-suspended in PBS, sonicated on ice, and then centrifuged. Supernatants, containing the TLA fractions (respectively named as RH-TLA and ME-TLA) were filtered through 0.22-µm filter membranes (Millipore Corp., Bedford, MA, USA). Proteins in the TLA fraction were quantified using a BCA commercial reagent (Pierce Biotechnology, Inc.) and stored at −80°C until used.

Flow Cytometry Analysis to Determine the Microglia Phenotype of BV-2 Cells after Treatment of the *T. gondii* Antigen

Antigens against *T. gondii* strain RH or ME49 tachyzoites (40 µg/mL) and/or recombinant IFN-γ (100 ng/mL; PeproTech, Rocky Hill, NJ, USA) were used for *in vitro* activation of BV-2 cells, a murine microglial cell line. BV-2 cells were cultured in Dulbecco's modified essential medium (Applied Scientific, San Francisco, CA, USA) supplemented with 10% heat-inactivated fetal calf serum (Hyclone, Ogden, UT, USA), 4 mM L-glutamine, 0.2 mM penicillin, 0.05 mM streptomycin, and 20 mM HEPES (Sigma-Aldrich Corporation, St. Louis, MO, USA) at 37°C under an atmosphere of 5% CO_2 (8). After incubation for 24 h, BV-2 cells were harvested for further fluorescence-activated cell sorting (FACS) analysis. The following anti-mouse antibodies were used for flow cytometry analysis of the cultured BV-2 microglial cells: fluorescein isothiocyanate (FITC)-conjugated anti-CD80 (eBioscience, Inc., San Diego, CA, USA), phycoerythrin (PE)-conjugated anti-CD86 (eBioscience, Inc.), FITC-conjugated anti-CD274 (PD-L1) (B7-H1; eBioscience, Inc.), PE-conjugated anti-CD273 (PD-L2) (B7-DC; eBioscience, Inc.), allophycocyanin (APC)-conjugated anti-major histocompatibility complex (MHC) II (CD74, eBioscience), PE-conjugated anti-CD40 (eBioscience, Inc.), and FITC-conjugated anti-CD206 (BioLegend, San Diego, CA, USA). All staining processes for FACS analysis were conducted in accordance with the manufacturer's protocols with FACS staining buffer (PBS containing 1% bovine serum albumin and 0.1% sodium azide). Samples were analyzed using a FACSCalibur flow cytometer (BD Immunocytometry Systems, San Jose, CA, USA) with forward/side scatter gates to exclude nonviable cells and the data were analyzed using FlowJo software (Tree Star, Inc., Ashland, OR, USA). Data are presented as the mean (±SD) fluorescence intensity (MFI). In this study, *in vitro* experiment of BV-2 cell culture was data obtained after conducting three individual experiments.

Western Blot Analysis

Total proteins were extracted from uninfected and infected whole mouse brains using the PRO-PREP™ Protein Extraction Kit (iNtRON Biotechnology, Seongnam-Si, Korea) and quantified with a NanoDrop spectrophotometer (NanoDrop Technologies, Oxfordshire, UK). Proteins were separated by sodium dodecyl sulfate-10% polyacrylamide gel electrophoresis at 100 V for 110 min and then transferred to a nitrocellulose membrane (Bio-Rad Laboratories) using the Mini Trans-Blot® Electrophoretic Transfer Cell (Bio-Rad Laboratories) at 80 V for 100 min. The membranes were then incubated with the primary antibodies goat anti-SOCS1 (ab9870; Abcam, Cambridge, UK) (1:200) and mouse anti-β-actin (sc-47778; dilution, 1:500; Santa Cruz Biotechnology, Dallas, TX, USA), followed by the secondary antibodies donkey anti-goat immunoglobulin (Ig)G-HRP (sc-2020; dilution, 1:2,000; Santa Cruz Biotechnology) and goat anti-mouse IgG-HRP (sc-2005; dilution, 1:4,000; Santa Cruz Biotechnology). Signals were detected by exposing the membrane to chemiluminescence HRP substrate (Thermo Fisher Scientific) using a Fuji LAS1000 Lumino Image Analyzer (Fujifilm Corporation, Tokyo, Japan).

Nitrite and Urea Production by BV-2 Cells Stimulated by Various Cytokines and Strain-Specific Tachyzoite Antigens (RH-TLA and ME-TLA)

BV-2 cells were incubated for 24 h in 6-well culture plates (SPL Lifesciences Co., Ltd., Pocheon, South Korea) with either 100 ng/mL of IFN-γ (PeproTech), 20 ng/mL of IL-4 (Prospec-Tany Technogene Ltd., Rehovot, Israel), and/or one of the *T. gondii* antigens (RH-TLA or ME-TLA) at a concentration of 20 or 40 µg/mL. Culture supernatants were collected and assayed to determine contents of nitrite and urea, which reflect NO production and Arg1 levels, respectively. NO production was determined using Griess reagent (Sigma-Aldrich Corporation). After 50 µL of culture supernatant was reacted with 50 µL of Griess reagent in each well of a 96-well plate (SPL Lifesciences Co., Ltd.), the reaction was measured using a microplate reader at an optical density (OD) of 540 nm (Biotech, VT, USA). Urea concentration was determined using a commercial urea kit (Abnova Corporation, Taipei, Taiwan) according to the manufacturer's protocol. In brief, 50 µL of culture supernatant was mixed with 50 µL of distilled water and the solution was reacted with 200 µL of a working reagent for 20 min. Then, the OD value of the sample was measured at 520 nm and the concentrations of nitrite and urea were calculated using standard curves. *In vitro* experiment of BV-2 cell culture was data obtained after conducting three individual experiments.

mRNA Levels of iNOS, COX-2, and Arg1 in *T. gondii*-Infected BV-2 Cells

BV-2 cells were infected with tachyzoites of *T. gondii* strain RH or ME49 *in vitro* at an effector to target ratio (E:T ratio; *T. gondii*:BV-2 cell) of 1:5 for 24 h. Total RNA of the cultured cells was extracted using the RNeasy kit (Qiagen). All samples were reverse transcribed using RT premix (Elpis Biotech Inc.) and the iQ5 real-time PCR detection system (Bio-Rad Laboratories) with SYBR green master mix (Enzynomics, Cheongju, South Korea) under the following condition: initial denaturation at 50°C for 5 min and 95°C for 10 min, followed by 40 amplification cycles of denaturation at 95°C for 10 s and annealing at 60°C for 30 s, with a final extension cycle at 72°C for 5 min. Specific amplification was verified by analysis of the melting curve and separation of the RT-PCR products on a 3% agarose gel. Data analysis was performed using iQ™5 optical system software (Bio-Rad Laboratories). The following primer sequences and amplicon sizes were retrieved from the PrimerBank database[2]: GAPDH (PrimerBank ID 6679937a1) forward 5′-AGG TCG GTG TGA ACG GAT TTG-3′ and reverse 5′-TGT AGA CCA TGT AGT TGA GGT CA-3′ (123 bp); Arg1 (PrimerBank ID7106255a1) forward 5′-CTC CAA GCC AAA GTC CTT AGA G-3′ and reverse 5′-AGG AGC TGT CAT TAG GGA CAT C-3′ (185 bp); Nos2 (iNOS) forward 5′-GTT CTC AGC CCA ACA ATA CAA GA-3′and reverse 5′-GTG GAC GGG TCG ATG TCA C-3′(127 bp); and Ptgs2 (COX-2) forward 5′-TGT GAC TGT ACC CGG ACT GG-3′ and reverse 5′-TGC ACA TTG TAA GTA GGT GGA C-3′(233 bp).

Statistical Analysis

All statistical analyses were performed using Microsoft Excel and GraphPad Prism 5 software (GraphPad Software, Inc., La Jolla, CA, USA). Data are presented as the mean ± SD. One-way ANOVA followed by the Bonferroni multiple-comparison test were used to assess differences between experimental groups. A probability (p) values of <0.05 was considered statistically significant. * indicates significant difference by one-way ANOVA compared with the control. # indicates significant difference between the experimental groups.

RESULTS

Histopathological Changes and Microglia Activation in the Hippocampal DG during the AI to CI Stage of *T. gondii*

To observe the neuronal cell damage caused by *T. gondii* infection, histopathologic changes in the hippocampal region were examined by H&E staining. As shown in **Figure 1A**, purple-colored normal and un-injured neurons were observed with a light microscopic throughout most of the hippocampal DG (**Figure 1A**, week 0), whereas *T. gondii* infection resulted in an increase the proportion of eosinophilic neurons, which were characterized by cell body shrinkage, intensely stained eosinophilic cytoplasm, and small/shrunken darkly stained nuclei

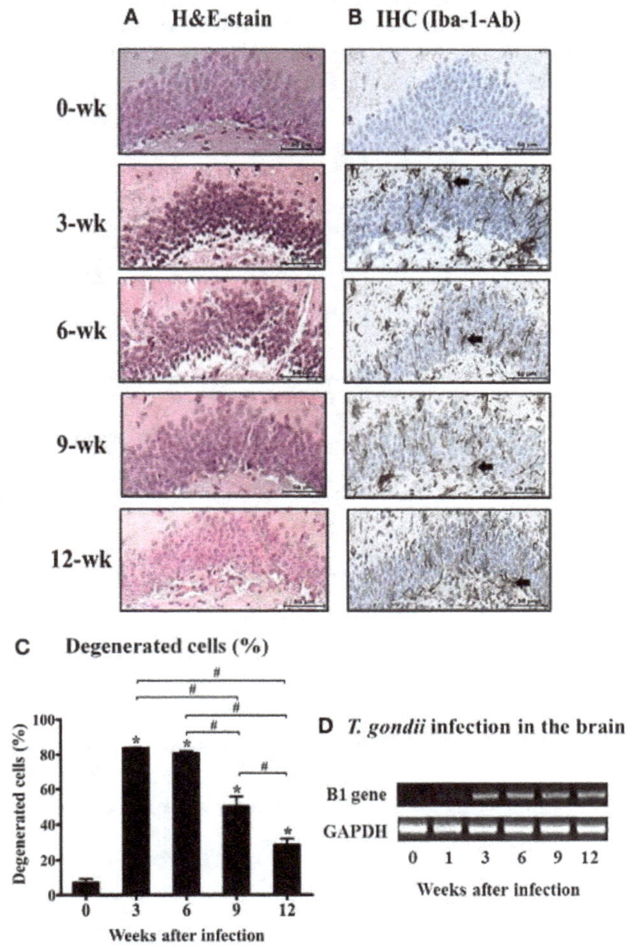

FIGURE 1 | Changes in neuronal degeneration and proliferation of microglial cells in the hippocampal dentate gyrus during *T. gondii* infection. The brain tissues were harvested at 0, 3, 6, 9, and 12 weeks postinfection, and subjected to histological staining. **(A)** hematoxylin and eosin staining, 400x. **(B)** Immunohistochemistry (IHC) results of the brain tissue stained with Iba-1-antibody (brown color), 400x. Scale bar = 50 μm. **(C)** Degenerated cells in the brain tissues after *T. gondii* infection were counted and are expressed by percentage (%).* indicates significant difference compared with the control. # indicates significant difference between the experimental groups. **(D)** *T. gondii*-specific B1 gene expression and RT-PCR products were loaded into 1% agarose gels (98 bp).

(**Figure 1A**, at 3 and 6 weeks PI). The appearance of eosinophilic neurons was increased during the AI stage and then significantly decreased during the CI stage from 6.7 ± 3.88% at week 0 to 83.8 ± 0.57% at week 3, 80.8 ± 2.38% at week 6, 50.1 ± 9.66 at week 9, and 28.5 ± 6.13% at week 12 PI (**Figure 1C**, $p < 0.05$). At this time, activation and infiltration of microglial cells in the DG were evaluated by immunohistochemical analysis with antibody against Iba-1, an activation marker of microglia (**Figure 1B**). The infiltration of Iba-1-positive cells (colored in brown) during hippocampal formation had increased from 3 weeks PI and was sustained during the 12-week experimental period (**Figure 1B**). These histopathological changes appeared after infection of *T. gondii*, which were detected by monitoring of the B1 gene (**Figure 1D**). Importantly, this result suggests that

[2]http://pga.mgh.harvard.edu/primerbank/.

neurodegeneration increases during the AI stage and decreases in the CI stage (9 weeks PI), despite the presence of harmful signs in the brain tissue, such as activation of inflammatory microglia and continuity of *T. gondii* infection. Accordingly, further analysis showed that neurodegeneration accompanying *T. gondii* infection had decreased during the CI stage.

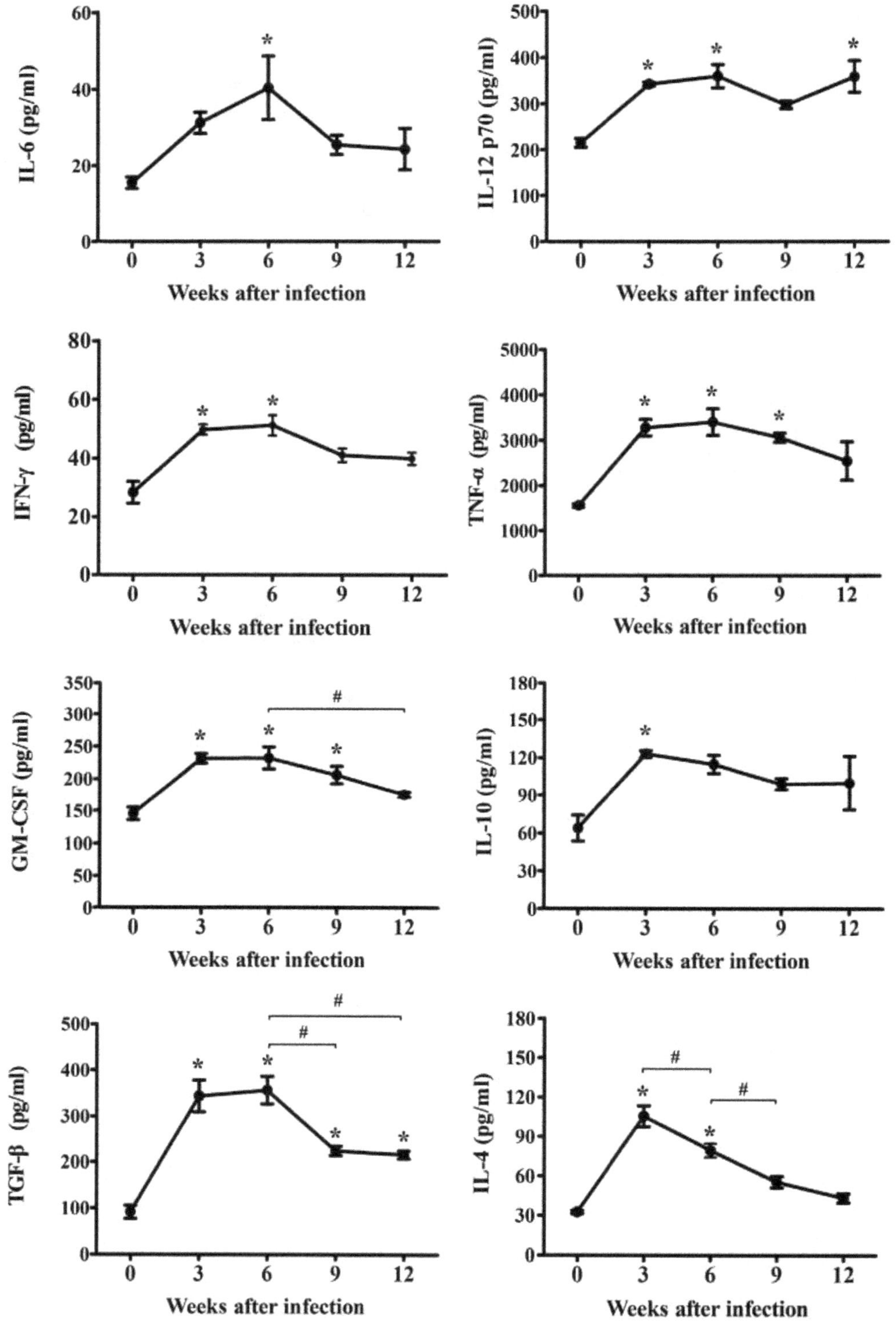

FIGURE 2 | Expression changes of cytokines in cerebral *Toxoplasma gondii* infection from the acute infection stage to the chronic infection stage. Brain tissues were harvested at 0, 3, 6, 9, and 12 weeks postinfection and analyzed for changes in cytokine levels due to infection. Levels of inflammatory cytokines [IL-6, IL-12p70, IFN-γ, tumor necrosis factor (TNF)-α, and granulocyte-macrophage colony-stimulating factor (GM-CSF)] and anti-inflammatory cytokines [IL-4, IL-10, and transforming growth factor-β (TGF-β)]. Cytokine levels are presented as the mean ± SD at each infection stage. *$p < 0.05$ (one-way analysis of variance). * indicates significant difference compared with the control. # indicates significant difference between the experimental groups.

Profiles of Inflammatory and Anti-inflammatory Cytokines in the Mouse Brain According to the Time of *T. gondii* Infection

To reveal the characteristics of the inflammatory mechanisms underlying microglia activation after *T. gondii* infection, inflammatory, and anti-inflammatory cytokines (IL-6, IL-12p70, IFN-γ, TNF-α, GM-CSF, IL-4, IL-10, and TGF-β) were examined at 0, 3, 6, 9, and 12 weeks PI. As show in **Figure 2**, the concentrations of inflammatory- (IL-6, IL-12p70, IFN-γ, TNF-α, and GM-CSF) and anti-inflammatory-cytokines (IL-4, IL-10, and TGF-β) had gradually and statistically increased during the AI stage (3–6 weeks PI, * $p < 0.05$ at every time point compared, as compared to week 0). Furthermore, the levels of inflammatory cytokines (IL-6, IL-12p70, IFN-γ, TNF-α, and GM-CSF) had peaked at 6 weeks PI, while those of the anti-inflammatory cytokines (IL-4 and IL-10) had peaked at 3 weeks PI, suggesting that levels of the anti-inflammatory cytokines had decreased immediately after the rapid increase during the early stage of infection (**Figure 2**). At this time, TGF-β, which is known to be associated with neuroprotection, continued to increase until 6 weeks PI. The peak level of each cytokine is shown in **Figure 2**. The abundance of the inflammatory cytokines IL-6, IL-12p70, IFN-γ, TNF-α, and GM-CSF had increased from baseline (week 0) to 6 weeks PI by 262, 167, 180, 218, and 160%, respectively, whereas the abundance of the anti-inflammatory cytokines IL-4 and IL-10 had increased by 324 and 192% at 3-weeks PI, respectively, and that of TGF-β had increased by 389% at 6 weeks PI. The cytokine IFN-γ, which produces a noxious cellular effect on the CNS and simultaneously activates the inflammatory cellular responses, had decreased at 6 weeks PI, whereas the levels of IL-12, which activates microglia, were sustained with no remarkable decrease during the experimental period. Moreover, levels of the cytokine TGF-β, which induces neuroprotective anti-inflammatory responses, were mostly sustained during the experimental period, but had decreased slightly. The levels of the anti-inflammatory cytokines IL-4 and IL-10 had decreased significantly during the CI stage (9–12 weeks). The results of the present study showed that levels of the inflammatory cytokines had continually increased to 6 weeks PI and were maintain at high levels even during the CI stage, although there were slight decreases, whereas levels of the anti-inflammatory cytokines had remarkably increased during the AI stage (3 weeks PI) and then decreased immediately thereafter during the CI stage. The most important finding was the significant increase and maintenance of IL-12 and TGF-β levels during the CI stage for 12 weeks PI (**Figure 2**, * $p < 0.05$).

Relative Cytokine mRNA Levels and Microglia Phenotype Markers for *T. gondii*-Infected Mouse Brain

Changes in gene expression levels of inflammatory and anti-inflammatory cytokines after *T. gondii* infection are shown in **Figure 3**. Gene expression levels of each cytokine at each time point of infection were compared to those of normal brain tissues (onefold at week 0 PI, a faint khaki color). Data are presented as heat maps (**Figure 3**), which depict the most commonly up- and downregulated transcripts from microarray analysis. The data presented in blue and yellow indicate reduced and increased cytokine expression levels. The present study analyzed gene expression patterns of inflammatory and anti-inflammatory cytokines (**Figure 3A**), as well as the microglia phenotype markers of the M1 and M2 types (**Figure 3B**). As compared with the anti-inflammatory cytokines (IL-4, IL-10 and TGF-β; 1.0- to 1.6-fold), transcript levels of the inflammatory cytokines (IL-12, IFN-γ, and TNF-α) had increased by 1.5- to 3.3-fold, as compared to log_2-values (onefold) of the transcript levels of control mice. Especially, IFN-γ was remarkably increased by 3.3-fold at 3 weeks PI and was constantly maintained at 2.2-fold at 12 weeks PI. Likewise, the inflammatory cytokine TNF-α and the anti-inflammatory cytokine TGF-β were relatively increased by 1.5- to 1.8-fold during the 12-week experimental period. Expression levels of the phenotype markers M1-type and M2-type were found to be polarized in the M1-type microglia (**Figure 3B**). Most importantly, Arg1 levels among M2-markers were consistently increased for 12 weeks PI at 1.7- to 3.4-fold, even though the increase in IFN-γ levels was 2.2- to 3.3-fold. Further examining of the 12 polarization markers in each type of microglial cell phenotype showed that nine markers of the M1-type (IL-1β, IL-12, TNF-α, IFN-γ, CCL5, CXCL1, CXCL10, CD16, and CD86) and four markers of the M2-type (IL-1Rα, TGF-β, Arg1, and YM1) were consistently expressed for the entire 12-week period after infection (**Figure 3B**). Most notably, there was no increase in iNOS, while Arg1 was remarkably increased even if polarization and activation of M1-type microglia were distinct during the CI stage (**Figure 3B**).

Kinetics of Microglia Activation and Phosphorylation of Stat1 in *T. gondii*-Infected Mouse Brain Tissues

The above results showed that the expression levels of the inflammatory cytokines (IL-12, IFN-γ, and TNF-α) had continuously increased during the CI stage. Among these cytokines, mRNA and protein levels of IL-12, a key cytokine of microglial cells activation, and IFN-γ, a key cytokine of Th1-helper T-cell activation, were maintained steadily with high levels during the CI stage (**Figures 2** and **3**). To comprehensively link changes between gene and protein expression levels, brain tissues were immunohistologically stained with Iba-1- and phosphorylated STAT-1 (pStat1) antibodies for microglial activation and to determine whether these molecules participate in the IFN-γ-mediated pathway, respectively (**Figures 4A,B**). Because IFN-γ plays a role in adaptive cellular immunity against *T. gondii* infection and STAT-1 is important for intracellular downregulation of IFN-γ, the increase in pStat1-stained cells in the brain indicates an increase in IFN-γ-mediated Th1-T-cell immune responses. However, pStat1-stained cells were observed around the cyst (red arrow) over a relatively short period of time at 6 weeks PI and, thereafter, were undetectably in the brain tissues (**Figure 4B**). At this time, the proportion of microglial cells had remarkably increased around the *T. gondii* cysts (red arrow) during the AI stage and

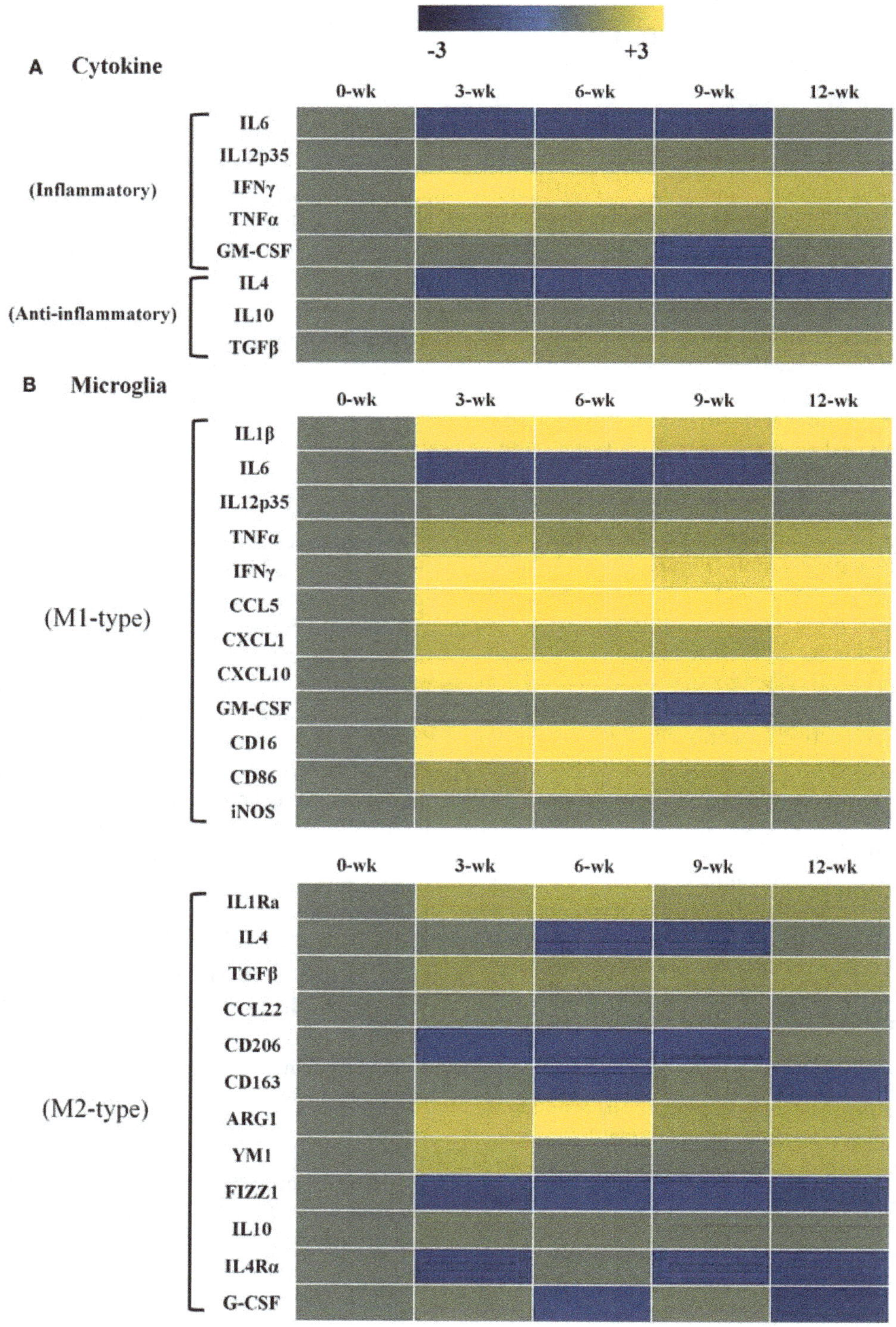

FIGURE 3 | Heat maps representing cytokine and chemokine concentrations in the inflammatory immune response and microglia phenotypes. Transcript levels of inflammatory and anti-inflammatory cytokines as well as microglia phenotype markers were measured in *Toxoplasma gondii*-infected mouse brains using microarray analysis. Each row of the heat map represents cytokines related with inflammatory and anti-inflammatory responses **(A)** as well as microglia phenotype markers related with the M1-type and M2-type **(B)**. Each column represents infection times from week 0 to 12 postinfection. The color scale corresponds to the relative expression of the cytokine for the minimum (−3) and maximum (+3) of all values.

was activated continuously during the CI stage (**Figure 4A**). This activation of microglial cells can be explained by morphological characteristics, such as hyper-ramification and long, thin processes extending from the cell body into the surrounding milieu (**Figure 4A**, colored in brown). The increase in activated microglia was greatest at 6–9 weeks PI and then had decreased

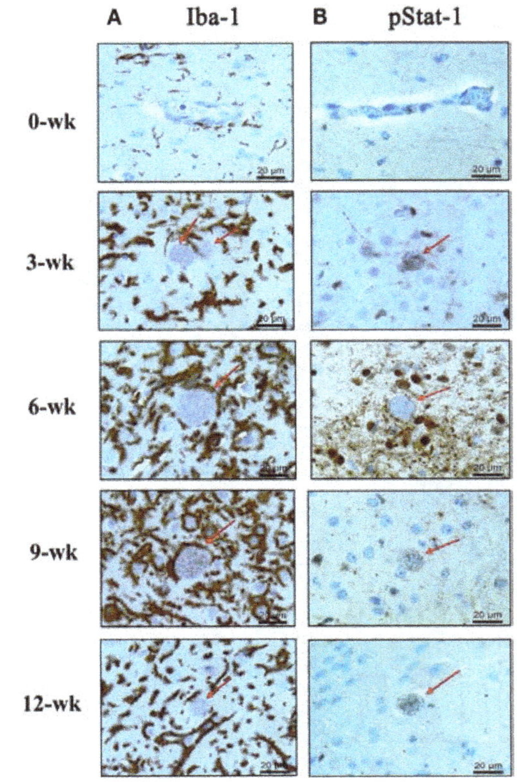

FIGURE 4 | Phosphorylation of Stat1 (pStat1) and Iba-1-stained microglia infiltrated and activated around *Toxoplasma gondii* cysts. *T. gondii*-infected mouse brains were harvested at 0, 3, 6, 9, and 12 weeks postinfection, embedded in paraffin, and immunostained with Iba-1- **(A)** and phosphorylated Stat-1 antibodies **(B)**. *T. gondii* cysts (arrow). Activated microglia [**(A)** brown color]. pStat1 immunoreactivity [**(B)** brown color]. Magnification, 400x. Scale bar = 20 μm.

slightly at 12 weeks PI (CI stage). These results strongly suggest microglia are activated throughout the infection period, whereas STAT1 phosphorylation was limited and no longer maintained during the CI stage.

Effects of TLA (RH- or ME-TLA) on the Polarization and Activation of Microglial Cells

Infection immunity in *T. gondii*-infected brain tissues can be explained by the immune characteristics regulated by the host–parasite relationship. Infectious immunity shown in the present study was characterized by an increase in microglial cells and the limited IFN-γ-mediated immune response. However, it remains unclear whether these immune responses were induced by immune regulation *via* the host–parasite relationship or by immunological triggering of *T. gondii* antigens as a PAMP. For this purpose, TLAs were prepared from RH- or ME49 tachyzoites to investigate the effects of TLA on the activation and polarization of microglia, which were further compared with transcript levels in the brain (**Figures 5A,B**). TLAs contain many PAMPs and stimulate toll-like receptor (TLR)-based immune responses. Moreover, because *T. gondii* strains (RH and ME49) have different modes of infectious immunity, the comparison of *T. gondii* antigens (RH-TLA or ME-TLA) on microglia activation is important to evaluate difference in immune responses between the AI and CI stages. As shown by the results, the MFI (FACS analysis) of the activation markers of BV-2 microglial cells [i.e., major histocompatibility complex II (MHCII), CD40, CD80, and CD86] had increased in response to IFN-γ stimulation (**Figure 5A**). Such an increase in MFI indicates an increase in target molecules in FACS. IFN-γ stimulation of BV-2 cells had increased the expression levels of these activation markers, which was accelerated by the presence of TLA (**Figure 5A**). At this time, ME-TLA had a greater effect on the increase in activation markers than RH-TLA. In contrast, expression of the M2 polarization marker CD206 was lower in ME-TLA than RH-TLA (**Figure 5A**). These results are consistent with the microarray results (**Figure 5B**). Subunit transcripts of MHC class II molecules (H2-Eb1, -Aa, and -Ab1), *Cd40*, *Cd80*, and *Cd86* were increased (16). In contrast, *Cd206* was decreased, as compared to the control (khaki) (**Figure 5B**). The M1 markers *Cd40*, *H2-EB1 (-Aa, -Ab1)* (MHCII), and *Cd86* (B7-2) were upregulated in activated microglial cell and acted as co-stimulatory molecules for further T- and B-cell immune responses. Both mRNA and protein levels of the representative M2 marker CD206 were decreased simultaneously in cells infected with *T. gondii* strain ME49, as well as by antigen treatment (ME-TLA) as PAMPs. Accordingly, our results showed that both *TLA* treatment and *T. gondii* infection induced the activation and M1 polarization of microglial cells compared with the control (no-treatment of IFN-γ and lysate antigens *in vitro* study as well as 0-week PI *in vivo* study).

Changes in Transcripts for T-Cell Differentiation- and T-Cell Exhaustion-Markers in the Brain during *T. gondii* Infection

CI of *T. gondii* in the brain may induce T-cell exhaustion and dysfunction. The results of this study showed a decrease in the IFN-γ-mediated immune response during CI even if microglial cell activation was maintained. To arrive at a possible explanation, markers of T-cell differentiation and dysfunction were examined, which showed that Th1 cell-specific transcription factor TBX21 that controls the expression of IFN-γ was mainly increased during CI, as compared to the Th2 cell-secreted cytokines *Gata3* and *Foxp3*, which promote the functions of regulatory T cells (**Figure 6A**). Nevertheless, markers of T-cell exhaustion, including *Tim3* and *Lag3*, were also increased simultaneously from the AI stage at 3 weeks PI (**Figure 6B**). *Tim3* and *Lag3* are known to negatively regulate T-cell proliferation, homeostasis, and Th1 immunity, and act as immune checkpoints. This result means that *T. gondii* infection actively influences the induction of the host immune response against infection. In other words, although these findings were limited to transcript profiles, *T. gondii* infection of the brain simultaneously induces both T-cell differentiation and exhaustion from the AI stage at 3 weeks PI, and maintains the immune environment during the entire the CI stage (**Figure 6**).

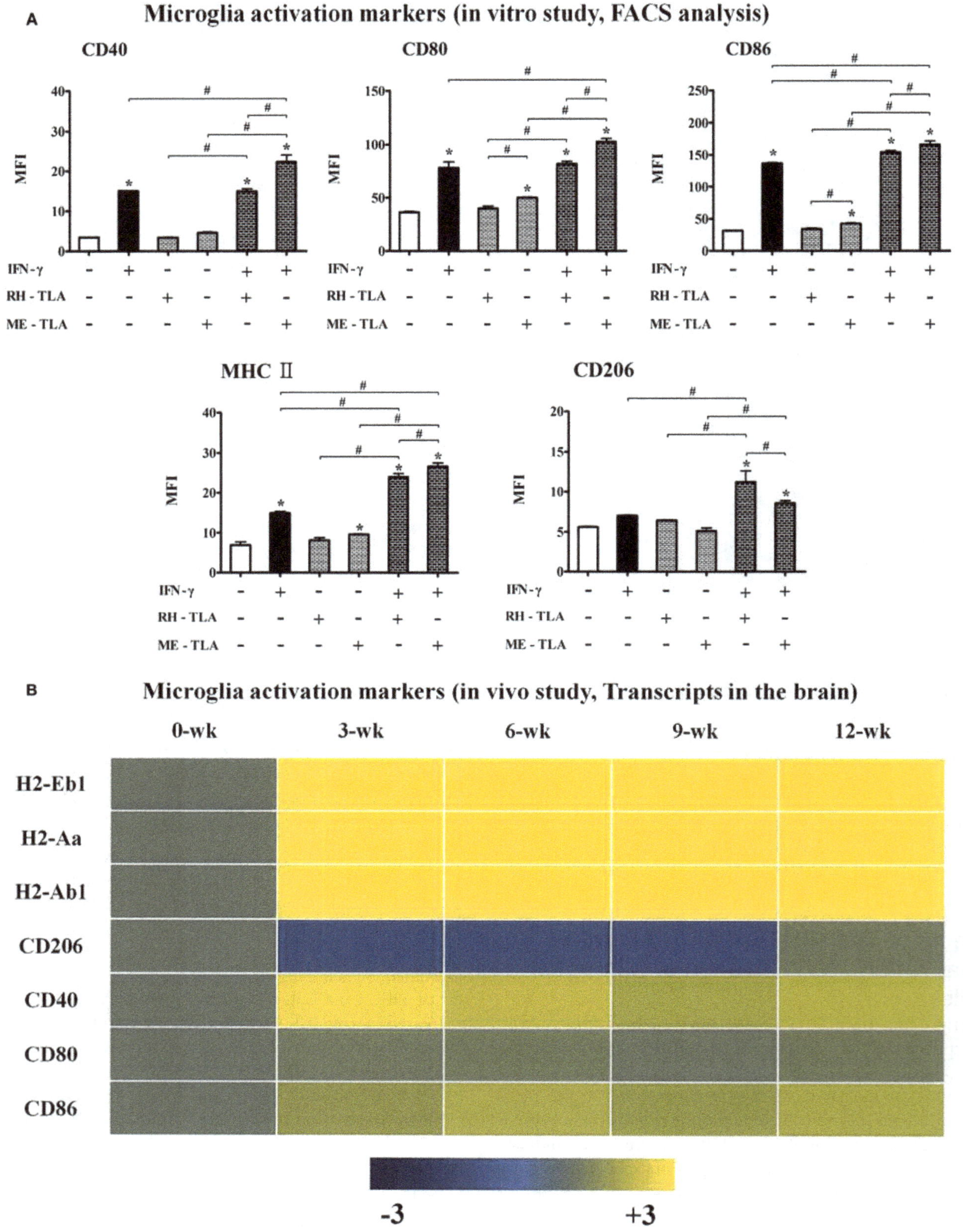

FIGURE 5 | Microglia activation in *Toxoplasma gondii*-infected brain and BV-2 cells stimulated with *T. gondii* lysate antigens (TLAs) (RH-TLA and ME-TLA). Expression levels of major histocompatibility complex II antigens (H2-Eb1, H2-Aa, and H2-Ab1), CD40, and CD86 by FACS analysis. **(A)** Heat map expression of cell surface markers related with microglia activation in *T. gondii*-infected brains, **(B)** results are expressed as the mean ± SD of the mean fluorescence intensity. *$p < 0.05$ (one-way analysis of variance). * indicates significant difference compared with the control. # indicates significant difference between the experimental groups.

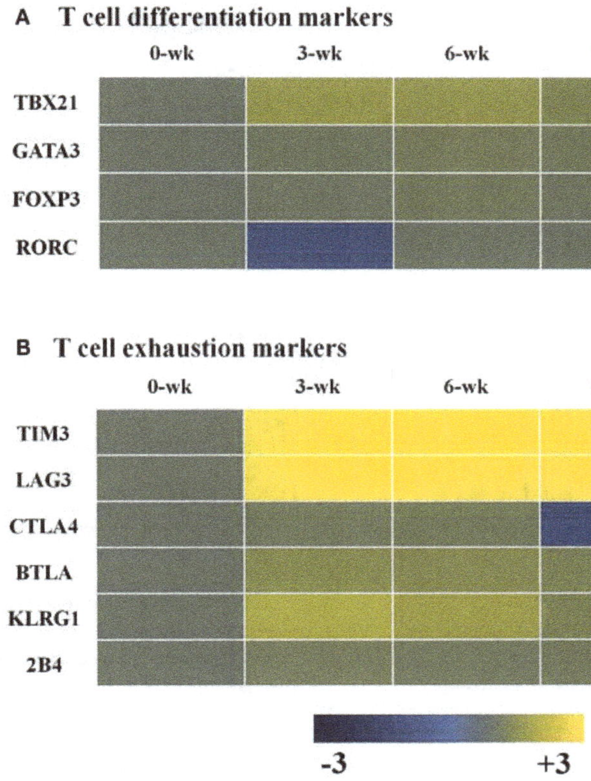

FIGURE 6 | Changes in T-cell differentiation **(A)** and exhaustion **(B)** markers in *Toxoplasma gondii*-infected brain tissues. Expression values represent the intensity of gene expression varying from −3 to +3 colored with blue or yellow.

Changes in mRNA Levels of Immune Effector and Checkpoint Molecules in *T. gondii*-Infected Brain Tissues

To investigate the expression of effector molecules associated with both inflammatory and anti-inflammatory responses, changes in transcripts and quantitative gene levels of Socs1, iNos, and Arg1 during the 12-week experimental period were compared to those at baseline (week 0 PI) (**Figure 7A**). Transcript levels of Socs1, which is thought to be an important immune regulatory factor in this study, was increased by 1.5-fold at 3-weeks PI and maintained during the CI stage (**Figure 7A**). Likewise, quantitative gene expression levels of Socs1 was the highest at 3 weeks PI (2.63-fold) with statistical significance and, thereafter, had slightly decreased during the CI stage. Similarly, the results of western blot analysis showed an increase in SOCS1 expression during the infection period. In contrast, there was no significant increase in iNOS mRNA levels, and quantitative gene expression levels of iNOS/Arg1 were decreased even during the AI stage (3 and 6 weeks PI). This result is also supported by transcript level of Arg1 (2.2- and 3.4-fold at 3 and 6 weeks PI, respectively) (**Figure 7A**). Expression levels of the of the immune inhibitory checkpoint molecules PD-1, PD-L1, and PD-L2, as related with T-cell dysfunction, were examined at the transcript level and by FACS analysis. As shown in **Figure 7B**, transcript levels of PD-1, an inhibitory receptor of T cells, were slightly increased by 1.1- to 1.4-fold at week 12 PI, whereas levels of PD-L1 were remarkably increased by 19.5-, 21.4-, 18.9-, and 23.0-fold at 3, 6, 9, and 12 weeks PI, respectively. This result was also strongly supported by the FACS results expressed as the MFI, suggesting strong activation of the M1-type microglia. When RH- or ME-TLA as PAMPs of *T. gondii* stimulate BV-2 microglial cells, the increase in the MFI of PD-L1 was greater than that of PD-L2 and the degree of increase was greater *via* stimulation of ME-TLA than RH-TLA. Accordingly, it is expected that the immune-triggering effect of *T. gondii* strain ME49 during CI seems to limit the expression of inflammatory effector molecules such as iNOS, even with activation of innate immunity by microglial cells.

Effects of *T. gondii* Antigens (RH- and ME-TLA) on Nitrite and Urea Production according to Microglia Polarization

For 12 weeks PI, iNOS production was decreased and Arg1 production was increased. As well, when BV-2 cells were treated with *T. gondii* antigens as a PAMPs, expression levels of the activation markers were increased. In this regard, an aim of this study was to investigate whether treatment of BV-2 microglial cells with *T. gondii* antigens (RH-TLA or ME-TLA) can induce changes in NO and urea production, as with *T. gondii*-infected brain tissues. In general, nitrite production is mainly increased as a result of M1-type activation, whereas urea production is increased by M2-type microglia activation. The results of the present study showed that the production of nitrite was increased by stimulation

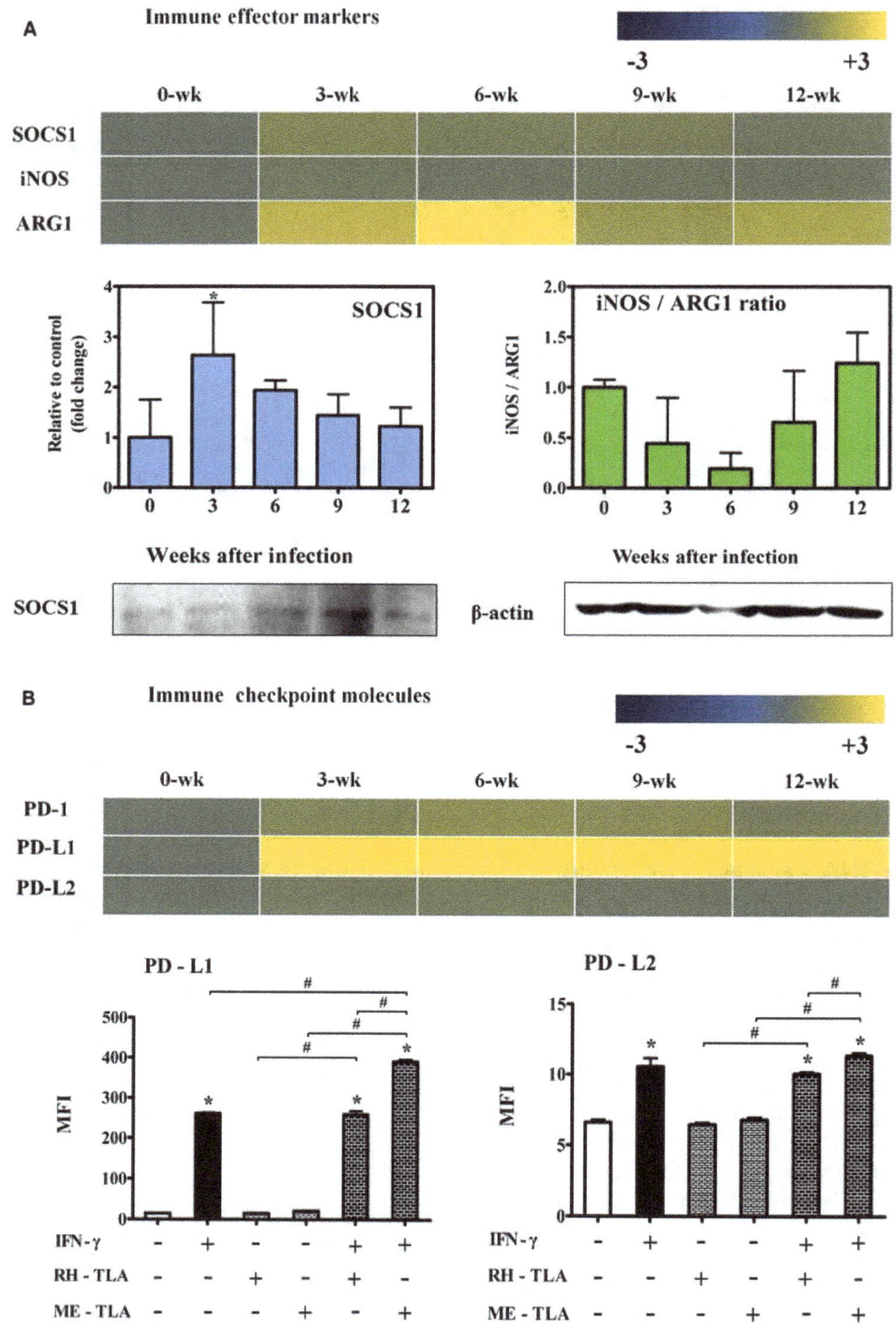

FIGURE 7 | Changes in immune effector and checkpoint molecules. Transcripts of immune effector markers [nitric oxide synthase (iNos) and Arg1] **(A)**, immune control marker (Socs1) **(A)** and immune checkpoint markers (PD-1, PD-L1 and PD-L2) **(B)**. RT-PCR results (SOCS1 and the iNos/Arg1 ratio) and western blot (SOCS1 and β-actin) **(A)**. Transcript expressions(PD-1, PD-L1, and PD-L2) and FACS analysis (PD-L1 and PD-L2) **(B)**. Results are expressed as the mean ± SD of the mean fluorescence intensity (MFI). $^{*}p < 0.05$ (one-way analysis of variance). * indicates significant difference compared with the control. # indicates significant difference between the experimental groups.

of IFN-γ alone (9.5 ± 0.3 μM) or IFN-γ with *T. gondii* antigen (6.6 ± 0.2 μM with RH-TLA and 17.1 ± 0.7 μM with ME-TLA), as compared to the control (4.3 ± 0.4 μM) (**Figure 8A**). At this time, nitrite concentration had significantly increased *via* stimulation with ME-TLA, as compared to RH-TLA, suggesting that ME-TLA itself is more preferable for the induction of M1-type

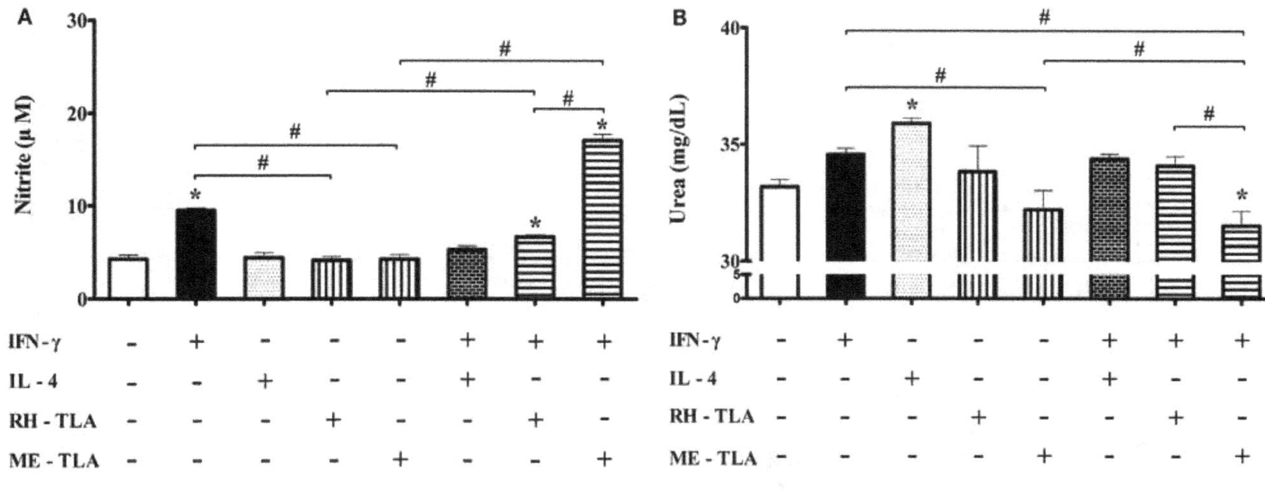

FIGURE 8 | Nitrite and urea production in BV-2 microglia stimulated with recombinant cytokines affecting microglia polarization (IFN-γ and IL-4) or *Toxoplasma gondii* antigens (RH-TLA or ME-TLA). Nitrite (μM) **(A)** and urea (mg/dL) concentrations **(B)**. Data are presented as the mean ± SD. *$p < 0.05$ (one-way analysis of variance). * indicates significant difference compared with the control. # indicates significant difference between the experimental groups.

microglial activation (*$p < 0.05$). In contrast, urea concentration was increased significantly by stimulation of IL-4, as compared to the control (36.0 ± 0.2 vs. 33.2 ± 0.3, respectively) (**Figure 8B**). As well, urea production was more decreased by ME-TLA than RH-TLA (32.2 ± 0.8 vs. 33.8 ± 1.1 mg/dL, respectively). Notably, treatment with IFN-γ + ME-TLA had decreased urea production even further than with treatment of IFN-γ + RH-TLA (31.5 ± 0.6 and 34.1 ± 0.4, respectively, *$p < 0.05$). These results clearly show that treatment of BV-2 cells with ME-TLA induced M1 polarization and M1-activation, which subsequently remarkably increased nitrite production and decreased urea production, suggesting that the immune induction of ME-TLA acts as a PAMP. However, this result is in contrast to the transcript results of the *T. gondii*-infected brain tissues. To clarify this difference, infection of BV-2 cells was performed *in vitro* (**Figure 9**).

Effects of *In Vitro T. gondii* Infection (RH- and ME-Strain) on mRNA Expression (iNOS, Cox-2, and Arg1) and Nitrite Production

To elucidate the differences in inflammatory responses and NO production between *T. gondii* infection in the brain and *in vitro* experiments with the *T. gondii* antigens (RH-TLA and ME-TLA), BV-2 cells were infected with *T. gondii* tachyzoites *in vitro*. As shown in **Figure 9**, the expression levels of the inflammatory response markers iNos and Cox-2 were significantly decreased after *T. gondii* infection *in vitro*, whereas that of Argl was significantly increased. Notably, Argl expression levels at 24 h after *in vitro* RH and ME49 infection were increased by 2.0 ± 0.3- and 2.9 ± 0.1-fold, respectively, as compared to control (*$p < 0.05$). Likewise, Argl induction was significantly greater after infection with strain ME49, as compared to strain RH. At this time, nitrite production was the highest with treatment of IFN-γ alone (39.6 ± 2.0 μM) and decreased significantly with IFN-γ + *T. gondii* infection (RH and ME49) (28.9 ± 1.4 and 24.0 ± 0.9 μM, respectively, *$p < 0.05$). As compared to IFN-γ alone, nitrite levels were 27% lower with IFN-γ + *T. gondii* strain RH infection and 39.4% lower with IFN-γ + *T. gondii* strain ME49 infection. Accordingly, these results emphasize that *in vitro T. gondii* infection induces polarization of microglial cells into the M1-type. However, simultaneous inhibition of harmful inflammatory factors, such as NO, had increased Argl expression for further immune regulation. This is an important result showing that *in vivo* and *in vitro* infection was consistent. In other words, TLAs acting as PAMPs had strongly induced polarization of M1-type microglial cells and inflammatory responses, while infection of *T. gondii* (*in vivo* and *in vitro*) induced polarization of M1-type microglial cells. However, it simultaneously inhibited a detrimental inflammatory response, such as NO production, *via* Argl induction. This host–parasite relationship seems to be a strategy of *T. gondii* to maintain a CI in the brain.

DISCUSSION

The results of our previous study demonstrated that *T. gondii* infection decreased the neurodegeneration in a Tg2576 mouse model of Alzheimer's disease (8). In that study, *T. gondii* infection of the brain inhibited neuronal degeneration, as well as learning and memory impairments in Tg2576 mice. As a possible reason, we proposed that the increase in the expression levels of the anti-inflammatory cytokines IL-10 and TGF-β, as well as decreased NO production had favorable effects of *T. gondii* infection and the pathogenesis and progression of Alzheimer's disease in mice (8). However, because inflammatory responses induced by IFN-γ and NO are essential for the control of *T. gondii* infection, NO regulation in the CNS is very important to control both parasitic proliferation and damage to the host tissues. As an extension of the above results, the aim of the present study was to address the progression of infection immunity to identify the appropriate timing to induce an anti-inflammatory response during CI. In

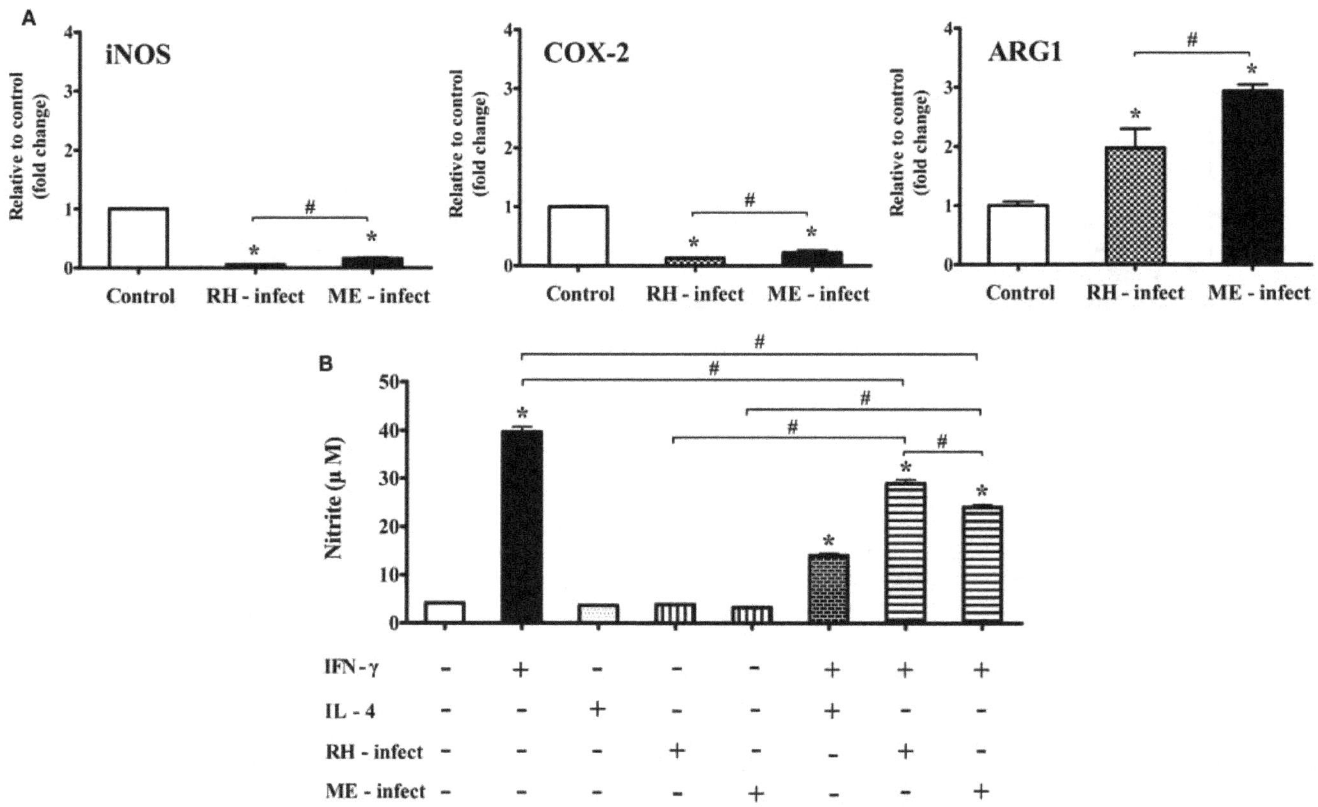

FIGURE 9 | mRNA levels of nitric oxide synthase (iNos), Cox-2, and Arg1, and nitrite production in *Toxoplasma gondii*-infected BV-2 microglial cells. **(A)** RT-PCR analysis of iNos, Cox-2, and Arg1 in *T. gondii* tachyzoites (strains RH and ME49)-infected BV-2 cells. **(B)** Nitrite concentration (μM) in culture supernatant treated with recombinant IFN-γ and/or IL-4, and/or *T. gondii* tachyzoites. Data are presented as the mean ± SD. $^{*}p < 0.05$ (one-way analysis of variance). * indicates significant difference compared with the control. # indicates significant difference between the experimental groups.

particular, because *T. gondii* is a pathogen that can lead to CI of the host, as well as induce encephalitis and neurodegeneration, it is very important to understand the infection immunity related with microglia polarization and harmful inflammatory responses.

Encephalitis is an important symptom of *T. gondii* infection, although the neuronal degeneration associated with neuroinflammation is not a common finding because immune modulation by *T. gondii* infection has been the focus of numerous previous studies (1–5, 8, 9). In the present study, neuronal cell death caused by *T. gondii* infection in the DG region of the hippocampus was increased in the AI stage at 3–6 weeks PI, which then decreased in the CI stage accompanied with slight decreases in the expression levels of the inflammatory cytokines IL-6, IFN-γ, TNF-α, and GM-CSF. Even in this case, the Iba-1 staining intensity of microglial cells was not significantly decreased during the entire 12-week experimental period. In fact, the microarray results of the *T. gondii*-infected brain and FACS analysis of *in vitro* cultured BV-2 microglial cells with lysate antigens (RH-TLA and ME-TLA) prepared from tachyzoites of *T. gondii* strains RH and ME49, showed M1 polarization of microglial cells both *in vivo* and *in vitro*. However, high levels of the inflammatory and anti-inflammatory cytokines remained during the 12-week experimental, even though the levels had slightly decreased from 6 weeks PI. Thus, it is necessary to consider why neuronal cell death was highest at 3 weeks PI and then decreased. Clearly, *T. gondii* infection induces a mixed immune response characterized by an increase in the expression levels of inflammatory cytokines and the activation and proliferation of microglial cells, as well as increases in the expression levels of the anti-inflammatory cytokines and Arg1 and decreased expression of iNOS and COX-2 accompanied with NO production.

The strategy of *T. gondii* intracellular parasitism involves the manipulation of an excessive response of immune cells and alterations in macrophage phenotypes to suppress inflammatory response and reduce damage to the host. According to the results of an earlier study, *T. gondii* infection is generally controlled by a strong Th1-type immune response *via* the cytokines IL-12p70, TNF-α, and IFN-γ. However, the recruited monocyte population is converted to an anti-inflammatory phenotype in order to restrain excessive immune responses during infection of *T. gondii* strain RH (3–6, 12, 14, 21, 22). On the other hand, the time of infection for the change in microglial cells and inflammatory responses as a cause of CI of the brain infected with strain ME49 it is not well defined. Some studies have provided important clues to prevent excessive activation of macrophages after *T. gondii* infection (3, 14). For example, *Toxoplasma* rhoptry and dense granule proteins play roles in the modulation of pro-inflammatory responses through the regulation in IFN-γ and NF-kB by GRA15 in addition to STAT3/6 activation by ROP16 (3, 14). ROP16 induces STAT1 tyrosine phosphorylation as well as *Socs1 via* STAT3 or 6 (23). As a result, the authors insisted that the infected hosts are able to induce a proper resistance against *T. gondii* infection as well as protection against excessive inflammatory immunity (3, 14, 23). However, these studies were limited by the failure to explain the promotion of immune modulation during *T. gondii* infection because the experiments employed Raw264.7, J447, DC2.4, or human foreskin fibroblast cells for *in vitro T. gondii* infection and *T. gondii*-infected peritoneal exudate cells for *in vivo* infection (3, 14). So, these studies do not reflect the entire infection process. On the contrary, the present study addressed the changes in the infection immunity during the CI stage. For example, the immune regulation for the control of parasitic proliferation without inducing harmful immunopathological events in the brain. Moreover, the present study provides some evidence of the immune regulation against *T. gondii* infection and protective immunity to prevent damage to host cells by an excessive inflammatory response.

The IFN-γ-mediated type 1 immune response with upregulation of the anti-parasitic factor NO is required to prevent the reactivation of *T. gondii* and TE in the brain (1). In the brain, microglia and infiltrating CD4 and CD8 T cells are the primary sources of IFN-γ, a cytokine leading noxious cellular effects in the CNS (1, 4). On the contrary, our earlier research also highlighted the importance of TGF-β in neuroprotection after *T. gondii* infection (8). In addition, the results of the present study suggest the importance of the interactions of various immunological factors between protective immunity and immunopathological effects by tracking of the immune response during the CI stage. First of all, changes in the immune response after *T. gondii* infection can be confirmed by microarray analysis of mRNA expression patterns, which can also predict the immunological phenotype. In the present study, there were increases in the mRNA levels of the T-cell exhaustion markers TIM3, LAG3, and KLRG1 without distinct increases in the mRNA levels of the T-cell differentiation markers TBX21, GATA3, FOXP3, and RORC during the AI stage, even though microglia activation was maintained in the M1-type. T-cell exhaustion markers are highly expressed by chronic antigen stimulation, but yet diminish the effector function of CD8 T cells (24). Accordingly, these results suggest that the inhibition of immune extension of adaptive T-cell immunity can accelerate neuronal cell death by expanding inflammatory cellular responses, although it is helpful for protective immunity of the host against *T. gondii* infection. Actually, pStat1, which is activated by IFN-γ and induces iNOS (25), was remarkably decreased at 6 weeks PI although the increase in IFN-γ expression was maintained for 12 weeks PI. Although IFN-γ-mediated activation of macrophages is critical for resistance against AI with *T. gondii*, *T. gondii* infection inhibits STAT1 transcriptional activity to allow the parasite to establish a CI (5, 23). Additionally, SOCS proteins, which can downregulate phosphorylation of JAK and STAT1, are actually induced by *T. gondii* infection (26). To understand the importance of microglia activation and further T-cell immune responses against *T. gondii* infection, transcript data of markers related to microglial cell polarization and T-cell-mediated adaptive immune responses were investigated. In particular, PD-L1 (B7-H1) was highly expressed in inflammatory macrophages, while PD-L2 (B7-DC) can be induced by alternative activation *via* IL-4 (27). Furthermore, PD-L1 might play a role in the downregulation of activated T cells and the expression of PD-L1 in a non-Stat1-dependent manner (27). Likewise, our results showed that PD-L1 expression was increased, as compared to PD-L2, at both transcript levels *in vivo* and *in vitro* ME-TLA stimulation (19.0–23.0- and 1.1–1.2-fold changes, respectively). At this time, M1-type activation of microglia and increases in the expression levels of the inflammatory cytokines IFN-γ, IL-12, and TNF-α were observed. However, these changes did not result in an increase in Stat-1 phosphorylation. This result provides a subtle balance for the control of parasitic proliferation and simultaneous inhibition of the increase in inflammatory cellular immune responses, which induce tissue damage during CI by altering the mRNA expression levels of PD-L1 and PD-1 because PD-1/PD-L1 interactions are required for the maturation of microglial cells and expansion of protective T-cell responses in *T. gondii* infection. However, excessive PD-1-mediated CD8 T-cell dysfunction plays a central role in immune tolerance, as well as *T. gondii* differentiation and reactivation (28–30). This is an important mechanism for the control of parasite expansion, even with the inhibition of iNOS, as in the present study.

The induction of iNOS, a M1-marker that leads to NO production, is generally elevated in the AI stage of *T. gondii* infection and in M1-like microglia (26, 31). Surprisingly, the results of the present showed that ME-TLA, a lysate antigen of *T. gondii* strain ME49, strongly induces the polarization of M1-type microglial cells and NO production. In other words, ME-TLA treatment of BV-2 microglial cells induced greater M1 polarization and NO production than treatment with IFN-γ. Simultaneously, urea production was decreased by treatment with the *T. gondii* antigens (RH and ME49) *in vitro*. TLA includes a variety of antigen pools, including TLR-based immune-triggering PAMPs (32). When soluble parasite TLA, as in the present study, stimulates dendritic cells and macrophages, the immune response resulted in TLR-signaling dependent production of IL-12 and NO (32). Accordingly, it is evident that the treatment of TLA as a PAMPs and parasite infection induce different immune triggering both *in vivo* and *in vitro*. To confirm this finding, NO production was compared between an *in vitro* infection model using *T. gondii* tachyzoites (strains RH and ME49) and an *in vitro* model using BV-2 microglial cell culture with TLA. As expected, the results were consistent with the *in vivo* infection study. NO production was decreased and mRNA expression levels of iNOS and COX-2 were lowered, while mRNA expression of Arg1 was increased by 2.9-fold. Based on these results, the authors insist that the host–parasite relationship in the regulation parasite control and host tissue damage by an excessive inflammatory response induces the control of effector molecules, which differs from the immune-triggering effect of TLA shown by the *in vitro* stimulation study. As a possible mechanism, increases in transcripts of SOCS and Arg1 during the CI stage are focused because of their immune regulatory functions.

Suppressor of cytokines signaling 1 protein is a known feedback inhibitor of IFN-γ receptor signaling and is induced directly by viable *T. gondii* parasites (26). In general, the SOCS proteins, especially SOCS1, are expressed by immune cells and cells of the CNS, and have the potential to impact immune processes within the CNS, including inflammatory cytokine and chemokine production, as well as activation of microglia (33). In this study, transcripts of SOCS1 were steadily expressed during the CI stage. It is known that SOCS induces a high Arg1:iNOS activity ratio and suppresses T-cell proliferation (34). Moreover, SOCS1 contributes to the inhibition of IFN-γ signaling and NO production without the dependency of TLR stimulation (35). In other words, due to upregulation of SOCS1 by IL-4-dependent M2 macrophage activation (34), the role of SOCS1 in the present study is sufficiently predictable for the direct increase in the Arg1:iNOS activity ratio, the decrease in transcripts of T-cell differentiation markers and Stat1 phosphorylation, and the increase in transcripts of T-cell exhaustion markers, suggesting modulations of the host–parasite relationship between parasite control and tissue damage in the brain.

Taken together, these results highlight the critical importance of M1-type microglia for the control of *T. gondii* as well as the limitation of STAT1 phosphorylation and the induc tion of SOCS1 to reduce detrimental inflammatory immune responses. Moreover, these results provide new insights into the characteristics of infection immunity through the host–parasite relationship during CI of *T. gondii*. In other words, *T. gondii* infection basically induces M1-type polarization of microglial cells, the limitation of IFN-γ-mediated inflammatory responses, including T-cell differentiation and Stat1 phosphorylation, and the reduction of iNOS/Arg1 ratio mediated by Socs1 induction. These phenomena are only expected by infection immunity due to the difference in the levels of effector molecules *via* the *in vitro* cellular response with TLA. In particular, this study revealed the characteristics of immune regulation in infection immunity by observing the persistent changes in the immune environment during a CI rather than at any one time.

AUTHOR CONTRIBUTIONS

YH and E-HS conceived and designed the experiments. J-HS and YH performed the experiments. J-HS, J-PY, and E-HS analyzed the data. B-KJ, SL, and E-HS contributed reagents/materials/analysis tools. E-HS wrote the paper.

REFERENCES

1. Wohlfert EA, Blader IJ, Wilson EH. Brains and Brawn: *Toxoplasma* infections of the central nervous system and skeletal muscle. *Trends Parasitol* (2017) 33:519–31. doi:10.1016/j.pt.2017.04.001
2. Mordue DG, Monroy F, La Regina M, Dinarello CA, Sibley LD. Acute toxoplasmosis leads to lethal overproduction of Th1 cytokines. *J Immunol* (2001) 167:4574–84. doi:10.4049/jimmunol.167.8.4574
3. Jensen KD, Wang Y, Wojno ED, Shastri AJ, Hu K, Cornel L, et al. *Toxoplasma* polymorphic effectors determine macrophage polarization and intestinal inflammation. *Cell Host Microbe* (2011) 9:472–83. doi:10.1016/j.chom.2011.04.015
4. Rozenfeld C, Martinez R, Seabra S, Sant'anna C, Goncalves JG, Bozza M, et al. *Toxoplasma gondii* prevents neuron degeneration by interferon-gamma-activated microglia in a mechanism involving inhibition of inducible nitric oxide synthase and transforming growth factor-beta1 production by infected microglia. *Am J Pathol* (2005) 167:1021–31. doi:10.1016/S0002-9440(10)61191-1
5. Suzuki Y. Host resistance in the brain against *Toxoplasma gondii*. *J Infect Dis* (2002) 185(Suppl 1):S58–65. doi:10.1086/337999
6. Jankovic D, Kugler DG, Sher A. IL-10 production by CD4+ effector T cells: a mechanism for self-regulation. *Mucosal Immunol* (2010) 3:239–46. doi:10.1038/mi.2010.8
7. Sarciron ME, Gherardi A. Cytokines involved in Toxoplasmic encephalitis. *Scand J Immunol* (2000) 52:534–43. doi:10.1046/j.1365-3083.2000.00817.x
8. Jung BK, Pyo KH, Shin KY, Hwang YS, Lim H, Lee SJ, et al. *Toxoplasma gondii* infection in the brain inhibits neuronal degeneration and learning and memory impairments in a murine model of Alzheimer's disease. *PLoS One* (2012) 7:e33312. doi:10.1371/journal.pone.0033312
9. Orihuela R, McPherson CA, Harry GJ. Microglial M1/M2 polarization and metabolic states. *Br J Pharmacol* (2016) 173:649–65. doi:10.1111/bph.13139
10. Nguyen TD, Bigaignon G, Van Broeck J, Vercammen M, Nguyen TN, Delmee M, et al. Acute and chronic phases of *Toxoplasma gondii* infection in mice modulate the host immune responses. *Infect Immun* (1998) 66:2991–5.
11. Hester J, Mullins J, Sa Q, Payne L, Mercier C, Cesbron-Delauw MF, et al. *Toxoplasma gondii* antigens recognized by IgG antibodies differ between mice with and without active proliferation of tachyzoites in the brain during the chronic stage of infection. *Infect Immun* (2012) 80:3611–20. doi:10.1128/IAI.00604-12
12. El Kasmi KC, Qualls JE, Pesce JT, Smith AM, Thompson RW, Henao-Tamayo M, et al. Toll-like receptor-induced arginase 1 in macrophages thwarts effective immunity against intracellular pathogens. *Nat Immunol* (2008) 9:1399–406. doi:10.1038/ni.1671
13. Guillemin GJ, Brew BJ. Microglia, macrophages, perivascular macrophages, and pericytes: a review of function and identification. *J Leukoc Biol* (2004) 75:388–97. doi:10.1189/jlb.0303114
14. Rosowski EE, Lu D, Julien L, Rodda L, Gaiser RA, Jensen KD, et al. Strain-specific activation of the NF-kappaB pathway by GRA15, a novel *Toxoplasma gondii* dense granule protein. *J Exp Med* (2011) 208:195–212. doi:10.1084/jem.20100717
15. Harris TH, Wilson EH, Tait ED, Buckley M, Shapira S, Caamano J, et al. NF-kappaB1 contributes to T cell-mediated control of *Toxoplasma gondii* in the CNS. *J Neuroimmunol* (2010) 222:19–28. doi:10.1016/j.jneuroim.2009.12.009
16. Rozenfeld C, Martinez R, Figueiredo RT, Bozza MT, Lima FR, Pires AL, et al. Soluble factors released by *Toxoplasma gondii*-infected astrocytes down-modulate nitric oxide production by gamma interferon-activated microglia and prevent neuronal degeneration. *Infect Immun* (2003) 71:2047–57. doi:10.1128/IAI.71.4.2047-2057.2003
17. Tait ED, Hunter CA. Advances in understanding immunity to *Toxoplasma gondii*. *Mem Inst Oswaldo Cruz* (2009) 104:201–10. doi:10.1590/S0074-02762009000200013

18. Christian DA, Koshy AA, Reuter MA, Betts MR, Boothroyd JC, Hunter CA. Use of transgenic parasites and host reporters to dissect events that promote interleukin-12 production during toxoplasmosis. *Infect Immun* (2014) 82:4056–67. doi:10.1128/IAI.01643-14
19. Lu F, Huang S, Kasper LH. Interleukin-10 and pathogenesis of murine ocular toxoplasmosis. *Infect Immun* (2003) 71:7159–63. doi:10.1128/IAI.71.12.7159-7163.2003
20. Kamerkar S, Davis PH. *Toxoplasma* on the brain: understanding host-pathogen interactions in chronic CNS infection. *J Parasitol Res* (2012) 2012:589295. doi:10.1155/2012/589295
21. Pyo KH, Jung BK, Xin CF, Lee YW, Chai JY, Shin EH. Prominent IL-12 production and tumor reduction in athymic nude mice after *Toxoplasma gondii* lysate antigen treatment. *Korean J Parasitol* (2014) 52:605–12. doi:10.3347/kjp.2014.52.6.605
22. Pyo KH, Lee YW, Lim SM, Shin EH. Immune adjuvant effect of a *Toxoplasma gondii* profilin-like protein in autologous whole-tumor-cell vaccination in mice. *Oncotarget* (2016) 7:74107–19. doi:10.18632/oncotarget.12316
23. Rosowski EE, Saeij JP. *Toxoplasma gondii* clonal strains all inhibit STAT1 transcriptional activity but polymorphic effectors differentially modulate IFNgamma induced gene expression and STAT1 phosphorylation. *PLoS One* (2012) 7:e51448. doi:10.1371/journal.pone.0051448
24. Legat A, Speiser DE, Pircher H, Zehn D, Fuertes Marraco SA. Inhibitory receptor expression depends more dominantly on differentiation and activation than "exhaustion" of human CD8 T cells. *Front Immunol* (2013) 4:455. doi:10.3389/fimmu.2013.00455
25. Gavrilescu LC, Butcher BA, Del Rio L, Taylor GA, Denkers EY. STAT1 is essential for antimicrobial effector function but dispensable for gamma interferon production during *Toxoplasma gondii* infection. *Infect Immun* (2004) 72:1257–64. doi:10.1128/IAI.72.3.1257-1264.2004
26. Zimmermann S, Murray PJ, Heeg K, Dalpke AH. Induction of suppressor of cytokine signaling-1 by *Toxoplasma gondii* contributes to immune evasion in macrophages by blocking IFN-gamma signaling. *J Immunol* (2006) 176:1840–7. doi:10.4049/jimmunol.176.3.1840
27. Loke P, Allison JP. PD-L1 and PD-L2 are differentially regulated by Th1 and Th2 cells. *Proc Natl Acad Sci U S A* (2003) 100:5336–41. doi:10.1073/pnas.0931259100
28. Bhadra R, Gigley JP, Weiss LM, Khan IA. Control of *Toxoplasma* reactivation by rescue of dysfunctional CD8+ T-cell response via PD-1-PDL-1 blockade. *Proc Natl Acad Sci U S A* (2011) 108:9196–201. doi:10.1073/pnas.1015298108
29. McBerry C, Dias A, Shryock N, Lampe K, Gutierrez FR, Boon L, et al. PD-1 modulates steady-state and infection-induced IL-10 production in vivo. *Eur J Immunol* (2014) 44:469–79. doi:10.1002/eji.201343658
30. Bhadra R, Gigley JP, Khan IA. PD-1-mediated attrition of polyfunctional memory CD8+ T cells in chronic toxoplasma infection. *J Infect Dis* (2012) 206:125–34. doi:10.1093/infdis/jis304
31. Lan X, Han X, Li Q, Yang QW, Wang J. Modulators of microglial activation and polarization after intracerebral haemorrhage. *Nat Rev Neurol* (2017) 13:420–33. doi:10.1038/nrneurol.2017.69
32. Denkers EY. From cells to signaling cascades: manipulation of innate immunity by *Toxoplasma gondii*. *FEMS Immunol Med Microbiol* (2003) 39:193–203. doi:10.1016/S0928-8244(03)00279-7
33. Baker BJ, Akhtar LN, Benveniste EN. SOCS1 and SOCS3 in the control of CNS immunity. *Trends Immunol* (2009) 30:392–400. doi:10.1016/j.it.2009.07.001
34. Whyte CS, Bishop ET, Ruckerl D, Gaspar-Pereira S, Barker RN, Allen JE, et al. Suppressor of cytokine signaling (SOCS)1 is a key determinant of differential macrophage activation and function. *J Leukoc Biol* (2011) 90:845–54. doi:10.1189/jlb.1110644
35. Stutz A, Kessler H, Kaschel ME, Meissner M, Dalpke AH. Cell invasion and strain dependent induction of suppressor of cytokine signaling-1 by *Toxoplasma gondii*. *Immunobiology* (2012) 217:28–36. doi:10.1016/j.imbio.2011.08.008

5

Trichinella spiralis Infection Mitigates Collagen-Induced Arthritis *via* Programmed Death 1-Mediated Immunomodulation

*Yuli Cheng[1], Xing Zhu[1], Xiaohuan Wang[1], Qinghui Zhuang[1], Xu Huyan[1], Ximeng Sun[1], Jingjing Huang[1], Bin Zhan[2] and Xinping Zhu[1]**

[1] Department of Medical Microbiology and Parasitology, School of Basic Medical Sciences, Capital Medical University, Beijing, China, [2] Department of Pediatrics, National School of Tropical Medicine, Baylor College of Medicine, Houston, TX, United States

***Correspondence:**
Xinping Zhu
zhuxping@ccmu.edu.cn

Helminth infection induces Th2-biased immune responses and inhibitory/regulatory pathways that minimize excessive inflammation to facilitate the chronic infection of helminth in the host and in the meantime, prevent host hypersensitivity from autoimmune or atopic diseases. However, the detailed molecular mechanisms behind modulation on inflammatory diseases are yet to be clarified. Programmed death 1 (PD-1) is one of the important inhibitory receptors involved in the balance of host immune responses during chronic infection. Here, we used the murine model to examine the role of PD-1 in $CD4^+$ T cells in the effects of *Trichinella spiralis* infection on collagen-induced arthritis (CIA). Mice infected with *T. spiralis* demonstrated higher expression of PD-1 in the spleen $CD4^+$ T cells than those without infection. Mice infected with *T. spiralis* 2 weeks prior to being immunized with type II collagen displayed lower arthritis incidence and significantly attenuated pathology of CIA compared with those of uninfected mice. The therapeutic effect of *T. spiralis* infection on CIA was reversed by blocking PD-1 with anti-PD-1 antibody, associated with enhanced Th1/Th17 pro-inflammatory responses and reduced Th2 responses. The role of PD-1 in regulating $CD4^+$ T cell differentiation and proliferation during *T. spiralis* infection was further examined in PD-1 knockout ($PD\text{-}1^{-/-}$) C57BL/6 J mice. Interestingly, *T. spiralis*-induced alteration of attenuated Th1 and enhanced Th2/regulatory T cell differentiation in wild-type (WT) mice was effectively diminished in $PD\text{-}1^{-/-}$ mice characterized by recovered Th1 cytokine levels, reduced levels of Th2 and regulatory cytokines and $CD4^+CD25^+Foxp3^+$ cells. Moreover, *T. spiralis*-induced $CD4^+$ T cell proliferation suppression in WT mice was partially restored in $PD\text{-}1^{-/-}$ mice. This study introduces the first evidence that PD-1 plays a critical role in helminth infection-attenuated CIA in a mouse model by regulating the $CD4^+$ T cell function, which may provide the new insights into the mechanisms of helminth-induced immunomodulation of host autoimmunity.

Keywords: *Trichinella spiralis*, rheumatoid arthritis, programmed death 1, $CD4^+$ T cell, immunomodulation

INTRODUCTION

After co-evolution with their hosts over a long period of time, helminths have developed the ability to induce host immune tolerance to facilitate their survival in the hosts. This helminth-induced immunomodulation may also benefit hosts to reduce pathological lesions caused by aberrant inflammatory responses that may underline many autoimmune disorders (1, 2). Rheumatoid arthritis

(RA) is a chronic autoimmune disease characterized by synovial inflammation and bone erosion, which affects up to 1% of the population worldwide. There is strong evidence that abnormally activated Th1 and Th17 cells and impaired $CD4^{+}CD25^{+}Foxp3^{+}$ regulatory T cell (Treg) contribute to the pathogenesis of RA (3). Helminth infections skew host immune response from Th1 to Th2/Treg characterized by stimulating the secretion of Th2 cytokine IL-4, IL-5, IL-10, and IL-13 (4) and induction of Treg development (5, 6). Th2 polarization and Treg-released IL-10, TGF-β downregulate the Th1 cell subset (6–8) that promotes the establishment of chronic infection (9). Immunomodulation by helminth infection has inspired to the idea of using helminthic therapy for atopic and autoimmune diseases in animal models and human trials which have provided convincing evidences for effectively alleviating a number of autoimmune diseases up to date (1). It has also been reported that helminth infection or helminth-derived products effectively alleviated the inflammatory arthritis by inducing Th2 responses or inducing $Foxp3^{+}$ T regulatory cells (10, 11). However, the detailed molecular mechanisms behind the modulation of inflammatory diseases are yet to be clarified.

Programmed death 1 (PD-1) is a member of the B7 family on the surface of T cells that delivers inhibitory signals to promote self-tolerance by suppressing T cell inflammatory activity and reduce immune-mediated tissue damage (12). PD-1 is an important immune checkpoint to keep immune balance and exerts critical inhibitory functions in the setting of persistent antigenic stimulation such as during encounter of self-antigens, chronic infections, and tumors (13, 14). There is evidence supporting a distinct role of PD-1 and its ligands (PD-L1/B7-H1 and PD-L2/B7-DC) in regulating T cell tolerance and autoimmunity (15). In humans, a role for PD-1 in the regulation of self-tolerance and autoimmunity was suggested to be associated with autoimmune diseases such as systemic lupus erythematosus, RA, multiple sclerosis, and type 1 diabetes mellitus (16–19). In animal models of collagen-induced arthritis (CIA), defective expression of PD-1 has been confirmed to contribute to T cell hyperactivity within the inflamed joint (20). In human investigations, blockade of PD-1 with anti-PD-1 increases the risk of developing RA (21).

In recent years, many studies indicated that helminths may exploit the PD-1 pathway to modulate host immune system to minimize excessive inflammation and promote the chronicity of helminth infection (22–24). *Trichinella spiralis* is an intestine- and tissue-dwelled nematode that secretes molecules to modulate hosts' immune system. Infection of this nematode or *Trichinella*-secreted proteins have been used for treatment of many hyperimmune-associated disorders in experimental studies such as asthma and allergic disorders (25), inflammatory bowel diseases (26, 27), encephalomyelitis (28), and type 1 diabetes (29), and significant alleviation of these diseases has been achieved.

It is well established that $CD4^{+}$ T cells play a central role in the pathogenesis of RA (30). In this study, we aim to investigate whether *T. spiralis* infection affects the PD-1 expression in $CD4^{+}$ T cells and its role in alleviation of arthritis using a CIA mouse model. We demonstrated for the first time that *T. spiralis* infection significantly alleviated CIA through activating the expression of PD-1 on $CD4^{+}$ T cells. Moreover, this study highlights the importance of PD-1 as a checkpoint for *T. spiralis*-induced Th2 polarization and Treg generation which may provide new insights into the mechanisms of helminths' immunomodulation on host autoimmunity.

MATERIALS AND METHODS

Ethics Statement

This study was carried out in accordance with the recommendations of "IRB of Capital Medical University." All animal experimental procedures were approved by the Animal Care and Use Committee of Capital Medical University (AEEI-2016-008) and comply with the National Institutes of Health Guidelines for the Care and Use of Experimental Animals.

Mice

Male DBA/1 mice with 6–8 weeks old were purchased from the Laboratory Animal Services Center of Capital Medical University (Beijing, China) for induction of arthritis and related experiments. Wild-type (WT) and $PD\text{-}1^{-/-}$ mice bred on the C57BL/6 background were purchased from the Jackson Laboratory (Stock no. 021157, USA). All mice were maintained under pathogen-free conditions with suitable humidity and temperature at the Animal Center of Capital Medical University.

Helminth Infection Model

The *T. spiralis* (ISS 533) strain used in this study was maintained in female ICR mice. Mice were each infected with 400 infective *T. spiralis* muscle larvae by oral gavage.

Induction of CIA

Experimental arthritis was induced in DBA/1 mice based on the method previously described (31). Bovine type II collagen (CII) purchased from Chondrex (Redmond, WA, USA) was dissolved in 0.01 M acetic acid at concentration of 2 mg/ml by stirring over night at 4°C and emulsified with the equal volume of complete Freund's adjuvant. Male DBA/1 mice were immunized intradermally at the base of the tail with 0.1 ml emulsion containing 100 μg CII. The mice were boosted once with the same amount of CII emulsified with incomplete Freund's adjuvant (Chondrex) 21 days after the first immunization. Induced arthritic mice were clinically assessed for redness and swelling of all limbs every other day up to 50 days. The clinical scores were assigned as previously described to evaluate disease (32) as follows: 0 = no signs of arthritis: 1 = swelling and/or redness of the paw or one digit; 2 = two joints involved; 3 = more than two joints involved and 4 = severe arthritis of the entire paw and digits. Each limb was graded, resulting in a maximal clinical score of 16 per animal.

Histopathologic Analysis

The paws of the mice were removed after being euthanized and fixed overnight in 4% paraformaldehyde, decalcified in 20% EDTA for 6 weeks, and then dehydrated and embedded in paraffin. The tissue serial paraffin sections (2 mm) were cut along longitudinal axis, mounted and sections were stained with hematoxylin and eosin or toluidine blue (TB). The severity of inflammatory cell infiltration in joint and cartilage destruction was scored using a semi-quantitative scale described previously (33, 34). The severity of inflammatory cell infiltration was scored 0–4 as follows: 0 = no infiltrate; 1 = minimal (few cells in perisynovial and synovial tissues); 2 = mild (infiltrating cells more numerous in perisynovial and synovial tissues, and/or in bone marrow beneath joints); 3 = moderate (inflammatory cell infiltrate more intense in perisynovial and synovial tissues, and often extending into adjacent periosseous tissues and/or in bone marrow beneath joints); and 4 = marked (increasing intensity of inflammatory cell infiltrate in synovial and perisynovial tissues, and extending into adjacent periosseous tissues and/or widely dispersed in bone marrow). Cartilage damage was scored 0–5 according to the following criteria: 0 = normal; 1 = minimal (loss of TB staining only); 2 = mild (loss of TB staining and mild cartilage thinning); 3 = moderate (moderate diffuse or multifocal cartilage loss); 4 = marked (marked diffuse or multifocal cartilage loss); and 5 = severe (severe diffuse or multifocal cartilage loss).

In Vivo Blockade of PD-1

In some experiments, the expression of PD-1 on immune cells in mice was blocked by injection of anti-mouse CD279 (PD-1) antibody (clone 29F.1A12, BioLegend, San Diego, CA, USA). Each mouse received 200 μg mAb intraperitoneally (i.p.) every 3 days, starting at 14 days post-infection until 3 days before the mice were sacrificed. For control mice, each was given the same amount of rat IgG2a isotype (clone RTK2758, BioLegend).

Isolation of Lymphocytes From Spleen and Lymph Nodes

Four weeks after second immunization, the draining inguinal lymph nodes (ILNs) and spleens were removed and minced through a 70-μm cell strainer. Lymphocytes were isolated using Ficoll density-gradient centrifugation for flow cytometry or released-cytokine measurement.

Spleen Cell Culture and Cytokine ELISA

Splenocytes were cultured in RPMI 1640 medium supplemented with 10% fetal bovine serum (FBS, Gibco, Grand Island, NY, USA), 100 U/ml penicillin, and 100 μg/ml streptomycin, at 2×10^6 cells/ml in 24-well culture plates. During culture, the cells were stimulated with anti-CD3 (1 μg/ml)/anti-CD28 (1 μg/ml) (Peprotech, NJ, USA). The supernatants were collected at 48 h and kept frozen at −80°C until used. Cytokines IFN-γ, IL-4, IL-5, IL-13, IL-10, IL-17A, and TNF-α in the culture supernatants were measured with Ready-Set Go! Kits or recombinant cytokine/antibody sets from eBioscience (San Diego, CA, USA) according to the manufacturer's instructions.

Anti-CII Antibody Measurement

Sera were collected from mice 4 weeks after the second immunization of CII and the anti-CII-specific IgG and subtype IgG1 and IgG2a were measured by using antibody assay kit according to the manufacturer's instructions (Chondrex, Redmond, WA, USA). Each sample was assayed in duplicate. OD values were measured at 490 nm using a Model 550 microplate reader and the results were analyzed using Microplate Manager III for Macintosh (Bio-Rad laboratories, Hercules, CA, USA).

$CD4^+$ T Cells Purification, CFSE Labeling, and Stimulation

$CD4^+$ T cells were isolated from spleen or ILNs by positive selection using a magnetic-activated cell sorting system with anti-CD4 mAb (Miltenyi Biotec, Bergisch Gladbach, Germany) according to the manufacturer's instructions. Isolated cells (5×10^6 cells) were suspended in 1 ml sterile PBS containing 3% FBS. Carboxyfluorescein succinimidyl amino ester (CFSE, Invitrogen, Carlsbad, CA, USA) was added into the culture up to 5 μM for 5 min to label the cells. Labeling reaction was stopped by diluting with 9 ml of PBS containing 3% FCS and cells were washed twice. The labeled $CD4^+$ T cells were used for the experiment of proliferation assessment and flow cytometry analysis. In experiment for determining non-specific T cell proliferation, the splenic $CD4^+$ T cells isolated from *T. spiralis*-infected mice were cultured in plates coated with anti-CD3 (5 μg/ml, BioLegend, San Diego, CA, USA) in the presence of anti-CD28 (5 μg/ml, BioLegend) for 72 h. In experiment for determining specific anti-CII T cell proliferation, mice were immunized with CII on day ≥35 after *T. spiralis* infection. Then $CD4^+$ T cells isolated from ILNs of mice on day 10 after CII immunization were cultured in the presence of CII for 72 h (20 μg/ml).

Flow Cytometry

To analyze PD-1 expression in $CD4^+$ T cells, the cells were stained with anti-mouse CD3-antigen-presenting cell (APC) (clone 17A2, eBioscience, Waltham, MA, USA), CD4-FITC (clone GK1.5, eBioscience), PD-1-PE (clone J43, eBioscience). To detect intracellular cytokine expression, T cells from each mouse were stimulated with 2 μl/ml. Cell Activation Cocktail (with Brefeldin) (BioLegend, San Diego, CA, USA) in complete RPMI 1640 medium for 6 h at 37°C in 5% CO_2, then collected and surface stained with CD3 and CD4. The cells were washed, fixed, and permeabilized with cytofix/cytoperm buffer (BD Pharmingen), then intracellularly stained with anti-IFN-γ PE-Cyanine7 (clone XMG1.2), IL-4 PE-Cyanine7 (clone 11B11), and IL-17A PE-Cyanine7 (clone eBio17B7), or rat IgG1 and IgG2a isotype antibody (clone eBRG1, all from eBioscience) as control, respectively. To determine Tregs, the $CD4^+$ cells were surface stained with anti-mouse CD3-PerCP (clone 17A2), CD4-FITC (clone RM4-5), and CD25-APC (clone PC61.5) in a Mouse Regulatory T cell Staining Kit (eBioscience). The cells were then permeabilized with cold Fix/Perm Buffer, and stained with anti-mouse Foxp3-PE (clone FJK-16s) or rat IgG2a isotype control antibody (clone eBR2a). Following immunofluorescence staining, samples were analyzed on a Flow cytometer (BD) using flowjo software (TreeStar). The cells were gated on $CD3^+$ $CD4^+$ T cells.

Statistical Analysis

Statistical analysis was performed using SPSS version 11.0. All data are expressed as mean ± SEM. To determine differences between multiple groups, analysis of variance was used with *post hoc* comparisons using Tukey's method. For comparison

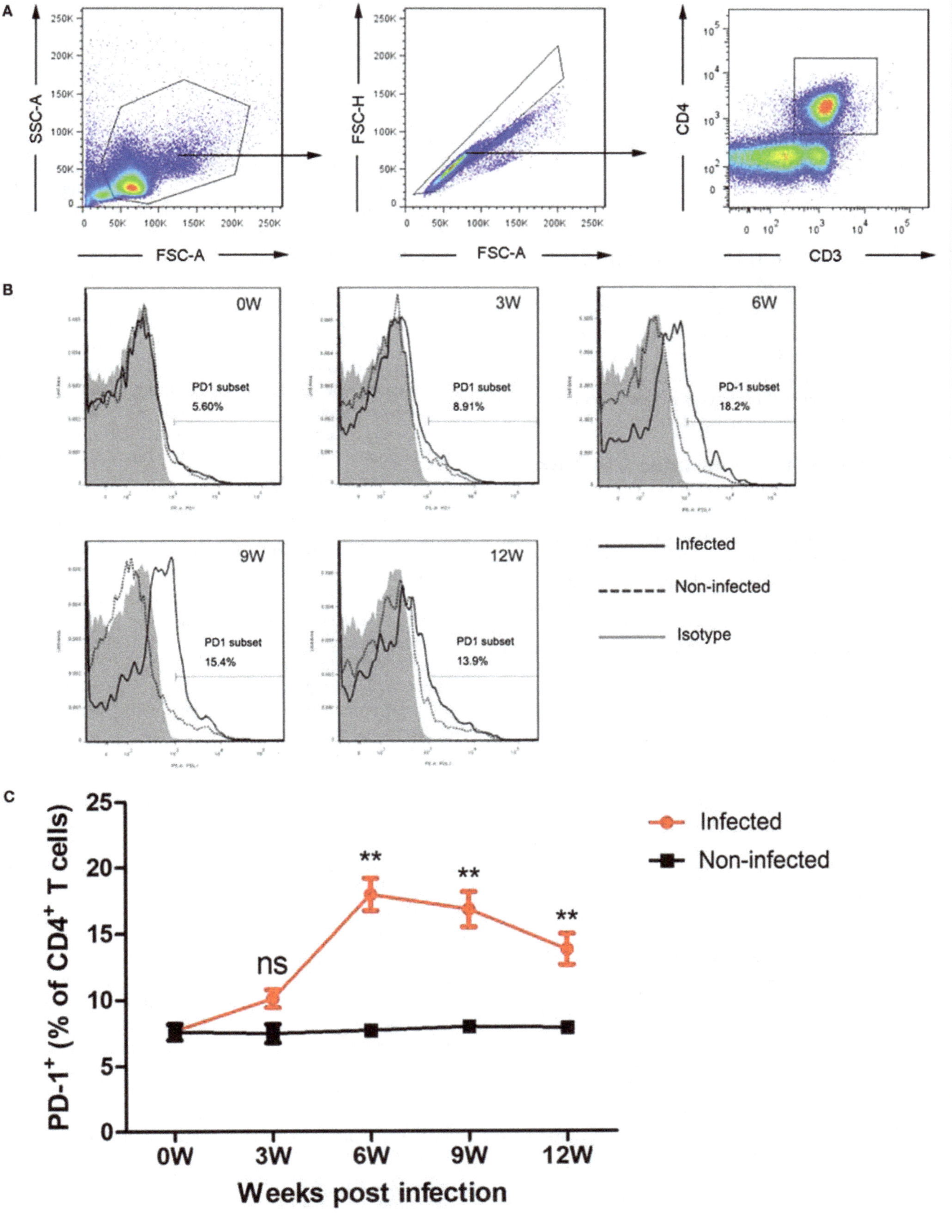

FIGURE 1 | Continued

FIGURE 1 | Dynamics of programmed death 1 (PD-1) expression in CD4$^+$ T cells from *Trichinella spiralis*-infected mice. **(A)** FACS gating strategy for CD4$^+$ T cells expressing PD-1. PD-1 gating was shown based on the PD-1 isotype control. **(B)** Flow cytometry showing the PD-1 subset in CD4$^+$ T cells from spleen of infected mice compared with those from non-infected mice. Non-specific isotype antibody was used as control. The representative PD-1 expression is represented in solid line in *T. spiralis*-infected mice and in dotted line in non-infected mice. Isotype control is illustrated in gray. **(C)** The dynamic expression of PD-1 in CD4$^+$ T cells of mice during *T. spiralis* infection. Data are expressed as mean ± SEM from three independent experiments ($n = 5$ mice per group).

between two groups, a Student's t-test was performed. A P-value <0.05 was considered significant.

RESULTS

T. spiralis Infection Upregulates PD-1 Expression in CD4$^+$ T Cells

Programmed death 1 expression in spleen CD4$^+$ T cells was upregulated in mice infected with *T. spiralis*. Increased expression of PD-1 in spleen CD4$^+$ T cells was observed in the initial acute stage of infection, peaked at week 6, and followed by a slight decline thereafter (**Figure 1**) with significant difference to the baseline expression level in the CD4$^+$ T cells of normal mice.

T. spiralis Infection Alleviates CIA Through PD-1 Pathway

To determine whether the infection of *T. spiralis* alleviates the severity of CIA in mice, mice were infected with *T. spiralis* 14 days prior to the first immunization of CII. The representative paw of mice with CIA was shown in **Figures 2A,B**. As shown in **Figures 2C,D**, *T. spiralis*-infected CIA mice displayed significant reduction in the incidence of induced CIA and alleviated arthritic score compared with uninfected CIA mice. PD-1 blockade with specific antibody significantly increased the incidence and severity of arthritis in *T. spiralis*-infected CIA mice (**Figures 2C,D**). Histologic analysis of the paws showed significantly decreased inflammation scores and cartilage destruction in *T. spiralis*-infected CIA mice compared with non-infected CIA mice. Similarly, the amelioration of inflammatory cell infiltration and cartilage destruction in *T. spiralis*-infected CIA mice was effectively reversed by the blockage of PD-1 with anti-PD-1 (**Figures 2E,F**). Isotype IgG2a control had no any effect on CIA (data not shown). These data suggested that PD-1 plays an important role in the inhibitory effect of *T. spiralis* infection on CIA in mouse.

Nematode-Induced Inhibition of Th1/Th17 Responses and Enhancement of Th2 Responses Were Abated by Blocking PD-1 in CIA Mice

To understand the mechanisms involved in the *T. spiralis* infection-attenuated CIA, the humoral and cellular immune responses were measured in the treated mice. It is well established that anti-CII antibody is involved in the pathogenesis of CIA (35). Serological levels of antigen-specific total IgG, and subtypes IgG2a and IgG1 were measured. As shown in **Figure 3A**, the anti-CII total IgG level in the sera of mice infected with *T. spiralis* was significantly lower than that in mice without infection. Subtype analysis demonstrated that the reduced IgG level mostly resulted from the reduction in the IgG2a (Th1) but not in IgG1 (Th2). The reduced levels of IgG and IgG2a in *T. spiralis*-infected mice were effectively restored when PD-1 was blocked using anti-PD-1 antibody. The cytokine profile of splenocytes stimulated by anti-CD3/anti-CD28 antibodies showed that *T. spiralis*-infected CIA mice produced significantly lower levels of pro-inflammatory cytokines including IFN-γ (Th1), IL-17 (Th17), and TNF-α, but higher level of Th2 cytokines IL-4, IL-5, IL-13, and regulatory cytokine IL-10 compared with CIA mice without infection (**Figure 3B**). However, the nematode-reduced pro-inflammatory cytokines and boosted Th2 cytokines in CIA mice were significantly abated when PD-1 was blocked using anti-PD-1 antibody. The above results indicate that alleviation of CIA by the infection of *T. spiralis* is associated with the reduced Th1/Th17, enhanced Th2 responses possibly through stimulating the expression of suppressive PD-1 in the immune cells.

PD-1 Knockout Offsets *T. spiralis*-Induced Anti-Inflammatory Modulation of CD4$^+$ T Cells

To further investigate whether *T. spiralis* infection-induced immunomodulation is PD-1 mediated, we profiled cytokines secreted by splenocytes upon stimulation of anti-CD3/anti-CD28 in WT and PD-1$^{-/-}$ C57BL/6 J mice infected with or without *T. spiralis*. As shown in **Figure 4A**, the inhibited IFN-γ and IL-17 production following *T. spiralis* infection in WT mice was recovered in PD-1$^{-/-}$ mice. By contrast, *T. spiralis*-enhanced IL-4, IL-5, IL-13, and IL-10 production in WT mice was abated in PD-1$^{-/-}$ mice. This result further suggests that *T. spiralis* may activate PD-1 pathway to inhibit Th1- and Th17-associated pro-inflammatory cytokine production and to boost Th2-associated anti-inflammatory cytokine and regulatory cytokine production. Flow cytometry also showed that *T. spiralis* infection decreased IFN-γ$^+$ (Th1), and increased IL-4$^+$ (Th2) CD4$^+$ T cells and CD25$^+$Foxp3$^+$ Tregs, but little effected on IL-17A$^+$ (Th17) CD4$^+$ T cells. However, these *T. spiralis*-induced attenuated Th1 and enhanced Th2/Treg differentiation in WT mice were effectively diminished in PD-1$^{-/-}$ mice (**Figures 4B–E**). These results with PD-1$^{-/-}$ mice further confirm that *T. spiralis*-induced differential control of CD4$^+$ T cell subsets is PD-1 mediated, suggesting that PD-1 play a critical role in *T. spiralis*-induced immunomodulation.

To determine the responsiveness of T cell in *T. spiralis*-infected mice, we examined the CD4$^+$ T cell proliferation upon non-specific (anti-CD3/anti-CD28) and antigen-specific stimulation in WT and PD-1$^{-/-}$ mice with or without infection. The proliferation of splenic CD4$^+$ T cells upon non-specific stimulation (anti-CD3/anti-CD28) was significantly inhibited in cells from *T. spiralis*-infected mice compared to those from non-infected mice. The inhibited CD4$^+$ T cell proliferation was partially restored in mice with PD-1 knockout (**Figure 5A**). We further analyzed the

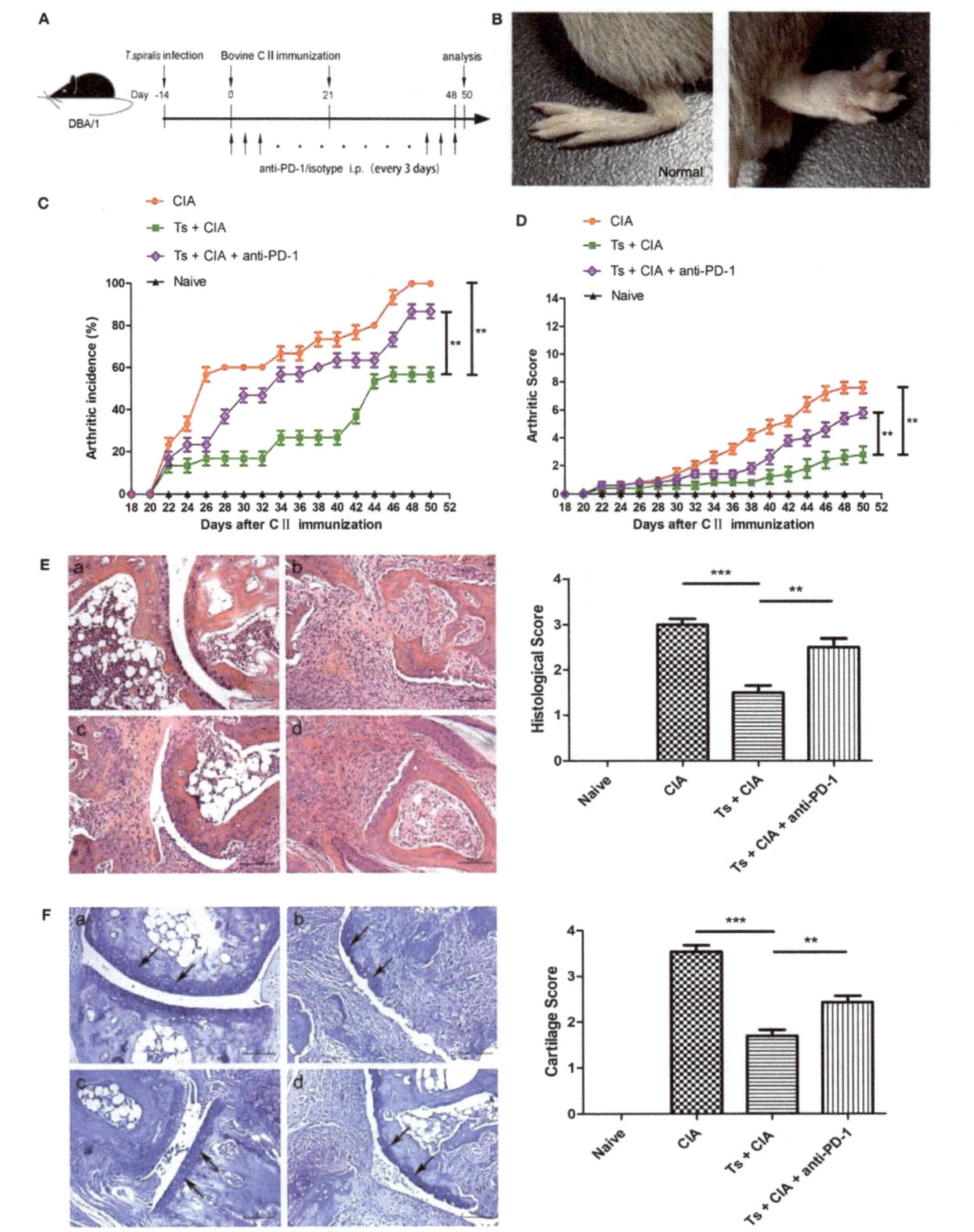

FIGURE 2 | Continued

FIGURE 2 | Programmed death 1 (PD-1) blockade abated *Trichinella spiralis* infection-induced attenuation of collagen-induced arthritis (CIA) in DBA/1 mice. **(A)** The regimen of study including the induction of CIA, treatment with infection of *T. spiralis* and anti-PD-1 antibody. **(B)** Hind paw of a mouse before and after induction of arthritis with bovine type II collagen (CII). Arthritic incidence **(C)** and total arthritic score **(D)** of mice from different groups ($n = 10$) at different time points. **(E)** Hematoxylin and eosin of the representative inflamed joints in the hind paw of mice from different groups at day 50 post first CII immunization, the histological score was shown on the right (mean ± SEM, $n = 6$). **(E)** The toluidine blue staining and cartilage score **(F)** of the representative inflamed joints in the hind paw of mice from different groups at day 50 post first CII immunization. (a) Naïve untreated control, (b) CIA, (c) Ts + CIA, (d) Ts + CIA + anti-PD-1. The bar graphs on the right side **(E,F)** show the histopathological scores for each group given as mean ± SEM ($n = 6$ mice per group). Statistical significance is determined by Student's *t*-test for single comparison. $^{**}P < 0.01$ and $^{***}P < 0.001$ (one-way analysis of variance).

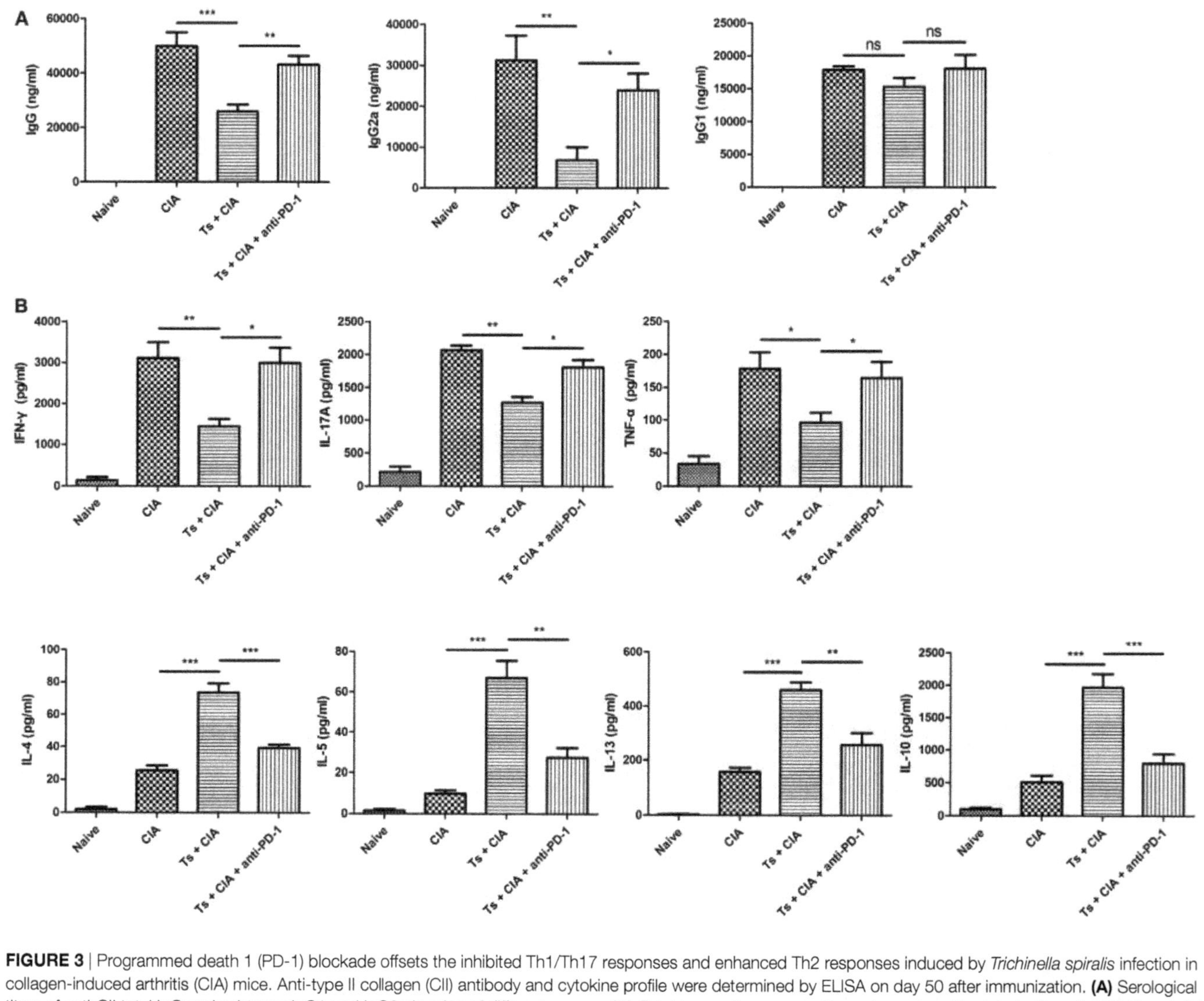

FIGURE 3 | Programmed death 1 (PD-1) blockade offsets the inhibited Th1/Th17 responses and enhanced Th2 responses induced by *Trichinella spiralis* infection in collagen-induced arthritis (CIA) mice. Anti-type II collagen (CII) antibody and cytokine profile were determined by ELISA on day 50 after immunization. **(A)** Serological titers of anti-CII total IgG and subtypes IgG1 and IgG2a in mice of different groups. **(B)** Cytokine profiles secreted by splenocytes stimulated with anti-CD3 (1 µg/ml)/anti-CD28 (1 µg/ml) for 48 h. Data are expressed as mean ± SEM for duplicate serum samples or cell cultures. Data are representative of results from two independent experiments ($n = 6$ mice per group). $^{*}P < 0.05$; $^{**}P < 0.01$; $^{***}P < 0.001$; ns, not significant (one-way analysis of variance).

antigen-specific T cell proliferation in $CD4^+$ T cells isolated from ILNs of CII-immunized mice upon CII stimulation. Similarly, the inhibition of $CD4^+$ T-cell proliferation upon re-stimulation of specific antigen CII in *T. spiralis*-infected mice was partially lifted in T cells from PD-$1^{-/-}$ mice (**Figure 5B**). These results suggest that PD-1 partially contributes to *T. spiralis*-induced hyposensitivity of $CD4^+$ T cells.

DISCUSSION

Immune responses are regulated by the balance of positive and negative regulatory pathways. Negative regulatory pathways are crucial for peripheral self-tolerance and preventing autoimmunity, and can function through signals delivered by cell surface inhibitory receptors, immunoregulatory cytokines, and Tregs (30).

Multiple co-inhibitory receptors such as lymphocyte activation gene 3 (LAG-3), B- and T-lymphocyte attenuator 4 (BTLA-4), cytotoxic T-lymphocyte antigen 4 (CTLA-4), and T cell membrane protein 3 (Tim-3), CD244, and CD160 are expressed in T cells to dampen immune activation and limit immune-mediated pathology (36, 37). Recent studies demonstrated that these inhibitory receptors also play an important role in the response to pathogens. It is reported that helminth infection drives the sustained expression of T cell inhibitory receptors, which may negatively regulate proliferation and the production of pro-inflammatory cytokines by helminth antigen-specific T cells (38–40). Because these molecules largely function to prevent over exuberant T cell activation, their essential role in preventing parasite-induced immunopathology have been confirmed in animal studies (38, 41). However, the impact of these parasite-induced inhibitory molecules on autoimmune pathology has not been clarified.

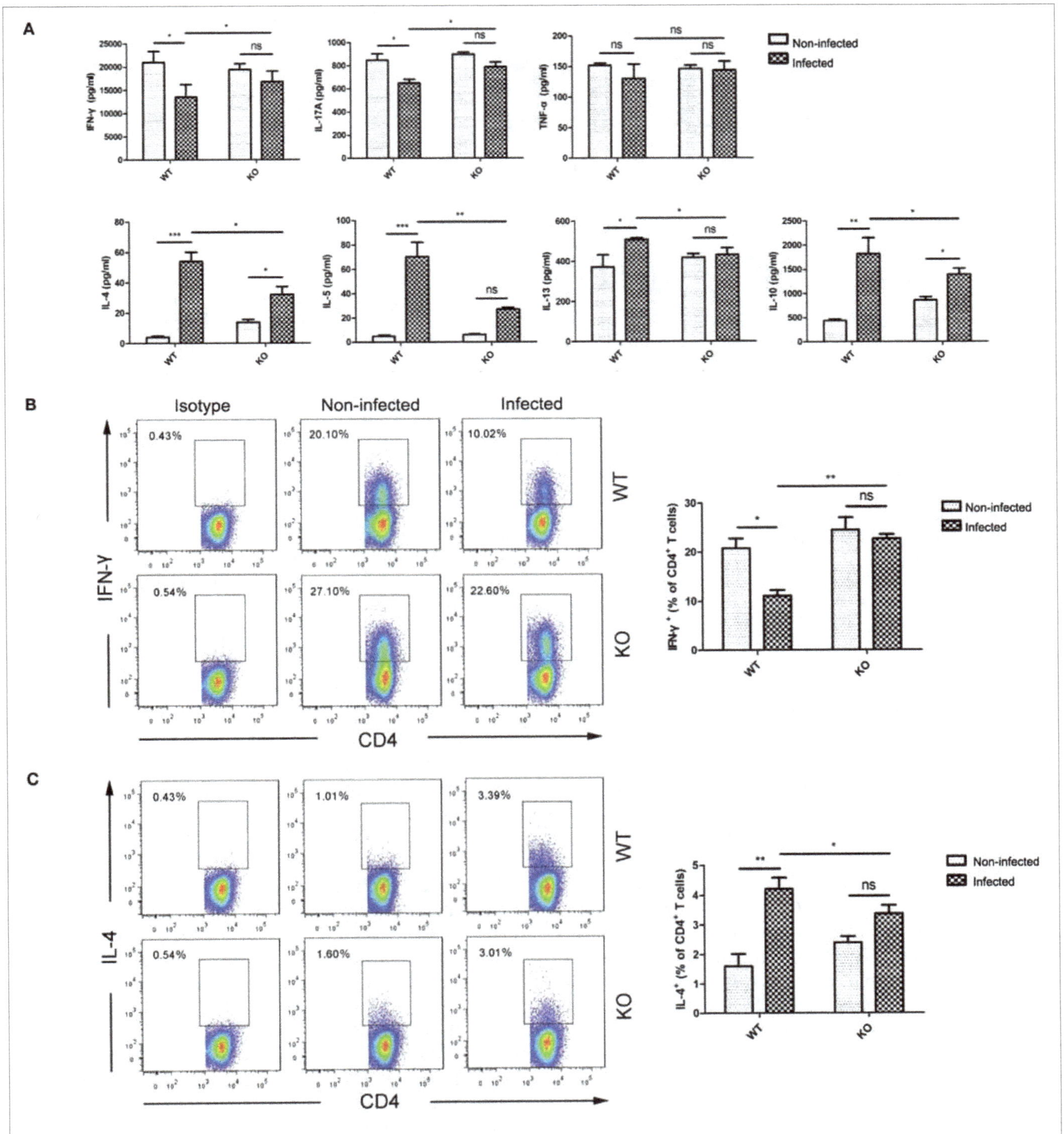

FIGURE 4 | Continued

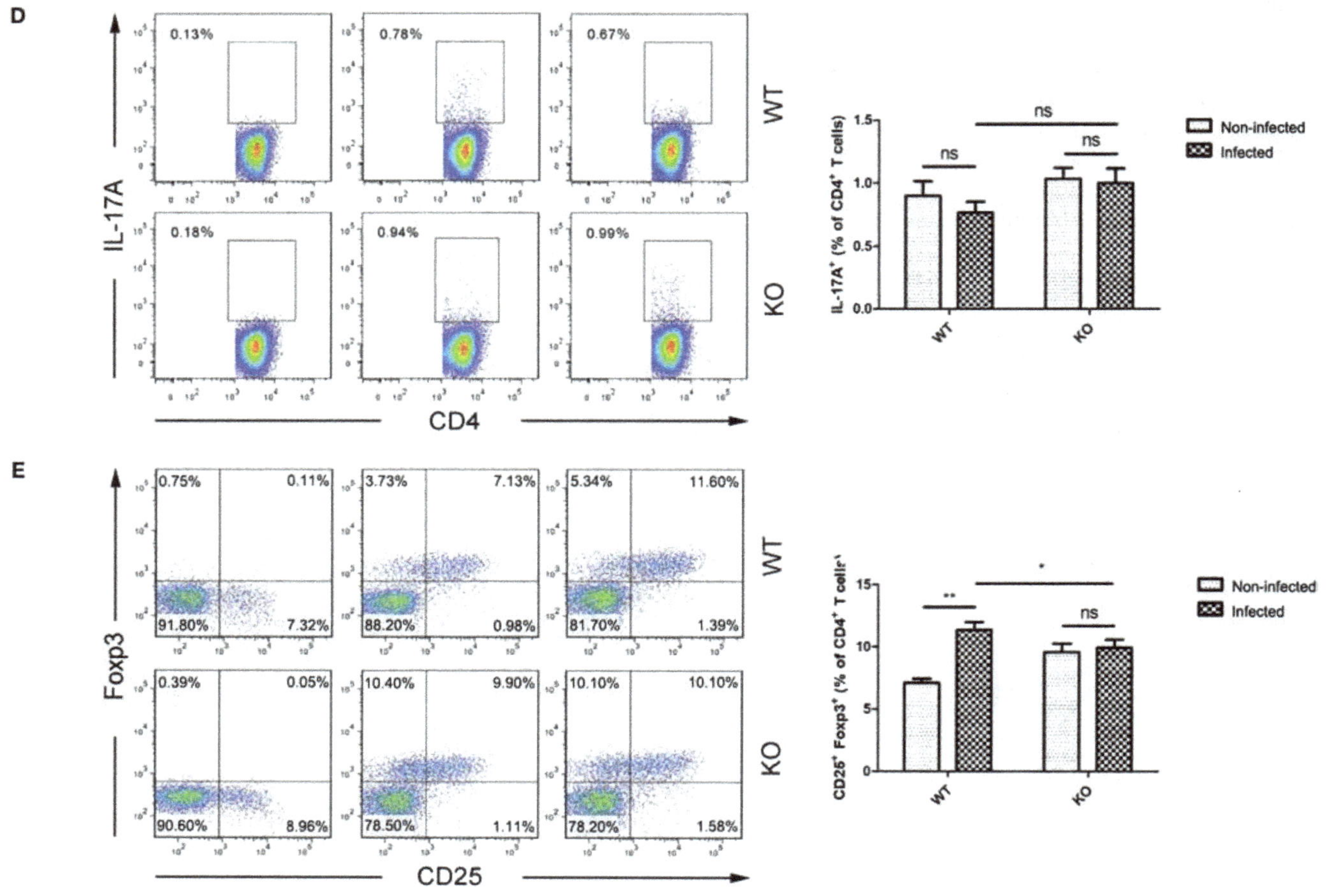

FIGURE 4 | Programmed death 1 (PD-1) knockout abated *Trichinella spiralis*-induced Th1/17 inhibition and Th2/regulatory T cell (Treg) enhancement. Single-cell suspensions of spleens from wild-type (WT) and PD-$1^{-/-}$ mice (KO) infected with or without *T. spiralis* were prepared. **(A)** Cytokine profiles secreted by splenocytes (IFN-γ, IL-17A, TNF-α, IL-10, IL-4, IL-5, and IL-13) upon stimulation with anti-CD3/CD28 for 48 h measured by ELISA. **(B–E)** Representative staining and percentages for IFN-γ-, IL-4-, IL-17-producing $CD4^+$ T cells and $CD4^+$ $CD25^+$ $Foxp3^+$ Treg cells by FACS. Data are expressed as mean ± SEM from three independent experiments ($n = 5$ mice per group). $^*P < 0.05$; $^{**}P < 0.01$; ns, not significant (paired Student's *t*-test).

Programmed death 1 plays a critical role in maintaining host immune homeostasis during chronic infection (42, 43). In this study, we observed upregulation of PD-1 in lymphocytes of mice infected with *T. spiralis*. The upregulation of PD-1 was also observed in the chronic infections of *Schistosoma japonicum* (24), *Fasciola hepatica* (44), *Taenia solium* (45), *Echinococcus multilocularis* (45) related to the survival of helminth in the host and reducing infection caused immunopathology.

To determine if the *T. spiralis* infection reduces the pathology of inflammatory arthritis, we established a collagen-induced mouse model (CIA). The CII-reactive $CD4^+$ T cells are the primary mediators of disease induction by driving autoantibody production in B cells and enhancing the chronic inflammatory response (46, 47). Our results demonstrated that *T. spiralis* infection significantly mitigated the pathology of CIA in mice mostly through reducing Th1/Th17 pro-inflammatory responses and boosting Th2 response. The results are in accordance with previous studies that showed increased Th1/Th17 cellular response played a key role in the CIA (48, 49). *T. spiralis* infection reduces these pro-inflammatory responses therefore alleviates pathology of CIA. It is well known that helminth chronic infection-induced Th2 polarization is also involved in the therapeutic effects on autoimmune diseases. *Nippostrongylus brasiliensi*-induced activation of Th2 axis effectively mitigates the course of inflammatory arthritis and this protective effect is dependent on IL-4/IL-13-induced STAT6 pathway (50). *F. hepatica* excretory–secretory products were reported to protect against experimental autoimmune encephalomyelitis *via* type 2 cytokines (51).

Given that the PD-1 expression is upregulated in the $CD4^+$ T cells of *T. spiralis*-infected mice and PD-1 is an important inhibitory and checkpoint receptor on immune cells, we postulated that *T. spiralis*-induced PD-1 expression may be involved in the alleviation of CIA by suppressing Th1 and Th17 responses and boosting Th2 response. Indeed, we observed that the reduced pathology of CIA in *T. spiralis*-infected mice was correlated with the increased expression of PD-1 in $CD4^+$ T cells. Blocking PD-1 with anti-PD-1 mAb seriously reversed the amelioration of CIA in *T. spiralis*-infected mice, correlating with recovered level of Th1/Th17 response and reduced Th2 response. PD-1 knockout also demonstrated its reversion to *T. spiralis* infection-involved Th1 and Th2 changes, however, it did not change much the frequency of Th17 within $CD4^+$ T cells at day 42 post-infection

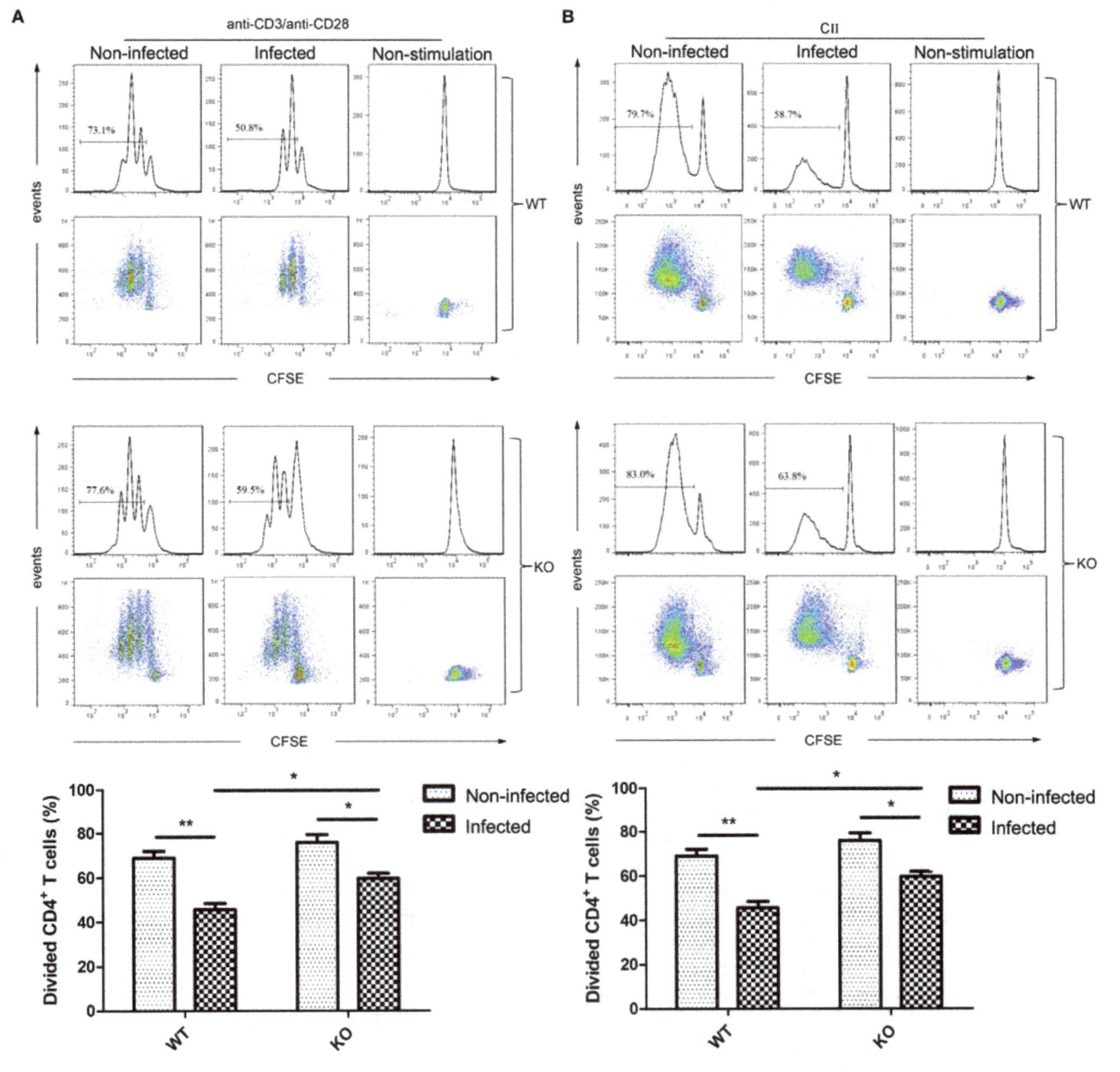

FIGURE 5 | Programmed death 1 (PD-1) knockout partially restored suppressed proliferation of CD4+ T cells in *Trichinella spiralis*-infected mice. CD4+ T cells were isolated from C57BL/6 wild-type (WT) and PD-1$^{-/-}$ mice and stained with CFSE. Decay of CFSE staining of CD4+ T cells was determined by flow cytometry. **(A)** FACS analysis of CD4+ T cell proliferation in response to non-specific stimulation. Purified CD4+ T cells from spleen of uninfected or *T. spiralis*-infected mice at day ≥35 of infection were stained with CFSE and incubated in the presence of anti-CD3/anti-CD28 for 72 h. **(B)** FACS analysis of CD4+ T cells proliferation in response to type II collagen (CII)-specific stimulation. Mice with or without *T. spiralis* infection (at day ≥35 of infection) were immunized with CII. CD4+ T cells were purified from LNCs of mice at day 10 post CII immunization and stained with CFSE, then incubated in the presence of CII (10 µg/ml) for 72 h. Irradiated naïve splenocytes were used as antigen-presenting cells (APCs). Data were expressed as mean ± SEM from two independent experiments ($n \geq 3$ mice per group). $^{**}P < 0.05$; $^{*}P < 0.01$ (paired Student's *t*-test).

(**Figure 4D**), possibly because the stage of chronic *T. spiralis* infection may not affect much on IL-17 expression (52). Th17 cells are known to be involved in the inflammatory immune responses and autoimmune diseases as shown in CIA induction in this study (**Figure 3B**). However, it is not well understood the role of Th17 cells in the helminth infections (53), even though it has been observed that *T. spiralis* infection really reduced the CIA-induced Th17 secretion (**Figure 3B**).

Our results provide strong evidences at the first time that PD-1 pathway is involved in immunomodulation induced by *T. spiralis* infection that attenuates autoimmune-related arthritis. We postulate that pre-infection with *T. spiralis* may induce an anti-inflammatory modulation ahead of the initiation of CIA *via* activating the PD-1 pathway.

The costimulatory pathway consists of the PD-1 and its ligands, PD-L1 and PD-L2, delivering inhibitory signals that regulate the balance among T-cell activation and immune-mediated tissue damage to prevent autoimmunity (13, 54, 55). Manipulation of PD-1:PD-L1/2 pathway is considered a potential therapeutic approach for treating autoimmune diseases (15). Impact of PD-L:PD-1 axis on differentiation of $CD4^+$ T cell subsets has been reported in previous studies (32, 56, 57). In this study, we also observed that the increased expression of PD-1 in $CD4^+$ T cells in *T. spiralis*-infected mice and knockout of PD-1 resulted in the recovery of inhibited $CD4^+$ T cell proliferation caused by nematode infection, indicating PD-1 is involved in the nematode infection caused regulation of $CD4^+$ T cells. At the meantime, we identified that the Th2 polarization and Treg generation induced by *T. spiralis* infection were effectively diminished in PD-$1^{-/-}$ mice. The results imply a critical role of PD-1 in modulating the balance of Th1/Th2 and Treg responses upon infection of *T. spiralis* that may outline the molecular mechanism behind the helminth-induced immunomodulation. Activation of PD-L1:PD-1 pathway may result in the enhanced Foxp3 expression and suppressive function of established induced regulatory T (iTreg) cells (12). $CD4^+CD25^+FoxP3^+$ Tregs are highly involved in the regulation of immune responses and preventing autoimmunity (58–60). *Schistosoma mansoni* and *T. spiralis* derived antigens have been demonstrated to exert protective effect against adjuvant arthritis by upregulation of the $Foxp3^+$ Tregs (10). Here, we confirmed that *T. spiralis*-induced expression of Foxp3 is highly dependent on PD-1 expression on immune cells, which implies that PD-1-mediated generation of $Foxp3^+$ Tregs may contribute to the *T. spiralis*-attenuated CIA. However, different helminth infection may modulate host immune regulation through different PD-L/PD-1 pathway. The conditional deletion of PD-L1 impaired Th2 polarization and cytokine production in mice following *N. brasiliensis* infection (56). By contrast, blockade of PD-1 results in recovery of hyporesponsive Th2 cell function which was mediated through PD-L2 during chronic infection with *Litomosoides sigmodontis* (22). While the reasons for the discrepancies regarding the role of PD-1 in regulating Th2 cytokine production remain unclear, it seems to be related to the types of PD-L which interact with PD-1 expressed in the $CD4^+$ T cells to control the function of Th subsets. It has been demonstrated that PD-L1 and PD-L2 have distinct roles in regulating host Th cell differentiation in response to leishmaniasis (61). Moreover, PD-1 has been suggested to enhance Th2 responses under conditions of sub-optimal TCR stimulation, which might be associated with the type of antigen (62).

In addition to activating Th2 cell-biased responses, helminths have also developed multiple mechanisms to regulate the host immune system. Humans with chronic infectious diseases, including helminth infection, experience sustained immune activation that is often accompanied by T cell hyporesponsiveness. Recent studies revealed that helminth infection induced T cell hyporesposiveness might contribute to suppression of autoimmune diseases. For example, infection with *Schistosome* regulates lymphocyte function *in vivo* by suppressing T cell activation (63, 64). Since PD-1 is described as a co-inhibitory receptor which induces T cell exhaustion, we examined the role of PD-1 in regulating T cell proliferation in *T. spiralis*-infected mice. Our study demonstrated a decreased T cell proliferation in *T. spiralis*-infected mice in response to both non-specific and CII-specific stimulation. However, PD-1 deletion only partially restored *T. spiralis*-suppressed $CD4^+$ T cells proliferation. Although blockage of PD-1 can reverse the hyporesponsiveness to *S. japonicum* (24) and *L. sigmodontis* (22), many possible mechanisms may underlie the incomplete recovery of the suppressed T-cell proliferation induced by *T. spiralis* infection after PD-1 deletion observed in this study. Helminth infection modulates host T cell function through multiple factors including induction of Tregs, IL-10/TGF-β regulatory cytokines (23, 64), PD-1/PD-L, and other co-inhibitory molecules such as LAG-3, BTLA-4, CTLA-4, Tim-3, etc. (9, 65). We postulate that synergetic effects from different inhibitory pathways may contribute to *T. spiralis*-induced $CD4^+$ T cells hyporesponsiveness besides PD-1/PD-L. Therefore, blocking PD-1/PD-L inhibitory pathway may not take away the whole inhibitory effects induced by *T. spiralis* infection.

In summary, this study demonstrates that *T. spiralis* infection significantly reduced the pathology of CIA in mice by inhibiting Th1/Th17 pro-inflammatory responses and inducing Th2/Treg polarization. PD-1 plays a critical role within the helminth-involved immunomodulation of $CD4^+$ T cell subsets which are central mediators of RA. However, the detailed molecular interaction between PD-1/PD-L pathway and the helminth-iTreg cell and cytokine IL-10 and TGF-β still remains unknown. Further studies are needed to explore the mechanism of PD-1-mediated regulation of immune response during helminth infection and autoimmune diseases.

AUTHOR CONTRIBUTIONS

YC and XPZ conceived and designed the experiments. YC, XZ, XW, QZ, XH, and JH performed the experiments. YC, XPZ, BZ, and XS analyzed the data. XPZ, YC, and BZ wrote the paper. All authors reviewed the manuscript.

ACKNOWLEDGMENTS

We thank Xiaoxue Xu (Core facility center, Capital Medical University) for her assistance with flow cytometry analysis. We thank Wenming Zhao and Huihui Yuan (Department of immunology, School of Basic Medical Sciences, Capital Medical University) for their technical assistance with induction of CIA in mouse model.

REFERENCES

1. Smallwood TB, Giacomin PR, Loukas A, Mulvenna JP, Clark RJ, Miles JJ. Helminth immunomodulation in autoimmune disease. *Front Immunol* (2017) 8:453. doi:10.3389/fimmu.2017.00453
2. Gieseck RR, Wilson MS, Wynn TA. Type 2 immunity in tissue repair and fibrosis. *Nat Rev Immunol* (2018) 18:62–76. doi:10.1038/nri.2017.90
3. Cope AP, Schulze-Koops H, Aringer M. The central role of T cells in rheumatoid arthritis. *Clin Exp Rheumatol* (2007) 25:S4–11.
4. Pritchard DI, Brown A. Is *Necator americanus* approaching a mutualistic symbiotic relationship with humans? *Trends Parasitol* (2001) 17:169–72. doi:10.1016/S1471-4922(01)01941-9
5. McSorley HJ, Maizels RM. Helminth infections and host immune regulation. *Clin Microbiol Rev* (2012) 25:585–608. doi:10.1128/CMR.05040-11
6. Ricci ND, Fiuza JA, Bueno LL, Cancado GG, Gazzinelli-Guimaraes PH, Martins VG, et al. Induction of CD4(+)CD25(+)FOXP3(+) regulatory T cells during human hookworm infection modulates antigen-mediated lymphocyte proliferation. *PLoS Negl Trop Dis* (2011) 5:e1383. doi:10.1371/journal.pntd.0001383
7. Maizels RM, Yazdanbakhsh M. Immune regulation by helminth parasites: cellular and molecular mechanisms. *Nat Rev Immunol* (2003) 3:733–44. doi:10.1038/nri1183
8. MacDonald AS, Loke P, Martynoga R, Dransfield I, Allen JE. Cytokine-dependent inflammatory cell recruitment patterns in the peritoneal cavity of mice exposed to the parasitic nematode *Brugia malayi*. *Med Microbiol Immunol* (2003) 192:33–40. doi:10.1007/s00430-002-0156-8
9. Zander RA, Butler NS. Dysfunctional adaptive immunity during parasitic infections. *Curr Immunol Rev* (2013) 9:179–89. doi:10.2174/1573395509666131126230832
10. Eissa MM, Mostafa DK, Ghazy AA, El AM, Boulos LM, Younis LK. Anti-arthritic activity of *Schistosoma mansoni* and *Trichinella spiralis* derived-antigens in adjuvant arthritis in rats: role of FOXP3+ Treg cells. *PLoS One* (2016) 11:e165916. doi:10.1371/journal.pone.0165916
11. Bashi T, Bizzaro G, Ben-Ami SD, Blank M, Shoenfeld Y. The mechanisms behind helminth's immunomodulation in autoimmunity. *Autoimmun Rev* (2015) 14:98–104. doi:10.1016/j.autrev.2014.10.004
12. Francisco LM, Sage PT, Sharpe AH. The PD-1 pathway in tolerance and autoimmunity. *Immunol Rev* (2010) 236:219–42. doi:10.1111/j.1600-065X.2010.00923.x
13. Sharpe AH, Wherry EJ, Ahmed R, Freeman GJ. The function of programmed cell death 1 and its ligands in regulating autoimmunity and infection. *Nat Immunol* (2007) 8:239–45. doi:10.1038/ni1443
14. Keir ME, Butte MJ, Freeman GJ, Sharpe AH. PD-1 and its ligands in tolerance and immunity. *Annu Rev Immunol* (2008) 26:677–704. doi:10.1146/annurev.immunol.26.021607.090331
15. Zamani MR, Aslani S, Salmaninejad A, Javan MR, Rezaei N. PD-1/PD-L and autoimmunity: a growing relationship. *Cell Immunol* (2016) 310:27–41. doi:10.1016/j.cellimm.2016.09.009
16. Mahmoudi M, Rezaiemanesh A, Salmaninejad A, Harsini S, Poursani S, Bahrami T, et al. PDCD1 single nucleotide genes polymorphisms confer susceptibility to juvenile-onset systemic lupus erythematosus. *Autoimmunity* (2015) 48:488–93. doi:10.3109/08916934.2015.1058370
17. Zou Y, Zhang Z, Liu Y, Liu D, Xu W. Are programmed cell death 1 gene polymorphisms correlated with susceptibility to rheumatoid arthritis? A meta-analysis. *Medicine (Baltimore)* (2017) 96:e7805. doi:10.1097/MD.0000000000007805
18. Pawlak-Adamska E, Nowak O, Karabon L, Pokryszko-Dragan A, Partyka A, Tomkiewicz A, et al. PD-1 gene polymorphic variation is linked with first symptom of disease and severity of relapsing-remitting form of MS. *J Neuroimmunol* (2017) 305:115–27. doi:10.1016/j.jneuroim.2017.02.006
19. Momin S, Flores S, Angel BB, Codner DE, Carrasco PE, Perez-Bravo F. Interactions between programmed death 1 (PD-1) and cytotoxic T lymphocyte antigen 4 (CTLA-4) gene polymorphisms in type 1 diabetes. *Diabetes Res Clin Pract* (2009) 83:289–94. doi:10.1016/j.diabres.2008.12.003
20. Raptopoulou AP, Bertsias G, Makrygiannakis D, Verginis P, Kritikos I, Tzardi M, et al. The programmed death 1/programmed death ligand 1 inhibitory pathway is up-regulated in rheumatoid synovium and regulates peripheral T cell responses in human and murine arthritis. *Arthritis Rheum* (2010) 62:1870–80. doi:10.1002/art.27500
21. Belkhir R, Burel SL, Dunogeant L, Marabelle A, Hollebecque A, Besse B, et al. Rheumatoid arthritis and polymyalgia rheumatica occurring after immune checkpoint inhibitor treatment. *Ann Rheum Dis* (2017) 76:1747–50. doi:10.1136/annrheumdis-2017-211216
22. van der Werf N, Redpath SA, Azuma M, Yagita H, Taylor MD. Th2 cell-intrinsic hypo-responsiveness determines susceptibility to helminth infection. *PLoS Pathog* (2013) 9:e1003215. doi:10.1371/journal.ppat.1003215
23. Hartmann W, Schramm C, Breloer M. Litomosoides sigmodontis induces TGF-beta receptor responsive, IL-10-producing T cells that suppress bystander T-cell proliferation in mice. *Eur J Immunol* (2015) 45:2568–81. doi:10.1002/eji.201545503
24. Zhou S, Jin X, Li Y, Li W, Chen X, Xu L, et al. Blockade of PD-1 signaling enhances Th2 cell responses and aggravates liver immunopathology in mice with *Schistosomiasis japonica*. *PLoS Negl Trop Dis* (2016) 10:e5094. doi:10.1371/journal.pntd.0005094
25. Park HK, Cho MK, Choi SH, Kim YS, Yu HS. *Trichinella spiralis*: infection reduces airway allergic inflammation in mice. *Exp Parasitol* (2011) 127:539–44. doi:10.1016/j.exppara.2010.10.004
26. Khan WI, Blennerhasset PA, Varghese AK, Chowdhury SK, Omsted P, Deng Y, et al. Intestinal nematode infection ameliorates experimental colitis in mice. *Infect Immun* (2002) 70:5931–7. doi:10.1128/IAI.70.11.5931-5937.2002
27. Yang X, Yang Y, Wang Y, Zhan B, Gu Y, Cheng Y, et al. Excretory/secretory products from *Trichinella spiralis* adult worms ameliorate DSS-induced colitis in mice. *PLoS One* (2014) 9:e96454. doi:10.1371/journal.pone.0096454
28. Gruden-Movsesijan A, Ilic N, Mostarica-Stojkovic M, Stosic-Grujicic S, Milic M, Sofronic-Milosavljevic L. Mechanisms of modulation of experimental autoimmune encephalomyelitis by chronic *Trichinella spiralis* infection in Dark Agouti rats. *Parasite Immunol* (2010) 32:450–9. doi:10.1111/j.1365-3024.2010.01207.x
29. Saunders KA, Raine T, Cooke A, Lawrence CE. Inhibition of autoimmune type 1 diabetes by gastrointestinal helminth infection. *Infect Immun* (2007) 75:397–407. doi:10.1128/IAI.00664-06
30. Kondo Y, Yokosawa M, Kaneko S, Furuyama K, Segawa S, Tsuboi H, et al. Transcriptional regulation of CD4+ T cell differentiation in experimentally-induced arthritis and rheumatoid arthritis. *Arthritis Rheumatol* (2018) 70(5):653–61. doi:10.1002/art.40398
31. Yuan H, Qian H, Liu S, Zhang X, Li S, Wang W, et al. Therapeutic role of a vaccine targeting RANKL and TNF-alpha on collagen-induced arthritis. *Biomaterials* (2012) 33:8177–85. doi:10.1016/j.biomaterials.2012.07.047
32. Bratke K, Fritz L, Nokodian F, Geissler K, Garbe K, Lommatzsch M, et al. Differential regulation of PD-1 and its ligands in allergic asthma. *Clin Exp Allergy* (2017) 47:1417–25. doi:10.1111/cea.13017
33. Stolina M, Schett G, Dwyer D, Vonderfecht S, Middleton S, Duryea D, et al. RANKL inhibition by osteoprotegerin prevents bone loss without affecting local or systemic inflammation parameters in two rat arthritis models: comparison with anti-TNFalpha or anti-IL-1 therapies. *Arthritis Res Ther* (2009) 11:R187. doi:10.1186/ar2879
34. Romas E, Sims NA, Hards DK, Lindsay M, Quinn JW, Ryan PF, et al. Osteoprotegerin reduces osteoclast numbers and prevents bone erosion in collagen-induced arthritis. *Am J Pathol* (2002) 161:1419–27. doi:10.1016/S0002-9440(10)64417-3
35. Nandakumar KS, Svensson L, Holmdahl R. Collagen type II-specific monoclonal antibody-induced arthritis in mice: description of the disease and the influence of age, sex, and genes. *Am J Pathol* (2003) 163:1827–37. doi:10.1016/S0002-9440(10)63542-0
36. Brown KE, Freeman GJ, Wherry EJ, Sharpe AH. Role of PD-1 in regulating acute infections. *Curr Opin Immunol* (2010) 22:397–401. doi:10.1016/j.coi.2010.03.007
37. Blackburn SD, Shin H, Haining WN, Zou T, Workman CJ, Polley A, et al. Coregulation of CD8+ T cell exhaustion by multiple inhibitory receptors during chronic viral infection. *Nat Immunol* (2009) 10:29–37. doi:10.1038/ni.1679
38. Wammes LJ, Hamid F, Wiria AE, May L, Kaisar MM, Prasetyani-Gieseler MA, et al. Community deworming alleviates geohelminth-induced immune hyporesponsiveness. *Proc Natl Acad Sci U S A* (2016) 113:12526–31. doi:10.1073/pnas.1604570113
39. Gagliani N, Magnani CF, Huber S, Gianolini ME, Pala M, Licona-Limon P, et al. Coexpression of CD49b and LAG-3 identifies human and mouse T regulatory type 1 cells. *Nat Med* (2013) 19:739–46. doi:10.1038/nm.3179

40. Hou N, Piao X, Liu S, Wu C, Chen Q. Tim-3 induces Th2-biased immunity and alternative macrophage activation during *Schistosoma japonicum* infection. *Infect Immun* (2015) 83:3074–82. doi:10.1128/IAI.00517-15
41. Prodjinotho UF, von Horn C, Debrah AY, Batsa DL, Albers A, Layland LE, et al. Pathological manifestations in lymphatic filariasis correlate with lack of inhibitory properties of IgG4 antibodies on IgE-activated granulocytes. *PLoS Negl Trop Dis* (2017) 11:e5777. doi:10.1371/journal.pntd.0005777
42. Jiang TT, Martinov T, Xin L, Kinder JM, Spanier JA, Fife BT, et al. Programmed death-1 culls peripheral accumulation of high-affinity autoreactive CD4 T cells to protect against autoimmunity. *Cell Rep* (2016) 17:1783–94. doi:10.1016/j.celrep.2016.10.042
43. Rao DA, Gurish MF, Marshall JL, Slowikowski K, Fonseka CY, Liu Y, et al. Pathologically expanded peripheral T helper cell subset drives B cells in rheumatoid arthritis. *Nature* (2017) 542:110–4. doi:10.1038/nature20810
44. Stempin CC, Motran CC, Aoki MP, Falcon CR, Cerban FM, Cervi L. PD-L2 negatively regulates Th1-mediated immunopathology during *Fasciola hepatica* infection. *Oncotarget* (2016) 7:77721–31. doi:10.18632/oncotarget.12790
45. Arce-Sillas A, Alvarez-Luquin DD, Cardenas G, Casanova-Hernandez D, Fragoso G, Hernandez M, et al. Interleukin 10 and dendritic cells are the main suppression mediators of regulatory T cells in human neurocysticercosis. *Clin Exp Immunol* (2016) 183:271–9. doi:10.1111/cei.12709
46. Son HJ, Lee SH, Lee SY, Kim EK, Yang EJ, Kim JK, et al. Correction: oncostatin M suppresses activation of IL-17/Th17 via SOCS3 regulation in CD4+ T cells. *J Immunol* (2017) 198:4879. doi:10.4049/jimmunol.1502314
47. Williams RO. Collagen-induced arthritis in mice. *Methods Mol Med* (2007) 136:191–9. doi:10.1007/978-1-59745-402-5_14
48. Kotake S, Yago T, Kobashigawa T, Nanke Y. The plasticity of Th17 cells in the pathogenesis of rheumatoid arthritis. *J Clin Med* (2017) 6:E67. doi:10.3390/jcm6070067
49. McInnes IB, Schett G. The pathogenesis of rheumatoid arthritis. *N Engl J Med* (2011) 365:2205–19. doi:10.1056/NEJMra1004965
50. Chen Z, Andreev D, Oeser K, Krljanac B, Hueber A, Kleyer A, et al. Th2 and eosinophil responses suppress inflammatory arthritis. *Nat Commun* (2016) 7:11596. doi:10.1038/ncomms11596
51. Finlay CM, Stefanska AM, Walsh KP, Kelly PJ, Boon L, Lavelle EC, et al. Helminth products protect against autoimmunity via innate type 2 cytokines IL-5 and IL-33, which promote eosinophilia. *J Immunol* (2016) 196:703–14. doi:10.4049/jimmunol.1501820
52. Kang SA, Cho MK, Park MK, Kim DH, Hong YC, Lee YS, et al. Alteration of helper T-cell related cytokine production in splenocytes during *Trichinella spiralis* infection. *Vet Parasitol* (2012) 186:319–27. doi:10.1016/j.vetpar.2011.12.002
53. Larkin BM, Smith PM, Ponichtera HE, Shainheit MG, Rutitzky LI, Stadecker MJ. Induction and regulation of pathogenic Th17 cell responses in schistosomiasis. *Semin Immunopathol* (2012) 34:873–88. doi:10.1007/s00281-012-0341-9
54. Nishimura H, Okazaki T, Tanaka Y, Nakatani K, Hara M, Matsumori A, et al. Autoimmune dilated cardiomyopathy in PD-1 receptor-deficient mice. *Science* (2001) 291:319–22. doi:10.1126/science.291.5502.319
55. Sage PT, Schildberg FA, Sobel RA, Kuchroo VK, Freeman GJ, Sharpe AH. Dendritic cell PD-L1 limits autoimmunity and follicular T cell differentiation and function. *J Immunol* (2018) 200(8):2592–602. doi:10.4049/jimmunol.1701231
56. Schwartz C, Khan AR, Floudas A, Saunders SP, Hams E, Rodewald HR, et al. ILC2s regulate adaptive Th2 cell functions via PD-L1 checkpoint control. *J Exp Med* (2017) 214:2507–21. doi:10.1084/jem.20170051
57. Han R, Luo J, Shi Y, Yao Y, Hao J. PD-L1 (programmed death ligand 1) protects against experimental intracerebral hemorrhage-induced brain injury. *Stroke* (2017) 48:2255–62. doi:10.1161/STROKEAHA.117.016705
58. Read S, Malmstrom V, Powrie F. Cytotoxic T lymphocyte-associated antigen 4 plays an essential role in the function of CD25(+)CD4(+) regulatory cells that control intestinal inflammation. *J Exp Med* (2000) 192:295–302. doi:10.1084/jem.192.2.295
59. Viglietta V, Baecher-Allan C, Weiner HL, Hafler DA. Loss of functional suppression by CD4+CD25+ regulatory T cells in patients with multiple sclerosis. *J Exp Med* (2004) 199:971–9. doi:10.1084/jem.20031579
60. Kukreja A, Cost G, Marker J, Zhang C, Sun Z, Lin-Su K, et al. Multiple immuno-regulatory defects in type-1 diabetes. *J Clin Invest* (2002) 109:131–40. doi:10.1172/JCI0213605
61. Liang SC, Greenwald RJ, Latchman YE, Rosas L, Satoskar A, Freeman GJ, et al. PD-L1 and PD-L2 have distinct roles in regulating host immunity to cutaneous leishmaniasis. *Eur J Immunol* (2006) 36:58–64. doi:10.1002/eji.200535458
62. McAlees JW, Lajoie S, Dienger K, Sproles AA, Richgels PK, Yang Y, et al. Differential control of CD4(+) T-cell subsets by the PD-1/PD-L1 axis in a mouse model of allergic asthma. *Eur J Immunol* (2015) 45:1019–29. doi:10.1002/eji.201444778
63. Prendergast CT, Sanin DE, Mountford AP. CD4 T-cell hyporesponsiveness induced by schistosome larvae is not dependent upon eosinophils but may involve connective tissue mast cells. *Parasite Immunol* (2016) 38:81–92. doi:10.1111/pim.12300
64. Prendergast CT, Sanin DE, Cook PC, Mountford AP. CD4+ T cell hyporesponsiveness after repeated exposure to *Schistosoma mansoni* larvae is dependent upon interleukin-10. *Infect Immun* (2015) 83:1418–30. doi:10.1128/IAI.02831-14
65. Said EA, Dupuy FP, Trautmann L, Zhang Y, Shi Y, El-Far M, et al. Programmed death-1-induced interleukin-10 production by monocytes impairs CD4+ T cell activation during HIV infection. *Nat Med* (2010) 16:452–9. doi:10.1038/nm.2106

6

Toxoplasma Effector TgIST Targets Host IDO1 to Antagonize the IFN-γ-Induced Anti-Parasitic Response in Human Cells

Hironori Bando[1,2†]*, Naoya Sakaguchi*[1†]*, Youngae Lee*[1,2]*, Ariel Pradipta*[1]*, Ji Su Ma*[1,2]*, Shun Tanaka*[1,2]*, De-Hua Lai*[3]*, Jianfa Liu*[4]*, Zhao-Rong Lun*[3]*, Yoshifumi Nishikawa*[5]*, Miwa Sasai*[1,2] *and Masahiro Yamamoto*[1,2*]

[1] *Department of Immunoparasitology, Research Institute for Microbial Diseases, Osaka University, Osaka, Japan,* [2] *Laboratory of Immunoparasitology, WPI Immunology Frontier Research Center, Osaka University, Osaka, Japan,* [3] *State Key Laboratory of Biocontrol, Center for Parasitic Organisms, School of Life Sciences, Guangzhou, China,* [4] *Department of Pathology and Pathogenic Biology, Medical College of Ningbo University, Ningbo, China,* [5] *National Research Center for Protozoan Diseases, Obihiro University of Agriculture and Veterinary Medicine, Obihiro, Japan*

***Correspondence:**
Masahiro Yamamoto
myamamoto@biken.osaka-u.ac.jp

† *These authors have contributed equally to this work*

Toxoplasma gondii is an important human and animal pathogen that causes life-threatening toxoplasmosis. Interferon-γ (IFN-γ) is critical for anti-*T. gondii* cell-autonomous immunity in both humans and mice. To proliferate efficiently within the hosts, virulent strains of *T. gondii* can suppress IFN-γ-dependent immunity. During parasite infection, it is well-characterized that various virulence effectors are secreted to transcriptionally or post-translationally target IFN-γ-inducible GTPases, which are essential for anti-parasite responses in mice. However, the role of IFN-γ-inducible GTPases in anti-*T. gondii* responses in human cells is controversial since they are non-functional or absent in humans. Instead, IFN-γ-induced tryptophan degradation by indole-2,3-dioxygenase (IDO) is important for the anti-*T. gondii* human response. To date, the *T. gondii* virulent mechanism targeting IDO in human cells remains elusive. Here we show that although humans possess two IDO isozymes, IDO1 and IDO2, human cells of various origins require IDO1 but not IDO2 for IFN-γ-induced cell-autonomous immunity to *T. gondii*. *T. gondii* secretes an effector TgIST to inhibit IDO1 mRNA expression. Taken together, the data suggests that *T. gondii* possesses virulence programs operated by TgIST to antagonize IFN-γ-induced IDO1-mediated anti-parasite cell-autonomous immunity in human cells.

Keywords: IFN-γ, IDO1, IDO2, virulence, human, TgIST

INTRODUCTION

Toxoplasma gondii is an intracellular apicomplexan protozoan that has a broad range of intermediate hosts, including humans (1, 2). Although it is estimated that at least one-third of the world's population is infected with *T. gondii*, most of these infections are asymptomatic. However, the parasite remains in a latent state and may reactivate and lead to severe diseases including hepatitis, encephalitis, and myocarditis if that individual becomes immunocompromised (3, 4). Moreover, toxoplasmosis caused by *T. gondii* infection may lead to congenital diseases in fetuses and newborn infants from primarily-infected pregnant women (5). Thus, *T. gondii* is one of the most important human and animal pathogens.

The host immune system plays a critical role in the course of *T. gondii* infection and in the progression of toxoplasmosis. In particular, the type I cytokine interferon-γ (IFN-γ), which is produced by CD4$^+$ T cells and natural killer cells (NK), is an essential host factor for anti-*T. gondii* responses in host cells (6). This is because IFN-γ activates the transcription factor STAT1 and induces the expression of hundreds of genes (7). In the mouse model, IFN-γ-induced anti-*T. gondii* responses have been extensively analyzed. Parasitocidal and parasitostatic effects mediated by IFN-γ-inducible gene products have been observed in mice. The parasitocidal effects are coordinated by IFN-γ-inducible GTPases such as p47 immunity-related GTPases (IRGs) and p65 guanylate-binding proteins (GBPs) (8, 9). These GTPases accumulate on parastitophorous vacuoles (PVs), leading to their destruction (10). In mice, the accumulation of IRGs and GBPs on *T. gondii* requires some essential autophagy-related (Atg) proteins such as Atg3, Atg5, Atg7, Atg16L1, and GABARAPs but not other Atg proteins such as Atg9, Atg14, FIP200, and LC3s (11), suggesting the non-autophagic role of these Atg proteins in IFN-γ-mediated anti-*T. gondii* responses in mice. Atg16L1-deficient murine cells are severely defective in the IFN-γ-induced clearance of *T. gondii* due to impaired recruitment of GBPs and IRGs to *T. gondii* (12, 13), suggesting the essential role of Atg16L1 in anti-*T. gondii* responses in mice. In addition, this parasitostatic mechanism involves nitric oxide (NO), which is produced by IFN-γ-inducible NO synthase (iNOS) (14). Mice lacking IRGs, GBPs, and iNOS are susceptible to *T. gondii* infection (8, 15–20). Thus, the significance of these IFN-γ-inducible factors for anti-*T. gondii* immune responses in mice has previously been established.

However, the importance of IFN-γ-inducible GTPase- and NO-mediated mechanisms in humans is less certain. For example, compared with more than 20 IRG members in mice, humans only possess one IRG, which is not inducible by IFN-γ (21). Furthermore, inhibition of NO production does not affect *T. gondii* growth in IFN-γ-stimulated human macrophages (22). Regarding GBPs, a human reprogrammed fibroblast-like cell line (HAP1) lacking all GBPs shows a normal IFN-γ-dependent reduction in *T. gondii* growth (12, 23). However, knockout of GBP1 in a human lung epithelial cell line (A549) and knockdown of GBP1 in human mesenchymal stem cells (MSCs) results in impaired restriction of *T. gondii* growth in response to IFN-γ (24, 25). Thus, the involvement of IFN-γ-inducible GTPases and NO in the human anti-*T. gondii* response is controversial (12, 23–26). Regarding the role of autophagy proteins in human cells, ATG16L1 is dispensable for IFN-γ-induced inhibition of *T. gondii* growth in HAP1 cells and HUVECs (12, 27), whereas ATG16L1 is required for anti-parasite responses in HeLa cells via IFN-γ-inducible ubiquitination of *T. gondii* PVs (23). Thus, the anti-*T. gondii* role of ATG16L1 in humans may be cell-type specific. By contrast, IFN-γ-dependent nutrient deprivation or cell death has been established as an anti-*T. gondii* response in human cells (28, 29). Regarding nutrient deprivation, IFN-γ stimulates the expression of indoleamine 2,3-dioxygenases (IDO) to degrade tryptophan, which is an essential amino acid for *T. gondii* intracellular growth (30, 31). The treatment of IFN-γ-activated human cells with a pharmacological inhibitor of IDO called 1-methyl-DL- tryptophan (1-DL-MT) leads to defects in the IFN-γ-induced reduction of *T. gondii* numbers (32), establishing the significance of IDO in the IFN-γ-induced anti-*T. gondii* response in human cells. IDO consists of two closely related family members, IDO1 and IDO2 (33). Previous studies using 1-DL-MT concluded that IDO is responsible for the IFN-γ-inducible anti-*T. gondii* response (32, 34). However, given that both IDO1 and IDO2 are sensitive to 1-DL-MT (35, 36), it remains unclear whether either IDO1 or IDO2 (or both) is more important.

To antagonize the IFN-γ-induced anti-parasitic host response, *T. gondii* secretes various effector molecules into host cells upon infection (37, 38). The effector mechanisms are also extensively analyzed in the mouse model. ROP5, ROP17, and ROP18 are secreted from the rhoptry organelles to suppress IRG/GBP-dependent immune responses at PV membranes, resulting in increased virulence in mice (39–43). In addition, a dense granule-derived effector GRA7 is also injected into host cells to enhance ROP18-mediated inhibition of IRGs in mice (44). Furthermore, *T. gondii* infection is shown to impede STAT1-mediated gene expression (45, 46). TgIST was recently shown to be secreted from dense granules and finally localized at the host nucleus, where TgIST associates with the remodeled host nucleosome and the deacetylase complex to inhibit the expression of STAT1-dependent genes including iNOS, chemokines, IRGs, and GBPs, leading to enhanced virulence in mice (47, 48). Although ROP5 and ROP18 are virulence factors in mice, these effectors do not affect the ability of *T. gondii* to survive in IFN-γ-stimulated human fibroblasts (49). Regarding TgIST, although TgIST-deficient parasites are defective in STAT1-depdendent gene expression in human cells (47, 48), whether TgIST affects parasite survival in IFN-γ-stimulated host cells and which, if any, of the STAT1-regulated human gene products is targeted by TgIST remains elusive, given the differences between humans and mice in terms of IFN-γ-induced anti-*T. gondii* cell-autonomous immunity.

In the present study, we first demonstrated that IDO1, but not IDO2, is required for IFN-γ-induced inhibition of *T. gondii* growth of human cell lines of various origins. In terms of *T. gondii* virulence mechanisms, we have shown that TgIST directly suppresses IDO1 gene expression to promote parasite growth in IFN-γ-activated human cells. Taken together, these data have revealed that *T. gondii* uses TgIST as a virulence mechanism to impede the IDO1-dependent cell-autonomous response in IFN-γ-activated human cells.

RESULTS

ATG16L1-Independent IFN-γ-Induced Reduction of *T. gondii* Numbers in the Human HAP1 Cell Line

We have previously shown that ATG16L1 plays an important role in the IFN-γ-induced reduction of type II *T. gondii* (ME49) in mouse cells (mouse embryonic fibroblasts; MEFs) but not in human HAP1 cells (**Figure 1A**), suggesting an ATG16L1-independent IFN-γ-induced anti-*T. gondii* response in human cells (12). To elucidate the molecular mechanism, we next challenged MEFs and HAP1 cells with type I (RH) or type II (ME49) parasites. As shown previously (12), MEFs showed more efficient IFN-γ-induced reduction of type II parasites than of type I parasites. By contrast, IFN-γ stimulation could similarly and efficiently reduce the numbers of both type I and II parasites in HAP1 cells (**Figure 1B**). IFN-γ-induced degradation of arginine by iNOS, or of tryptophan by IDO, which consists of two members, IDO1 and IDO2, have been shown to be important for the anti-*T. gondii* response in mouse or human cells (18, 30, 31). To test whether iNOS or IDO (or both) are involved in the process in HAP1 cells, we examined iNOS, IDO1, or IDO2 mRNA expression in HAP1 cells (**Figure 1C**). Stimulation of IFN-γ led to strong induction of IDO1 and IDO2 mRNAs and weak induction of iNOS mRNA. Second, we tested the expression levels of these mRNAs in IFN-γ-stimulated cells followed by *T. gondii* infection (**Figure 1C**). *T. gondii* infection at 24 hours after IFN-γ stimulation did not interfere with the expression of iNOS, IDO1, and IDO2 mRNAs in HAP1 cells (**Figure 1C**). Furthermore, we treated HAP1 cells with a pharmacological inhibitor of iNOS known as aminoguanidine or an inhibitor of IDO known as 1-methyl-DL-tryptophan (1-DL-MT), and compared the parasite numbers. 1-DL-MT but not aminoguanidine treatment abolished the IFN-γ-induced reduction of *T. gondii* numbers in HAP1 cells (**Figure 1D**), strongly suggesting the anti-*T. gondii* function of IDO in the human HAP1 cell line.

IDO1 but Not IDO2 Plays a Critical Role in the Anti-*T. gondii* Response in HAP1 Cells

Both IDO1 and IDO2 could be inhibited by 1-DL-MT (35, 36). Although both IDO1 and IDO2 mRNAs were highly induced by IFN-γ stimulation in HAP1 cells (**Figure 1C**), it remained to be seen which was more important for the IFN-γ-induced response in HAP1 cells. To clarify the contribution of IDOs in HAP1 cells, we generated IDO1 singly deficient (IDO1-KO), IDO2 singly deficient (IDO2-KO), and doubly deficient (IDO1/IDO2-DKO) HAP1 cells by CRISPR/Cas9 genome editing (**Figures 2A,B, Figure S1A**) and tested the IFN-γ-induced reduction of type II parasite numbers. Although IDO2-KO HAP1 cells functioned normally, IDO1-KO cells as well as IDO1/IDO2-DKO cells were completely defective in IFN-γ-induced parasite reduction (**Figure 2C**), suggesting that IDO1 but not IDO2 is essential for the IFN-γ-induced anti-*T. gondii* response in the human cell line. Kynurenine is a tryptophan metabolite of IDOs (50). Therefore, we measured kynurenine concentrations in HAP1 cells lacking IDOs (**Figure S1B**). Whereas, the kynurenine concentrations were increased upon IFN-γ treatment in wild-type HAP1 cells, such an increment was not observed in IDO1-KO or IDO1/IDO2-DKO HAP1 cells (**Figure S1B**). By contrast, IDO2-KO cells showed normal induction of kynurenine after IFN-γ stimulation (**Figure S1B**), correlating with the importance of IDO1 in the IFN-γ-induced reduction of parasite numbers and the degree of tryptophan degradation. In mouse cells, a *T. gondii* strain-dependent difference was observed in the IFN-γ-induced anti-*T. gondii* response (**Figure 1B**) (12, 13). By contrast, although wild-type cells exhibited greatly reduced numbers of type I parasites after IFN-γ stimulation, this IFN-γ-mediated reduction was not observed in IDO1-KO HAP1 cells (**Figure S1C**), suggesting the lack of strain dependence in this human cell line. Next, we analyzed whether IDO1 expression could rescue the defective anti-*T. gondii* response of IDO1-KO cells. To achieve this, IDO1-KO cells were transfected with a doxycycline-inducible IDO1 or the empty control vectors and the IFN-γ-induced anti-*T. gondii* response was tested (**Figure 2D, Figure S1D**). The doxycycline-inducible IDO1 expression led to a reduction of parasite numbers in the IFN-γ-stimulated IDO1-KO cells (**Figure 2D**). Next we tested whether IDO1 plays a role in the inhibition of *T. gondii* replication or in parasite elimination. The parasite numbers per vacuole in IFN-γ-stimulated IDO1-KO HAP1 cells were significantly higher than those of wild-type cells (**Figures 2E,F**). Whereas, the rates of *T. gondii*-infected wild-type or IDO1-KO cells were comparable 3 and 24 h post infection (**Figures 2E,G**), indicating that IDO1 inhibits *T. gondii* replication in IFN-γ-stimulated HAP1 cells. Taken together, these data suggest that IDO1 plays a critical role in the IFN-γ-induced anti-*T. gondii* response in HAP1 cells.

IDO1 Is Required for the Anti-*T. gondii* Response in Various Human Cell Lines

Next we assessed whether IDO1 is important for the IFN-γ-induced anti-*T. gondii* response in other human cells. IDO1 mRNAs were highly induced in foreskin fibroblasts (HFFs), a hepatocyte cell line (Huh7), and an epithelial cell line (HeLa) upon IFN-γ stimulation regardless of the subsequent *T. gondii* infection (**Figure 3A**). Then we generated IDO1-KO HFFs, Huh7, or HeLa cells by CRISPR/Cas9-genome editing (**Figure 3B, Figure S2A**) and analyzed the IFN-γ-induced reduction in *T. gondii* numbers. Among all of the cell types tested, IDO1-KO cells were defective in the IFN-γ-mediated anti-*T. gondii* response (**Figure 3C**). However, compared with IDO1-KO HAP1 cells or HFFs, both of which displayed complete loss of an anti-parasite response (**Figures 2C, 3C**), IDO1 deficiency in Huh7 or HeLa cells resulted in severely impaired or modest defects (**Figure 3C**), suggesting an IDO1-independent anti-*T. gondii* response in Huh7 and HeLa cells. In addition, Tryptophan 2,3-dioxygenase (TDO) was not involved to IFN-γ induced anti-*T. gondii* responses in Huh7 cells (**Figure S2B**).

ATG16L1 Is Required for the Anti-*T. gondii* Response in a Cell Type-Specific Manner

A previous study demonstrated that ATG16L1 is involved in the IFN-γ-induced anti-*T. gondii* response in HeLa cells (23). Therefore, we hypothesized that ATG16L1 plays a role in the IDO1-independent response in Huh7 and HeLa cells. To examine this possibility, we generated ATG16L1-deficient (ATG16L1-KO) HFFs, Huh7, and HeLa cells by CRISPR/Cas9 genome editing (**Figure 4A**). Although ATG16L1-KO HFFs and Huh7 cells showed no increment of parasite

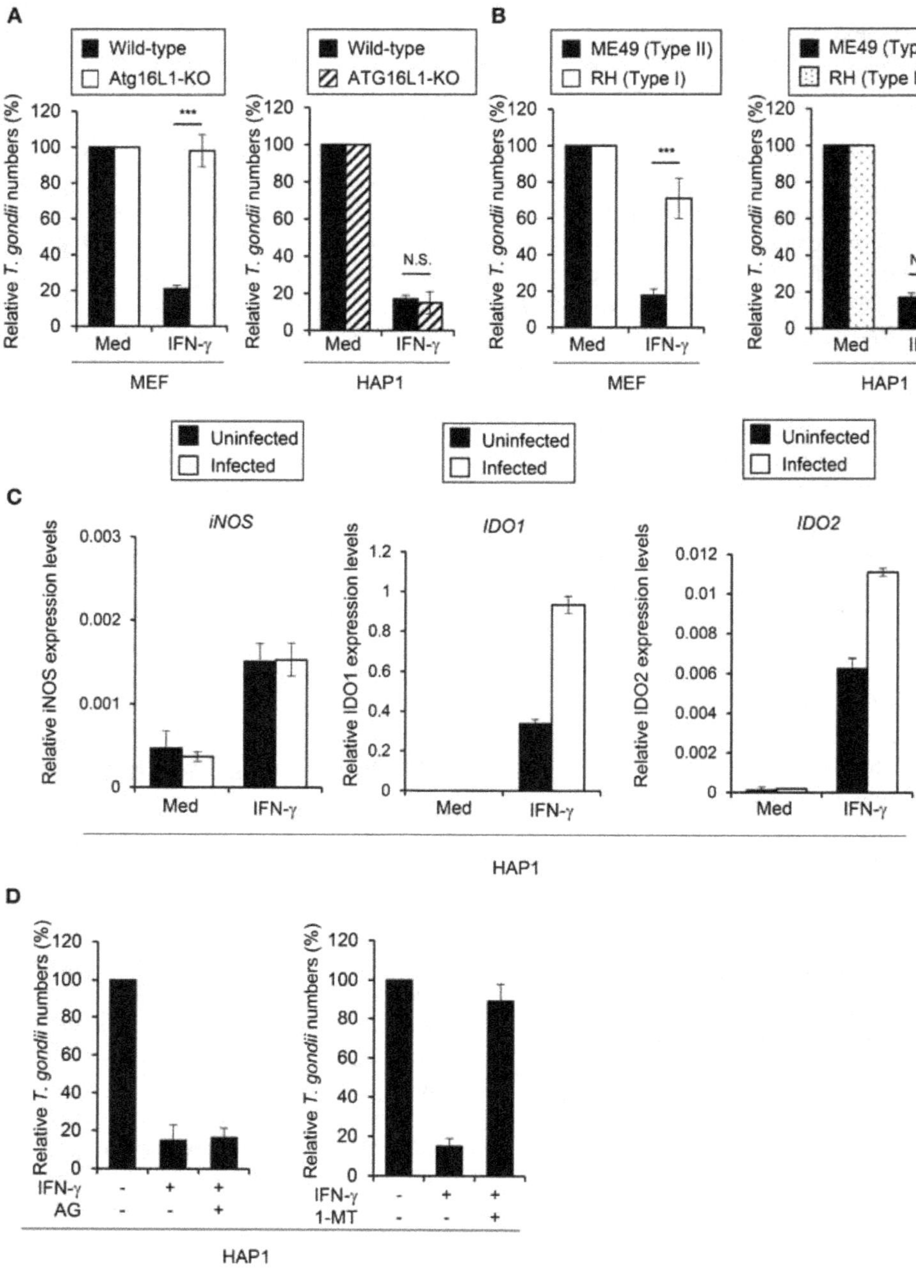

FIGURE 1 | IDO plays a critical role in anti *T. gondii* response in HAP1 cells. **(A)** WT or Atg16L1-KO MEFs or HAP1 cells were untreated or pre-treated with IFN-γ for 24 h, and then infected with *T. gondii*. The parasite survival rate after 24 h post infection was measured by luciferase assay. **(B)** MEFs or HAP1 cells were untreated or pre-treated with IFN-γ for 24 h, and then infected with Type I or Type II *T. gondii*. The parasite survival rate after 24 h post infection was measured by luciferase assay. **(C)** Quantitative RT-PCR analysis of iNOS, IDO1 or IDO2 mRNA level in HAP1 cells that were untreated or treated with IFN-γ for 24 h, and then infected with or without *T. gondii* was performed. **(D)** HAP1 cells were untreated or treated with IFN-γ and/or Aminoguanidine and/or 1-DL-MT for 24 h, and then infected with *T. gondii*. The parasite survival rate after 24 h post infection was measured by luciferase assay. Indicated values are means of ± s.d. (three biological replicates per group from three independent experiments) **(A–D)**. ***$p < 0.001$; N.S., not significant; (Student's *t*-test).

numbers (**Figure 4B**) or parasite numbers per vacuole upon IFN-γ stimulation (**Figures 4C,D**), ATG16L1-KO HeLa cells exhibited modest defects (**Figures 4C,D**). Furthermore, 1-DL-MT treatment in ATG16L1-KO HeLa cells resulted in a less efficient IFN-γ-mediated response than in non-treated control cells (**Figure S2C**), suggesting that ATG16L1 is involved in the IFN-γ-induced anti-parasite response in a cell type-specific manner. Thus, IDO1 is involved in the IFN-γ-induced anti-*T. gondii* response in human cells of various origins (**Figure 6A**). However, given the dispensable role of IDO in HUVECs (51), the degree of importance of IDO1 in the anti-*T. gondii* response depends on cell type.

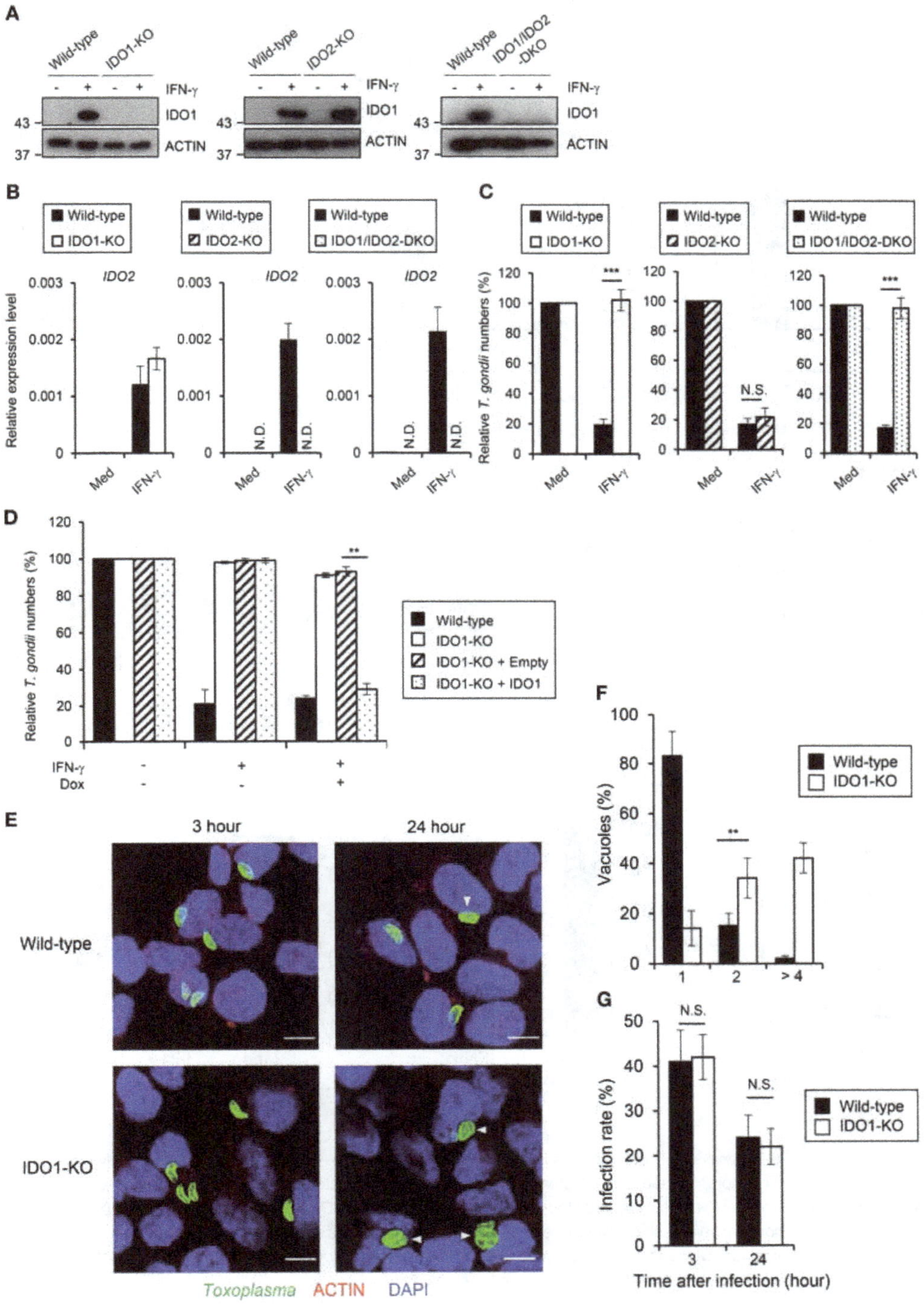

FIGURE 2 | IDO1 but not IDO2 has a critical role in anti-*T. gondii* response in HAP1 cells. **(A)** WT, IDO1-KO, IDO2-KO, or IDO1/IDO2-DKO HAP1 cells were stimulated with IFN-γ for 24 h, and then lysates were detected by Western blot. **(B)** Quantitative RT-PCR analysis of IDO2 mRNA level in IDO1-KO, IDO2-KO, or IDO1/IDO2-DKO HAP1 cells that were untreated or treated with IFN-γ for 24 h was performed. **(C)** WT, IDO1-KO, IDO2-KO, or IDO1/IDO2-DKO HAP1 cells were untreated or treated with IFN-γ for 24 h, and then infected with *T. gondii*. The parasite survival rate after 24 h post infection was measured by luciferase assay. **(D)** WT, IDO1-KO, IDO1-KO+empty, or IDO1-KO+IDO1 HAP1 cells were untreated or treated with IFN-γ for 24 h, and then infected with *T. gondii*. The parasite survival rate after 24 h post infection was measured by luciferase assay. **(E)** Fluorescence confocal microscopy of WT and IDO1-KO HAP1 cells stimulated by IFN-γ for 24 h, subsequently infected with *T. gondii* for 3 or 24 h, and immunostained for ACTIN (red) and *T. gondii* GAP45 (green). The nucleus was stained with DAPI (blue). Arrow heads show vacuoles containing 2 or more parasites. Scale bars correspond to 5 μm. **(F,G)** WT or IDO1-KO HAP1 cells were stimulated with IFN-γ for 24 h, and then infected with *T. gondii*. The parasite number per vacuole after 24 h post infection **(F)** or the parasite infection rate after 3 or 24 h post infection **(G)** was measured by IFA. Western blot and immunofluorescence images are representative of three independent experiments **(A,E)**. Indicated values are means of ± s.d. (three biological replicates per group from three independent experiments) **(B,C,D,F,G)**. $^{***}p < 0.001$, $^{**}p < 0.01$; N.S., not significant; (Student's *t*-test). N.D., not detected.

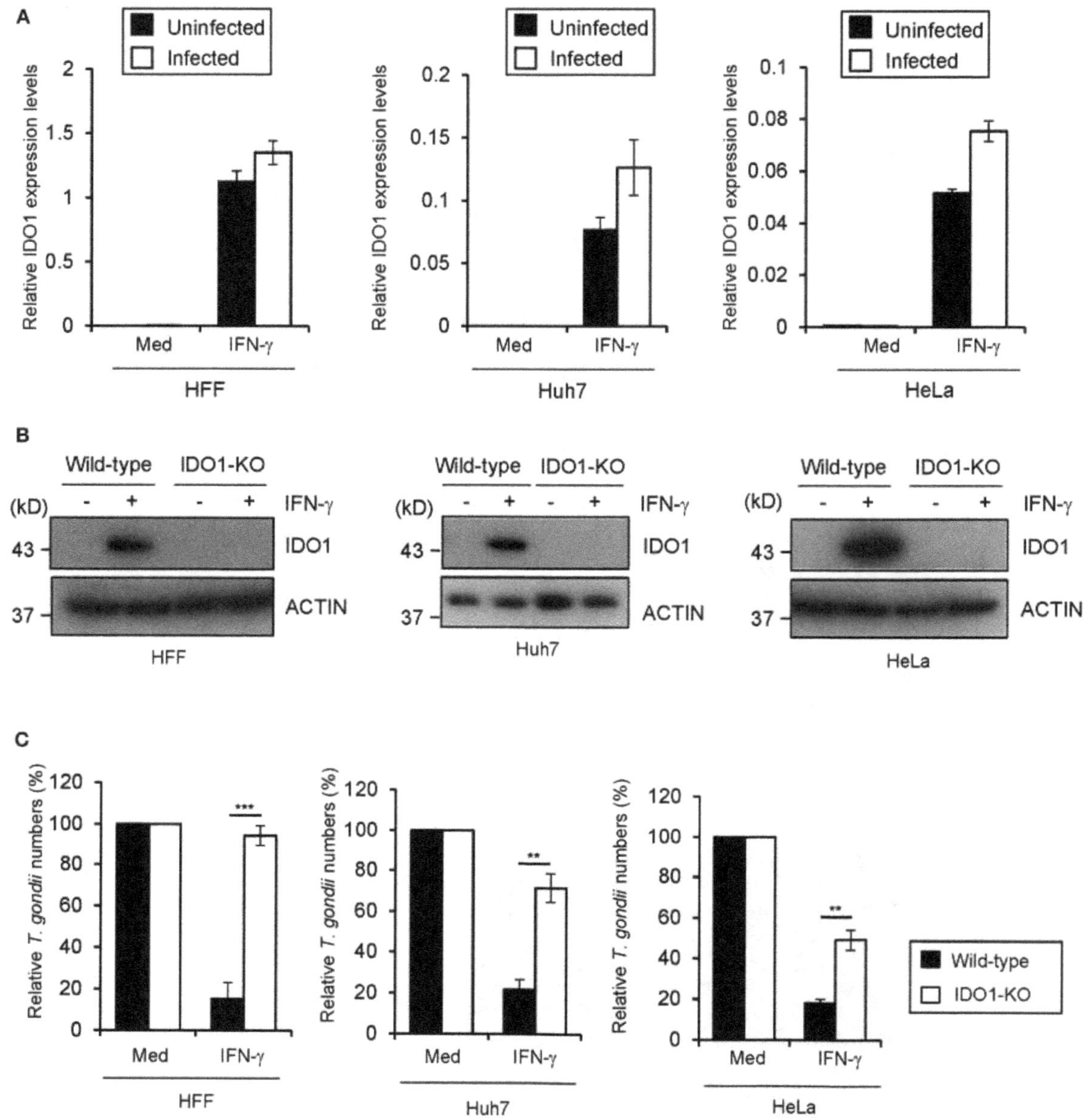

FIGURE 3 | IDO1 has a critical role in anti-*T. gondii* response in various human cells. **(A)** Quantitative RT-PCR analysis of IDO1 mRNA level in HFFs, Huh7 or HeLa cells that were untreated or treated with IFN-γ for 24 h, and then infected with or without *T. gondii* was performed. **(B)** WT or IDO1-KO HFFs, Huh7 or Hela cells were untreated or treated with IFN-γ for 24 h, and then lysates were detected by Western blot. **(C)** WT or IDO1-KO HFFs, Huh7 or Hela cells were untreated or treated with IFN-γ for 24 h, and then infected with *T. gondii*. The parasite survival rate after 24 h post infection was measured by luciferase assay. Western blot image is representative of three independent experiments **(B)**. Indicated values are means of ± s.d. (three biological replicates per group from three independent experiments) **(A,C)**. ***$p < 0.001$, **$p < 0.01$; N.S., not significant; (Student's *t*-test). N.D., not detected.

TgIST Directly Suppresses IDO1 Expression to Inhibit the IFN-γ-Induced Anti-*T. gondii* Response in Human Cell Lines

Since IDO1 plays a critical role in the IFN-γ-induced anti-*T. gondii* response in various human cells, we next explored the possible *T. gondii* virulence mechanisms targeting IDO1 in human cells. We selected TgIST, a *T. gondii* secreting effector molecule, as the candidate (47, 48), since the regulation of IDO1 expression by IFN-γ was shown to be regulated by STAT1 (52). To assess this possibility, we generated TgIST-KO type II parasites by CRISPR/Cas9 genome editing (**Figures S3A,B**) and asked whether TgIST deficiency affects *T. gondii* virulence in human cells (**Figure 5A**). As previously reported (47, 48), we also confirmed that TgIST-dependent suppression of the anti-*T. gondii* effect could be detected only when *T. gondii*-infected cells were subsequently stimulated with IFN-γ but not when IFN-γ-pre-treated cells were followed by *T. gondii* infection (**Figure 5A**, **Figure S4A**). By contrast, we observed

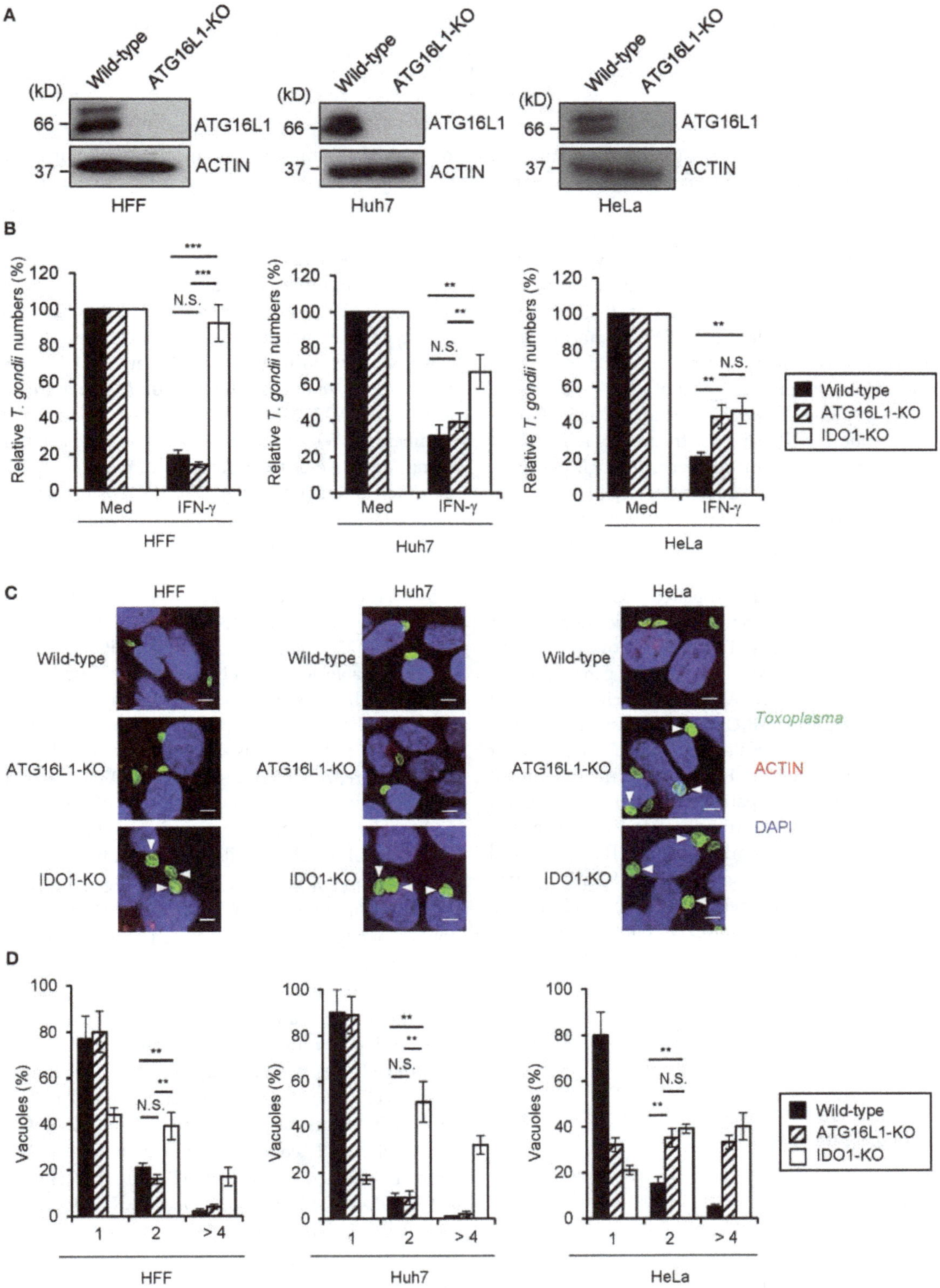

FIGURE 4 | IDO1 but not ATG16L1 extensively participate in anti-*T. gondii* response in human cell lines. **(A)** WT or ATG16L1-KO HFFs, Huh7 or Hela cells were untreated or treated with IFN-γ for 24 h, and then lysates were detected by Western blot. **(B)** WT, IDO1-KO, or ATG16L1-KO HFFs, Huh7 or Hela cells were untreated or treated with IFN-γ for 24 h, and then infected with *T. gondii*. The parasite survival rate after 24 h post infection was measured by luciferase assay. **(C)** Fluorescence confocal microscopy of WT, ATG16L1-KO and IDO1-KO HFF, Huh7 or HeLa cells stimulated by IFN-γ for 24 h, subsequently infected with *T. gondii* for 24 h, and immunostained for ACTIN (red) and *T. gondii* GAP45 (green). The nucleus was stained with DAPI (blue). Arrow heads show vacuoles containing 2 or more parasites.

(Continued)

FIGURE 4 | Scale bars correspond to 5 μm. **(D)** WT, IDO1-KO or ATG16L1-KO HFFs, Huh7 or Hela cells were untreated or treated with IFN-γ for 24 h, and then infected with *T. gondii*. The number of parasites per vacuole after 24 h post infection was measured by IFA. Western blot and immunofluorescence images representative of three independent experiments **(A,C)**. Indicated values are means of ± s.d. (three biological replicates per group from three independent experiments) **(B,D)**. $^{***}p < 0.001$, $^{**}p < 0.01$; N.S., not significant; (Student's *t*-test). N.D., not detected.

an IFN-γ-dependent reduction in TgIST-KO parasite numbers (**Figure 5A**), suggesting that TgIST promotes parasite growth in the IFN-γ-post-stimulated cells. Phosphorylation of the Y701 residue of STAT1 (STAT1 Y701-p) was previously shown to be induced by *T. gondii* infection without IFN-γ stimulation and STAT1 Y701-p proteins were translocated to the nucleus (48). TgIST directly binds to STAT1 and recruits the chromatin-modifying Mi-2/NuRD complex to STAT1 transcriptional complexes. As a result, chromatin is remodeled and interferon-stimulated gene expression, including that of IRF-1, is decreased (47, 48). We tested whether *T. gondii* infection inhibits STAT1-dependent transcription in IFN-γ-post-treated HFF, Huh7, or HAP1 cells in a TgIST-dependent manner. Although phospho-STAT1 (STAT1 Y701-p) proteins were not detected in the nucleus in unstimulated cells, STAT1 Y701-p proteins were translocated to the nucleus upon IFN-γ-treatment. As previously reported (47, 48), wild-type *T. gondii* infection caused STAT1 Y701-p nuclear translocation even in unstimulated cells (**Figure 5B**). The subsequent IFN-γ-stimulation further induced translocation of STAT1 Y701-p to the nucleus (**Figure 5B**); however, STAT1 Y701-p was not active since STAT1-regulated gene products such as IRF1 and IDO1 mRNAs and proteins were not induced (**Figure 5C, Figures S4B,C**). By contrast, infection of TgIST-KO *T. gondii* did not result in STAT1 Y701-p nuclear translocation in unstimulated cells. Furthermore, the subsequent IFN-γ stimulation in TgIST-KO parasite-infected cells normally induced STAT1 Y701-p nuclear translocation in comparison with uninfected cells. Moreover, normal levels of IFN-γ-induced IRF1 and IDO1 expression suggested that the STAT1 activity in TgIST-KO *T. gondii*-infected cells was normal (**Figure 5C, Figures S4B,C**). Furthermore, IDO1-KO cells did not exhibit an IFN-γ-induced reduction in TgIST-KO parasites (**Figure 5D**). Conversely, growth of TgIST-intact wild-type *T. gondii* as well as TgIST-KO parasite growth was strongly inhibited by doxycycline-induced (thereby, STAT1-independent) IDO1 overexpression (**Figure 5E**), indicating that the pro-parasitic role of TgIST for *T. gondii* growth in IFN-γ-post-stimulated human cells is mainly due to inhibition of IDO1 but not other IFN-γ-inducible proteins (**Figure 6B**).

DISCUSSION

In the present study, we have demonstrated that IDO1 but not IDO2 plays an essential role in the IFN-γ-induced anti-*T. gondii* response in several human cell lines and primary fibroblasts. This finding is further strengthened by subsequent findings that treatment of an IDO inhibitor 1-DL-MT, consisting of 1-D-MT and 1-L-MT, reverses IFN-γ-dependent growth inhibition (32). However, IDO2 as well as IDO1 are possibly inhibited by both 1-D-MT and 1-L-MT (35, 36). Thus, whether the inhibitory effect of 1-DL-MT is on IDO1 or/and IDO2 remained unclear. Here we found that, by complete genetic deletion of IDO1 or/and IDO2 in HAP1 cells, IDO2-KO cells were able to reduce parasite numbers similarly to wild-type cells. By contrast, IDO1-KO cells as well as IDO1/IDO2-DKO cells could not control the parasite in response to IFN-γ. In addition, *T. gondii* numbers per vacuole at 24 h post infection in IDO1-KO cells were higher than in wild-type cells, whereas the infection rates were comparable. Thus, we have formally clarified that IDO1 is more important for the IFN-γ-induced inhibition of *T. gondii* growth in human cells than IDO2. Moreover, given that assessment in *T. gondii* numbers in PVs and the infection rate have been established as being indicative of the restriction of parasite replication and of parasite elimination/killing (20), IDO1 is required for *T. gondii* replication control rather than parasite elimination.

The ATG16L1-dependent cell-autonomous response mediated by IFN-γ-inducible GTPases such as IRGs and GBPs is important for the IFN-γ-mediated anti-*T. gondii* response in mice (12, 13). However, humans lack most of the IRGs (21). Moreover, human GBPs have been shown to be dispensable for the IFN-γ-inducible response (12, 24, 29). Recently, the IFN-γ-induced ubiquitination of *T. gondii* PVs has been shown to be required for the anti-*T. gondii* response in human cells such as HeLa cells and HUVECs (23, 27). Furthermore, ATG16L1 together with ATG7 are also important for the ubiquitin-mediated reduction of parasite numbers in HeLa cells (23). We have confirmed the anti-parasitic role of ATG16L1 in HeLa cells in this study. Moreover, although ATG16L1 is dispensable for the IFN-γ-induced reduction of *T. gondii* numbers in HAP1 cells, HFFs, and Huh7 cells, this autophagy protein is required in HeLa cells. The specific participation of ATG16L1 in the anti-*T. gondii* response in HeLa cells might be partly due to constitutively high levels of basal autophagy in HeLa cells (53, 54). Although the involvement of ATG16L1 in the human IFN-γ-induced anti-*T. gondii* response may be cell type-specific, complete genetic deletion of IDO1 in all human cells tested led to the impaired control of *T. gondii* growth by IFN-γ, suggesting that IDO1 is mainly used for the IFN-γ-mediated anti-*T. gondii* response in normal cells and various human cell lines. Given that ATG16L1-KO HeLa cells treated with 1-DL-MT still exhibit a modest IFN-γ-dependent reduction of *T. gondii* numbers, an ATG16L1 and IDO-independent anti-*T. gondii* response may exist in HeLa cells. It has been shown that IFN-γ stimulates cell death before parasite replication, reducing the parasite number in HFFs. In addition, IFN-γ-inducible cell death is independent of ATG5 and IDOs (29). Although we have not tested cell death in 1-DL-MT-treated ATG16L1-KO HeLa cells, it is possible that IFN-γ-dependent cell death might be responsible for the ATG16L1 and IDO-independent response.

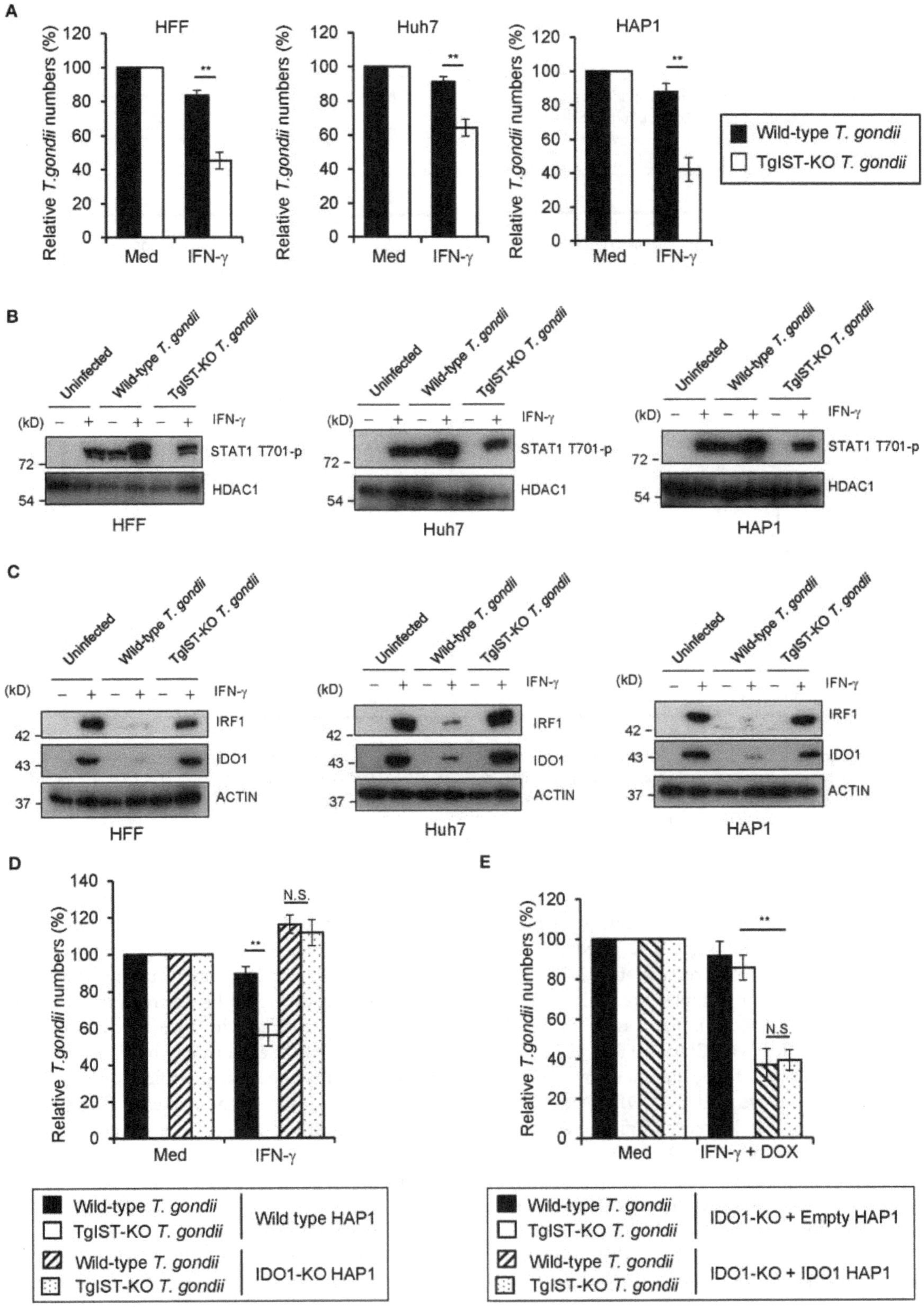

FIGURE 5 | TgIST directly inhibits IDO1 mRNA induction in IFN-γ-post-treated human cells **(A)** HFFs, Huh7, or HAP1 cells were infected with WT or TgIST-KO *T. gondii* for 8 h, and subsequently treated with IFN-γ for 24 h or untreated. The parasite survival rate after 24 h post IFN-γ treatment was measured by luciferase assay. **(B,C)** HFFs, Huh7 or HAP1 cells infected with WT or TgIST-KO *T. gondii* for 8 h or uninfected, and subsequently treated with IFN-γ for 24 h or untreated. Cell lysates

(Continued)

FIGURE 5 | were detected by Western blot to detect phospho-STAT1 and HDAC1 **(B)** or IRF1, IDO1, and Actin **(C)**. **(D)** WT or IDO1-KO HAP1 cells were infected with WT or TgIST-KO *T. gondii* for 8 h, and subsequently treated with IFN-γ for 24 h or untreated. The parasite survival rate after 24 h post IFN-γ treatment was measured by luciferase assay. **(E)** IDO1-KO + Empty or IDO1-KO + IDO1 HAP1 cells were infected with WT or TgIST-KO *T. gondii* for 8 h, and subsequently treated with IFN-γ and doxycycline for 24 h or untreated. The parasite survival rate 24 h post treatment was measured by luciferase assay. Western blot image is representative of three independent experiments **(B,C)**. Indicated values are means of ± s.d. (three biological replicates per group from three independent experiments) **(A,D,E)**. $^{**}p < 0.01$; N.S., not significant; (Student's *t*-test).

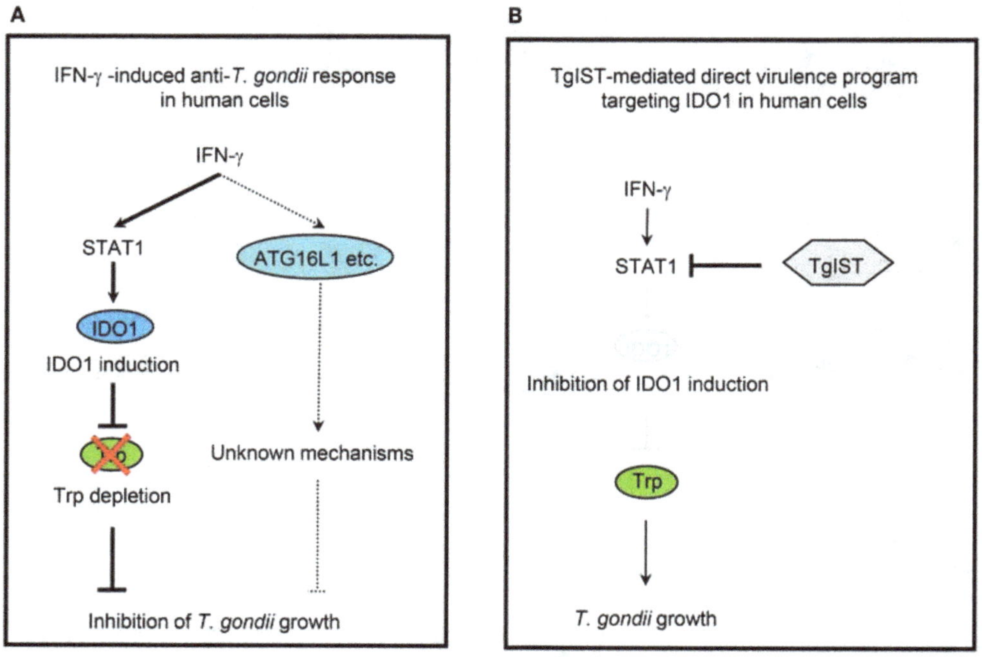

FIGURE 6 | Simplified scheme of IFN-γ-induced anti-*T. gondii* host immune response and *T. gondii* virulence programs in human cells. **(A)** IFN-γ-induced anti-*T. gondii* response in human cells. IFN-γ induce the expression of IDO1, which results in depletion of L-tryptophan (Trp), leading to inhibition of *T. gondii* growth in various human cells. IFN-γ also induce ATG16L1-dependent cell—autonomous response, but the involvement of ATG16L1 in the human IFN-γ-induced anti-*T. gondii* response is cell type-specific manner. **(B)** TgIST-mediated direct virulence program targeting IDO1 in human cells. *T. gondii* secrete effector TgIST in the infected human cells, which results in the inhibition of host STAT1-dependent gene expression, leading to directly inhibition of IDO1 mRNA induction and allowing the *T. gondii* growth.

We report a novel *T. gondii* virulence strategy in human cells, where IDO1 mRNA transcription is targeted by TgIST that directly binds to STAT1 and recruits the Mi-2/NuRD chromatin remodeling repressor complex to inhibit STAT1-dependent gene expression (47, 48). Expression of STAT1-regulated genes such as IRF1, CXCL9, CIITA, MX, GBP2, SOCS1, and ICAM1 is shown to be inhibited by TgIST in human cells (47, 48). Here we added IDO1 to the list of genes down-regulated by TgIST. Moreover, TgIST-independent (STAT1-independent) expression of IDO1 fully recovered the IFN-γ-induced growth inhibition by TgIST-sufficient parasite infection. In addition, TgIST-KO parasites can proliferate in IDO1-KO cells. Given that mRNA and protein levels of IRF1 as well as IDO1 were also inhibited in a TgIST-dependent manner, *T. gondii* may secrete TgIST to directly target STAT1 and non-specifically suppress expression of STAT1-regulated genes including IDO1 and IRF1 in the infected human cells.

In summary, we have demonstrated that IDO1 plays an important role in IFN-γ-inducible anti-*T. gondii* responses in various human cell types. Furthermore, TgIST suppresses the IFN-γ-induced anti-*T. gondii* response by directly targeting IDO1, which plays an important role in various human cells. By focusing on the difference between human and mouse immune responses, unidentified virulence mechanisms by known or unknown *T. gondii* effectors might be discovered in the future. In addition, STAT1-independent artificial induction of IDO1 could evade the TgIST-dependent virulence mechanism and offer a novel therapeutic strategy for treating human toxoplasmosis.

MATERIALS AND METHODS

Cells and Parasites

All *T. gondii* strains were maintained in Vero cells in RPMI (Nacalai Tesque) supplemented with 2% heat-inactivated FBS (JRH Bioscience), 100 U/ml penicillin, and 0.1 mg/ml streptomycin (Nacalai Tesque), as previously described (55). HAP1 cells were maintained in IMDM (Nacalai Tesque) containing 10% heat-inactivated FBS, and 100 U/ml penicillin, and 0.1 mg/ml streptomycin. HFFs, Huh7 cells were maintained in RPMI (Nacalai Tesque) containing 10% heat-inactivated FBS, and 100 U/ml penicillin, and 0.1 mg/ml streptomycin. HeLa cells and MEF cells were maintained in DMEM (Nacalai Tesque) containing 10% heat-inactivated FBS, 100 U/ml penicillin, and 0.1 mg/ml streptomycin.

Reagents

Antibodies against IDO1 (13268-1-AP), HDAC1 (10197-1-AP), and IRF1 (11335-1-AP) was obtained from Proteintech. Antibodies against Phospho-Stat1 (Tyr701) (#9167) was obtained from Cell Signaling. Antibodies against ATG16L1 (PM040) was obtained from MBL. Anti-β-actin antibody (A1978) was obtained from Sigma. Antibodies against GAP45 was described previously (56). Recombinant human and mouse IFN-γ were obtained from Peprotech. 1-Methyl-DL-tryptophan (sc-224746) was obtained from Santa Cruz Biotechnology, Inc. Aminoguanidine hydrochloride (396494) was obtained from Sigma.

Plasmid Construction for Generation of Human Cell Lines

All genomic deficient cell lines were generated with the px330 plasmid CRISPR/Cas9 system. The insert fragment of IDO1, IDO2 ATG16L1 gRNA were generated by annealing primers. All the primers used in this study are listed in **Table S1**. These insert fragments were inserted into the BbsI site of the cloning vector containing U6 promoter to generate gRNA expressing plasmids pIDO1_gRNA1, pIDO1_gRNA2, pIDO2_gRNA1, pIDO2_gRNA2, pATG16L1_gRNA1, and pATG16L1_gRNA2, respectively. The insert fragment was cut out by XhoI and SalI from the pIDO1_gRNA2, pIDO2_gRNA2, and pATG16L1_gRNA2 vector, and ligated into the XhoI site of the pIDO1_gRNA1, pIDO2_gRNA1, and pATG16L1_gRNA1 vector to generate plasmids pIDO1_gRNA1/2, pIDO2_gRNA1/2, and pATG16L1_gRNA1/2. The insert fragment was cut out by KpnI and MluI from pIDO1_gRNA1/2, pIDO2_gRNA1/2, and pATG16L1_gRNA1/2 vector, respectively, and ligated into the KpnI and MluI site of the pEF6-hCas9-Puro vector.

Generation of Gene-Targeted Human Cell Lines by CRISPR/Cas9 Genome Editing

Human cells were electroporated with the pEF6-hCas9-Puro vector containing target gRNA1/2 using NEPA21 (nepa gene). And then 24 h post-electroporation, 0.5–5 μg/ml puromycin was added for 5–10 days to select for cells with a stably integrated. Cells were plated in limiting dilution in 96-well plates to isolate single cell clones. To confirm complete target gene deficient, the IDO1, IDO2 and ATG16L1 protein expression were analyzed by Western blot. Atg16L1 KO MEF cells were described previously (12).

Plasmid Construction for Generation of Knockout *T. gondii* Strain

Plasmid pSAG1::Cas9-U6::sgUPRT that encoding Cas9 nuclease (GFP fusion) under control of the *T. gondii* SAG1 promotor was obtained from addgene (plasmid 54467). The primer sequences are listed in **Table S1**. The TgIST-targeting CRISPR/Cas9 plasmid (pSAG1::Cas9-U6::sgTgIST-1 or pSAG1::Cas9-U6::sgTgIST-2) was constructed in two steps. First, the overlap PCR method was used to generate gRNA expressing plasmids. The U6 promoter from ME49 driving expression of the TgIST specific sgRNA (pgTgIST-1 or pgTgIST-2) was amplified from pSAG1::Cas9-U6::sgUPRT. For first-step PCR, primer pairs TgU6_F and TgISTgRNA1-R, TgISTgRNA1-F and TgU6_R, TgU6_F and TgISTgRNA2-R, TgISTgRNA2-F and TgU6_R were used. For second-step PCR primer pairs TgU6_F and TgU6_R were used, and cloning it into the NotI and SacI sites of the pBluescript II SK(+) (plasmid 54467). Second, the Cas9-Ds-Red monomer cassette under the SAG1 promoter was cut out from pSAG1::Cas9-U6::sgUPRT (Ds-Red monomer fusion), and ligated into the KpnI and NotI site of the pgTgIST-1 or pgTgIST-2. To generate a construct for deleting the entire coding sequence of TgIST, flanking regions of 5′ outside the sgTgIST-1 and 3′ outside the sgTgIST-2 regions were used to surround the TgIST cassette. To generate a plasmid for inserting HXGPRT into the TgIST gene, upstream regions of sgTgIST-1 (894-bp) and downstream regions of sgTgIST-2 (670-bp) were amplified from ME49 genomic DNA by using primers TgIST targeting 5′_F and TgIST targeting 5′_R or TgIST targeting 3′_F and TgIST targeting 3′_R. These two fragments were ligated into the KpnI and XhoI or BamHI and NotI sites of pHXGPRT vector.

Generation of TgIST-KO *T. gondii* by CRISPR/Cas9 Genome Editing

Prugniaud (Pru) *T. gondii*-expressing luciferase were filtered, washed and resuspended in Cytomix (10 mM KPO_4, 120 mM KCl, 0.15 mM $CaCl_2$, 5 mM $MgCl_2$, 25 mM HEPES, 2 mM EDTA). Parasites were mixed with 50 μg of sgTgIST-1 and sgTgIST-2 CRISPR plasmid along with 40 μg of the targeting vector linearized by KpnI and SacI, and supplemented with 2 mM ATP, 5 mM GSH. Parasites were electroporated by GENE PULSER II (Bio-Rad Laboratories). Selection by growth for 14 days in 25 μg/ml mycophenolic acid (Sigma) and 25 μg/ml xanthine (Wako) were used to obtain stably resistant clone. And then parasites were plated in limiting dilution in 96-well plates to isolate single clones. To confirm the disruption of the gene encoding TgIST, we analyzed messenger RNA of TgIST from WT and TgIST-KO parasites by quantitative RT-PCR. In addition, we observed comparable *in vitro* growth and *in vivo* virulence to each other and to the parental line.

Quantitative RT-PCR

Total RNA was extracted, and cDNA was synthesized using Verso Reverse transcription (Thermo Fisher Scientic). Quantitative RT-PCR was performed with a CFX connect real-time PCR system (Bio-Rad Laboratories) using the Go-Taq Real-Time PCR system (Promega). The values were normalized to the amount of beta actin (β-actin) for human cells or tubulin for *T. gondii* in each sample. The primer sequences are listed in **Table S1**.

Western Blot Analysis

Cells were lysed in a lysis buffer (0.5% Nonidet P-40, 150 mM NaCl, and 20 mM Tris-HCl, pH 7.5) containing a protease inhibitor cocktail (Roche) and phosphatase inhibitor cocktail

(Nacalai Tesque). The cell lysates were separated by SDS-PAGE and transferred to polyvinylidene uoride membranes and subjected to Western blot analysis using the indicated antibodies as described previously (57).

Luciferase Assay

For the experiment using IFN-γ pre-stimulated cells, HFFs (6×10^5), HAP1 (2×10^6), HeLa (8×10^5), or Huh7 (6×10^5) cells were untreated or treated with 10 ng/ml IFN-γ for 24 h, and subsequently infected with the luciferase-expressing *T. gondii* (MOI = 0.5) for 24 h. For the experiment using IFN-γ post-stimulation cells, HFFs (6×10^5), HAP1 (2×10^6), HeLa (8×10^5), or Huh7 (6×10^5) cells were infected with the luciferase-expressing *T. gondii* (MOI = 0.5) for 8 h, and subsequently untreated or treated with 10 ng/ml IFN-γ for 24 h. To measure the number of *T. gondii*, all infected cells were collected and lysed by 100 µl of lysis buffer (Promega) and sonicated. After centrifugation at 20,000 × g at 4°C, the luciferase activity of the supernatant was measured using the Dual Luciferase Reporter Assay System (Promega) and GLOMAX 20/20 luminometer (Promega). The percentages of the activities in cytokines stimulated cells over those in unstimulated cells were shown as "Relative *T. gondii* numbers" in figures.

Immunofluorescence Assays

HFFs, Huh7, or HeLa cells were cultured on glass coverslips, and infected with *T. gondii* (MOI = 2) for the indicated time, and fixed in PBS containing 3.7% paraformaldehyde for 10 min at room temperature. Cells were permeabilized with PBS containing 0.002% Digitonin for 5 min and then blocked with 8% FBS in PBS for 1 h at room temperature. And then, cells were incubated with the indicated primary antibodies for 1 h at 37°C, followed by incubation with Alexa 488-, Alexa 594-, or Alexa 647-conjugated secondary antibodies (Molecular Probes) and DAPI for 1 h at 37°C in the dark. Finally, coverslips were mounted onto glass slides with PermaFluor (Thermo Scientific) and analyzed using confocal laser microscopy (FV1200 IX-83, Olympus).

IDO Activity Assay

The enzymatic IDO activity was evaluated by the calculation of the kynurenine concentration in the cell culture supernatant as previously described (58). Cells were cultured in 12-well plates and untreated or treated with 10 ng/ml IFN-γ for 24 h. The concentration of kynurenine in culture supernatant was measured using Ehrlich reagent method (59). Seventy microliters of culture supernatant was mixed with 35 µl of 30% trichloroacetic acid, and centrifuged at 8,000 x g for 5 min. Then 75 µl of the supernatant was added to an equal volume of Ehrlich reagent (0.8% p-dimethylaminobenzaldehyde in acetic acid) in a 96-well plate, and the absorbance was read at 490 nm. The values were compared with a standard curve with defined concentrations of kynurenine (Sigma Aldrich).

Statistical Analysis

All statistical analyses were performed using Excel (Microsoft). All the experimental points and n values represent an average of each three biological replicates (three independent experiments). The statistical significance of differences in mean values was analyzed by using an unpaired two-tailed Student's *t*-test. *P*-values less than 0.05 were considered to be statistically significant.

AUTHOR CONTRIBUTIONS

HB, NS, ST, YN, and MY designed the experiments. AP, JM, ST, and MS prepared the materials. HB, NS, JL, Z-RL, and MY analyzed the data. HB, NS, DL, Z-RL, and MY wrote the paper. All authors listed contributed to revised work and approved the final manuscript.

FUNDING

This work was Supported by the Research Program on Emerging and Re-emerging Infectious Diseases (18fk0108047h0002) and Japanese Initiative for Progress of Research on Infectious Diseases for global Epidemic (18fm0208018h0002) from Agency for Medical Research and Development (AMED), Grant-in-Aid for Scientific Research on Innovative Areas (17K15677) from Ministry of Education, Culture, Sports, Science and Technology, Cooperative Research Grant of the Institute for Enzyme Research, Joint Usage/Research Center, Tokushima University, Takeda Science Foundation, Mochida Memorial Foundation on Medical and Pharmaceutical Research, Uehara Memorial Foundation and Research Foundation for Microbial Diseases of Osaka University for MY and National Science Foundation of China (#31772445) for DL and Z-RL.

ACKNOWLEDGMENTS

We thank Mari Enomoto (Osaka University) for secretarial and technical assistance.

REFERENCES

1. Dubey JP. *Toxoplasmosis of Animals and Humans*. Boca; Raton, FL: CRC Press (2010).
2. Boothroyd JC. *Toxoplasma gondii*: 25 years and 25 major advances for the field. *Int J Parasitol.* (2009) 39:935–46. doi: 10.1016/j.ijpara.2009.02.003
3. Weitberg AB, Alper JC, Diamond I, Fligiel Z. Acute granulomatous hepatitis in the course of acquired toxoplasmosis. *N Engl J Med.* (1979) 300:1093–96. doi: 10.1056/NEJM197905103001907
4. Frenkel JK, Remington JS. Hepatitis in toxoplasmosis. *N Engl J Med.* (1980) 302:178–9.
5. Montoya JG, Remington JS. Management of *Toxoplasma gondii* infection during pregnancy. *Clin Infect Dis.* (2008) 47:554–66. doi: 10.1086/590149
6. Suzuki Y, Orellana MA, Schreiber RD, Remington JS. Interferon-gamma: the major mediator of resistance against *Toxoplasma gondii*. *Science* (1988) 240:516–8. doi: 10.1126/science.3128869

7. Platanias LC. Mechanisms of type-I- and type-II-interferon-mediated signalling. *Nat Rev Immunol.* (2005) 5:375–86. doi: 10.1038/nri1604
8. Yamamoto M, Okuyama M, Ma JS, Kimura T, Kamiyama N, Saiga H, et al. A cluster of interferon-gamma-inducible p65 GTPases plays a critical role in host defense against *Toxoplasma gondii*. *Immunity* (2012) 37:302–13. doi: 10.1016/j.immuni.2012.06.009
9. Gazzinelli RT, Mendonca-Neto R, Lilue J, Howard J, Sher A. Innate resistance against Toxoplasma gondii: an evolutionary tale of mice, cats, and men. *Cell Host Microbe* (2014) 15:132–8. doi: 10.1016/j.chom.2014.01.004
10. MacMicking JD. Interferon-inducible effector mechanisms in cell-autonomous immunity. *Nat Rev Immunol.* (2012) 12:367–82. doi: 10.1038/nri3210
11. Sasai M, Sakaguchi N, Ma JS, Nakamura S, Kawabata T, Bando H, et al. Essential role for GABARAP autophagy proteins in interferon-inducible GTPase-mediated host defense. *Nat Immunol.* (2017) 18:899–910. doi: 10.1038/ni.3767
12. Ohshima J, Lee Y, Sasai M, Saitoh T, Su Ma J, Kamiyama N, et al. Role of mouse and human autophagy proteins in IFN-gamma-induced cell-autonomous responses against *Toxoplasma gondii*. *J Immunol.* (2014) 192:3328–35. doi: 10.4049/jimmunol.1302822
13. Choi J, Park S, Biering SB, Selleck E, Liu CY, Zhang X, et al. The parasitophorous vacuole membrane of *Toxoplasma gondii* is targeted for disruption by ubiquitin-like conjugation systems of autophagy. *Immunity* (2014) 40:924–35. doi: 10.1016/j.immuni.2014.05.006
14. Sibley LD, Adams LB, Fukutomi Y, Krahenbuhl JL. Tumor necrosis factor-alpha triggers antitoxoplasmal activity of IFN-gamma primed macrophages. *J Immunol.* (1991) 147:2340–5.
15. Ling YM, Shaw MH, Ayala C, Coppens I, Taylor GA, Ferguson DJ, et al. Vacuolar and plasma membrane stripping and autophagic elimination of *Toxoplasma gondii* in primed effector macrophages. *J Exp Med.* (2006) 203:2063–71. doi: 10.1084/jem.20061318
16. Selleck EM, Fentress SJ, Beatty WL, Degrandi D, Pfeffer K, Virgin HWT, et al. Guanylate-binding protein 1 (Gbp1) contributes to cell-autonomous immunity against *Toxoplasma gondii*. *PLoS Pathog.* (2013) 9:e1003320. doi: 10.1371/journal.ppat.1003320
17. Degrandi D, Kravets E, Konermann C, Beuter-Gunia C, Klumpers V, Lahme S, et al. Murine guanylate binding protein 2 (mGBP2) controls Toxoplasma gondii replication. *Proc Natl Acad Sci USA.* (2013) 110:294–9. doi: 10.1073/pnas.1205635110
18. Scharton-Kersten TM, Yap G, Magram J, Sher A. Inducible nitric oxide is essential for host control of persistent but not acute infection with the intracellular pathogen *Toxoplasma gondii*. *J Exp Med.* (1997) 185:1261–73. doi: 10.1084/jem.185.7.1261
19. Collazo CM, Yap GS, Sempowski GD, Lusby KC, Tessarollo L, Woude GF, et al. Inactivation of LRG-47 and IRG-47 reveals a family of interferon gamma-inducible genes with essential, pathogen-specific roles in resistance to infection. *J Exp Med.* (2001) 194:181–8. doi: 10.1084/jem.194.2.181
20. Zhao Y, Ferguson DJ, Wilson DC, Howard JC, Sibley LD, Yap GS. Virulent Toxoplasma gondii evade immunity-related GTPase-mediated parasite vacuole disruption within primed macrophages. *J Immunol.* (2009) 182:3775–81. doi: 10.4049/jimmunol.0804190
21. Bekpen C, Hunn JP, Rohde C, Parvanova I, Guethlein L, Dunn DM, et al. The interferon-inducible p47 (IRG) GTPases in vertebrates: loss of the cell autonomous resistance mechanism in the human lineage. *Genome Biol.* (2005) 6:R92. doi: 10.1186/gb-2005-6-11-r92
22. Murray HW, Teitelbaum RF. L-arginine-dependent reactive nitrogen intermediates and the antimicrobial effect of activated human mononuclear phagocytes. *J Infect Dis.* (1992) 165:513–7. doi: 10.1093/infdis/165.3.513
23. Selleck EM, Orchard RC, Lassen KG, Beatty WL, Xavier RJ, Levine B, et al. A Noncanonical autophagy pathway restricts *Toxoplasma gondii* growth in a strain-specific manner in IFN-gamma-activated human cells. *MBio* (2015) 6:e01157-01115. doi: 10.1128/mBio.01157-15
24. Johnston AC, Piro A, Clough B, Siew M, Virreira Winter S, Coers J, et al. Human GBP1 does not localize to pathogen vacuoles but restricts *Toxoplasma gondii*. *Cell Microbiol.* (2016) 18:1056–64. doi: 10.1111/cmi.12579
25. Qin A, Lai DH, Liu Q, Huang W, Wu YP, Chen X, et al. Guanylate-binding protein 1 (GBP1) contributes to the immunity of human mesenchymal stromal cells against *Toxoplasma gondii*. *Proc Natl Acad Sci USA.* (2017) 114:1365–70. doi: 10.1073/pnas.1619665114
26. Gomez-Marin JE. No NO production during human Toxoplasma infection. *Parasitol Today* (2000) 16:131. doi: 10.1016/S0169-4758(99)01614-2
27. Clough B, Wright JD, Pereira PM, Hirst EM, Johnston AC, Henriques R, et al. K63-linked ubiquitination targets *Toxoplasma gondii* for endo-lysosomal destruction in IFNgamma-stimulated human cells. *PLoS Pathog.* (2016) 12:e1006027. doi: 10.1371/journal.ppat.1006027
28. Pfefferkorn ER. Interferon gamma blocks the growth of *Toxoplasma gondii* in human fibroblasts by inducing the host cells to degrade tryptophan. *Proc Natl Acad Sci USA.* (1984) 81:908–12. doi: 10.1073/pnas.81.3.908
29. Niedelman W, Sprokholt JK, Clough B, Frickel EM, Saeij JP. Cell death of gamma interferon-stimulated human fibroblasts upon *Toxoplasma gondii* infection induces early parasite egress and limits parasite replication. *Infect Immun.* (2013) 81:4341–9. doi: 10.1128/IAI.00416-13
30. Pfefferkorn ER, Eckel M, Rebhun S. Interferon-gamma suppresses the growth of *Toxoplasma gondii* in human fibroblasts through starvation for tryptophan. *Mol. Biochem. Parasitol.* (1986) 20:215–24.
31. Pfefferkorn ER, Rebhun S, Eckel M. Characterization of an indoleamine 2,3-dioxygenase induced by gamma-interferon in cultured human fibroblasts. *J Interferon Res.* (1986) 6:267–79. doi: 10.1089/jir.1986.6.267
32. Heseler K, Spekker K, Schmidt SK, MacKenzie CR, Daubener W. Antimicrobial and immunoregulatory effects mediated by human lung cells: role of IFN-gamma-induced tryptophan degradation. *FEMS Immunol Med Microbiol.* (2008) 52:273–81. doi: 10.1111/j.1574-695X.2007.00374.x
33. Ball HJ, Sanchez-Perez A, Weiser S, Austin CJ, Astelbauer F, Miu J, et al. Characterization of an indoleamine 2,3-dioxygenase-like protein found in humans and mice. *Gene* (2007) 396:203–13. doi: 10.1016/j.gene.2007.04.010
34. Murakami Y, Hoshi M, Hara A, Takemura M, Arioka Y, Yamamoto Y, et al. Inhibition of increased indoleamine 2,3-dioxygenase activity attenuates *Toxoplasma gondii* replication in the lung during acute infection. *Cytokine* (2012) 59:245–51. doi: 10.1016/j.cyto.2012.04.022
35. Qian F, Liao J, Villella J, Edwards R, Kalinski P, Lele S, et al. Effects of 1-methyltryptophan stereoisomers on IDO2 enzyme activity and IDO2-mediated arrest of human T cell proliferation. *Cancer Immunol Immunother.* (2012) 61:2013–20. doi: 10.1007/s00262-012-1265-x
36. Yuasa HJ, Ball HJ, Austin CJ, Hunt NH. 1-L-methyltryptophan is a more effective inhibitor of vertebrate IDO2 enzymes than 1-D-methyltryptophan. *Comp Biochem Physiol. B Biochem Mol Biol.* (2010) 157:10–5. doi: 10.1016/j.cbpb.2010.04.006
37. Hunter CA Sibley LD. Modulation of innate immunity by *Toxoplasma gondii* virulence effectors. *Nat Rev Microbiol.* (2012) 10:766–78. doi: 10.1038/nrmicro2858
38. Hakimi MA, Olias P, Sibley LD. Toxoplasma effectors targeting host signaling and transcription. *Clin Microbiol Rev.* (2017) 30:615–45. doi: 10.1128/CMR.00005-17
39. Steinfeldt T, Konen-Waisman S, Tong L, Pawlowski N, Lamkemeyer T, Sibley LD, et al. Phosphorylation of mouse immunity-related GTPase (IRG) resistance proteins is an evasion strategy for virulent *Toxoplasma gondii*. *PLoS Biol.* (2010) 8:e1000576. doi: 10.1371/journal.pbio.1000576
40. Reese ML, Zeiner GM, Saeij JP, Boothroyd JC, Boyle JP. Polymorphic family of injected pseudokinases is paramount in Toxoplasma virulence. *Proc Natl Acad Sci USA.* (2011) 108:9625–30. doi: 10.1073/pnas.1015980108
41. Fentress SJ, Behnke MS, Dunay IR, Mashayekhi M, Rommereim LM, Fox BA, et al. Phosphorylation of immunity-related GTPases by a *Toxoplasma gondii*-secreted kinase promotes macrophage survival and virulence. *Cell Host Microbe* (2010) 8:484–95. doi: 10.1016/j.chom.2010.11.005
42. Behnke MS, Khan A, Wootton JC, Dubey JP, Tang K, Sibley LD. Virulence differences in Toxoplasma mediated by amplification of a family of polymorphic pseudokinases. *Proc Natl Acad Sci USA.* (2011) 108:9631–6. doi: 10.1073/pnas.1015338108
43. Etheridge RD, Alaganan A, Tang K, Lou HJ, Turk BE, Sibley LD. The Toxoplasma pseudokinase ROP5 forms complexes with ROP18 and ROP17 kinases that synergize to control acute virulence in mice. *Cell Host Microbe* (2014) 15:537–50. doi: 10.1016/j.chom.2014.04.002

44. Alaganan A, Fentress SJ, Tang K, Wang Q, Sibley LD. Toxoplasma GRA7 effector increases turnover of immunity-related GTPases and contributes to acute virulence in the mouse. *Proc Natl Acad Sci USA.* (2014) 111:1126–31. doi: 10.1073/pnas.1313501111
45. Rosowski EE, Saeij JP. *Toxoplasma gondii* clonal strains all inhibit STAT1 transcriptional activity but polymorphic effectors differentially modulate IFNgamma induced gene expression and STAT1 phosphorylation. *PLoS ONE* (2012) 7:e51448. doi: 10.1371/journal.pone.0051448
46. Rosowski EE, Nguyen QP, Camejo A, Spooner E, Saeij JP. *Toxoplasma gondii* Inhibits gamma interferon (IFN-gamma)- and IFN-beta-induced host cell STAT1 transcriptional activity by increasing the association of STAT1 with DNA. *Infect Immun.* (2014) 82:706–19. doi: 10.1128/IAI.01291-13
47. Olias P, Etheridge RD, Zhang Y, Holtzman MJ, Sibley LD. Toxoplasma effector recruits the Mi-2/NuRD complex to repress STAT1 transcription and block IFN-gamma-dependent gene expression. *Cell Host Microbe* (2016) 20:72–82. doi: 10.1016/j.chom.2016.06.006
48. Gay G, Braun L, Brenier-Pinchart MP, Vollaire J, Josserand V, Bertini RL, et al. *Toxoplasma gondii* TgIST co-opts host chromatin repressors dampening STAT1-dependent gene regulation and IFN-gamma-mediated host defenses. *J Exp Med.* (2016) 213:1779–98. doi: 10.1084/jem.20160340
49. Niedelman W, Gold DA, Rosowski EE, Sprokholt JK, Lim D, Farid Arenas A, et al. The rhoptry proteins ROP18 and ROP5 mediate *Toxoplasma gondii* evasion of the murine, but not the human, interferon-gamma response. *PLoS Pathog.* (2012) 8:e1002784. doi: 10.1371/journal.ppat.1002784
50. Yamamoto S, Hayaishi O. Tryptophan pyrrolase of rabbit intestine. D- and L-tryptophan-cleaving enzyme or enzymes. *J Biol Chem.* (1967) 242:5260–6.
51. Woodman JP, Dimier IH, Bout DT. Human endothelial cells are activated by IFN-gamma to inhibit *Toxoplasma gondii* replication. Inhibition is due to a different mechanism from that existing in mouse macrophages and human fibroblasts. *J Immunol.* (1991) 147:2019–23.
52. Sotero-Esteva WD, Wolfe D, Ferris M, Taylor MW. An indoleamine 2,3-dioxygenase-negative mutant is defective in stat1 DNA binding: differential response to IFN-gamma and IFN-alpha. *J Interferon Cytokine Res.* (2000) 20:623–32. doi: 10.1089/107999000414790
53. Mizushima N, Yoshimori T, Levine B. Methods in mammalian autophagy research. *Cell* (2010) 140:313–26. doi: 10.1016/j.cell.2010.01.028
54. Klionsky DJ, Abdelmohsen K, Abe A, Abedin MJ, Abeliovich H, Acevedo Arozena A, et al. Guidelines for the use and interpretation of assays for monitoring autophagy (3rd edition). *Autophagy* (2016) 12:1–222. doi: 10.1080/15548627.2015.1100356
55. Ma JS, Sasai M, Ohshima J, Lee Y, Bando H, Takeda K, et al. Selective and strain-specific NFAT4 activation by the *Toxoplasma gondii* polymorphic dense granule protein GRA6. *J Exp Med.* (2014) 211:2013–32. doi: 10.1084/jem.20131272
56. Terkawi MA, Kameyama K, Rasul NH, Xuan X, Nishikawa Y. Development of an immunochromatographic assay based on dense granule protein 7 for serological detection of *Toxoplasma gondii* infection. *Clin Vaccine Immunol.* (2013) 20:596–601. doi: 10.1128/CVI.00747-12
57. Yamamoto M, Standley DM, Takashima S, Saiga H, Okuyama M, Kayama H, et al. A single polymorphic amino acid on *Toxoplasma gondii* kinase ROP16 determines the direct and strain-specific activation of Stat3. *J Exp Med.* (2009) 206:2747–60. doi: 10.1084/jem.20091703
58. Daubener W, Wanagat N, Pilz K, Seghrouchni S, Fischer HG, Hadding U. A new, simple, bioassay for human IFN-gamma. *J Immunol Methods* (1994) 168:39–47. doi: 10.1016/0022-1759(94)90207-0
59. Braun D, Longman RS, Albert ML. A two-step induction of indoleamine 2,3 dioxygenase (IDO) activity during dendritic-cell maturation. *Blood* (2005) 106:2375–81. doi: 10.1182/blood-2005-03-0979

7

Trypanosoma cruzi Exploits Wnt Signaling Pathway to Promote its Intracellular Replication in Macrophages

*Ximena Volpini[1,2], Laura F. Ambrosio[1,2], Laura Fozzatti[1,2], Constanza Insfran[1,2], Cinthia C. Stempin[1,2], Laura Cervi[1,2] and Claudia Cristina Motran[1,2]**

[1] Departamento de Bioquímica Clínica, Facultad de Ciencias Químicas, Universidad Nacional de Córdoba, Córdoba, Argentina, [2] Centro de Investigaciones en Bioquímica Clínica e Inmunología (CIBICI), CONICET, Haya de la Torre y Medina Allende, Ciudad Universitaria, Córdoba, Argentina

***Correspondence:**
Claudia Cristina Motran
cmotran@fcq.unc.edu.ar

During the acute phase of *Trypanosoma cruzi* infection, macrophages can act as host cells for the parasites as well as effector cells in the early anti-parasitic immune response. Thus, the targeting of specific signaling pathways could modulate macrophages response to restrict parasite replication and instruct an appropriate adaptive response. Recently, it has become evident that Wnt signaling has immunomodulatory functions during inflammation and infection. Here, we tested the hypothesis that during *T. cruzi* infection, the activation of Wnt signaling pathway in macrophages plays a role in modulating the inflammatory/tolerogenic response and therefore regulating the control of parasite replication. In this report, we show that early after *T. cruzi* infection of bone marrow-derived macrophages (BMM), β-catenin was activated and Wnt3a, Wnt5a, and some Frizzled receptors as well as Wnt/β-catenin pathway's target genes were upregulated, with Wnt proteins signaling sustaining the activation of Wnt/β-catenin pathway and then activating the Wnt/Ca^{+2} pathway. Wnt signaling pathway activation was critical to sustain the parasite's replication in BMM; since the treatments with specific inhibitors of β-catenin transcriptional activation or Wnt proteins secretion limited the parasite replication. Mechanistically, inhibition of Wnt signaling pathway armed BMM to fight against *T. cruzi* by inducing the production of pro-inflammatory cytokines and indoleamine 2,3-dioxygenase activity and by downregulating arginase activity. Likewise, *in vivo* pharmacological inhibition of the Wnts' interaction with its receptors controlled the parasite replication and improved the survival of lethally infected mice. It is well established that *T. cruzi* infection activates a plethora of signaling pathways that ultimately regulate immune mediators to determine the modulation of a defined set of effector functions in macrophages. In this study, we have revealed a new signaling pathway that is activated by the interaction between protozoan parasites and host innate immunity, establishing a new conceptual framework for the development of new therapies.

Keywords: ***Trypanosoma cruzi*** **infection, Wnt proteins, beta-catenin, macrophages, cytokines, indoleamine 2,3-dioxygenase**

INTRODUCTION

Chagas' disease, caused by the protozoan parasite *Trypanosoma cruzi*, represents a major cause of heart disease and cardiovascular-related deaths in endemic areas and causes a significant economic burden on the affected countries. Approximately 8 million people are infected with *T. cruzi* in Central and South America, and at least 120 million are at risk of infection (1). Currently, there are no vaccines available to prevent Chagas disease, and treatment options are limited to anti-parasitic drugs that are expensive, not well tolerated, and effective only during short periods of the acute phase (2).

The entry of metacyclic trypomastigotes (Tps) of *T. cruzi* into the mammalian host initiates the invasion by these parasites of several host cell types where they are converted into amastigotes, which are the replicative form of this parasite (3). During the acute phase of the infection macrophages represent an important target of *Trypanosoma cruzi* and therefore, these cells are central for the control of this pathogen. Within macrophages, the replication of *T. cruzi* can be either inhibited or favored leading to the dissemination of the parasite (4). Thus, it has been reported that during the early phase of infection, the control *T. cruzi* parasitism is dependent on macrophage activation through toll-like receptors (TLRs) and their subsequent activation by pro-inflammatory cytokines. Activated macrophages upregulate inducible nitric oxide synthase (iNOS) and indoleamine 2,3-dioxygenase (IDO) enzymes, leading to the production of nitric oxide (NO) and kynurenines, with both being important effector molecules that induce death of the amastigotes (5–9). The protective mechanisms of cell-mediated immunity (Th1 cells) are required for the resistance during this infection; nevertheless, unbalanced Th1 cells can also orchestrate a deleterious response that can cause tissue damage and fibrosis, since high levels of NO, IFN-γ, and tumor necrosis factor (TNF) have been associated with the pathogenesis of chronic Chagas disease (10–14). Therefore, a better understanding of the cellular and molecular mechanisms that orchestrate the different signals that promote the effective macrophage activation (able to restrict parasite replication) followed by its opportune contraction to prevent immunopathology is mandatory to design improved therapeutic strategies.

The Wnt pathway is an evolutionarily highly conserved signaling system that plays a critical role in cellular development, motility, polarization, survival, and proliferation (15, 16). In the last years, emerging studies have highlighted that the Wnt signaling pathway, particularly in dendritic cells (DC) and macrophages, plays a major role in regulating tolerance versus immunity. Members of the Wnt family are lipid-modified glycoproteins secreted by different cell types that bind to G-protein-coupled receptors of the Frizzled (Fzd) family and different coreceptors to activate a signaling cascade involved in complex mechanisms of gene regulation. In mice and human, 19 ligands secreted glycoproteins of the Wnt family, 10 seven-transmembrane receptors of the Fzd family, as well as several coreceptors or alternative receptors are known (16, 17). Depending on the composition of the Wnt–Fzd-coreceptor complex and the cellular context, Wnt proteins can initiate at least three different intracellular signaling cascades that regulate many cellular events: the Wnt/β-catenin called canonical pathway, the Wnt/Planar cell polarity pathway, and the Wnt/Ca^{+2} pathway (18, 19). In resting state, cytosolic/nuclear β-catenin is maintained at a very low level through rapid turnover of free β-catenin. This turnover is executed through a multi-protein complex, termed the β-catenin destruction complex, integrated by AXIN1/2, adenomatous polyposis coli, casein kinase I-alpha, and glycogen synthase kinase 3 beta (GSK-3β). GSK-3β sequentially phosphorylates β-catenin with β-catenin hyperphosphorylated subjected to ubiquitination and proteasomal degradation. Activation of Wnt/β-catenin signaling pathway results in the inhibition of the activity of GSK-3β, which leads to the accumulation of β-catenin in the cytoplasm and its translocation to the nucleus, where it interacts with T-cell factor/lymphoid enhancer factor family members and regulates the transcription of several target genes (16, 17). While canonical Wnt signaling has been extensively studied from the view point of innate and adaptive immune response, the non-canonical Wnt/Ca^{+2} signaling cascade has been less focused on. The binding of Wnt ligand to cognate Fzd receptor leads to the activation of calcium/calmodulin-dependent kinase II (CaMKII) and protein kinase C (PKC). Both CaMKII and PKC activate many nuclear transcription factors as NF-κB and CREB. Similarly, calcium ions can activate widely expressed protein phosphatase calcineurin that can activate cytoplasmic protein nuclear factor associated with T cells (NFAT) *via* dephosphorylation. This event results in accumulation, nuclear translocation and transcription of several NFAT target genes, including pro-inflammatory genes in lymphocytes (20).

Human and murine DC and macrophages express various receptors and Wnt proteins and are susceptible to both canonical and non-canonical signaling, and recently, several studies have emphasized the important role of DC and macrophages Wnt/β-catenin pathway in regulating inflammatory responses to microbial infections (21, 22). In DC, the activation of canonical and Wnt/Ca^{+2} pathways is associated with the development of a tolerogenic profile, secretion of anti-inflammatory cytokines, induction of Treg cells, and the inhibition of the adaptive immune response (23–28). However, Wnt pathways activation in macrophages may have both pro- and anti-inflammatory consequences, and different Wnt proteins may effectively cross-regulate each other in macrophages [reviewed in Ref. (21, 29)]. Wnt proteins and Fzd receptors are induced by STAT3-, TLR2-, TLR4-, and NF-κB-mediated signaling and, in addition to direct activation of β-catenin by Wnt proteins, TLR-mediated signals can also directly activate β-catenin (21, 26, 28, 30–37). Considering that TLR2 and TLR4 are involved in the recognition of different *T. cruzi* components (38–40), here we tested the hypothesis that during *T. cruzi* infection, the activation of Wnt signaling pathway in macrophages plays a role modulating the inflammatory/tolerogenic response and therefore regulating the control of intracellular parasite replication.

MATERIALS AND METHODS

Mice and Parasites

All animal experiments were approved by and conducted in accordance with guidelines of the Animal Care and Use Committee of the Facultad de Ciencias Químicas, Universidad

Nacional de Córdoba (Approval Number HCD 831/15). C57BL/6 (B6) was obtained from School of Veterinary, La Plata National University (La Plata, Argentina). All animals were housed in the Animal Facility of the Facultad de Ciencias Químicas, Universidad Nacional de Córdoba (OLAW Assurance number A5802-01). The Tulahuen strain of *T. cruzi* was used, which was maintained by weekly i.p. inoculations in mice.

Reagents

Macrophages were cultured in complete medium: RPMI 1640 (Gibco, ThermoFisher Scientific) supplemented with 2 mM GlutaMAX (Gibco, ThermoFisher Scientific), 10% heat-inactivated fetal calf serum (Gibco, Thermo Fisher), and 50 μg/mL Gentamicin (Gibco, ThermoFisher Scientific). PBS was purchased from Gibco (ThermoFisher Scientific); bovine serum albumin and DMSO were obtained from Sigma-Aldrich.

Cells

Bone marrow-derived macrophages (BMM) were generated as described previously (41). Peritoneal macrophages (PM) were obtained as described previously (42). J774 murine macrophages and the human monocytic THP-1 cell lines were obtained from the American Type Culture Collection (Manassas, VA, USA). THP-1 cell line was differentiated into macrophages by culture in complete medium supplemented with of 50 nM phorbol 12-myristate 13-acetate (Sigma-Aldrich) for 24 h followed by 24 h of incubation in complete medium.

In Vitro Infections and Treatments

Mo were incubated with LiCl (10 mM, #746460 Sigma-Aldrich), BIO (5 μM, #3194 TOCRIS), iCRT14 (50 μM, #4299, TOCRIS), CCT036477 (20 μM, #BML-WN114, ENZO), IWP-L6 (20 μM, #504819, Calbiochem), IFN-γ (10 ng/mL, Sigma-Aldrich) plus LPS (10 μg/mL, from *Escherichia coli* serotype 0111:B4, Sigma-Aldrich), 1-methyl-D-tryptophan (1-MT, #860646, Sigma-Aldrich) or complete medium before being infected with *T. cruzi* Tps (Mo:Tps = 1:3). Culture medium with PBS or DMSO was used as vehicle control for LiCl and 1-MT or iCRT14, CCT036477, and IWP-L6, respectively. MeBIO (5 μM, #3873, TOCRIS) was used as control of BIO.

In Vitro Trypanocidal Activity Assay

The growth of parasites in Mos was evaluated by counting the intracellular amastigotes by immunofluorescence assay using serum of patient with chronic Chagas disease as described previously (8). The number of intracellular amastigotes was calculated by dividing intracellular parasites (*n*/200 cells) in differentially treated cultures by number of intracellular parasites (*n*/200 cells) in the corresponding vehicle-treated cultures, and expressed as relative units.

Western Blotting

Spleen cells or BMM treated with RIPA buffer were analyzed by 10% SDS-PAGE and transferred to a nitrocellulose membrane. After blocking with 5% milk the membranes were incubated with the following antibodies: anti-β-catenin (15B8, eBioscience), anti-p-Ser552-β-catenin (D8E11, Cell Signaling), anti-NFATc1 (7A6, Santa Cruz Biotechnology), anti-p-Thr286-CaMKII (D21E4, Cell Signaling), anti-p-Ser9-GSK-3β (37F11, Cell Signaling), anti-Wnt3a (ab19925-100 polyclonal, Abcam), anti-Wnt5a (ab72583 polyclonal, Abcam), anti-IDO antibody (Santa Cruz Biotechnology) followed by anti-rabbit or -mouse fluor-coupled secondary antibody. Anti-β-actin (mAbcam8226, Abcam) was used as loading control. The blots were revealed by incubation with corresponding IRD Fluor 800-labeled IgG or IRD Fluor 680-labeled IgG secondary antibody (LI-COR Inc., Lincoln, NE, USA) for 1 h at room temperature. After washing, the membranes were scanned with the Odyssey infrared imaging system (LI-COR, Lincoln, NE, USA) at a wavelength of 700–800 nm. Densitometric analysis was performed using ImageJ software.

β-Catenin and NFATc1 Immunofluorescence

The cells were fixed in 4% formaldehyde and perm with 10% TritonX-100 for 15 min, washed three times with 0.01 M PBS, and incubated with 5% bovine serum albumin (Sigma-Aldrich) for 1 h for blocking. The sections were then incubated overnight at 4°C with anti-β-catenin (15B8, eBioscience) or anti-NFATc1 (7A6, Santa Cruz Biotechnology) primary antibodies. Next, the cells were washed three times with 0.01 M PBS, incubated with secondary antibody Alexa Fluor 488-conjugated Goat anti-Mouse IgG (#A11001, Invitrogen) for 4 h and washed three times with 0.01 M PBS. For nuclear counterstaining, the cells were incubated with 4′,6-diamidino-2-phenylindone (Cell Signaling Technology, #4083) for 10 min, washed in 1× PBS, and the slides were set with FluorSave™ reagent (EMD Millipore). Expression and localization of beta-catenin were observed with an Olympus FV1200 laser scanning confocal microscope (Olympus Corporation) with fixed exposure time for all samples. Colocalization was quantified as a ratio of overlapping pixels to the total number of pixels by Threshold Mander's coefficient and expressed as nuclear percentage (% nuclear). The preparations were visualized using confocal microscopy (Olympus FV1200), and the analyses of images were carried out using FIJI/ImageJ.

Measurement of Cytokine Production

Cytokines were measured in culture supernatants of BMM 24 h post-infection (pi) by capture ELISA using antibodies and protocols suggested by the manufacturer (eBioscience). The cytokine concentration was expressed as index of cytokine release (Index) obtained by dividing the cytokine release of inhibitors/activators-treated BMM by the cytokine release of vehicle-treated BMM.

Quantitative Real-Time-PCR (q-PCR)

RNA was extracted from BMM by the Trizol reagent (Invitrogen, ThermoFisher Scientific) and reverse-transcribed into cDNA by using Revert Aid First Strand cDNA Synthesis (Fermentas). Transcripts were quantified by real-time quantitative PCR on an StepOnePlus™ Real-Time System (ThermoFisher Scientific) using SYBR Green (ThermoFisher Scientific) with the following primers (all primers listed in the 5′ to 3′ orientation): *Wnt3a* TTC TTA CTT GAG GGC GGA GA (forward) and CTG TCG GGT CAA GAG AGG AG (reverse); *Wnt5a* GCA GGA CTT TCT CAA

GGA CA (forward) and CCC TGC CAA AGA CAG AAG TA (reverse); *Ctnnb1* AGC CGA GAT GGC CCA GAA T (forward) and AAG GGC AAG GTT TCG AAT CAA (reverse); *Ccnd1* AGT GCG TGC AGA AGG AGA TT (forward) and CAC AAC TTC TCG GCA GTC AA (reverse); *Axin1* CTG GGC TTG TAT CCC ACT GT (forward) and ACC AAG CTG GTG GCT AGA GA (reverse); *Wisp1* CTG GAC AGA AAA GGG CAT GT (forward) and AGG AAG GAG GGG AAA TCT CA (reverse); *Fzd4* CTG CAG CAT GCC TAA TGA GA (forward) and CGT CTG CCT AGA TGC AAT CA (reverse); *Fzd6* TCC GAC GCT TGA AGA AAA CT (forward) and CAA CCC CAG GTC CTC AAG TA (reverse); *Fzd8* GCA GCA TGT TCG CTA TGA AA (forward) and AGT AGC CTG CTA TGG CCT CA (reverse); *Fzd9* AGA GCC TGT GCT ACC GAA AA (forward) and CAA GGA GGG AGC AAC CAT AA (reverse); *Actb* CGC CAC CAG TTC GCC ATG GA (forward) and TAC AGC CCG GGG AGC ATC GT (reverse). Relative expression was normalized to β-actin (*Actb*) and expressed as mRNA relative levels. The cycling conditions included a hot start at 95°C for 10 min, followed by 40 cycles at 95°C for 15 s and 60°C for 1 min. Specificity was verified by melting curve analysis and agarose gel electrophoresis.

Arginase and IDO Activity

Arginase and IDO assays were performed as described previously (8, 43) with cell lysates that had been cultured in different conditions as indicated in the figure legends.

NO Assay

The production of NO was measured indirectly by assaying nitrites in the culture supernatant using the Griess reaction as described previously (8).

Lactate Dehydrogenase (LDH) Assay

Lactate dehydrogenase release was measured in the supernatant of BMM using LDH colorimetric assay kit (Wiener Lab) following the manufacturer's protocol and expressed as international units (I/U).

IWP-L6 Treatment

Groups of 6 mice (6–8 weeks old) maintained under standard conditions were infected with 5,000 bloodstream *T. cruzi* Tps by the i.p. route. On days 5, 8, 11, and 14 pi, mice were treated with IWP-L6 (7.5 mg/kg/dose) by the i.p. route. We resuspended IWP-L6 in DMSO (10 mg/mL) and then injected diluted in PBS, with this vehicle also being employed as a negative control. The levels of parasitemia were monitored every 2 days as described earlier, and the number of deaths was recorded daily. Determination of tissue parasitism was assessed in heart and liver obtained from 180-day-infected IWP-L6 or control mice as described previously (7).

Statistical Analysis

Statistical analyses were performed using Student's *t*-test, and two-way ANOVA followed by Bonferroni's post-test for comparing more than two groups. The Kaplan–Meier analysis test was used for comparing survival of control and treated mice. Percent survival at each time was also compared by using the log-rank and Gehan–Breslow–Wilcoxon tests. The results were considered significantly different when $P < 0.05$.

RESULTS

T. cruzi Infection Promotes Wnt Signaling Pathway Activation in Spleen Cells

Trypanosoma cruzi-infected B6 mice have great difficulty in controlling inflammatory response, resulting in the premature death of these animals by liver failure. Interestingly, we have observed that B6, unlike BALB/c mice, did not expand the population of Treg cells in parallel with the large expansion undergone by the T cell compartment resulting in an increased ratio of T effector/Treg cells (not shown). These results suggest that, as observed in patients with severe chronic Chagas disease cardiomyopathy (12, 44), the fatal outcome in B6 mice may be linked to an unbalanced inflammatory response. For that, although in *T. cruzi*-infected B6 mice the main target organ of pathological inflammatory response is the liver, and not the heart as in infected human patients, we performed the experiments in B6 mice to evaluate both parasite replication and inflammatory pathology.

To study whether experimental infection with *T. cruzi* induces the production of Wnt pathway proteins, the expression of the most common inflammation-linked Wnt proteins such as Wnt3a and Wnt5a, and β-catenin was evaluated in spleen cells from infected B6 mice at different times pi. **Figure 1** shows that, as *T. cruzi* infection progresses, the expression of Wnt3a, Wnt5a, and β-catenin is positively regulated in spleen cells. These results suggest that *T. cruzi* recognition induces in spleen cells the expression of Wnt proteins that could signal for the activation of the Wnt/β catenin canonical pathway, taking into account the accumulation of β-catenin.

T. cruzi Infection Induces Expression of Wnt Proteins and Fzd Receptors in Macrophages

To evaluate whether *T. cruzi* experimental infection induces the expression of proteins involved in Wnt signaling in macrophages, BMM were *in vitro* infected with *T. cruzi* Tps and the expression of Wnt3a and Wnt5a transcripts and proteins determined by q-PCR and Western blot. **Figures 2A,B** show that *in vitro* infection of BMM with *T. cruzi* induced the expression of Wnt5a and Wnt3a transcripts and proteins. The evaluation by means of q-PCR of the transcripts corresponding to Fzd receptors that most strongly interact with Wnt3a and Wnt5a, such as Fzd4, Fzd6, Fzd8, and Fzd9 (45), revealed that as early as 5 min pi, there is an increase in the transcription of these genes (**Figure 2C**), suggesting that after the recognition of *T. cruzi* by innate immune receptors start the transcription of Wnt proteins that could signal through Fzd receptors to activate the Wnt signaling pathways.

T. cruzi Infection Induces First β-Catenin Activation and Then Activates Wnt/Ca^{+2} Pathway in Macrophages

To evaluate whether *T. cruzi* infection activates β-catenin in BMM, the kinetics of expression of β-catenin (mRNA and protein) and

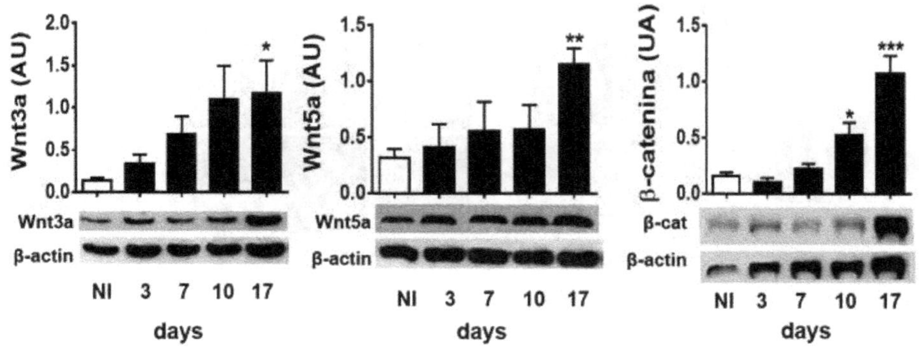

FIGURE 1 | Experimental *Trypanosoma cruzi* infection induces the expression of Wnt pathway proteins. Western blot analysis of Wnt3a, Wnt5a, and β-catenin expression in spleen mononuclear cell homogenates derived from uninfected (NI) or *T. cruzi*-infected B6 mice at different times post-infection. Images show one representative NI and one infected mice by time point. Each bar represents the mean ± SEM of protein relative expression levels quantified by scanning the intensity of bands areas in the homogenates normalized to β-actin ($n = 5$ mice per time point) (*$P < 0.05$; **$P < 0.01$; and ***$P < 0.001$).

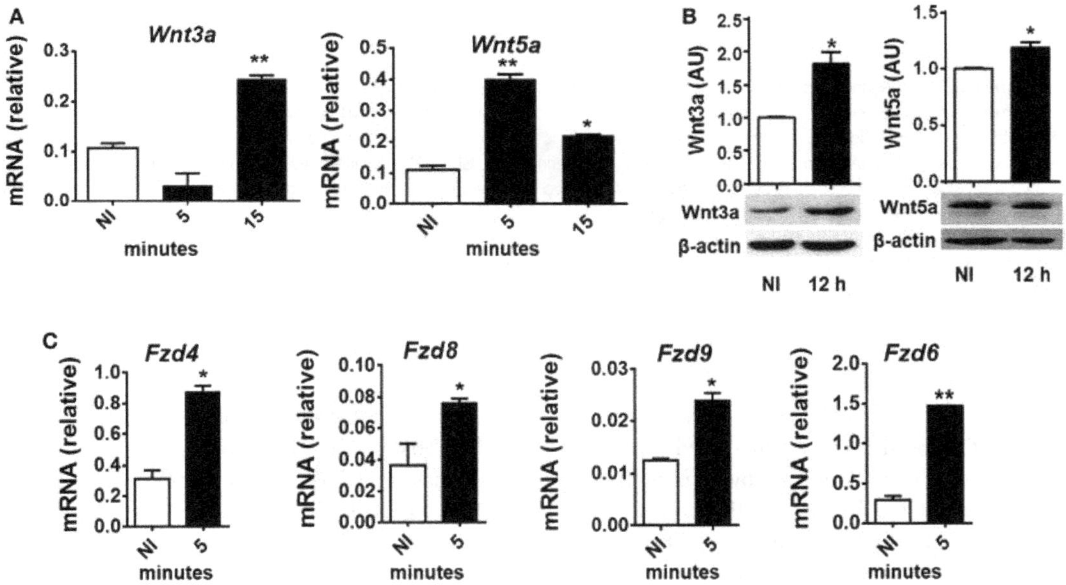

FIGURE 2 | *In vitro Trypanosoma cruzi* infection induces expression of Wnt proteins, Frizzled (Fzd) receptors, and β-catenin macrophages. Bone marrow-derived macrophages were *in vitro* infected with *T. cruzi* trypomastigotes or left uninfected (NI) and then evaluated for expression of Wnt proteins and Fzd receptors at different times post-infection (pi). **(A)** Expression of Wnt3a and Wnt5a mRNA (relative to β-actin) was determined by quantitative real-time-PCR. **(B)** The relative abundance of Wnt3, Wnt5a, and β-actin in the cell lysates were determined by Western blot and densitometry at 12 h pi. Representative Western blot and the ratio of Wnt3a or Wnt5a to β-actin are shown. **(C)** Expression of Fzd4, Fzd8, Fzd9, and Fzd6 mRNA (relative to β-actin) was determined by q-PCR. The results are expressed as the average of three independent experiments ± SEM. Abbreviation: AU, arbitrary units (*$P < 0.05$ and **$P < 0.01$).

its translocation to the nucleus were evaluated in *in vitro*-infected BMM at different times pi. At very short times after the infection (5 min), a significant increase in the transcription of the gene coding for β-catenin (*Ctnnb1*) was detected (**Figure 3A**), while the protein expression and translocation to the nucleus began at 2 h pi and reached the maximum between 8 and 12 h pi (**Figures 3A,B**). Moreover, the upregulation of Wnt/β-catenin pathway-target genes transcription, such as *Wisp1*, *Axin1*, and *Ccnd1*, correlates with β-catenin accumulation and nucleus translocation (**Figure 3C**). In addition, accumulation of β-catenin was observed in PM from B6-infected mice obtained at 24 h pi (**Figure 3D**). Taken together, our results showed that *in vitro* and *in vivo T. cruzi* infection was associated with significant activation of the genes and proteins involved in the canonical Wnt signaling pathway in macrophages.

Next, we tested whether *T. cruzi* infection is also able to activate Wnt/Ca^{+2} pathway by analyzing the expression of CaMKII phosphorylated at Thr286 [phosphorylated CAMKII (p-CAMKII)] and the activation and nuclear translocation of NFATc1. As shown in **Figure 4A**, *T. cruzi* infection led to an increase in the phosphorylation of CaMKII at Thr286 from 12 h pi. We also detected an induced NFATc1 activation after 18 h pi as measured

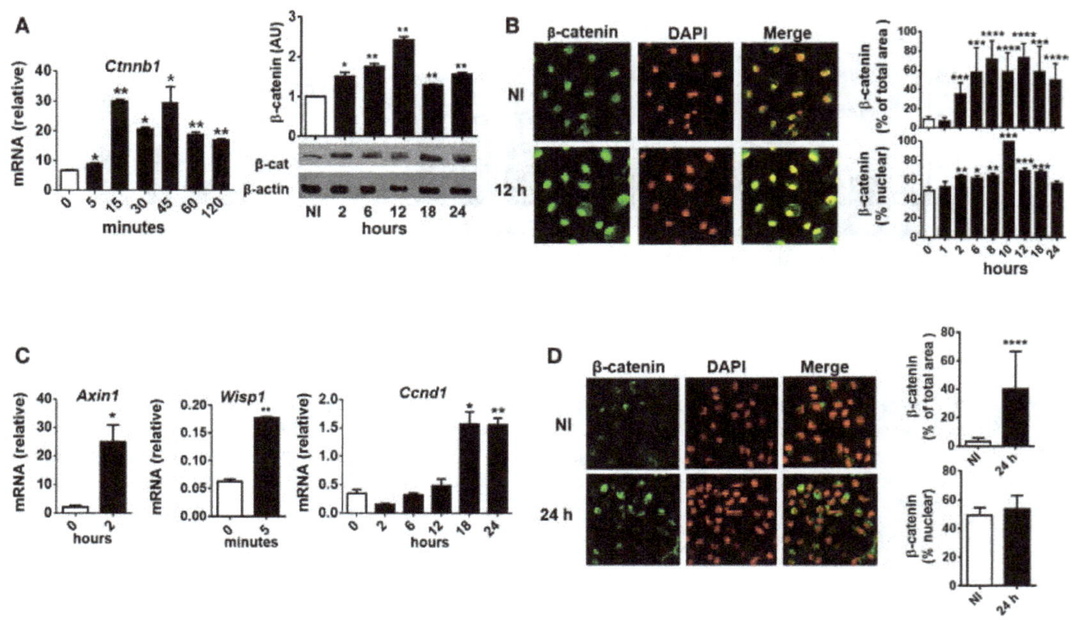

FIGURE 3 | *Trypanosoma cruzi* infection induces early β-catenin activation in macrophages. Bone marrow-derived macrophages were *in vitro* infected with trypomastigotes of *T. cruzi* or left uninfected (NI) and then evaluated for β-catenin activation. **(A)** mRNA and protein expression levels of β-catenin by q-PCR and Western blot at different times post-infection (pi). β-Catenin mRNA relative to β-actin is shown. A representative Western blot and the ratio of β-catenin to β-actin are shown. The results are expressed as the average of three independent experiments ± SEM. Abbreviation: AU, arbitrary units. **(B)** Expression and localization of β-catenin by immunofluorescence and confocal microscopy. **(C)** mRNA relative expression of β-catenin target genes Axin1, Wisp1, and Ccnd1 by q-PCR. mRNA expression levels normalized over the expression of β-actin are expressed as the average of three independent experiments ± SEM. **(D)** Peritoneal macrophages were obtained from uninfected or infected mice at 24 h pi, and the levels of expression and localization of β-catenin were evaluated by immunofluorescence and confocal microscopy. In panels **(B,D)**, a representative field for each group is shown [**(B,D)**, 1,200×]. Nuclear staining was detected with 4′,6-diamidino-2-phenylindone (DAPI), and the levels of expression of β-catenin (% of total area) and the threshold Mander's colocalization (% nuclear) coefficients calculated using FIJI/ImageJ program as described in Section "Materials and Methods." Green, β-catenin; red, DAPI (*$P < 0.05$; **$P < 0.01$; ***$P < 0.001$; and ****$P < 0.0001$).

by faster migrating, dephosphorylated, active NFATc1 bands on Western blot (arrows; **Figure 4B**) and the increased expression and nuclear translocation of NFATc1 detected by immunofluorescence (**Figure 4C**). Interestingly, the upregulation of p-CaMKII and activation of NFATc1 were dependent on the secretion of Wnt proteins; since the use of IWP-L6, a porcupine inhibitor that is the *O*-acetyltransferase membrane involved in the palmitoylation of Wnt proteins, a critical modification for its secretion, was able to inhibit both p-CaMKII upregulation and NFATc1 activation (**Figures 4D,E**). Treatment of BMM with the calcium ionophore ionomycin was used as positive control of Ca^{+2} pathway activation (46). Moreover, we were unable to detect NFATc1 upregulation or translocation to the nucleus in PM obtained at 24 h pi (Figure S1 in Supplementary Material), even though it's upregulation was evident in PM obtained from infected mice at 18 days pi (Figure S2 in Supplementary Material).

The Inhibition of Wnt/β-Catenin Signaling Pathway Limits the Replication of *T. cruzi* in Macrophages

To evaluate the role of the Wnt/β-catenin pathway activation in the control of *T. cruzi* intracellular replication, BMM were pretreated with LiCl or BIO, both inhibitors of GSK-3β activity which mimics activation of Wnt/β catenin signaling, or specific inhibitors of β-catenin-responsive transcription such as iCRT14 and CCT036477 for 24 h before being infected. Then, the intracellular amastigotes were counted by IF assay, with the results shown in **Figures 5A,B**. Treatment of BMM with IFN-γ plus LPS was used to activate BMM to control *T. cruzi* replication as described previously (8). β-Catenin-responsive transcription blockade with iCRT14 and CCT036477 was shown to result in a strong inhibitory effect on intracellular parasite growth. Similar results were obtained by inhibiting the secretion of Wnt proteins with IWP-L6 (**Figures 5A,B**). The inhibition of parasite replication observed by β-catenin transcription blockade was even more significant than those observed after the activation of BMM with IFN-γ plus LPS, and these results were not due to drugs-induced cytotoxicity, as revealed by using LDH release assay to determine cell membrane integrity (**Figure 5C**). In addition, the treatment with IWP-L6 inhibited both β-catenin accumulation and nucleus translocation at 12 h pi (**Figure 5D**). Similar results were obtained when the drugs were added to the culture at the same time as the parasites (not shown). Likewise, inhibition of Wnt/β-catenin pathway or Wnt protein secretion in human monocyte-derived THP-1 macrophages and J774 cell line (macrophages derived from BALB/c mice) resulted in the suppression of intracellular parasite replication (Figure S3 in Supplementary Material). On the other hand, treatments with β-catenin activators (LiCl and BIO) were unable to significantly increase the intracellular parasite growth (**Figures 5A,B**).

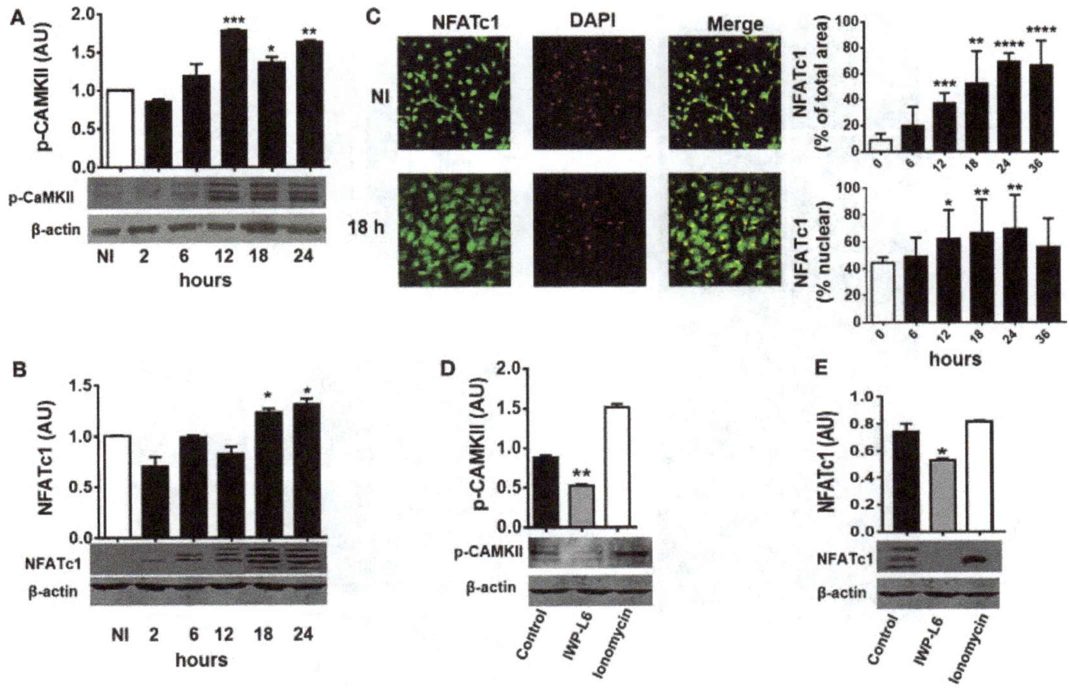

FIGURE 4 | *Trypanosoma cruzi* infection induces late Wnt/Ca^{+2} pathway activation in macrophages. Bone marrow-derived macrophages were *in vitro* infected with trypomastigotes (Tps) of *T. cruzi* or left uninfected (NI) and then evaluated for calcium/calmodulin-dependent kinase II (CaMKII) phosphorylated at Thr286 expression and NFATc1 expression and localization at different times post-infection (pi). Phosphorylated CAMKII (p-CAMKII) expression **(A)** and NFATc1 expression **(B)** were assessed by Western blot and normalized to β-actin. **(C)** Expression and localization of β-catenin by immunofluorescence and confocal microscopy. A representative field for each group is shown (1,200×). Nuclear staining was detected with 4′,6-diamidino-2-phenylindone (DAPI), and the levels of expression of NFATc1 (% of total area) and the threshold Mander's colocalization (% nuclear) coefficients calculated using FIJI/ImageJ program as described in Section "Materials and Methods." Green, NFATc1; red, DAPI. **(D,E)** Bone marrow-derived macrophages (BMM) were treated for 24 h with the PORCN inhibitor (IWP-L6) or left untreated (control), infected with *T. cruzi* Tps and assayed for p-CaMKII and NFATc1 expression at 24 h pi. Ionomycin-activated BMM (20 min, 1 μM) were used as a positive control. In panels **(A,B,D,E)**, a representative Western blot and the ratio of protein expression to β-actin are shown. The results are expressed as the average of three independent experiments ± SEM. Abbreviation: AU, arbitrary units (*$P < 0.05$; **$P < 0.01$; ***$P < 0.001$; and ****$P < 0.0001$).

Then, we studied whether the inhibition of canonical Wnt signaling regulates macrophages function by modulating the secretion of pro-inflammatory and anti-inflammatory cytokines. **Figure 6A** shows that inhibition of Wnt/β-catenin signaling induced the secretion of the pro-inflammatory cytokines IFN-γ, IL-12, IL-6, and TNF while inhibited the production of TGF-β (**Figure 6A**; Table S1 in Supplementary Material), an effect that correlates with the control of parasite replication observed in iCRT14-, CCT036477-, or IWP-L6-treated BMM (**Figures 5A,B**). In addition, canonical signaling activation using LiCl or BIO induced a slightly upregulation of TGF-β while only LiCl increased IL-10 production by *T. cruzi*-infected BMM (**Figure 6A**).

Nitric oxide production is counteracted by the expression of arginase, an enzyme that competes with iNOS for L-arginine that leads to L-ornithine and urea production (47). *T. cruzi* antigens can upregulate arginase activity with this type of activation profile associated with the ability to promote the intracellular growth of *T. cruzi* (48). Interestingly, although the pharmacological inhibition of Wnt/β-catenin pathway did not affect NO production (**Figure 6B**), the treatments with CCT036477 and IWP-L6 significantly downregulated arginase activity in infected BMM (**Figure 6C**).

Because IDO activity is also critical for the control of *T. cruzi* amastigote growth in macrophages (7–9), we analyzed the effect of the inhibition of Wnt/β-catenin signaling on the activity and expression of IDO and their role in the intracellular parasite replication control. The inhibition of both β-catenin-responsive gene transcription as well as Wnt secretion induced upregulation of IDO expression and activity in infected BMM (**Figures 6C,D**). Remarkably, the inhibitory effect of intracellular amastigote growth induced by pharmacological inhibitors of the Wnt/β-catenin pathway was reversed when IDO activity was blocked using 1-MT (**Figure 6E**). In addition, as it was previously demonstrated, 1-MT exacerbated the intracellular parasite replication in untreated BMM (**Figure 6E**). Taken together, these results demonstrated that pharmacological inhibition of Wnt/β-catenin pathway activates macrophages to fight against *T. cruzi*.

In Vivo Inhibition of Wnt Signaling Improves the Resistance to *T. cruzi* Infection

Next, we evaluated whether the inhibition of Wnt proteins secretion *in vivo* would result in the control of the parasite load. Five

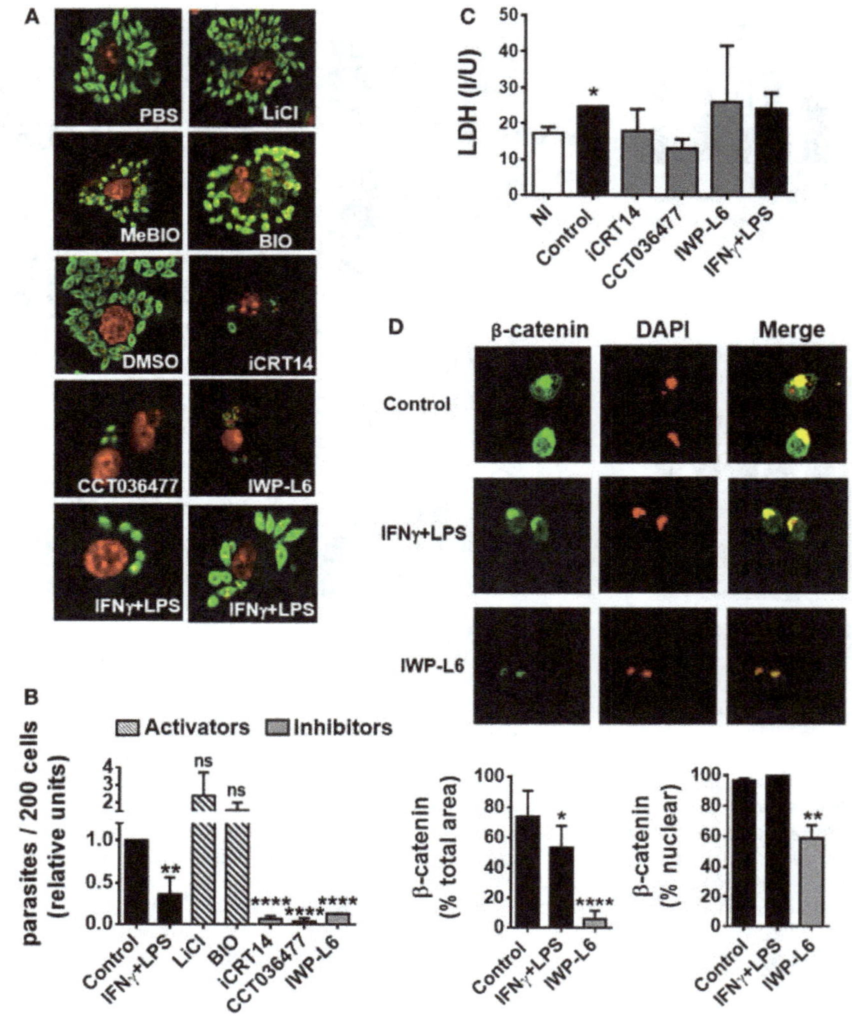

FIGURE 5 | The activation of Wnt signaling pathway promotes the replication of *Trypanosoma cruzi* in macrophages. Bone marrow-derived macrophages (BMM) were treated for 24 h with β-catenin activators (LiCl or BIO), specific β-catenin transcriptional inhibitors (iCRT14 and CCT036477), PORCN inhibitor (IWP-L6), or IFNγ plus LPS as BMM activation control. Then, the cells were infected with trypomastigotes of *T. cruzi*, and intracellular parasites were counted by immunofluorescence assay. **(A)** A representative field for each group is shown (2,000×). PBS or DMSO was used as vehicle for LiCl or iCRT14, CCT036477, and IWP-L6, respectively. MeBIO was used as control of BIO treatment. **(B)** The number of intracellular amastigotes was determined by confocal microscopy. Bars represent relative units, calculated by dividing number of intracellular parasites (*n*/200 cells) in differentially treated cultures by number of intracellular parasites (*n*/200 cells) in the corresponding vehicle-treated cultures. **(C)** Lactate dehydrogenase (LDH) levels were determined in the culture supernatant of uninfected (NI) or differentially treated infected BMM at 24 h post-infection. **(D)** Effect of IWP-L6 treatment on β-catenin activation. Accumulation and nuclear translocation of β-catenin in untreated (control), IFNγ plus LPS- or IWP-L6-treated *T. cruzi*-infected BMM was calculated as described in Section "Materials and Methods." A representative field for each group is shown (1,200×). Bars in panels **(B–D)** represent averages ± SEM from three **(C)** or four **(B,D)** independent experiments (*$P < 0.05$; **$P < 0.01$; ***$P < 0.001$; and ****$P < 0.0001$).

days after *T. cruzi* infection with a lethal dose 50 (DL50) of Tps, the mice were treated every 3 days with IWP-L6 (**Figure 7A**). The dose of IWP-L6 used has been previously assayed to examine the effect of Wnt proteins in an experimental model of cancer (49). As expected, *in vivo* IWP-L6 treatment could maintain inhibited both Wnt/β-catenin as well as Wnt/Ca^{+2} signaling pathways until 18 days pi, as denoted by the lack of β-catenin or NFATc1 accumulation in PM from treated versus control mice (Figure S2 in Supplementary Material). Mice infected with *T. cruzi* and injected with vehicle presented high levels of parasitemia, causing death of ~50% of mice between 18 and 30 days pi (**Figure 7B**). By contrast, although only four doses of IWP-L6 were given, 100% of treated mice survived to acute infection and displayed lower parasitemia than control mice during the acute phase of the infection (**Figure 7C**). In addition, IWP-L6-treated mice showed significantly lower parasite load in liver and heart than control mice during the chronic phase of the disease (**Figure 7D**).

DISCUSSION

Given that during the acute phase of *T. cruzi* infection macrophages can act as host cells for the parasites as well as effector cells in the early anti-parasitic immune response, the targeting of specific signaling pathways in macrophages could modulate its response

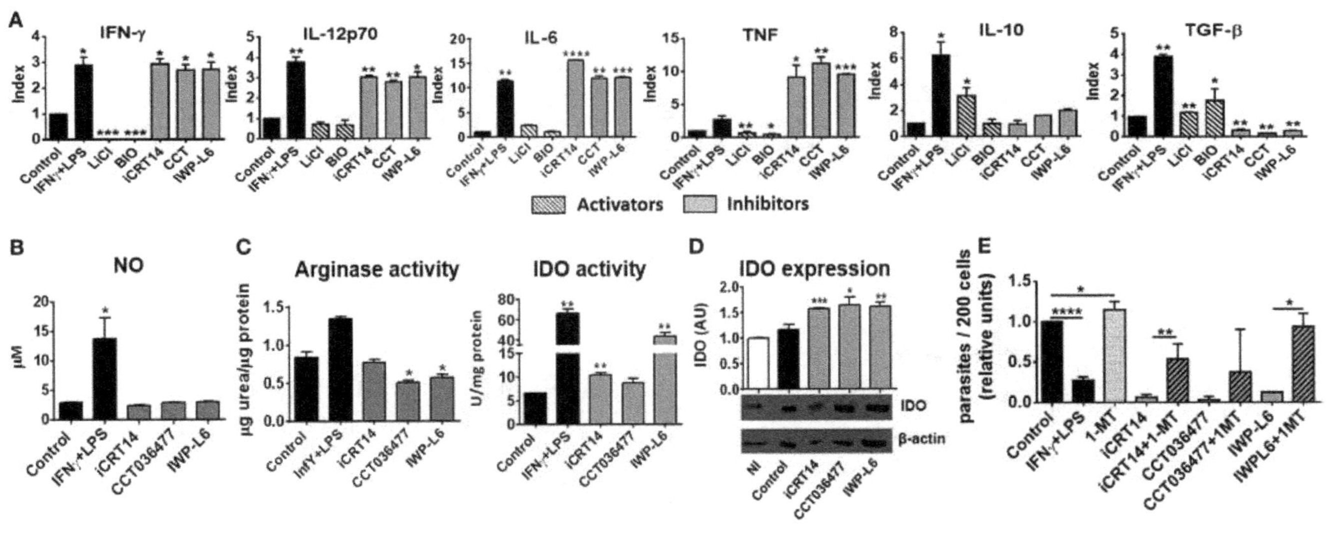

FIGURE 6 | Pharmacological inhibition of Wnt pathway enhances anti-*Trypanosoma cruzi* activity of macrophages. Bone marrow-derived macrophages (BMM) were treated for 24 h with β-catenin activators (LiCl or BIO), specific β-catenin transcriptional inhibitors (iCRT14 and CCT036477), IWP-L6, 1-MT, IFNγ plus LPS or vehicle before being infected with *T. cruzi* trypomastigotes. **(A)** Cytokine levels assayed in 24 h post-infection (pi)-supernatants represented as Index obtained by dividing the cytokine release of inhibitors/activators-treated BMM for the cytokine release of the corresponding vehicle-treated BMM. The bars represent averages ± SEM from three independent experiments. **(B)** Nitrite concentration in 24 h pi-supernatant. **(C)** Arginase and indoleamine 2,3-dioxygenase (IDO) activity assayed in 24 h pi-cell **(D)** IDO expression. One representative experiment out of three performed for each condition is shown. The ratio of protein expression to β-actin is shown, and the results are expressed as the average of three independent experiments ± SEM. Abbreviation: AU, arbitrary units. Data points of nitric oxide (NO) concentrations, arginase, and IDO activity represent means ± SEM of data pooled from three cultures of the same experiment. All data are from one experiment representative of three in total. **(E)** Number of intracellular amastigotes determined by confocal microscopy at 72 h pi. The bars represent relative units, calculated as described in **Figure 5B** (*$P < 0.05$; **$P < 0.01$; ***$P < 0.001$; and ****$P < 0.0001$).

to restrict parasite replication and instruct an appropriate adaptive immune response. In recent years, it has become apparent that Wnt signaling pathway, known for its essential participation in embryonic development and tissue homeostasis, exerts immunomodulatory functions during inflammation and infection.

In this study, we have demonstrated that early after the recognition of *T. cruzi* by innate immune receptors in BMM, β-catenin was activated and Wnt3a, Wnt5a, some Fzd receptors as well as target genes of Wnt/β-catenin pathway as *Axin1*, *Wisp1*, and *Ccnd1* were upregulated. Subsequently to canonical pathway activation, Wnt/Ca^{+2} pathway was activated; since we have demonstrated an Wnt proteins-dependent upregulated of p-CaMKII-Thr286 and activated NFATc1 expression after infection. Many studies have demonstrated that *T. cruzi* utilize the host Ca^{+2} signaling to establish the infection (50) and several mechanisms have been proposed to explain the intracellular Ca^{+2} influx that occurs during *T. cruzi* infection (51). In addition, Kayama et al. (52) have reported that NFATc1 is activated in response to *T. cruzi* infection in a TLR-independent manner, but the critical molecules and signaling pathways that lead to NFATc1 activation during *T. cruzi* infection have not yet been identified. Wnt3a and Wnt5a are more commonly associated with canonical and non-canonical Wnt signaling, respectively (19). However, Wnt5a can also activate discrete β-catenin signaling (53, 54), and recent reports have suggested that the activity of Wnt ligands and their binding to Fzd receptors depend on the cellular context; therefore, Wnt and Fzd proteins cannot be rigorously subdivided according to the pathways they induce (55). Thus, considering that we found that *T. cruzi* infection-induced β-catenin, p-CaMKII-Thr286, and activated NFATc1 upregulation were suppressed by IWP-L6 treatment, these results suggest that both Wnt3a and Wnt5a proteins, and others Wnt proteins not evaluated in this paper, could be the responsible for the activation and maintenance of both canonical and non-canonical signaling pathways during *T. cruzi* infection which allows the parasite to spread in the host.

Resistance to *T. cruzi* infection has been associated with the capacity of NK cells and T lymphocytes to generate IFN-γ which can, in turn, activate macrophages to kill the obligate intracellular amastigote form of *T. cruzi*. The trypanocidal activity of pro-inflammatory cytokines-activated macrophages is mediated at least by the upregulation of the enzymes iNOS and IDO which lead to the production of NO and kynurenines, respectively (5–9, 56). On the other hand, susceptibility to infection is associated with the production of IL-10 and transforming growth factor beta (TGF-β) (5, 56). Here, we have demonstrated that while the activation of Wnt/β-catenin pathway did not promote the intracellular parasite replication, the treatments of macrophages with specific inhibitors of β-catenin transcriptional activity or the inhibition of Wnt proteins secretion were able to inhibit the parasite replication by modifying macrophages activity. Inhibition of Wnt signaling pathway enhanced production of the pro-inflammatory cytokines IFN-γ, IL-12, TNF and IL-6 and suppressed production of TGF-β, results that are in agreement

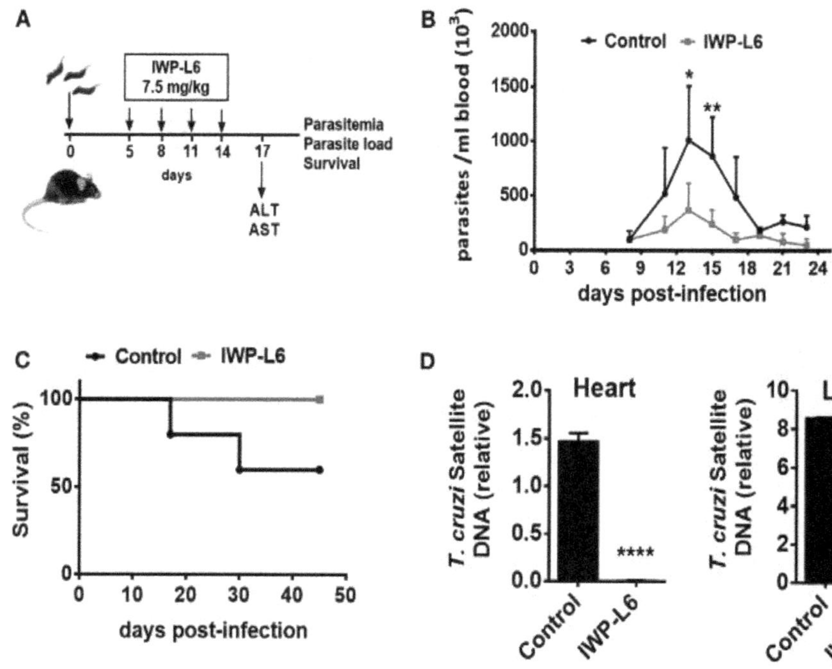

FIGURE 7 | *In vivo* inhibition of Wnt signaling improves the resistance to *Trypanosoma cruzi* infection. **(A)** B6 mice infected with 5,000 *T. cruzi* trypomastigotes were treated with IWP-L6. Vehicle-treated mice were used as control. **(B)** Parasitemia. Results are means ± SD of 5–6 animals/group and are representative of three independent experiments. **(C)** Survival rate. Data are representative of one of three independent experiments. **(D)** Relative amount of *T. cruzi* satellite DNA in heart and liver from 180-day *T. cruzi*-infected IWP-L6 and control mice. Murine GAPDH was used for normalization. Data are shown as mean ± SD of triplicates (control, $n = 4$; IWP-L6, $n = 6$) mice per group ($^*P < 0.05$; $^{**}P < 0.001$; and $^{****}P < 0.0001$).

with previous reports showing that the activation of the canonical pathway in macrophages and DC controls the inflammatory response (28). In addition, these treatments induced down-regulation of arginase activity, an enzyme that counteracts iNOS activity, but failed to upregulate iNOS activity, suggesting that the resulting treated-macrophages do not fully fit in the classically activated/inflammatory macrophage phenotype. Interestingly, and despite the fact that there is a close relationship between the activation of the Wnt/β-catenin pathway and the induction of IDO and *vice versa* (27, 57, 58), in our experimental model the inhibition of β-catenin-induced transcription or Wnt proteins secretion upregulated IDO expression and activity. In addition, IDO activity proved to be critical for the control of *T. cruzi* replication in BMM, as denoted by the recovery of *T. cruzi* replication observed in cultures where the inhibitors were combined with 1-MT. Expression of IDO and activation of β-catenin within macrophages and DC under tolerogenic conditions are particularly important mechanisms that limits inflammation within the gastrointestinal tract and tumor cell microenvironment (28, 59). The IDO promoter has been shown to exhibit LEF-1 binding sites, and kynurenine and quinolinic acid, produced by IDO activity, can activate the Wnt/β-catenin pathway (60, 61). However, as IDO gene expression is induced not only in tolerogenic conditions but also by IFNs and TNF during inflammatory conditions (62, 63), in our experimental settings the upregulation of IDO could be induced by the milieu of pro-inflammatory cytokines generated in inhibitors-treated *T. cruzi*-infected macrophages. Thus, our results suggest that the anti-*T. cruzi* activity of inhibitor-treated macrophages is due to the production of pro-inflammatory cytokines-inducible antimicrobial molecules, with IDO being one of the most important.

In summary, in this study, we have revealed a new signaling pathway that is activated by the interaction between protozoan parasites and host innate immunity. In this context, it is well founded that *T. cruzi* infection activates a plethora of signaling pathways that ultimately regulate the immune mediators to determine the modulation of a defined set of effector functions in macrophages and thus establishes a conceptual framework for the development of novel therapeutics.

AUTHOR CONTRIBUTIONS

XV, LF, and CM designed the experiments. XV, LA, LF, and CI performed the experiments. XV, LF, LC, CS, and CM analyzed the data. XV, LC, and CM wrote the manuscript.

ACKNOWLEDGMENTS

XV, LA, and CI thank Consejo Nacional de Investigaciones Científicas y Técnicas from Argentina for the fellowships granted.

CM, LF, CS, and LC are members of the Scientific Career of Consejo Nacional de Investigaciones Científicas y Técnicas from Argentina. We thank Eva Acosta Rodriguez for providing us with various reagents and technical support and David Rojas Marquez for their skillful technical assistance. We thank F. Navarro, D. Lutti, V. Blanco, and C. Florit for animal care.

REFERENCES

1. Salvatella R, Irabedra P, Sánchez D, Castellanos LG, Espinal M. South-south cooperation for Chagas disease. *Lancet* (2013) 382(9890):395–6. doi:10.1016/S0140-6736(13)61671-2
2. Le Loup G, Pialoux G, Lescure FX. Update in treatment of Chagas disease. *Curr Opin Infect Dis* (2011) 24(5):428–34. doi:10.1097/QCO.0b013e32834a667f
3. Sosa-Estani S, Segura E. Etiological treatment in patients infected by *Trypanosoma cruzi*: experiences in Argentina. *Curr Opin Infect Dis* (2006) 19(6):583–7. doi:10.1097/01.qco.0000247592.21295.a5
4. Tanowitz HB, Kirchhoff LV, Simon D, Morris SA, Weiss LM, Wittner M. Chagas' disease. *Clin Microbiol Rev* (1992) 5(4):400–19. doi:10.1128/CMR.5.4.400
5. Gazzinelli RT, Oswald IP, Hieny S, James SL, Sher A. The microbicidal activity of interferon-gamma-treated macrophages against *Trypanosoma cruzi* involves an L-arginine-dependent, nitrogen oxide-mediated mechanism inhibitable by interleukin-10 and transforming growth factor-beta. *Eur J Immunol* (1992) 22(10):2501–6. doi:10.1002/eji.1830221006
6. Silva JS, Vespa GN, Cardoso MA, Aliberti JC, Cunha FQ. Tumor necrosis factor alpha mediates resistance to *Trypanosoma cruzi* infection in mice by inducing nitric oxide production in infected gamma interferon-activated macrophages. *Infect Immun* (1995) 63(12):4862–7.
7. Knubel CP, Martinez FF, Acosta Rodriguez EV, Altamirano A, Rivarola HW, Diaz Lujan C, et al. 3-Hydroxy kynurenine treatment controls *T. cruzi* replication and the inflammatory pathology preventing the clinical symptoms of chronic Chagas disease. *PLoS One* (2011) 6(10):e26550. doi:10.1371/journal.pone.0026550
8. Knubel CP, Martinez FF, Fretes RE, Lujan CD, Theumer MG, Cervi L, et al. Indoleamine 2,3-dioxygenase (IDO) is critical for host resistance against *Trypanosoma cruzi*. *FASEB J* (2010) 24(8):2689–701. doi:10.1096/fj.09-150920
9. Knubel CP, Insfran C, Martinez FF, Diaz Lujan C, Fretes RE, Theumer MG, et al. 3-hydroxykynurenine, a tryptophan metabolite generated during the infection, is active against *Trypanosoma cruzi*. *ACS Med Chem Lett* (2017) 8(7):757–61. doi:10.1021/acsmedchemlett.7b00169
10. Martin D, Tarleton R. Generation, specificity, and function of CD8+ T cells in *Trypanosoma cruzi* infection. *Immunol Rev* (2004) 201(1):304–17. doi:10.1111/j.0105-2896.2004.00183.x
11. Lúcia CJA, Luiz VR, Bárbara I, Fabiana A, Fernando B, Dirceu C, et al. Chronic Chagas' disease cardiomyopathy patients display an increased IFN-γ response to *Trypanosoma cruzi* infection. *J Autoimmun* (2001) 17(1):99–107. doi:10.1006/jaut.2001.0523
12. Gomes JAS, Bahia-Oliveira LMG, Rocha MOC, Martins-Filho OA, Gazzinelli G, Correa-Oliveira R. Evidence that development of severe cardiomyopathy in human Chagas' disease is due to a Th1-specific immune response. *Infect Immun* (2003) 71(3):1185–93. doi:10.1128/IAI.71.3.1185-1193.2003
13. Jacqueline Araújo F, Ricardo Toshio F, Juliana Assis Silva G, Manoel Otávio das Costa R, Ana Thereza C, Fernanda Fortes de A, et al. Profile of central and effector memory T cells in the progression of chronic human Chagas disease. *PLoS Negl Trop Dis* (2009) 3(9):e512. doi:10.1371/journal.pntd.0000512
14. Gomes JAS, Bahia-Oliveira LMG, Rocha MOC, Busek SCU, Teixeira MM, Silva JS, et al. Type 1 chemokine receptor expression in Chagas' disease correlates with morbidity in cardiac patients. *Infect Immun* (2005) 73(12):7960–6. doi:10.1128/IAI.73.12.7960-7966.2005
15. van Amerongen R, Nusse R. Towards an integrated view of Wnt signaling in development. *Development* (2009) 136(19):3205–14. doi:10.1242/dev.033910
16. Clevers H, Nusse R. Wnt/β-catenin signaling and disease. *Cell* (2012) 149(6):1192–205. doi:10.1016/j.cell.2012.05.012
17. Staal FJ, Luis TC, Tiemessen MM. WNT signalling in the immune system: WNT is spreading its wings. *Nat Rev Immunol* (2008) 8(8):581–93. doi:10.1038/nri2360
18. Angers S, Moon RT. Proximal events in Wnt signal transduction. *Nat Rev Mol Cell Biol* (2009) 10(7):468–77. doi:10.1038/nrm2717
19. Kikuchi A, Yamamoto H, Sato A, Matsumoto S. Chapter 2 – new insights into the mechanism of Wnt signaling pathway activation. In: Kwang WJ, editor. *International Review of Cell and Molecular Biology*. (Vol. 291), Netherlands: Academic Press (2011). p. 21–71.
20. Feske S, Okamura H, Hogan PG, Rao A. Ca 2+/calcineurin signalling in cells of the immune system. *Biochem Biophys Res Commun* (2003) 311(4):1117–32. doi:10.1016/j.bbrc.2003.09.174
21. Schaale K, Neumann J, Schneider D, Ehlers S, Reiling N. Wnt signaling in macrophages: augmenting and inhibiting mycobacteria-induced inflammatory responses. *Eur J Cell Biol* (2011) 90(6–7):553–9. doi:10.1016/j.ejcb.2010.11.004
22. Silva-Garcia O, Valdez-Alarcon JJ, Baizabal-Aguirre VM. The Wnt/beta-catenin signaling pathway controls the inflammatory response in infections caused by pathogenic bacteria. *Mediators Inflamm* (2014) 2014:310183. doi:10.1155/2014/310183
23. Jiang A, Bloom O, Ono S, Cui W, Unternaehrer J, Jiang S, et al. Disruption of E-cadherin-mediated adhesion induces a functionally distinct pathway of dendritic cell maturation. *Immunity* (2007) 27(4):610–24. doi:10.1016/j.immuni.2007.08.015
24. Oderup C, LaJevic M, Butcher EC. Canonical and noncanonical Wnt proteins program dendritic cell responses for tolerance. *J Immunol* (2013) 190(12):6126–34. doi:10.4049/jimmunol.1203002
25. Reuter S, Martin H, Beckert H, Bros M, Montermann E, Belz C, et al. The Wnt/beta-catenin pathway attenuates experimental allergic airway disease. *J Immunol* (2014) 193(2):485–95. doi:10.4049/jimmunol.1400013
26. Valencia J, Hernández-López C, Martínez V, Hidalgo L, Zapata A, Vicente Á, et al. Wnt5a skews dendritic cell differentiation to an unconventional phenotype with tolerogenic features. *J Immunol* (2011) 187(8):4129–39. doi:10.4049/jimmunol.1101243
27. Holtzhausen A, Zhao F, Evans KS, Tsutsui M, Orabona C, Tyler DS, et al. Melanoma-derived Wnt5a promotes local dendritic-cell expression of IDO and immunotolerance: opportunities for pharmacologic enhancement of immunotherapy. *Cancer Immunol Res* (2015) 3(9):1082–95. doi:10.1158/2326-6066.CIR-14-0167
28. Manicassamy S, Reizis B, Ravindran R, Nakaya H, Salazar-Gonzalez R, Wang Y-C, et al. Activation of beta-catenin in dendritic cells regulates immunity versus tolerance in the intestine. *Science* (2010) 329(5993):849–53. doi:10.1126/science.1188510
29. Sen M, Ghosh G. Transcriptional outcome of Wnt-frizzled signal transduction in inflammation: evolving concepts. *J Immunol* (2008) 181(7):4441–5. doi:10.4049/jimmunol.181.7.4441
30. Katoh M, Katoh M. STAT3-induced WNT5A signaling loop in embryonic stem cells, adult normal tissues, chronic persistent inflammation, rheumatoid arthritis and cancer (Review). *Int J Mol Med* (2007) 19(2):273–8. doi:10.3892/ijmm.19.2.273
31. Manoharan I, Hong Y, Suryawanshi A, Angus-Hill ML, Sun Z, Mellor AL, et al. TLR2-dependent activation of beta-catenin pathway in dendritic cells induces regulatory responses and attenuates autoimmune inflammation. *J Immunol* (2014) 193(8):4203–13. doi:10.4049/jimmunol.1400614
32. Brown JB, Cheresh P, Goretsky T, Managlia E, Grimm GR, Ryu H, et al. Epithelial phosphatidylinositol-3-kinase signaling is required for beta-catenin activation and host defense against *Citrobacter rodentium* infection. *Infect Immun* (2011) 79(5):1863–72. doi:10.1128/IAI.01025-10
33. Bansal K, Trinath J, Chakravortty D, Patil SA, Balaji KN. Pathogen-specific TLR2 protein activation programs macrophages to induce Wnt-β-catenin signaling. *J Biol Chem* (2011) 286(42):37032–44. doi:10.1074/jbc.M111.260414
34. Bergenfelz C, Medrek C, Ekström E, Jirström K, Janols H, Wullt M, et al. Wnt5a induces a tolerogenic phenotype of macrophages in sepsis and breast cancer patients. *J Immunol* (2012) 188(11):5448–58. doi:10.4049/jimmunol.1103378
35. Neumann J, Schaale K, Farhat K, Endermann T, Ulmer AJ, Ehlers S, et al. Frizzled1 is a marker of inflammatory macrophages, and its ligand Wnt3a is involved in reprogramming *Mycobacterium tuberculosis*-infected macrophages. *FASEB J* (2010) 24(11):4599–612. doi:10.1096/fj.10-160994
36. Blumenthal A, Ehlers S, Lauber J, Buer J, Lange C, Goldmann T, et al. The Wingless homolog WNT5A and its receptor frizzled-5 regulate inflammatory responses of human mononuclear cells induced by microbial stimulation. *Blood* (2006) 108(3):965–73. doi:10.1182/blood-2005-12-5046

37. Pereira C, Schaer DJ, Bachli EB, Kurrer MO, Schoedon G. Wnt5A/CaMKII signaling contributes to the inflammatory response of macrophages and is a target for the antiinflammatory action of activated protein C and interleukin-10. *Arterioscler Thromb Vasc Biol* (2008) 28(3):504–10. doi:10.1161/ATVBAHA.107.157438
38. Ouaissi A, Guilvard E, Delneste Y, Caron G, Magistrelli G, Herbault N, et al. The *Trypanosoma cruzi* Tc52-released protein induces human dendritic cell maturation, signals via toll-like receptor 2, and confers protection against lethal infection. *J Immunol* (2002) 168(12):6366–74. doi:10.4049/jimmunol.168.12.6366
39. Oliveira AC, Peixoto JR, de Arruda LB, Campos MA, Gazzinelli RT, Golenbock DT, et al. Expression of functional TLR4 confers proinflammatory responsiveness to *Trypanosoma cruzi* glycoinositolphospholipids and higher resistance to infection with *T. cruzi*. *J Immunol* (2004) 173(9):5688–96. doi:10.4049/jimmunol.173.9.5688
40. Oliveira AC, de Alencar BC, Tzelepis F, Klezewsky W, da Silva RN, Neves FS, et al. Impaired innate immunity in Tlr4(-/-) mice but preserved CD8+ T cell responses against *Trypanosoma cruzi* in Tlr4-, Tlr2-, Tlr9- or Myd88-deficient mice. *PLoS Pathog* (2010) 6(4):e1000870. doi:10.1371/journal.ppat.1000870
41. Hsu YM, Zhang Y, You Y, Wang D, Li H, Duramad O, et al. The adaptor protein CARD9 is required for innate immune responses to intracellular pathogens. *Nat Immunol* (2007) 8(2):198–205. doi:10.1038/ni1426
42. Motran CC, Diaz FL, Montes CL, Bocco JL, Gruppi A. In vivo expression of recombinant pregnancy-specific glycoprotein 1a induces alternative activation of monocytes and enhances Th2-type immune response. *Eur J Immunol* (2003) 33(11):3007–16. doi:10.1002/eji.200323993
43. Motran CC, Diaz FL, Gruppi A, Slavin D, Chatton B, Bocco JL. Human pregnancy-specific glycoprotein 1a (PSG1a) induces alternative activation in human and mouse monocytes and suppresses the accessory cell-dependent T cell proliferation. *J Leukoc Biol* (2002) 72(3):512–21. doi:10.1189/jlb.72.3.512
44. Araujo F, Vitelli-Avelar D, Teixeira-Carvalho A, Antas P, Gomes J, Sathler-Avelar R, et al. Regulatory T cells phenotype in different clinical forms of Chagas' disease. *PLoS Negl Trop Dis* (2011) 5(5):e992. doi:10.1371/journal.pntd.0000992
45. Dijksterhuis JP, Baljinnyam B, Stanger K, Sercan HO, Ji Y, Andres O, et al. Systematic mapping of WNT-FZD protein interactions reveals functional selectivity by distinct WNT-FZD pairs. *J Biol Chem* (2015) 290(11):6789–98. doi:10.1074/jbc.M114.612648
46. Dejmek J, Safholm A, Kamp Nielsen C, Andersson T, Leandersson K. Wnt-5a/Ca2+-induced NFAT activity is counteracted by Wnt-5a/Yes-Cdc42-casein kinase 1alpha signaling in human mammary epithelial cells. *Mol Cell Biol* (2006) 26(16):6024–36. doi:10.1128/MCB.02354-05
47. Munder M, Eichmann K, Modolell M. Alternative metabolic states in murine macrophages reflected by the nitric oxide synthase/arginase balance: competitive regulation by CD4+ T cells correlates with Th1/Th2 phenotype. *J Immunol* (1998) 160(11):5347–54.
48. Stempin C, Giordanengo L, Gea S, Cerban F. Alternative activation and increase of *Trypanosoma cruzi* survival in murine macrophages stimulated by cruzipain, a parasite antigen. *J Leukoc Biol* (2002) 72(4):727–34. doi:10.1189/jlb.72.4.727
49. Hong Y, Manoharan I, Suryawanshi A, Shanmugam A, Swafford D, Ahmad S, et al. Deletion of LRP5 and LRP6 in dendritic cells enhances anti-tumor immunity. *Oncoimmunology* (2015) 5(4):e1115941. doi:10.1080/2162402X.2015.1115941
50. Yoshida N. Molecular basis of mammalian cell invasion by *Trypanosoma cruzi*. *An Acad Bras Cienc* (2006) 78(1):87–111. doi:10.1590/S0001-37652006000100010
51. Burleigh BA, Andrews NW. The mechanisms of *Trypanosoma cruzi* invasion of mammalian cells. *Annu Rev Microbiol* (1995) 49:175–200. doi:10.1146/annurev.mi.49.100195.001135
52. Kayama H, Koga R, Atarashi K, Okuyama M, Kimura T, Mak TW, et al. NFATc1 mediates toll-like receptor-independent innate immune responses during *Trypanosoma cruzi* infection. *PLoS Pathog* (2009) 5(7):e1000514. doi:10.1371/journal.ppat.1000514
53. Mikels AJ, Nusse R. Purified Wnt5a protein activates or inhibits beta-catenin-TCF signaling depending on receptor context. *PLoS Biol* (2006) 4(4):e115. doi:10.1371/journal.pbio.0040115
54. Pukrop T, Binder C. The complex pathways of Wnt 5a in cancer progression. *J Mol Med (Berl)* (2008) 86(3):259–66. doi:10.1007/s00109-007-0266-2
55. Niehrs C. The complex world of WNT receptor signalling. *Nat Rev Mol Cell Biol* (2012) 13(12):767–79. doi:10.1038/nrm3470
56. Silva JS, Morrissey PJ, Grabstein KH, Mohler KM, Anderson D, Reed SG. Interleukin 10 and interferon gamma regulation of experimental *Trypanosoma cruzi* infection. *J Exp Med* (1992) 175(1):169–74. doi:10.1084/jem.175.1.169
57. Thomas SR, Mohr D, Stocker R. Nitric oxide inhibits indoleamine 2,3-dioxygenase activity in interferon-gamma primed mononuclear phagocytes. *J Biol Chem* (1994) 269(20):14457–64.
58. von Bergwelt-Baildon MS, Popov A, Saric T, Chemnitz J, Classen S, Stoffel MS, et al. CD25 and indoleamine 2,3-dioxygenase are up-regulated by prostaglandin E2 and expressed by tumor-associated dendritic cells in vivo: additional mechanisms of T-cell inhibition. *Blood* (2006) 108(1):228–37. doi:10.1182/blood-2005-08-3507
59. Munn DH, Mellor AL. IDO and tolerance to tumors. *Trends Mol Med* (2004) 10(1):15–8. doi:10.1016/j.molmed.2003.11.003
60. Soichot M, Hennart B, Al Saabi A, Leloire A, Froguel P, Levy-Marchal C, et al. Identification of a variable number of tandem repeats polymorphism and characterization of LEF-1 response elements in the promoter of the IDO1 gene. *PLoS One* (2011) 6(9):e25470. doi:10.1371/journal.pone.0025470
61. Thaker AI, Rao MS, Bishnupuri KS, Kerr TA, Foster L, Marinshaw JM, et al. IDO1 metabolites activate β-catenin signaling to promote cancer cell proliferation and colon tumorigenesis in mice. *Gastroenterology* (2013) 145(2):416–25.e4. doi:10.1053/j.gastro.2013.05.002
62. Hassanain HH, Chon SY, Gupta SL. Differential regulation of human indoleamine 2,3-dioxygenase gene expression by interferons-gamma and -alpha. Analysis of the regulatory region of the gene and identification of an interferon-gamma-inducible DNA-binding factor. *J Biol Chem* (1993) 268(7):5077–84.
63. Robinson CM, Hale PT, Carlin JM. The role of IFN-gamma and TNF-alpha-responsive regulatory elements in the synergistic induction of indoleamine dioxygenase. *J Interferon Cytokine Res* (2005) 25(1):20–30. doi:10.1089/jir.2005.25.20

8

Oral Versus Intragastric Inoculation: Similar Pathways of *Trypanosoma cruzi* Experimental Infection? From Target Tissues, Parasite Evasion and Immune Response

*Juliana Barreto de Albuquerque[1], Danielle Silva dos Santos[2], Jens V. Stein[1] and Juliana de Meis[2,3]**

[1] Theodor Kocher Institute, University of Bern, Bern, Switzerland, [2] Laboratory on Thymus Research, Oswaldo Cruz Institute, Oswaldo Cruz Foundation, Rio de Janeiro, Brazil, [3] National Institute of Science and Technology on Neuroimmunomodulation (INCT-NIM), Rio de Janeiro, Brazil

***Correspondence:**
Juliana de Meis
jdemeis@ioc.fiocruz.br

Currently, oral infection is the most frequent transmission mechanism of Chagas disease in Brazil and others Latin American countries. This transmission pathway presents increased mortality rate in the first 2 weeks, which is higher than the calculated mortality after the biting of infected insect vectors. Thus, the oral route of *Trypanosoma cruzi* infection, and the consequences in the host must be taken into account when thinking on the mechanisms underlying the natural history of the disease. Distinct routes of parasite entry may differentially affect immune circuits, stimulating regional immune responses that impact on the overall profile of the host protective immunity. Experimental studies related to oral infection usually comprise inoculation in the mouth (oral infection, OI) or gavage (gastrointestinal infection, GI), being often considered as similar routes of infection. Hence, establishing a relationship between the inoculation site (OI or GI) with disease progression and the mounting of *T. cruzi*-specific regional immune responses is an important issue to be considered. Here, we provide a discussion on studies performed in OI and GI in experimental models of acute infections, including *T. cruzi* infection.

Keywords: *Trypanosoma cruzi*, oral cavity, intragastric infection, immune response, T cell activation

INTRODUCTION

Chagas disease, or American trypanosomiasis, caused by the hemoflagellate protozoan *Trypanosoma cruzi*, is a tropical neglected illness *Trypanosoma cruzi* (*T. cruzi*). Infection was initially enzooty and maintained among wild animals and insect vectors of the *Reduviidae* family. Deforestation in rural areas allowed vectors to invade human homes (1, 2).

Chagas disease transmission to humans can be classified in primary (vectorial, blood transfusion, congenital, and orally) and secondary (less frequent, such as laboratory accident, handling of infected animals, organ transplantation from infected donors, and hypothetically through sexual) routes of *T. cruzi* infection (3, 4). Different transmission routes present variable incubation period, such as oral, 3–22 days; vector feces near the bite, 4–15 days; blood transfusion, 8–120 days; and organ transplantation, 23–420 days (5–9). Besides the transmission pathway, mortality rates depend also on the patients' clinical condition and on the time between disease diagnosis and beginning of treatment. Oral transmission results in a higher mortality, estimated between 8 and 35%, than the classical vector-borne infection (<5–10%) (5, 7–10).

From 1990 to 1993, the Brazilian Health Minister started to insert the Notifiable Diseases System of Information-SINAN (DATASUS) to control the number of acute cases in the country. Although underestimated, from 2002 to 2006 Brazil registered 2510 cases of acute Chagas disease according to the DATASUS system. Number of notifications decreased at the time that the pan-American Health Organization registered the interruption of *Triatoma infestans* population in the area in 2006 (11); however, numbers still reached 1,539 new cases in the DATASUS from 2007 to 2014. Nowadays, oral transmission of Chagas disease is the most frequent transmission route in the Brazilian Amazon region (12). Food/beverages contamination with *T. cruzi*-infected insect excreta, macerate, or reservoir meal is responsible for oral transmission in one to more than a hundred cases (outbreaks). It is noteworthy that oral transmission has been associated with high mortality and morbidity, including increased prevalence and severity of the cardiac pathology (myocarditis) (13–16). Argentina, Bolivia, Colombia, Ecuador, French Guiana, and Venezuela have also reported acute Chagas disease outbreaks associated with contaminated food consumption [revised in Ref. (11, 17)]. Fruits pasteurization is the appropriate pathway to kill the parasite, and it has been shown that outbreaks of oral infection in Brazilian Amazonia increase with seasonal months of higher açaí pulp production. Moreover, epidemiological data suggest that in the Pará state most of the cases are caused by consumption of artisanal açaí. Therefore, good practices of quality control could avoid the transmission, such as good agricultural practice and "bleaching" or "whitening" of the fruits (12, 18).

The infection is presently considered as a worldwide health problem with deficiencies in treatment, absence of vaccines, and world spreading (19–22).

PARASITE–HOST INTERACTION AND TARGET TISSUES

T. cruzi presents one of the most complex life cycles among the trypanosomatids, alternating between vertebrate hosts, which comprises a wide range of mammals including humans and invertebrate hematophagous insects from the Reduviidae family (23, 24). Mammalian cell invasion by the *T. cruzi* is critical to its survival in the host. Once inside the vertebrate host, the metacyclic trypomastigotes are able to infect several nucleated mammalian cells at the inoculation site, such as macrophages, fibroblasts, epithelial cells, and others. The intracellular cycle in a mammalian cell presents different steps and begins at the moment that infective forms of *T. cruzi* interact with phagocytic or non-phagocytic surface molecules. These processes lead to cell signaling and internalization of the parasite through multiple endocytic pathways (25–27). *T. cruzi* proteins such as gp82, gp80, gp35/50, gp85, trans-sialidase, and host cell adhesion molecules such as mucins, VLA (very late antigen), and extracellular matrix proteins (ECM) such as laminin and fibronectin have been reported to contribute to parasite infection (23, 25, 28–33). In addition, *T. cruzi* proteases as cruzipain, oligopeptidase B, and Tc80 have been implicated in *T. cruzi* internalization (23, 31). In addition to presenting a large variety of surface molecules that can participate in host–parasite interaction, strain and forms (metacyclic trypomastigotes, tissue culture-derived trypomastigotes, and amastigotes) of the parasite differently express these molecules in the membrane. The capacity of trypomastigotes to interact with a diverse number of molecules on cell surface is determinant to improve invasion processes and allows the parasite to explore survival and multiplicative strategies in the host (23, 31, 34).

It is believed that any mammalian host cell class of molecules in the membrane are potential partners for *T. cruzi* recognition, and the expression of these molecules can vary depending on the cell type involved. Well-characterized groups of receptor are carbohydrates that contain galactosyl, mannosyl, and sialyl residues and lectin-like proteins (23, 26). Interestingly, *T. cruzi* is either able to use and increase expression of ECM in the host cell during the initial process of infection. Regarding *T. cruzi* surface molecules, it has been shown that trypomastigote forms present motifs that bind to cytokeratin 18, fibronectin, laminin, heparan sulfate proteoglycans, and integrins (35, 36).

The components involved in *T. cruzi* oral infection were suggested in experimental models. Hoft and colleagues demonstrated by histological analysis that after oral infection, *T. cruzi* invades and replicates inside epithelial cells within the gastric mucosa. This initial invasion is followed by the establishment of a progressive gastritis and further systemic dissemination of the parasite. Furthermore, hypertrophy and the presence of parasites in adjacent lymph nodes of stomach and inflammatory infiltrates in various organs (pancreas, liver, spleen, bone marrow, heart, duodenum, adrenal, brain, and/or skeletal muscle) were also described. Amastigote nests were detected in the gastric mucosal epithelium, but not in the upper gastrointestinal tract, like esophagus and oropharynx after oral infection. These data suggested that oral infection initiates in gastric mucosal followed by systemic dissemination (37).

Analysis of molecular mechanisms involved in *T. cruzi* interaction with host cells during oral infection is under investigation. It has been suggested that gastric epithelium express mucins that interacts with *T. cruzi* glycoproteins, such as gp82 and gp30, triggering a cascade of intracellular signaling in the parasite and at the host cell, leading to the mobilization of intracellular Ca^{2+} that is essential for parasite internalization (32, 34, 38, 39).

In line with this, previous studies of intrapharyngeal infection in mice, and *in vitro* studies of human epithelial cells have demonstrated the key role of glycoprotein gp82 during *T. cruzi* invasion in gastric of mucosal (40). Gp82 is present in metacyclic trypomastigotes forms, but not in amastigotes, epimastigotes, or tissue culture-derived trypomastigotes forms (41, 42). Interestingly, gp82 expressed in different *T. cruzi* strains is resistant to degradation by pepsin or proteinase K (43, 44). Metacyclic forms of *T. cruzi* recovered from the stomach 1 h after an intrapharyngeal inoculation in mice preserve the gp82 intact, and the parasite infectivity was not altered. Furthermore, *T. cruzi* $gp82^{-/-}$ metacyclic forms have reduced gastric mucin-binding capacity, less efficient migration through the gastric mucin-coated and low infectivity in mice by the intrapharyngeal route when compared with metacyclic forms that express gp82 (44, 45).

GP30 is another glycoprotein involved in *T. cruzi* interaction with the gastric epithelium, binding the target cells in a receptor-dependent manner, inducing Ca^{2+} response and lysosome exocytosis, both required for the parasite internalization in the cell (44, 45). Interestingly, gp30 shows a lower affinity to gastric mucin-binding proteins as compared to gp82, and this seems to be associated with low infective capacity of gp82-deficient strains *in vivo* (45, 46). Different isolates of Y strain differ in the expression of gp82 and gp30 surface molecules and the ability to infect mice by the intragastric/intrapharyngeal inoculation (46).

The infection process is also influenced by gp90, a metacyclic stage-specific molecule, that binds to mammalian cells in receptor-dependent manner but, differently from gp82, this protein is unable to trigger Ca^{2+} signal and downmodulates the parasite cell invasion capacity (47). It has been shown that *T. cruzi* strains that express high levels of gp90 on the surface, in addition to gp82 and gp30, have low cellular infection capacity *in vitro*. However, recent *in vivo* studies indicated that infectivity of *T. cruzi* is also influenced by the susceptibility of g90 molecules to peptic digestion. *T. cruzi* strains expressing pepsin-resistant gp90 isoform show a low capacity to invade gastric mucosal epithelium after intrapharyngeal inoculation in mice, resulting in subpatent or low parasitemia. By contrast, *T. cruzi* strains expressing pepsin-susceptible gp90 produced high parasitemia and high mortality when given to mice by the intrapharyngeal route (43). In addition, analysis of extracellular vesicles and soluble proteins released by metacyclic trypomastigotes forms of *T. cruzi* has revealed presence of gp82 and gp90 surface molecules in these compartments (48, 49).

A variety number of molecules involved in parasite–host cell interactions are potential candidates in oral infection. During the oral infection, parasites come across different cells throughout the gastrointestinal tract, from tissues as the mouth to intestines. In previous data, Diaz-Ungría and Bracho showed signs of a possible *T. cruzi* penetration in the oral, esophageal, gastric, and intestinal mucosa with local eosinophilia, infiltrated lymphocytes and monocytes in histological sections from dogs after oral infection (50). We have recently demonstrated that the site of parasite entrance, through the mouth (oral infection—OI), which is more similar to natural infection, versus gastrointestinal infection (GI) promotes different host immune response and mortality. Thus, compared with GI mice, OI mice presented elevated infection rate, parasitemia, and higher Th1 cytokines (51) (**Figures 1A,B**). This distinct immunological response and infection severity according to the different mucosal pathways highlighted important considerations concerning the primary site of *T. cruzi* infection in the oral route and indicated that the pathophysiology in this model may not be the same when parasites are administrated into the oral cavity or by gavage into the stomach (intrapharyngeal/intragastric).

In a recent study, the site of parasite entry in OI mice, inoculating *T. cruzi* directly in the mouth and analyzing by bioluminescence imaging corroborates the hypothesis that oral cavity is a potential critical site of initial *T. cruzi* infection before spreading to other organs in the acute phase. Moreover, OI leads to *T. cruzi* entrance in the palate, multiplication at the nasal cavity and dissemination to central nervous system and peripheral tissues. These evidences suggest that oral cavity is the primary site of infection and the nasal cavity comprises most of the parasite replication (52) (**Figures 1C,D**). Interestingly, facial edema and paresthesia of the tongue were already described in patients infected with *T. cruzi* by the oral route (53).

The mouth/oral cavity is also a target tissue for different viral, bacterial, and fungal infections disease, such as Herpes virus type 1 and 2, *Helicobacter pylori*, *Candida albicans*, and others disease (54–56). The oral cavity contains distinct mucosal surfaces and molecules expression, such as mucins, in which microorganisms can bind and, consequently colonize this anatomical region (57). The oral mucosa is coated by a film of mucus consisting of lipids, glycosylated proteins, such as mucin immunoglobulins, as well as growth factors and others. The mucins are considered as the first line of defense in the oral cavity, preventing the attachment of certain pathogens to the epithelium or forming aggregates facilitating the elimination of pathogens by the organism. However, some pathogens can bind in the carbohydrate structures present in the mucins, such as sialic acids, which favors access to epithelial cells and cell invasion (57–59).

Previous data demonstrated that *Streptococcus* sp. binds to salivary mucins on the surface of the tooth, being one of the first steps in the formation of dental plaque (60). Studies using *Tannerella forsythia*, one of the major bacterial pathogens associated with periodontitis, uncovered that glycoprotein-associated sialic acid in terminal sugars on the surface of oral cavity epithelium is important for the adhesion and invasion of these bacteria. In this study, parasite inactivation by mutation or inhibition of NanH sialidase decreased the adhesion and invasion of *T. forsythia* in human gingival epithelial cell culture lines (OBA-9). The NanH sialidase activity is specific for α-2,3 sialic acid present on the surface of gingival epithelial cells, suggesting its role in parasite adhesion and invasion (61, 62).

In line with these findings, Lakdawala and colleagues demonstrated that the soft palate is a relevant focus of influenza viruses' infection. The soft palate is a mucin-rich environment, which favors the infection and may contribute to airborne transmission. Furthermore, the expression of α-2,3 sialic acids, the viral hemagglutinin ligands, is detected on the soft palate, in the regions of the oral surface and the nasopharyngeal tissues from humans and ferret (63).

Interestingly, α-2,3 sialic acids are the main molecule involved in *T. cruzi* trans-sialidase-mediated binding. Trans-sialidase are considered as an important virulence factor, since this enzyme is able to reduce host cell immune response and mediates *T. cruzi* and host cells adhesion (33). It has been shown that trans-sialidase binds to host sialoglycans, generating "eat me" signals in epithelial cells, which facilitates parasite entry into non-phagocytic cells (64). Notably, the mouth seems to be a potential source of infection and this knowledge contributes to the elucidation of the target tissue/organs and the molecular components regulating the establishment of *T. cruzi* oral infection and its pathogenesis.

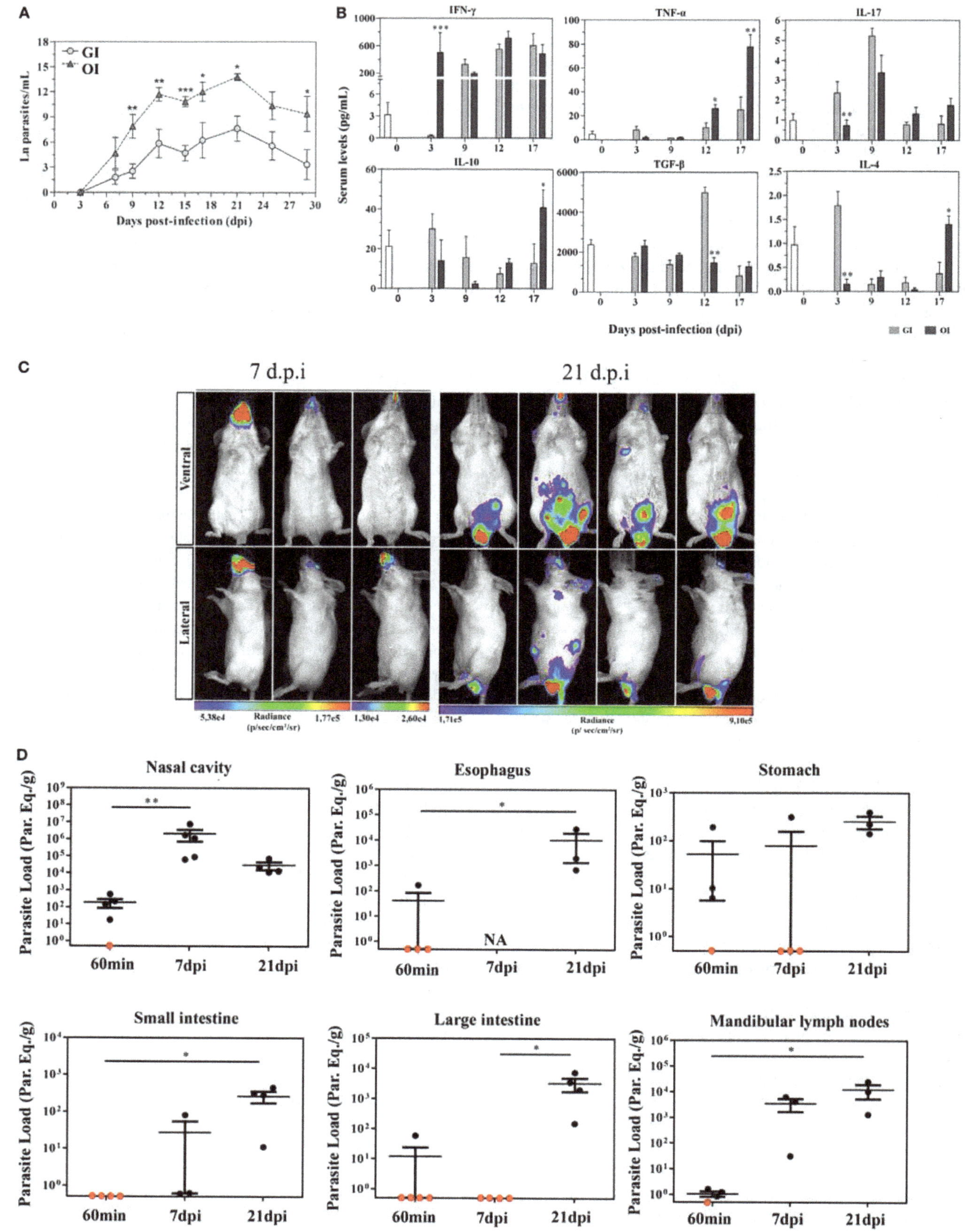

FIGURE 1 | Continued

FIGURE 1 | Severity and target tissues during acute phase of *Trypanosoma cruzi* orally infected mice. **(A)** Male BALB/c mice were infected with 5×10^4 tissue culture-derived trypomastigotes forms of *T. cruzi* (Tulahuén strain) through gavage [gastrointestinal infection (GI)] or oral cavity (OI). Parasitemia (mean and SEM) was assessed during the acute phase and expressed as ln parasites per milliliter for statistical analysis. Parasites were counted by light microscopy, and parasitemia calculated by the Brenner method. Parasitemia comparisons were performed at different days post-infection (dpi), Kruskal–Wallis, Dunn's post-test (until 15 dpi), and one-tailed Mann–Whitney (after 15 dpi) tests were used. **(A)** *n*: GI, 3 dpi = 7; 7 dpi = 22; 9 dpi = 29; 12 dpi = 17; 15 dpi = 45; 17 dpi = 10; 21 dpi = 24; 25 dpi = 16; 29 dpi = 11 and OI, 3 dpi = 4; 7 dpi = 9; 9 dpi = 14; 12 dpi = 22; 15 dpi = 40; 17 dpi = 12; 21 dpi = 14; 25 dpi = 8; 29 dpi = 6. Lower numbers represent early stages, when parasitemia was still undetectable and final stages, when mortality rates were too high. **(B)** Cytokine analysis in GI and OI mice. Male BALB/c mice were infected with 5×10^4 tissue culture-derived trypomastigotes forms of *T. cruzi* (Tulahuén strain) through gavage (GI) or within oral cavity (OI). In the course of acute infection, serum was isolated and levels of cytokines (IFN-γ, TNF, IL-17, IL-10, and TGF-β) were quantified in uninfected control and infected mice by a multiplex analysis. The results are expressed as the mean values (±SEM) for each group/day post-infection. *n*: IFN-γ, uninfected (0) = 12; 3 dpi GI = 11, OI = 5; 9 dpi GI = 8, OI = 5; 12 dpi GI = 9, OI = 4; 17 dpi GI = 4, OI = 6. TNF, uninfected (0) = 11; 3 dpi GI = 10, OI = 10; 9, 12 dpi, GI = 3, OI = 3; 17 dpi, GI = 6, OI = 11. IL-17, uninfected (0) = 12; 3 dpi, GI = 10, OI = 10; 9 dpi, GI = 3, OI = 3; 12 dpi, GI = 5, OI = 5; 17 dpi, GI = 6, OI = 14. TGF-β, uninfected (0) = 6; 3 dpi, GI = 4, OI = 4; 9 dpi, GI = 5, OI = 5; 12 dpi, GI = 5, OI = 4; 17 dpi, GI = 2, OI = 5. IL-10 and IL-4, uninfected (0) = 6; 3, 9, 12 dpi, GI = 6, OI = 6; 17 dpi, GI = 3, OI = 8. Statistical analysis was performed using GraphPad Prism 5. **p* = 0.05; ***p* = 0.01; ****p* = 0.001. **(C)** Course of parasite distribution in oral infection. Male BALB/c mice were infected in the oral cavity (OI) with 1×10^6 trypomastigotes forms of *T. cruzi* expressing luciferase (Dm28c-luc). Representative *in vivo* bioluminescence images were acquired in the same mice (*n* = 6), at 7 and 21 dpi, after 15 min of D-luciferin intraperitoneal administration (150 mg/kg), using IVIS® Lumina image system (Xenogen). **(D)** *T. cruzi* loads in orally infected mice. Male BALB/c mice were infected in the oral cavity (OI) with 1×10^6 trypomastigotes forms of *T. cruzi* expressing luciferase (Dm28c-luc). Organs and tissues were harvested for qPCR analysis to determine the parasite load (parasite equivalent/g) at 60 min, 7, and 21 dpi. The qPCR was performed in multiplex, targeting *T. cruzi* nuclear satellite DNA (Sat DNA) and IAC (internal amplification control), as a quality control. Parasite load in the nasal cavity (*n*: 60 min and 7 dpi = 5; 21 dpi = 4), esophagus (*n*: 60 min = 4; 21 dpi = 3), stomach (*n*: 60 min and 7 dpi = 4; 21 dpi = 3), small intestine (*n*: 60 min = 5; 7 dpi = 3; 21 dpi = 4), large intestine (*n*: 60 min = 5; 7 and 21 dpi = 4), and mandibular lymph nodes (*n*: 60 min = 4; 7 and 21 dpi = 3). Red dots: no parasite detection. Values present mean ± SEM. Kruskal–Wallis (Dunn's post-test) for group kinetics. Statistical analysis was performed using Graph Pad Prism 5. **p* < 0.05, ***p* < 0.01. Adapted from Barreto-de-Albuquerque et al. (51) and Silva-dos Santos et al. (52).

IMMUNE RESPONSE AND DISEASE OUTCOME IN EXPERIMENTAL MODELS

The most widely used experimental model to study *T. cruzi* infection has been for years the intraperitoneal (IP) inoculation of the parasite in mice, in which 10^2 trypomastigotes are able to promote functional alterations in the immune system from 14 days post-infection (dpi) (65). However, this pathway does not mimic the natural infection through contaminated excreta left by the vector after biting. More importantly, especially in Brazil and other endemic countries, the most frequent transmission route has been reported to be by ingestion of contaminated food and beverages (7, 17, 66, 67). Several approaches to address oral infection in mice have been described in the literature, such as intrapharyngeal, intragastric, and in the oral cavity inoculation (37, 44, 45, 51, 68–70).

Comparing mucosal routes through the digestive tube with systemic inoculation, differences in disease outcome and immune response can be observed. Intraperitoneally infected mice present higher parasitemia and mortality than intragastric or oral cavity-inoculated mice with the same inoculum (51, 69, 71). Besides, IP-infected mice also start to die earlier than GI/OI-infected and present 80–100% mortality, while GI/OI results in higher survival rates. Still, OI leads to parasitemia and mortality levels higher than in GI models. Infection through gavage (intragastrically) presents less percentage of mice with patent parasitemia, parasitemia, and mortality than IP injection (51, 70). Despite intermediate parasitemia and mortality levels between GI and IP, OI infection leads to a percentage of mice with patent parasitemia similar to IP (49.3% for GI and 97.5% for OI) (51). These temporal and quantitative differences in parasitemia might be related to the distinct barriers the parasite needs to cross after these inoculation routes. As it has been discussed in the literature, the route of parasite inoculation affects the pathogenesis and disease outcome of experimental *T. cruzi* infection (72).

After oral infection, parasites have been detected in several tissues, and even where they are not detected, inflammatory infiltrates are found (37, 52). Systemic *versus* mucosal *T. cruzi* infection leads to distinct disease patterns. Systemic infections with Peruvian strain, such as IP, IV (intravenous), or SC (subcutaneous) promote higher infection rates (67–100%) and mortality than mucosal, such as OI, GI, intrarectal, genitalia, or conjunctival infection (17–67%) (73). By contrast, the study by Caradonna and Pereiraperrin (74), mice infected with Tulahuén strain through intranasal (IN) route present higher mortality than SC. In addition, after an oral inoculation (oropharynx), insect-derived metacyclic trypomastigotes are more infective when compared to cutaneous challenge (over puncture wound that is not the same as the SC) (75).

Inoculation route can also lead to preferential tropism, as well as distinct local and systemic immune responses (51, 52, 72, 74) (**Table 1**). Inflammatory infiltrates can be found in the heart and the severity is not necessarily the main cause of death (37, 51, 69). Infiltration of immune cells is observed in several organs regardless the presence of parasite (37). The literature shows that Tulahuén strain of *T. cruzi* induces TNF production and apoptosis of hepatocytes (76). In this regard, OI and GI infection leads to apoptosis in the liver and in the heart of acute infected mice and the macrophages are the main source of TNF. These different pathways can also lead to elevated serum IFN-γ levels and TNF, especially in OI (51). Also in the heart higher levels of TNF mRNA is detected in OI when compared with GI. This elevated TNF levels in OI may be associated with cardiac, spleen, and hepatic damage, as well as toxic shock in mice, as reported in studies with other models (51, 77, 78). Besides, it can be considered one of the factors for death in mice, since blockage of this cytokine improves the survival (51).

After OI or GI, different cell types can be found within the heart and liver, such as $CD4^+$ and $CD8^+$ cells, neutrophils, and macrophages. Among them, macrophages constitute the main source

TABLE 1 | Cytokines are differentially expressed according to the infection route.

	GI	Reference	OI	Reference
CCL3	↑ stomach (a; c)/spleen (c)	(79)	N.A.	–
CCL5	↑ stomach (c)/heart (c)	(79)	N.A.	–
CXCL1	↑ stomach (c)/heart (c)	(79)	N.A.	–
CXCL10	↑ stomach (c)/heart (c)/ spleen (c)	(79)	N.A.	–
CXCL9	↑ stomach (c)/heart (c)/ spleen (c)	(79)	N.A.	–
G-CSF	↑ stomach (c)	(79)	N.A.	–
IFN-γ	↑ stomach (a; c)/spleen (c)/ serum (a)	(51, 79)	↑ IEL (a)/ LP (a)/↑↑ serum (a)	(37, 51)
IL-10	↑ stomach (a; c)/heart (c)/ spleen (a)	(79)	↑ serum (a)	(51)
IL-12	↑ stomach (a; c)/heart (c)/ spleen (a)	(79)	N.A.	
IL-17	↑ serum (a)	(51, 79)	↑↑ serum (a)	(51)
IL-2	↑ stomach (c)/spleen (c)	(79)	N.A.	–
IL-3	↑ stomach (a; c)	(79)	N.A.	–
IL-4	↑ stomach (a; c)/spleen (c)	(79)	↑ serum (a)	(51)
IL-6	↑ spleen (c)	(79)	N.A.	–
IL-7	↑ stomach (c)/spleen (c)	(79)	N.A.	–
IL-9	↑ spleen (c)	(79)	N.A.	–
M-CSF	↑ stomach (c)	(79)	N.A.	–
TGF-β	↑↑ serum (a)	(51)	↑ serum (a)	(51)
TNF	↑ stomach (c)/spleen (c)/liver (a)/heart (a)/↑ serum (a)	(51, 79)	↑ liver/ heart/↑↑ serum (a)	(51)
GM-CSF	↑ spleen (a; c)	(79)	N.A.	–

GI, gastrointestinal infection; OI, oral infection; a, acute phase; c, chronic phase; N.A., not analyzed; IEL, intraephitelial lymphocytes; LP, lamina propria.

of tissue TNF (51). In acute and chronic phase, inflammation can be detected in the stomach and heart after GI infection, followed by alterations in cytokine production. An increase of IL-12, IFN-γ, IL-4, IL-10, CCL3/4, and IL-3 is observed in the stomach during the acute phase of the disease and IL-12, TNF-α, CCL3/4, CXCL1, CCL5, CXCL9, CXCL10, G-CSF, M-CSF, IL-2, and IL-7 in the chronic phase. Hoft and collaborators demonstrated that after oral inoculation, *T. cruzi* infection within the gastric epithelium is able to stimulate B cell responses with parasite-specific IgA and IgG, suggesting activation of these cells in mucosal inductive sites, such as Peyer's patches, although the presence of parasite was not proven there. Furthermore, gastric intraepithelial lymphocytes and from lamina propria produce IFN-γ (37). In the heart, IL-10 and CXCL1 increase in animals GI-infected with the CL strain, in addition to IL-12, IL-10, CXCL9, and CXCL10 during the chronic phase. Of note, this profile can vary according to strain (79). Yet, little is known after oral inoculation of the parasite.

It was already described after IP infection, alterations in secondary lymphoid organs are observed in acute infection with an increase in total cell numbers and individual subsets as well as cytokine production in the subcutaneous lymph nodes and spleen, and a decrease in mesenteric lymph nodes and thymus (65, 80). After GI, there is an increase of neutrophils, lymphocytes, and monocytes and a reduction of the number of eosinophils in GI- and IP-infected mice. As demonstrated in Domingues and colleagues study, the peak of parasitemia in GI at 18 dpi is correlated with an increase in monocytes in the blood. The spleen also increases in GI, mainly CD8$^+$ cells and double-positive CD8$^+$CD4$^+$, but at a later time and the thymus is slightly increased instead of the atrophy observed after IP (70). High levels of IL-12, IL-10, and GM-CSF are expressed in the spleen during the acute phase of CL strain-infected mice, while IFN-γ, TNF-α, IL-6, IL-4, IL-9, CCL3/4, CXCL9, CXCL10, GM-CSF, IL-2, and IL-7 are elevated during chronic infection (79). The mesenteric lymph nodes decrease in GI with reduction of CD4$^+$ cells (70). Of note, the only study addressing lymphoid organ alteration after oral infection (oral cavity inoculation) reports an increase of gastric lymph nodes (37).

Regarding systemic cytokines GI and OI mice have a high concentration of serum IL-4, while OI leads to lower amounts of the regulatory cytokine IL-10 and TGF-β. These cytokines are known to inhibit macrophage microbicidal function, protecting the host from tissue damage (77, 81). Furthermore, inoculation of parasite through digestive mucosa (oral and more in GI) triggers IL-17 production, which is reflected in the serum. IL-17-producing cells have also been described to contribute to the formation of the gastrointestinal barrier (82). Moreover, mucosal infections (IN or OI/GI) with bacteria, such as *Listeria monocytogenes* (Lm), *Streptococcus pyogenes*, and *Francisella tularensis* leads to Th17 responses, while the systemic routes (IV or SC) trigger a Th1 response (83).

For different infection models systemic inoculations, IP, IV, and SC have been widely used. Although these approaches do not always necessarily mimic the natural transmission pathway. Our group and others have already demonstrated that the route of parasite administration is relevant for the disease outcome in infections by different pathogens (72, 84). Besides as ideal experimental model should mimic all phases of infection, including the transmission pathway (84). In this regard, for food-borne diseases, oral inoculation is an essential issue to consider.

Considering the human counterpart in Chagas disease, oral transmission has become more epidemiologically relevant and the outbreaks are related to contaminated food ingestion (85). Interestingly, facial edema is frequently observed in these patients (53). In experimental models, we described that host response is distinct when parasites are delivered into the oral cavity or by gavage (51). As it has been discussed also in non-infectious models, the oral cavity represents the first contact with the organism after ingestion and presents an underexplored environment. Thus, it should really be considered as more than just the entrance for the gastrointestinal tract (86). Tolerogenic dendritic cells producing IL-10 and IL-12 (regulatory and inflammatory profiles) can capture parasite/antigens within the mucosa in the oral cavity and in the gastrointestinal tract from where they can also be drained to the liver by the portal system (87, 88). Thus, regarding oral infections, parasite delivery into the oral cavity or by gavage (intrapharyngeal/gastrointestinal) should not be assumed as equivalent processes.

The importance to standardize the nomenclature and the choice among different approaches to address "oral" infection, such as *ad libitum*, oral gavage and in the oral cavity has been discussed also in the context of other food-borne diseases, such as Listeriosis, caused by the bacteria Lm (84). After GI Lm inoculation, high amounts of Lm and specific T cells are found in the intestinal mucosa, mesenteric lymph nodes, spleen, and liver, whereas ingestion of Lm-contaminated bread promotes increased and phenotypically distinct intestinal resident memory cells (T_{RM}) compared with other routes of infection (89–91). Moreover, IV and IN routes are able to induce T_H1 and T_H17 $CD4^+$ cells, respectively, but T_H1 cells from IV were are more likely to originate a memory cell pool than T_H17 from IN (92).

CONCLUSION AND PERSPECTIVES

Nowadays, *T. cruzi* oral transmission is an important route of infection in Latin American countries. Despite its relevance, significant studies about this form of parasite infection are largely lacking. Experimental studies related to oral *T. cruzi* and other infective agents usually comprise inoculation in the mouth (OI) or intragastrically/intrapharyngeal (GI), being roughly considered as similar routes of infection. In this review, we unraveled the intrinsic importance of specific (and distinct) tissues involved in the primary site of an infective agent entrance, resulting in regional immune response and differential disease outcome. New studies investigating the influence of target tissues and host–parasite interactions in OI and GI must be performed.

AUTHOR CONTRIBUTIONS

JM, JBA, DSS, and JS contributed with text writing and review construction.

REFERENCES

1. Schofield CJ, Diotaiuti L, Dujardin JP. The process of domestication in Triatominae. *Mem Inst Oswaldo Cruz* (1999) 94(Suppl 1):375–8. doi:10.1590/S0074-02761999000700073
2. Coura JR, Vinas PA, Junqueira AC. Ecoepidemiology, short history and control of Chagas disease in the endemic countries and the new challenge for non-endemic countries. *Mem Inst Oswaldo Cruz* (2014) 109(7):856–62. doi:10.1590/0074-0276140236
3. Dorn P, Buekens P, Hanford E. Whac-a-mole: future trends in Chagas transmission and the importance of a global perspective on disease control. *Future Microbiol* (2007) 2:365–7. doi:10.2217/17460913.2.4.365
4. Tarleton RL, Reithinger R, Urbina JA, Kitron U, Gurtler RE. The challenges of Chagas disease – grim outlook or glimmer of hope. *PLoS Med* (2007) 4:e332. doi:10.1371/journal.pmed.0040332
5. Wendel S. Transfusion transmitted Chagas disease: is it really under control? *Acta Trop* (2010) 115:28–34. doi:10.1016/j.actatropica.2009.12.006
6. Bern C, Kjos S, Yabsley MJ, Montgomery SP. *Trypanosoma cruzi* and Chagas' disease in the United States. *Clin Microbiol Rev* (2011) 24:655–81. doi:10.1128/CMR.00005-11
7. Shikanai-Yasuda MA, Carvalho NB. Oral transmission of Chagas disease. *Clin Infect Dis* (2012) 54:845–52. doi:10.1093/cid/cir956
8. Noya BA, Diaz-Bello Z, Colmenares C, Ruiz-Guevara R, Mauriello L, Munoz-Calderon A, et al. Update on oral Chagas disease outbreaks in Venezuela: epidemiological, clinical and diagnostic approaches. *Mem Inst Oswaldo Cruz* (2015) 110:377–86. doi:10.1590/0074-02760140285
9. Alarcón de Noya B, Noya González O, Robertson LJ. *Trypanosoma cruzi* as a foodborne pathogen. *SpringerBriefs in Food, Health, and Nutrition*. New York, Heidelberg, Dordrecht, London: Springer (2016). 92 p.
10. Rassi A Jr, Rassi A, Marin-Neto JA. Chagas disease. *Lancet* (2010) 375: 1388–402. doi:10.1016/S0140-6736(10)60061-X
11. Sanchez LV, Ramirez JD. Congenital and oral transmission of American trypanosomiasis: an overview of physiopathogenic aspects. *Parasitology* (2013) 140:147–59. doi:10.1017/S0031182012001394
12. Santos V, Meis J, Savino W, Andrade JAA, Vieira J, Coura JR, et al. Acute Chagas disease in the state of para, Amazon region: is it increasing? *Mem Inst Oswaldo Cruz* (2018) 113:e170298. doi:10.1590/0074-02760170298
13. Barbosa-Ferreira JM, Nobre AF, Maldonado JG, Borges-Pereira J, Zauza PL, Coura JR. [Stroke in a chronic autochthonous chagasic patient from the Brazilian Amazon]. *Rev Soc Bras Med Trop* (2010) 43:751–3. doi:10.1590/S0037-86822010000600034
14. Pinto AY, Harada GS, Valente V, Abud JE, Gomes F, Souza GC, et al. [Cardiac attacks in patients with acute Chagas disease in a family micro-outbreak, in Abaetetuba, Brazilian Amazon]. *Rev Soc Bras Med Trop* (2001) 34:413–9. doi:10.1590/S0037-86822001000500003
15. Vinas Albajar P, Laredo SV, Terrazas MB, Coura JR. [Dilated cardiomyopathy in patients with chronic chagasic infection: report of two fatal autochthonous cases from Rio Negro, state of Amazonas, Brazil]. *Rev Soc Bras Med Trop* (2003) 36:401–7. doi:10.1590/S0037-86822003000300013
16. Ianni BM, Mady C. [The sugarcane juice was delicious, but...]. *Arq Bras Cardiol* (2005) 85:379–81. doi:10.1590/S0066-782X2005001900001
17. de Noya BA, Gonzalez ON. An ecological overview on the factors that drives to *Trypanosoma cruzi* oral transmission. *Acta Trop* (2015) 151:94–102. doi:10.1016/j.actatropica.2015.06.004
18. Barbosa RL, Pereira KS, Dias VL, Schmidt FL, Alves DP, Guaraldo AM, et al. Virulence of *Trypanosoma cruzi* in Acai (*Euterpe oleraceae* Martius) pulp following mild heat treatment. *J Food Prot* (2016) 79:1807–12. doi:10.4315/0362-028X.JFP-15-595
19. Hotez PJ, Molyneux DH, Stillwaggon E, Bentwich Z, Kumaresan J. Neglected tropical diseases and HIV/AIDS. *Lancet* (2006) 368:1865–6. doi:10.1016/S0140-6736(06)69764-X
20. Savino W, Villa-Verde DM, Mendes-Da-Cruz DA, Silva-Monteiro E, Perez AR, Aoki Mdel P, et al. Cytokines and cell adhesion receptors in the regulation of immunity to *Trypanosoma cruzi*. *Cytokine Growth Factor Rev* (2007) 18:107–24. doi:10.1016/j.cytogfr.2007.01.010
21. Malik LH, Singh GD, Amsterdam EA. Chagas heart disease: an update. *Am J Med* (2015) 128(1251):e1257–9. doi:10.1016/j.amjmed.2015.04.036
22. Thakare R, Dasgupta A, Chopra S. An update on benznidazole for the treatment of patients with Chagas disease. *Drugs Today (Barc)* (2018) 54:15–23. doi:10.1358/dot.2018.54.1.2753402
23. de Souza W, de Carvalho TM, Barrias ES. Review on *Trypanosoma cruzi*: host cell interaction. *Int J Cell Biol* (2010) 2010:295394. doi:10.1155/2010/295394
24. Coura JR, Junqueira AC. Ecological diversity of *Trypanosoma cruzi* transmission in the Amazon basin. The main scenaries in the Brazilian Amazon. *Acta Trop* (2015) 151:51–7. doi:10.1016/j.actatropica.2015.04.029
25. Maeda FY, Cortez C, Yoshida N. Cell signaling during *Trypanosoma cruzi* invasion. *Front Immunol* (2012) 3:361. doi:10.3389/fimmu.2012.00361
26. Barrias ES, de Carvalho TM, De Souza W. *Trypanosoma cruzi*: entry into mammalian host cells and parasitophorous vacuole formation. *Front Immunol* (2013) 4:186. doi:10.3389/fimmu.2013.00186
27. Cardoso MS, Reis-Cunha JL, Bartholomeu DC. Evasion of the immune response by *Trypanosoma cruzi* during acute infection. *Front Immunol* (2015) 6:659. doi:10.3389/fimmu.2015.00659
28. Schenkman S, Jiang MS, Hart GW, Nussenzweig V. A novel cell surface trans-sialidase of *Trypanosoma cruzi* generates a stage-specific epitope required for invasion of mammalian cells. *Cell* (1991) 65:1117–25. doi:10.1016/0092-8674(91)90008-M
29. Buscaglia CA, Campo VA, Frasch AC, Di Noia JM. *Trypanosoma cruzi* surface mucins: host-dependent coat diversity. *Nat Rev Microbiol* (2006) 4:229–36. doi:10.1038/nrmicro1351

30. Yoshida N, Cortez M. *Trypanosoma cruzi*: parasite and host cell signaling during the invasion process. *Subcell Biochem* (2008) 47:82–91. doi:10.1007/978-0-387-78267-6_6
31. Villalta F, Scharfstein J, Ashton AW, Tyler KM, Guan F, Mukherjee S, et al. Perspectives on the *Trypanosoma cruzi*-host cell receptor interactions. *Parasitol Res* (2009) 104:1251–60. doi:10.1007/s00436-009-1383-3
32. Yoshida N. Molecular mechanisms of *Trypanosoma cruzi* infection by oral route. *Mem Inst Oswaldo Cruz* (2009) 104(Suppl 1):101–7. doi:10.1590/S0074-02762009000900015
33. Freire-de-Lima L, Fonseca LM, Oeltmann T, Mendonca-Previato L, Previato JO. The trans-sialidase, the major *Trypanosoma cruzi* virulence factor: three decades of studies. *Glycobiology* (2015) 25:1142–9. doi:10.1093/glycob/cwv057
34. Yoshida N. *Trypanosoma cruzi* infection by oral route: how the interplay between parasite and host components modulates infectivity. *Parasitol Int* (2008) 57:105–9. doi:10.1016/j.parint.2007.12.008
35. Ortega-Barria E, Pereira ME. A novel *T. cruzi* heparin-binding protein promotes fibroblast adhesion and penetration of engineered bacteria and trypanosomes into mammalian cells. *Cell* (1991) 67:411–21. doi:10.1016/0092-8674(91)90192-2
36. Calvet CM, Melo TG, Garzoni LR, Oliveira FO Jr, Neto DT, Meirelles MNSL, et al. Current understanding of the *Trypanosoma cruzi*-cardiomyocyte interaction. *Front Immunol* (2012) 3:327. doi:10.3389/fimmu.2012.00327
37. Hoft DF, Farrar PL, Kratz-Owens K, Shaffer D. Gastric invasion by *Trypanosoma cruzi* and induction of protective mucosal immune responses. *Infect Immun* (1996) 64:3800–10.
38. Staquicini DI, Martins RM, Macedo S, Sasso GR, Atayde VD, Juliano MA, et al. Role of GP82 in the selective binding to gastric mucin during oral infection with *Trypanosoma cruzi*. *PLoS Negl Trop Dis* (2010) 4:e613. doi:10.1371/journal.pntd.0000613
39. Yoshida N, Tyler KM, Llewellyn MS. Invasion mechanisms among emerging food-borne protozoan parasites. *Trends Parasitol* (2011) 27:459–66. doi:10.1016/j.pt.2011.06.006
40. Neira I, Silva FA, Cortez M, Yoshida N. Involvement of *Trypanosoma cruzi* metacyclic trypomastigote surface molecule gp82 in adhesion to gastric mucin and invasion of epithelial cells. *Infect Immun* (2003) 71:557–61. doi:10.1128/IAI.71.1.557-561.2003
41. Teixeira MM, Yoshida N. Stage-specific surface antigens of metacyclic trypomastigotes of *Trypanosoma cruzi* identified by monoclonal antibodies. *Mol Biochem Parasitol* (1986) 18:271–82. doi:10.1016/0166-6851(86)90085-X
42. Araya JE, Cano MI, Yoshida N, Da Silveira JF. Cloning and characterization of a gene for the stage-specific 82-kDa surface antigen of metacyclic trypomastigotes of *Trypanosoma cruzi*. *Mol Biochem Parasitol* (1994) 65:161–9. doi:10.1016/0166-6851(94)90124-4
43. Cortez M, Silva MR, Neira I, Ferreira D, Sasso GR, Luquetti AO, et al. *Trypanosoma cruzi* surface molecule gp90 downregulates invasion of gastric mucosal epithelium in orally infected mice. *Microbes Infect* (2006) 8:36–44. doi:10.1016/j.micinf.2005.05.016
44. Cortez C, Yoshida N, Bahia D, Sobreira TJ. Structural basis of the interaction of a *Trypanosoma cruzi* surface molecule implicated in oral infection with host cells and gastric mucin. *PLoS One* (2012) 7:e42153. doi:10.1371/journal.pone.0042153
45. Cortez M, Neira I, Ferreira D, Luquetti AO, Rassi A, Atayde VD, et al. Infection by *Trypanosoma cruzi* metacyclic forms deficient in gp82 but expressing a related surface molecule, gp30. *Infect Immun* (2003) 71:6184–91. doi:10.1128/IAI.71.11.6184-6191.2003
46. Cortez C, Martins RM, Alves RM, Silva RC, Bilches LC, Macedo S, et al. Differential infectivity by the oral route of *Trypanosoma cruzi* lineages derived from Y strain. *PLoS Negl Trop Dis* (2012) 6:e1804. doi:10.1371/journal.pntd.0001804
47. Malaga S, Yoshida N. Targeted reduction in expression of *Trypanosoma cruzi* surface glycoprotein gp90 increases parasite infectivity. *Infect Immun* (2001) 69:353–9. doi:10.1128/IAI.69.1.353-359.2001
48. Bayer-Santos E, Cunha-E-Silva NL, Yoshida N, Franco Da Silveira J. Expression and cellular trafficking of GP82 and GP90 glycoproteins during *Trypanosoma cruzi* metacyclogenesis. *Parasit Vectors* (2013) 6:127. doi:10.1186/1756-3305-6-127
49. Clemente TM, Cortez C, Novaes Ada S, Yoshida N. Surface molecules released by *Trypanosoma cruzi* metacyclic forms downregulate host cell invasion. *PLoS Negl Trop Dis* (2016) 10:e0004883. doi:10.1371/journal.pntd.0004883
50. Diaz-Ungría C, Bracho JS. Camino que sigue el *Trypanosoma cruzi* en perros infectados por vía bucal: nuevos estudios. *Rev Vet Venezuelana* (1970) 44:114–9.
51. Barreto-de-Albuquerque J, Silva-dos-Santos D, Perez AR, Berbert LR, de Santana-Van-Vliet E, Farias-de-Oliveira DA, et al. *Trypanosoma cruzi* infection through the oral route promotes a severe infection in mice: new disease form from an old infection? *PLoS Negl Trop Dis* (2015) 9:e0003849. doi:10.1371/journal.pntd.0003849
52. Silva-dos-Santos D, Barreto-de-Albuquerque J, Guerra B, Moreira OC, Berbert LR, Ramos MT, et al. Unraveling Chagas disease transmission through the oral route: gateways to *Trypanosoma cruzi* infection and target tissues. *PLoS Negl Trop Dis* (2017) 11:e0005507. doi:10.1371/journal.pntd.0005507
53. Pinto AY, Ferreira AG Jr, Valente Vda C, Harada GS, Valente SA. Urban outbreak of acute Chagas disease in Amazon region of Brazil: four-year follow-up after treatment with benznidazole. *Rev Panam Salud Publica* (2009) 25:77–83. doi:10.1590/S1020-49892009000100012
54. Stoopler ET, Sollecito TP. Oral mucosal diseases: evaluation and management. *Med Clin North Am* (2014) 98:1323–52. doi:10.1016/j.mcna.2014.08.006
55. Salvatori O, Puri S, Tati S, Edgerton M. Innate immunity and saliva in *Candida albicans*-mediated oral diseases. *J Dent Res* (2016) 95:365–71. doi:10.1177/0022034515625222
56. Yee JK. Helicobacter pylori colonization of the oral cavity: a milestone discovery. *World J Gastroenterol* (2016) 22:641–8. doi:10.3748/wjg.v22.i2.641
57. Wu RQ, Zhang DF, Tu E, Chen QM, Chen W. The mucosal immune system in the oral cavity—an orchestra of T cell diversity. *Int J Oral Sci* (2014) 6:125–32. doi:10.1038/ijos.2014.48
58. Tabak LA. In defense of the oral cavity: structure, biosynthesis, and function of salivary mucins. *Annu Rev Physiol* (1995) 57:547–64. doi:10.1146/annurev.ph.57.030195.002555
59. Derrien M, van Passel MW, van de Bovenkamp JH, Schipper RG, de Vos WM, Dekker J. Mucin-bacterial interactions in the human oral cavity and digestive tract. *Gut Microbes* (2010) 1:254–68. doi:10.4161/gmic.1.4.12778
60. Murray PA, Prakobphol A, Lee T, Hoover CI, Fisher SJ. Adherence of oral streptococci to salivary glycoproteins. *Infect Immun* (1992) 60:31–8.
61. Honma K, Mishima E, Sharma A. Role of *Tannerella forsythia* NanH sialidase in epithelial cell attachment. *Infect Immun* (2011) 79:393–401. doi:10.1128/IAI.00629-10
62. Roy S, Honma K, Douglas CW, Sharma A, Stafford GP. Role of sialidase in glycoprotein utilization by *Tannerella forsythia*. *Microbiology* (2011) 157:3195–202. doi:10.1099/mic.0.052498-0
63. Lakdawala SS, Jayaraman A, Halpin RA, Lamirande EW, Shih AR, Stockwell TB, et al. The soft palate is an important site of adaptation for transmissible influenza viruses. *Nature* (2015) 526:122–5. doi:10.1038/nature15379
64. Butler CE, de Carvalho TM, Grisard EC, Field RA, Tyler KM. Trans-sialidase stimulates eat me response from epithelial cells. *Traffic* (2013) 14:853–69. doi:10.1111/tra.12078
65. de Meis J, Morrot A, Farias-de-Oliveira DA, Villa-Verde DM, Savino W. Differential regional immune response in Chagas disease. *PLoS Negl Trop Dis* (2009) 3:e417. doi:10.1371/journal.pntd.0000417
66. Benchimol Barbosa PR. The oral transmission of Chagas' disease: an acute form of infection responsible for regional outbreaks. *Int J Cardiol* (2006) 112:132–3. doi:10.1016/j.ijcard.2005.11.087
67. Dias JC. [Notes about of *Trypanosoma cruzi* and yours bio-ecology characteristics with agents of the transmission by meals]. *Rev Soc Bras Med Trop* (2006) 39:370–5. doi:10.1590/S0037-86822006000400010
68. Kirchhoff LV, Hoft DF. Immunization and challenge of mice with insect-derived metacyclic trypomastigotes of *Trypanosoma cruzi*. *Parasite Immunol* (1990) 12:65–74. doi:10.1111/j.1365-3024.1990.tb00936.x
69. Camandaroba EL, Pinheiro Lima CM, Andrade SG. Oral transmission of Chagas disease: importance of *Trypanosoma cruzi* biodeme in the intragastric experimental infection. *Rev Inst Med Trop Sao Paulo* (2002) 44:97–103. doi:10.1590/S0036-46652002000200008
70. Domingues CS, Hardoim DJ, Souza CS, Cardoso FO, Mendes VG, Previtalli-Silva H, et al. Oral Outbreak of Chagas disease in Santa Catarina, Brazil: experimental evaluation of a patient's strain. *PLoS One* (2015) 10:e0122566. doi:10.1371/journal.pone.0122566

71. Dias GB, Gruendling AP, Araujo SM, Gomes ML, Toledo MJ. Evolution of infection in mice inoculated by the oral route with different developmental forms of *Trypanosoma cruzi* I and II. *Exp Parasitol* (2013) 135:511–7. doi:10.1016/j.exppara.2013.08.013
72. de Meis J, Barreto de Albuquerque J, Silva dos Santos D, Farias-de-Oliveira DA, Berbert LR, Cotta-de-Almeida V, et al. *Trypanosoma cruzi* entrance through systemic or mucosal infection sites differentially modulates regional immune response following acute infection in mice. *Front Immunol* (2013) 4:216. doi:10.3389/fimmu.2013.00216
73. Marsden PD. *Trypanosoma cruzi* infections in CFI mice. II. Infections induced by different routes. *Ann Trop Med Parasitol* (1967) 61:62–7. doi:10.1080/00034983.1967.11686458
74. Caradonna K, Pereiraperrin M. Preferential brain homing following intranasal administration of *Trypanosoma cruzi*. *Infect Immun* (2009) 77:1349–56. doi:10.1128/IAI.01434-08
75. Eickhoff CS, Dunn BA, Sullivan NL, Hoft DF. Comparison of the infectivity of *Trypanosoma cruzi* insect-derived metacyclic trypomastigotes after mucosal and cutaneous contaminative challenges. *Mem Inst Oswaldo Cruz* (2013) 108:508–11. doi:10.1590/S0074-02762013000400018
76. Ronco MT, Frances DE, Ingaramo PI, Quiroga AD, Alvarez ML, Pisani GB, et al. Tumor necrosis factor alpha induced by *Trypanosoma cruzi* infection mediates inflammation and cell death in the liver of infected mice. *Cytokine* (2010) 49:64–72. doi:10.1016/j.cyto.2009.09.012
77. Holscher C, Mohrs M, Dai WJ, Kohler G, Ryffel B, Schaub GA, et al. Tumor necrosis factor alpha-mediated toxic shock in *Trypanosoma cruzi*-infected interleukin 10-deficient mice. *Infect Immun* (2000) 68:4075–83. doi:10.1128/IAI.68.7.4075-4083.2000
78. Andrade SG, Magalhaes Ldos A, Pessina DH. Importance of TNF-alpha in the course of acute infection with *Trypanosoma cruzi*: influence of its inhibition by pentoxifylline treatment. *Mem Inst Oswaldo Cruz* (2008) 103:21–6. doi:10.1590/S0074-02762008005000006
79. Rodrigues AA, Notario AF, Teixeira TL, Silva E, Quintal RT, Alves AP. A high throughput analysis of cytokines and chemokines expression during the course of *Trypanosoma cruzi* experimental oral infection. *Acta Trop* (2016) 157:42–53. doi:10.1016/j.actatropica.2016.01.025
80. de Meis J, Ferreira LM, Guillermo LV, Silva EM, Dosreis GA, Lopes MF. Apoptosis differentially regulates mesenteric and subcutaneous lymph node immune responses to *Trypanosoma cruzi*. *Eur J Immunol* (2008) 38:139–46. doi:10.1002/eji.200737582
81. Reed SG, Brownell CE, Russo DM, Silva JS, Grabstein KH, Morrissey PJ. IL-10 mediates susceptibility to *Trypanosoma cruzi* infection. *J Immunol* (1994) 153:3135–40.
82. Blaschitz C, Raffatellu M. Th17 cytokines and the gut mucosal barrier. *J Clin Immunol* (2010) 30:196–203. doi:10.1007/s10875-010-9368-7
83. Hu W, Pasare C. Location, location, location: tissue-specific regulation of immune responses. *J Leukoc Biol* (2013) 94:409–21. doi:10.1189/jlb.0413207
84. D'Orazio SE. Animal models for oral transmission of *Listeria monocytogenes*. *Front Cell Infect Microbiol* (2014) 4:15. doi:10.3389/fcimb.2014.00015
85. Toso MA, Vial UF, Galanti N. [Oral transmission of Chagas' disease]. *Rev Med Chil* (2011) 139:258–66. doi:10.4067/S0034-98872011000200017
86. Novak N, Haberstok J, Bieber T, Allam JP. The immune privilege of the oral mucosa. *Trends Mol Med* (2008) 14:191–8. doi:10.1016/j.molmed.2008.03.001
87. Weiner HL, Da Cunha AP, Quintana F, Wu H. Oral tolerance. *Immunol Rev* (2011) 241:241–59. doi:10.1111/j.1600-065X.2011.01017.x
88. Moingeon P, Mascarell L. Induction of tolerance via the sublingual route: mechanisms and applications. *Clin Dev Immunol* (2012) 2012:623474. doi:10.1155/2012/623474
89. Kursar M, Bonhagen K, Kohler A, Kamradt T, Kaufmann SH, Mittrucker HW. Organ-specific CD4+ T cell response during *Listeria monocytogenes* infection. *J Immunol* (2002) 168:6382–7. doi:10.4049/jimmunol.168.12.6382
90. Kursar M, Kohler A, Kaufmann SH, Mittrucker HW. Depletion of CD4+ T cells during immunization with nonviable *Listeria monocytogenes* causes enhanced CD8+ T cell-mediated protection against listeriosis. *J Immunol* (2004) 172:3167–72. doi:10.4049/jimmunol.172.5.3167
91. Sheridan BS, Pham QM, Lee YT, Cauley LS, Puddington L, Lefrancois L. Oral infection drives a distinct population of intestinal resident memory CD8(+) T cells with enhanced protective function. *Immunity* (2014) 40:747–57. doi:10.1016/j.immuni.2014.03.007
92. Pepper M, Linehan JL, Pagan AJ, Zell T, Dileepan T, Cleary PP, et al. Different routes of bacterial infection induce long-lived TH1 memory cells and short-lived TH17 cells. *Nat Immunol* (2010) 11:83–9. doi:10.1038/ni.1826

9

Silent Witness: Dual-Species Transcriptomics Reveals Epithelial Immunological Quiescence to Helminth Larval Encounter and Fostered Larval Development

Friederike Ebner[1], Mathias Kuhring[2,3,4,5], Aleksandar Radonić[6], Ankur Midha[1], Bernhard Y. Renard[2] and Susanne Hartmann[1]*

[1] Department of Veterinary Medicine, Institute of Immunology, Freie Universität Berlin, Berlin, Germany, [2] Bioinformatics Unit (MF1), Department for Methods Development and Research Infrastructure, Robert Koch Institute, Berlin, Germany, [3] Core Unit Bioinformatics, Berlin Institute of Health (BIH), Berlin, Germany, [4] Berlin Institute of Health Metabolomics Platform, Berlin Institute of Health (BIH), Berlin, Germany, [5] Max Delbrück Center (MDC) for Molecular Medicine, Berlin, Germany, [6] Center for Biological Threats and Special Pathogens: Highly Pathogenic Viruses (ZBS 1), Robert Koch Institute, Berlin, Germany

***Correspondence:**
Friederike Ebner
friederike.ebner@fu-berlin.de

Gastrointestinal nematodes are among the most prevalent parasites infecting humans and livestock worldwide. Infective larvae of the soil-transmitted nematode *Ascaris* spp. enter the host and start tissue migration by crossing the intestinal epithelial barrier. The initial interaction of the intestinal epithelium with the parasite, however, has received little attention. In a time-resolved interaction model of porcine intestinal epithelial cells (IPEC-J2) and infective *Ascaris suum* larvae, we addressed the early transcriptional changes occurring simultaneously in both organisms using dual-species RNA-Seq. Functional analysis of the host response revealed an overall induction of metabolic activity, without induction of immune responsive genes or immune signaling pathways and showing suppression of chemotactic genes like CXCL8/IL-8 or CHI3L1. *Ascaris* larvae, when getting in contact with the epithelium, showed induction of genes that orchestrate motor activity and larval development, such as myosin, troponin, myoglobin, and protein disulfide isomerase 2 (PDI-2). In addition, excretory-secretory products that likely facilitate parasite invasion were increased, among them, aspartic protease 6 or hyaluronidase. Integration of host and pathogen data in an interspecies gene co-expression network indicated links between nematode fatty acid biosynthesis and host ribosome assembly/protein synthesis. In summary, our study provides new molecular insights into the early factors of parasite invasion, while at the same time revealing host immunological unresponsiveness. Reproducible software for dual RNA-Seq analysis of non-model organisms is available at https://gitlab.com/mkuhring/project_asuum and can be applied to similar studies.

Keywords: host–pathogen, parasitic nematode, IPEC-J2, *Ascaris suum*, dual-species, RNA sequencing, transcriptomics, epithelial communication

INTRODUCTION

The large roundworms *Ascaris (A.) lumbricoides* and *Ascaris suum* are the most prevalent soil-transmitted helminths worldwide and parasitize the gastrointestinal tract of humans and pigs, respectively. With an estimated 800 million people currently infected, typically in the most impoverished populations, Ascariasis belongs to the group of neglected tropical diseases (1–3). Among pigs, the prevalence of *A. suum* in high intensity production farms remains high all over the world and *A. suum* infections are known to cause major economic losses in the pig industry due to reduced growth performance, liver condemnation, and reduced vaccination responses (4, 5). Due to the genetic closeness of *A. lumbricoides* and *A. suum* (6, 7), studying host–parasite interactions in pigs is not only of veterinary importance but also represents an ideal research model for the human condition (8).

Ascariasis is caused by ingesting infective eggs containing L3 larvae from contaminated food and water, or with regard to pigs, coprophagy (9). The eggs hatch in the intestine and parasites undergo larval migration through the body before developing into adult worms that inhabit the small intestine. The early, intestinal migratory path involves newly hatched L3 larvae penetrating the walls of the distal small intestine, cecum, and proximal colon (10, 11) and migrating toward the liver.

Given the initial invasion and chronic infestation at gastrointestinal barriers, the mucosal immune response is of fundamental importance for defending against the parasite. The first cells to encounter invading *Ascaris* larvae are epithelial cells. The intestinal epithelium represents a tight barrier that prevents pathogen invasion. However, rather than being just a physical barrier, epithelial cells are equipped with microbial-detection mechanisms, signaling circuits, and both homeostatic and inflammatory mediators (12, 13). At the interface between host and environment, the epithelium defends the host against infection to the one side while fostering innate immune recognition and transmission of danger signals to the other side (12). While many types of pattern recognition receptors (PRRs) facilitate sensing of microbes, it is less clear how enteric parasites like *Ascaris* spp., which do not express known PAMPs, are sensed and detected by the epithelium. Conversely, whether a targeted host–pathogen interaction at the epithelial barrier drives larval tissue migration is not yet known.

The site-specific mucosal penetration of invading *Ascaris* L3 occurs within 3–6 h after oral infection (11) and restricts the window for an early intervention. Infection and challenge studies have greatly contributed to our understanding of hepatic- and pulmonary immune responses against *A. suum* (11, 14, 15); however, not much is known concerning the initial steps of immune recognition and modulation during early larval migration. Understanding to what extend host and parasite might sense, interact, regulate, or harm each other at the epithelial interface might clarify how mucosal immunity is initiated and reveal possible intervention strategies.

Therefore, we performed a time-resolved transcriptional analysis of infective *A. suum* third-stage larvae (AscL3) co-incubated with porcine intestinal-epithelial cells (IPEC-J2), an *in vitro* model widely used to study microbial pathogen–host interaction (16, 17). In that context, RNA-Seq is extremely useful for addressing non-model organisms such as a parasitic nematode (*A. suum*) and the pig. Addressing the limitations of most current dual RNA-Seq pathogen–host studies, pointed out by Westerman and colleagues (18) in a recent review, we do not restrict our analysis to pairwise differential comparisons of sets of time points, but account for the complete temporal behavior. By contrasting splines fitted across the time lines to baseline models rather than individual time point comparisons, statistical power can be increased (19) and the statistical model can capture trends that otherwise may be missed due to the restricted temporal granularity of individual time points (18).

In contrast to intracellular microbial pathogens, the possibility of separating larvae and host tissue after incubation enables purer sequencing and thus transcriptome analysis is unaffected by asymmetric read coverage as well as cross read mappings. In addition, we complement annotation of the non-model *A. suum* transcriptome for functional analysis by implementing a unique iterative annotation strategy favoring transfer from closely related species. This workflow builds upon continuously increasing the search space of species, thereby favoring results from closely related species were available, but still annotating sequences were no hits on closely related species can be found.

While many software solutions for individual steps are available, we are not aware of any interconnected analysis pipeline for dual RNA-Seq studies of non-model organisms. Here, we rely on Snakemake (20) as a current bioinformatics community standard to provide workflows at https://gitlab.com/mkuhring/project_asuum/. These workflows not only allow full reproduction of our analyses but are provided for reusage in related experiments and capture all relevant steps. Particularly, we integrated and primarily automated the annotation steps for both non-model organisms with the differential expression and functional analysis.

Our time-resolved, dual-species whole-transcriptome approach provides molecular insights into host–parasite interactions during direct physical interaction and in the absence of surrounding microbes, their metabolites and second line immune cells, enabling us to focus exclusively on parasite-epithelial cross-talk. Our results demonstrate that *Ascaris* larvae invade the host soft-footed without initiating immune alarming responses while expressing genes ensuring invasion and their further development.

MATERIALS AND METHODS

Generation of Infective *A. suum* L3 Stage Larvae and Hatching

Infective third-stage larvae of *A. suum* were generated as previously described (21). In brief, secreted *A. suum* eggs were collected from the culture fluid of female worms obtained from a local slaughter house. Eggs were decoated in 0.5 M sodium hydroxide, washed, and embryonated in 0.1 N H_2SO_4 for 6–8 weeks under weekly aeration. For hatching, embryonated eggs were treated with 5.25% sodium hypochlorite to remove the chitinous layer from the eggs. Hypochlorite-treated eggs were further layered below slowly moving sterile glass beads (4 mm) to facilitate hatching. Subsequently, intact and motile *A. suum* larvae were collected, washed, counted, and adapted to mammalian cell culture media (IMDM, 5% FCS, 1% P/S) over night.

Parasite and Epithelial Cell Co-Incubation

Porcine intestinal epithelial cells (IPEC-J2 cell line) were cultured as monolayers for complete confluence in 35 mm Petri dishes [IMDM, 5% FCS, 1% P/S (all from PAN-Biotech, Aidenbach, Germany)]. L3 stage *A. suum* worms (50,000/dish, resulting in a larva to cell ratio of 1:10) were layered on top of epithelial cells and co-incubated for the indicated time points at 37°C, 5% CO_2. Three biological replicates of a time-resolved co-incubation series of pathogen and epithelial cells were performed, with five time points (0, 1, 2, 3, and 9 h) being interrogated with regard to the early migratory pathway of *A. suum* (10, 11). Monocultures of either worms or epithelial cells served as controls (referred to as time point 0 h). Following co-incubation, *A. suum* larvae were removed from the epithelial layer and worms and epithelial cells were processed separately for RNA isolation. Viability of IPEC-J2 cells following larval coculture was verified in separate experiments by vital cell counting, measuring ATP as indicator for metabolically active cells and by documenting the monolayer appearance using Giemsa staining (Figures S6A–C in Supplementary Material). Asc L3 were visually inspected for larval motility throughout the entire coculture period and assayed for migration capacity and viability [excretory-secretory (ES) production] after 9 h of coculture (Figures S6E,F in Supplementary Material).

RNA Isolation and Quality Check

Worm samples were homogenized using shredder columns filled with 200 mg sterile sea sand and the FastPrep®-24 instrument (MP Biomedicals) at 5 m/s for 35 s. Supernatants of homogenized worms and epithelial cell lysates were further processed for RNA isolation (InnuPREP RNA isolation, Analytik Jena AG, Germany), DNase treatment (Analytik Jena AG, Germany), and RNA quality control (Agilent 2100 Bioanalyzer, RNA 6000 Nano Kit, Agilent Technologies, Waldbronn, Germany). RNA sample RIN values ranged between 7.9 and 10 for porcine epithelial cells and 7.3 and 9.5 for AscL3, respectively.

Sequencing and Mapping

For transcriptome sequencing on an Illumina platform a TruSeq RNA library generation was utilized. The library was generated by using the TruSeq RNA Sample Prep Kit v2 (Illumina, San Diego, CA, USA) following the manufacturer's instructions. The library was quantified by using the KAPA Library Quantification Kit for Illumina (Kapa Biosystems, Wilmington, MA, USA). The library size was determined by using the High Sensitivity DNA Analysis Kit for the 2100 Bioanalyzer Instrument (Agilent Technologies, Waldbronn, Germany). Libraries were adjusted to a concentration of 12 pM and sequenced on a HiSeq 1500 instrument (Illumina, San Diego, CA, USA) in high-output mode. For cluster generation, the TruSeq PE Cluster Kit v3 was used. Cluster generation was performed on a cBot instrument. For sequencing, the TruSeq SBS Kit v3 was used to sequence 100 + 100 bases.

Sequence data processing and analysis were conducted as illustrated in **Figure 1B**. We sequenced 15 (resulting in three replicates for each of the five time points) AscL3 and IPEC-J2 samples each, with a mean library size of 45.5 million paired-end reads and a SD of 25.4. Raw reads were subjected to quality control and trimming *via* the QCumber pipeline (version 1.0.0)[1] utilizing FastQC (v0.11.5)[2], Trimmomatic (0.33) (22), and Kraken (0.10.5-beta) (23). On average, 88.21% of reads remained after trimming.

Preprocessed reads were mapped to reference genomes as specified below and corresponding sequence features using the TopHat split-read mapper (v2.1.1) (24) and reference as well as novel features were extracted and merged with the aid of Cufflinks (25) and Cuffmerge (25) (v2.2.1) to obtain one integrated and unified transcriptome for AscL3 and IPEC-J2 samples,

[1]https://gitlab.com/RKIBioinformaticsPipelines/QCumber (Accessed: March 17, 2018).

[2]https://www.bioinformatics.babraham.ac.uk/projects/fastqc/ (Accessed: March 17, 2018).

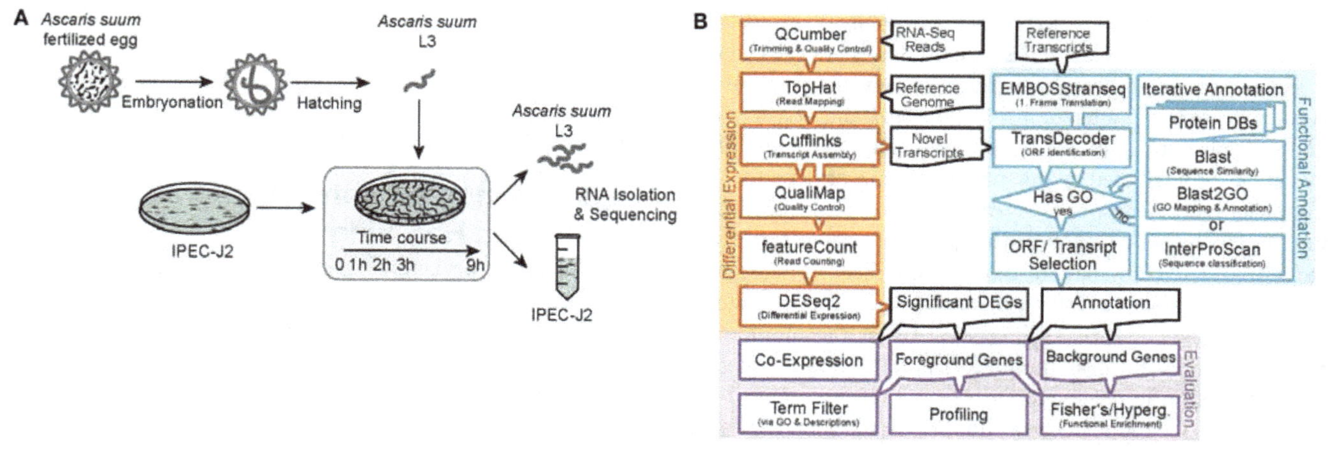

FIGURE 1 | Experimental design and RNA-Seq data processing. **(A)** Analysis of the early host–parasite interaction of *Ascaris suum* L3 and porcine epithelial cells (IPEC-J2) by studying dual-species gene expression dynamics over a time course (0–9 h). **(B)** Paired RNA samples were Illumina sequenced, preprocessed, mapped to reference genomes, annotated, and differential gene expression and functional analysis was performed using the illustrated bioinformatics pipeline.

respectively. Reference genomes used included the original *A. suum* draft genome from Jex et al. (26) as available from the WormBase ParaSite (27) FTP server (ftp.wormbase.org/pub/wormbase/species/a_suum/assemblies/v1/) and the *Sus scrofa* genome assembly from Ensembl (28) (Sscrofa10.2, release 85).

Differential Expression

For each sample, raw expression values were created by counting uniquely mapped reads on gene level using featureCounts (v1.5.0-p3) (29). To identify differentially expressed genes (DEGs) within AscL3 and IPEC-J2 samples, respectively, DESeq2 (1.12.4) (19) was adjusted for a time series design model based on natural splines to account for the time points in the experiment. A likelihood-ratio test against fits of a reduced null model including only intercept and the batch variable was applied to infer significant DEGs. However, pairwise fold-changes for each time point greater than 0 h were extracted *via* a classic DESeq2 model and pairwise contrasts with the base time point 0 h (indicating expression changes in comparison to 0 h). In addition, normalized and transformed expression values were extracted from DESeq2 (regularized log transformation) and corrected for batch effects *via* Limma (3.28.21, removeBatchEffect) (30) to allow for sample quality control with clustered heatmaps and principal component analysis (PCA).

Functional Annotation

Reference as well as novel transcripts were functionally annotated with focus on Gene Ontology (GO) terms (31, 32) using a novel iterative annotation strategy. First, transcripts were either first-frame translated (reference) or examined for ORFs (novels, Cuffcompare class code "u") using EMBOSS transeq (6.6.0.0) (33) and TransDecoder (v2.1)[3], respectively. Next, resulting protein sequences were passed through a series of database searches until successfully annotated with GO, either *via* blastp (2.6.0+) (34) and Blast2GO (4.0.7) (35) or by a final InterProScan classification (5.23–62.0 for *A. suum*, 5.22–61.0 for *S. scrofa*) (36). Databases used for *A. suum* sequences annotation included (in this order) the UniProt (37) *A. suum* proteome (UP000017900), UniProt Swiss-Prot Nematoda proteins, UniProt TrEMBL Nematoda proteins as well as the complete Swiss-Prot database and the complete TrEMBL database (all downloaded at 16.02.2017). For *S. scrofa* sequences, Ensembl reference annotations were obtained *via* the Ensembl BioMart server (38, 39) (with date of 30.10.2016). In addition, remaining non-annotated transcripts were searched against the UniProt *S. scrofa* proteome (UP000008227), Swiss-Prot Mammalia proteins, TrEMBL Mammalia proteins (all downloaded at 27.02.2017) as well as the complete Swiss-Prot database and the complete TrEMBL database (both downloaded at 16.02.2017).

In addition to GO terms, protein sequences were annotated with KEGG Orthology terms (KO) (40) *via* the BlastKOALA web interface (2.1) (41) using the "family_eukaryotes" and "genus_prokaryotes" databases for *A. suum* sequences and the "genus_eukaryotes" database for *S. scrofa* sequences, respectively (database builds 02.05.2017). However, for *S. scrofa*, reference annotations obtained *via* biomaRt (2.28.0) (42) and KEGGREST (1.12.3)[4] were preferred if available. KO terms were then mapped to KEGG pathways *via* KEGGREST. Furthermore, *A. suum* sequences were examined for potential excretory and secretory proteins as previously described by others (43). In brief, ES proteins were annotated as classical or non-classical secretory proteins by combining SignalP (4.1 Server, organism group "Eukaryotes") (44) and SecretomeP (2.0 Server, organism groups "Gram-negative bacteria," "Gram-positive bacteria," and "Mammalian") (45, 46). Mitochondrial proteins were excluded from that list using TargetP (1.1 Server, organism group "Non-plant") (47) as well as proteins predicted for transmembrane regions by TMHMM (Server v. 2.0) (48). The remaining predicted ES proteins were further categorized by KEGG ENZYME enzyme codes derived from KO-terms with the use of KEGGREST.

Functional Analysis

Functional profiles and enrichment analysis of significant DEGs were calculated based on GO term annotations (projected onto level 2) of the three classes of molecular function (MF), cellular component (CC), and biological process (BP) as well as on KEGG Pathways. For enrichment analysis, significant DEGs were tested against background gene sets representing the expression potential in the experiment, i.e., all expressed and sufficiently annotated genes in the AscL3 and IPEC-J2 samples, respectively. Significantly over- and underrepresented GO terms were determined by the two-sided Fisher's Exact test in Blast2GO (adjusted $p < 0.05$) while enriched KEGG pathways were determined with a hypergeometric test in clusterProfiler (3.0.5) (49) (adjusted $p < 0.05$). In addition to global analysis, significant DEGs were mined for specific functions of particular interest *via* filters based on specifically selected GO terms, free-text searched GO term collections, as well as gene description analysis. Thereby, GO term filters were recursively extended with corresponding child terms to account for descending functionality using GO.db (3.3.0)[5]. Target functions as well as corresponding GO-terms and description filter are found in Table S3 in Supplementary Material.

Co-Expression Analysis

The normalized, transformed, and batch-corrected expression values were used to infer an interspecies gene co-expression network (GEN) between *A. suum* and *S. scrofa*. The AscL3 and IPEC-J2 expression matrices were combined (excluding replicate C of time point 2 h due to quality issues) and subjected to pairwise Spearman rank correlation tests using the psych R package (1.7.5) (50) with FDR *p*-value adjustment for multiple testing. Resulting gene pairs (edges in the GEN) were filtered by significance (adjusted $p < 0.05$) and correlation strength (rho > 0.95) before further analysis and visualization within Cytoscape (3.2.1) (51). In Cytoscape, duplicated edges and self-loops were removed and the network was reduced to nodes participating in interspecies interactions (GEN1). Node degrees were calculated based once on all edges and once on interspecies edges alone (GEN2) to identify highly interacting genes between species. In addition, node (resp. gene) clusters were calculated on GEN1 with the MCODE plugin (v1.4.1) (52).

[3] https://github.com/TransDecoder/TransDecoder (Accessed: March 17, 2018).

[4] http://bioconductor.org/packages/KEGGREST/ (Accessed: March 17, 2018).

[5] http://bioconductor.org/packages/GO.db/ (Accessed: March 17, 2018).

RESULTS AND DISCUSSION

Transcriptional Response Reveals Temporal Dynamics of Early Host–Pathogen Interaction

A critical event during initial invasion of *Ascaris* parasites is crossing the intestinal epithelial barrier of their mammalian hosts. The initial dialog of host epithelium and parasite before the parasite starts tissue migration has, however, received little attention. We thus performed a time-resolved RNA-Seq transcriptional profiling of both, *A. suum* L3 larvae and porcine epithelial cells (IPEC-J2) to examine the early and comprehensive transcription of genes potentially involved in sensing, attachment, barrier disruption, and immune response early after initial parasite–host contact.

We sequenced *A. suum* larvae (AscL3) and IPEC-J2 at five different time points during co-incubation (0, 1, 2, 3, and 9 h) with $n = 3$ biological replicates each (**Figure 1A**). Mapping quality control of raw reads using QualiMap (v.2.2.1, **Figure 1B**) (53) indicated one sample (IPEC-J2, 2 h, replicate C) being inconsistent

TABLE 1 | Numbers of differentially expressed and annotated genes.

	Total DEG	FC ≥ 1.5[a]	FC ≥ 1.8[a]	FC ≥ 2[a]
Complete				
Ascaris suum ($\alpha = 0.05$)	146	74	17	9
Sus scrofa ($\alpha = 0.01$)	1,423	763	181	56
GO-annotated				
A. suum	87	34	11	5
S. scrofa	1,214	621	121	33

[a]*abs(log(fold-change)) ≥ log(n).*

Total and gene ontology (GO) annotated numbers of differentially expressed genes (DEG) and DEG numbers for distinct fold-change cut-offs (with respect to the maximal pairwise fold-change) are depicted for A. suum L3 and S. scrofa epithelial cell (IPEC-J2) expression data.

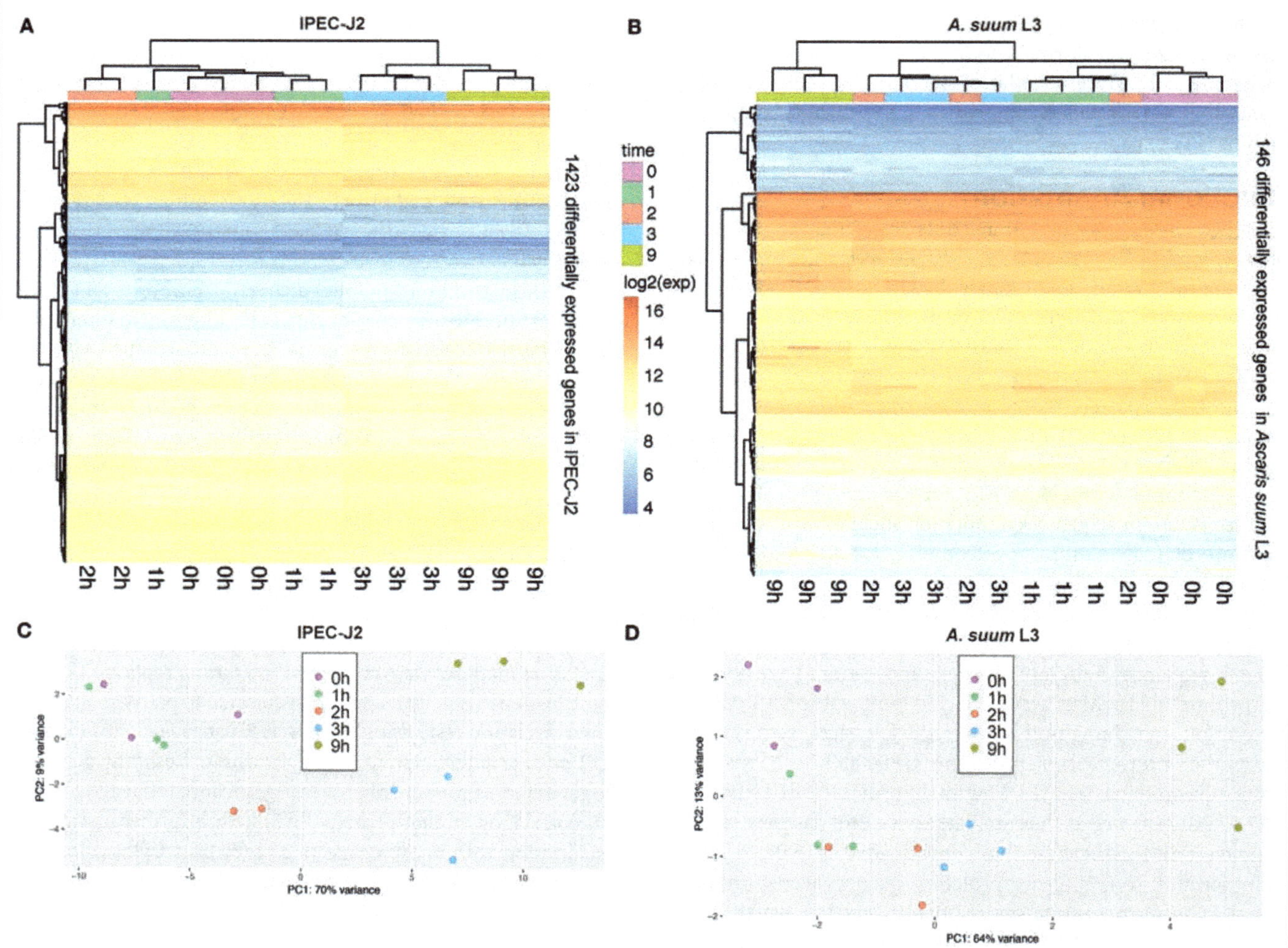

FIGURE 2 | Principal component analysis (PCA) of porcine epithelial cells (IPEC-J2) and *Ascaris suum* L3 expression data and clustering of differentially expressed genes (DEGs). **(A)** Unsupervised clustering heatmap of DEG in porcine epithelial cells ($n = 1,423$, IPEC-J2) and **(B)** *A. suum* L3 ($n = 146$). Red intensity indicates high gene expression during the time-course of host–parasite co-incubation, whereas blue intensity indicates low gene expression. PCA of RNA-Seq samples of **(C)** porcine epithelial cells and **(D)** *A. suum* L3 reveals that 79% (IPEC-J2) and 77% (*A. suum*) of the data variation is explained by the first two PCs, respectively. The five time points are color-coded (● 0, ● 1, ● 2, ● 3, and ● 9 h) and comprise $n = 3$ biological replicates (exception: $n = 2$ for IPEC-J2; ● 2 h, due to RNA-Seq quality control exclusion).

in comparison to all the other samples in the experiment, which consequently was excluded from further analysis.

In total, our exploratory study identified 146 *A. suum* genes and 1,423 *S. scrofa* genes with significant differential expression over time (**Table 1**, with adjusted p-value < 0.05 for *A. suum* and 0.01 for *S. scrofa*, respectively). Normalized expression values of both IPEC-J2 and *A. suum* L3 genes demonstrated successful clustering of replicates by time with minor exceptions of earlier time points for IPEC-J2 (**Figure 2A**) and median time points for AscL3 (**Figure 2B**). Clustering analysis indicates that most distinct changes in expression occur in later time points, additionally confirmed by the pairwise fold-changes (Table S1 in Supplementary Material). PCA of IPEC-J2 (**Figure 2C**) and *A. suum* L3 (**Figure 2D**) expression data indicate a relation of the first principal component with time direction and thus confirms that most of the variance and, therefore, change in expression is occurring over time.

Particularly for genes of the non-model nematode *A. suum*, available GO annotation was limited. We, therefore, implemented an iterative annotation strategy, depicted in **Figure 1B** and Figure S1 in Supplementary Material, which enabled us to assign GO terms to 13,683 reference and 410 novel *A. suum* genes as well as to 21,265 reference and 890 novel *S. scrofa* genes (including Ensembl reference GO-annotations). Regarding our co-incubation experiment, 59.6% of the *A. suum* DEGs (87 of the 146) and 85.3% of the *S. scrofa* DEGs (1,214 of the 1,423) were adequately annotated and thereby eligible for further functional analysis (**Table 1**). In parallel, a total of 8,034 *A. suum* genes could be annotated with KEGG Orthology (KO) identifiers including 7,306 reference and 728 novel genes. Furthermore, 9,711 *S. scrofa* genes could be annotated with KOs comprising 8,954 reference and 757 novel genes. KEGG pathways were assigned to 59 *A. suum* and 471 *S. scrofa* DEGs, respectively. These data highlight the GO annotation gap for *A. suum* genes and point out a need for improving methods to functional annotate nematode genes in general. A complete list of all *A. suum* L3 and IPEC-J2 genes (annotated and not annotated) is provided as Table S4 in Supplementary Material.

The Epithelial Cell Response to Worm Invasion

Epithelial Cells Are Not Intensely "Alarmed"

The IPEC-J2 cell line is a non-transformed, porcine epithelial cell line derived from the small intestine and currently the most convincing model for porcine infection studies (16, 54). The initial contact of *A. suum* larvae with the intestinal epithelial cells over 9 h results in a transcriptomic response of 1,423 *S. scrofa* genes (982 upregulated/441 downregulated, with respect to the maximal pairwise fold-change). To functionally describe the regulated *S. scrofa* genes, level 2 GO term profiles are illustrated (**Figure 3A**), categorizing MF, CC, and BP. To gain insight into the biological significance of alterations in gene expression levels, GO enrichment analysis was used to determine whether certain GO terms are over- or underrepresented within the gene set of interest. GO terms significantly overrepresented (adjusted $p < 0.05$) among *S. scrofa* DEGs were *binding* (as part of MF), *CC organization* or *biogenesis and cellular process* (BP) as well as several CC including *cell, cell part, macromolecular complex, membrane-enclosed lumen, organelle, organelle part*, and *supramolecular fiber* (**Figure 3A**). Surprisingly, the few underrepresented terms are almost exclusively attributed to extracellular matrix (ECM), membrane, and membrane part (CC), a group of terms that we expected to be specifically addressed while being co-incubated with a comparably large and motile extracellular parasite. Further global analysis as subcellular location of *S. scrofa* DEGs and KEGG pathway annotation are depicted in **Figures 3B,C**. *S. scrofa* KEGG profiling features several significantly enriched pathways (hypergeometric test, adjusted $p < 0.05$) including induced cell cycle activity, FoxO signaling, homologous recombination and RNA degradation as well as a suppressed ribosome pathway. In addition, though not significant, oxidative phosphorylation and purine metabolism show distinct repression (**Figure 3C**). Genes of the FoxO family that are central for the here enriched *FoxO signaling* pathway regulate transcriptional responses including apoptosis, cell-cycle control, glucose metabolism, oxidative stress resistance, and longevity. A recent study revealed that intestinal FoxO-mediated signaling is required for epithelial antimicrobial response and AMP synthesis by enterocytes (55). Factors inducing FoxO signaling include oxidative and nutrient stress stimuli, such as insulin or several growth factors. The induced oxidative stress response is in line with the repression of the oxidative phosphorylation pathway, and together imply increased nutrient consumption or even nutritional competition between IPEC-J2 and *A. suum* larvae.

KEGG pathway analysis further highlights that pathways linked to extracellular recognition such as TLR signaling are not regulated (**Figure 3C**). This is supported by several other studies showing that host PRRs such as TLR are modulated by nematode species to limit inflammation (56–58) but TLR signaling in generating an anti-helminth immune response remains controversial (59). Since epithelial cells are known to express all kinds of PRRs, we more specifically considered the role of C-type lectin receptors such as mannose receptor, DC-sign, ICAM-3, collectins, or selectins (59, 60) to be addressed, but found no transcriptional evidence that these receptors or corresponding receptor signaling pathways are affected by the presence of *A. suum* larvae. Interestingly, we observe a generally low presence of *S. scrofa* DEGs in several other signal transduction pathways, such as HIF-1, MAPK, mTOR, NF-kappa B, Rap1, TGF-ß, or RAS indicating that IPEC-J2 cells overall were not in an "alarmed state" as expected.

Although we hypothesized that epithelial cells somehow sense incoming *Ascaris* larvae and might orchestrate an appropriate response, we were surprised to find such a low magnitude of response (indicated by fold-change values) and the lack of conclusive activation signatures. We then specifically looked for genes involved in inflammatory responses (**Figure 4A**, GO declination in Table S3 in Supplementary Material) and chemotactic responses (**Figure 4B**, GO declination in Table S3 in Supplementary Material) and found chemokine transcripts (CCL5, IL8, and CXCL18), the chitinase 3 like 1 protein, and the cytokines genes for IL17D to be suppressed. Interleukin-8, one

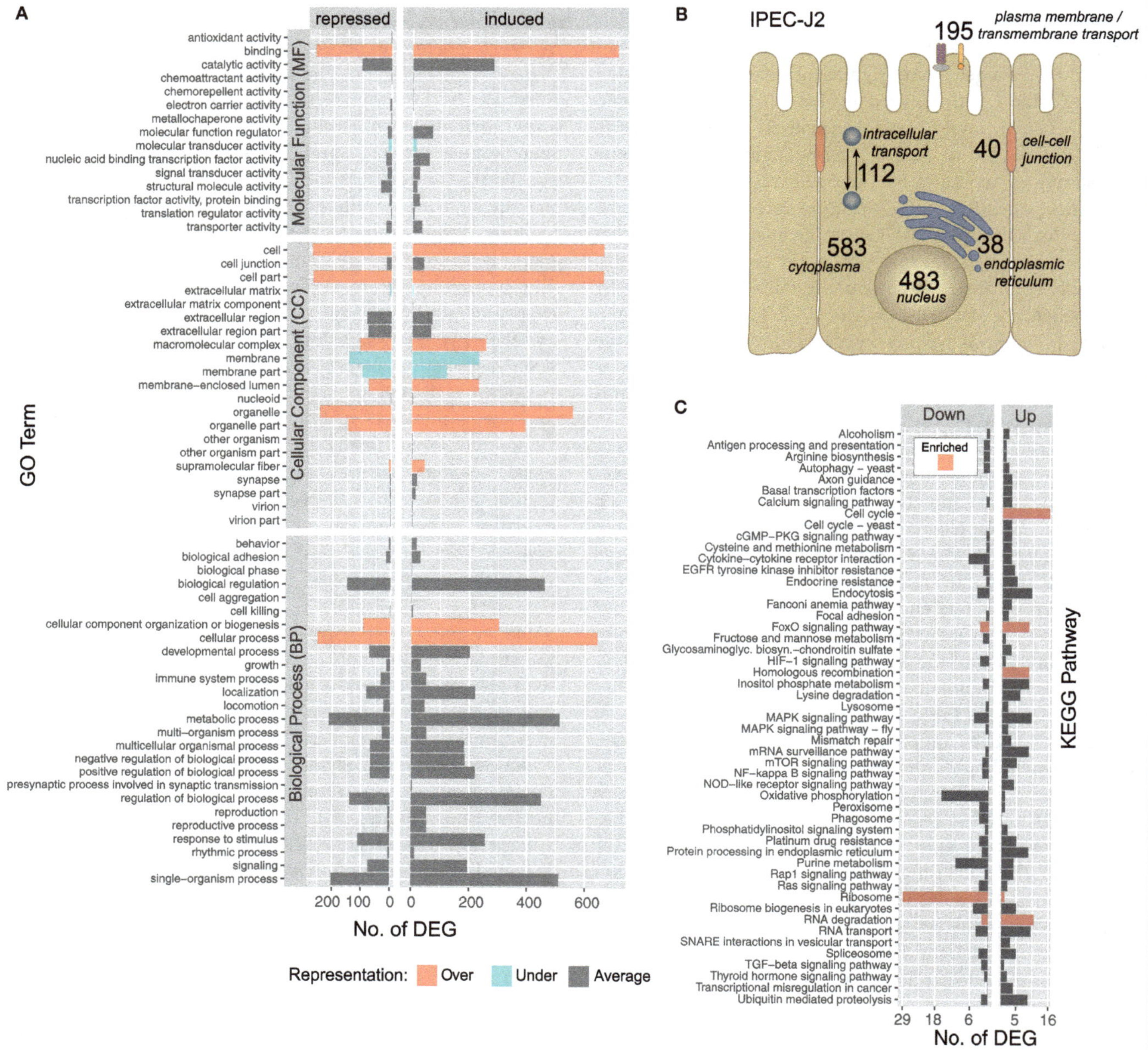

FIGURE 3 | Gene ontology (GO) and pathway profiling of porcine intestinal epithelial cell differentially expressed genes (DEGs). An iterative annotation strategy was used to assign GO terms to reference and novel porcine transcripts. **(A)** For 1,214 GO-annotated porcine DEGs, the level 2 of GO hierarchy is illustrated and classified into Molecular Function (MF), Cellular Component (CC) and Biological Process (BP). GO terms significantly enriched among differentially expressed *S. scrofa* genes (Fischer's Exact Test, two-sided, $p < 0.05$) are highlighted as over-( ) and under-( ) represented terms alongside with averagely represented terms ( ) with regard to the reference genome. **(B)** Subcellular localization of DEG encoding proteins deduced from binning relevant GO terms (Table S3 in Supplementary Material) and offsprings [*nucleus* (CC, 483), *endoplasmic reticulum* (CC, 38), *cytoplasm* (CC, 583*), intracellular transport* (BP, 112), *plasma membrane* (CC, 128), *transmembrane transport* (BP, 34), *transmembrane transporter activity* (MF, 33), *cell–cell-junction* (CC, 31), and *cell–cell junction organization* (BP, 9)]. **(C)** Sequences were annotated with KEGG pathways and pathways with three or more assigned DEGs are visualized including color-coded ( ) enrichment analysis (hypergeometric test, $p < 0.05$).

of the repressed immunity genes, is a potent chemoattractant for primary neutrophils but also other granulocytes, and is secreted by epithelial cells in response to bacterial stimuli (61). Upon LPS stimulation, also porcine IPEC-J2 cells rapidly upregulate IL-8 transcripts (Figure S6D in Supplementary Material). Intriguingly, Aprianto and colleagues (62) showed that a highly adherent, unencapsulated form of *S. pneumoniae* suppressed IL-8 production from epithelial cells compared to a free-floating, non-adherent form of the same strain early during infection. Their RNA-Seq study thereby links repression of epithelial innate immune response with the adherence mechanisms of the invading pathogen and provides evidence for targeted immune evasion. Hence, active suppression of the innate chemokine response combined with restricted epithelial recognition of AscL3 larvae,

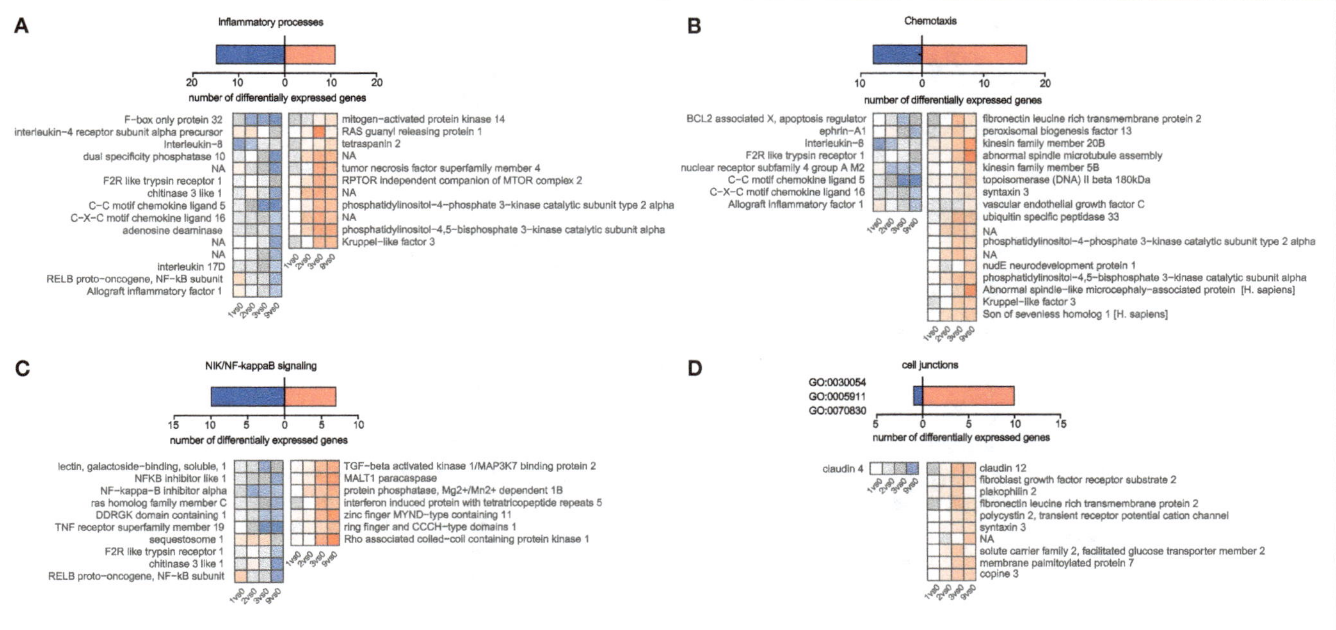

FIGURE 4 | Temporal gene expression changes in porcine intestinal epithelial cells in response to *A. suum* larvae. Blastp, Blast2GO, and InterProScan were used to identify *S. scrofa* differentially expressed genes associated with distinct immune responses or cell junction for **(A)** "Inflammatory processes," **(B)** "Chemotaxis," and **(C)** "NIK/NF-kappaB signaling." For **(D)** "Cell junctions," the cell–cell junction localization filter was manually selected for GO:0030054, GO:0005911, and GO:0070830.

weak induction and even suppression of NIK/NF kappaB signaling (**Figure 4C**), could explain the poor response of immune-related genes that we observed. Following this line, mice lacking NF kappaB signaling specifically in epithelial cells are incapable of mounting protective type 2 cell-mediated immunity to the nematode *Trichuris muris* in its rodent host (63). The initiation of protective type 2 responses against helminth typically begins with production of epithelial cell-derived cytokines (IL-25, IL-33, and thymic stromal lymphopoietin), but none of them was found to be regulated in porcine IPEC-J2 cells early after *A. suum* co-incubation. However, it has to be taken into account that it was recently found that rather than every epithelial cell, a very rare epithelial cell type, intestinal tuft cells, initiated mucosal type 2 responses to helminth parasites through IL-25 secretion after TRMP5 taste chemoreception (64, 65).

Studies in the mouse model parasitic nematode *Heligmosomoides polygyrus* showed that factors secreted by the nematodes directly suppressed IL-33 release (66), but the upstream mechanisms of IL-33 release are somewhat controversial and suggest that IL-33 might also be released from intracellular stores when cells undergo necrosis or even after mechanical stress (67). However, from our data, we cannot conclude that IL-33 is not released. We, therefore, speculated that during co-incubation, worms cause epithelial barrier damage and induce mechanical stress responses or cell death, but the latter was only poorly reflected in the epithelial transcriptome response [no wound healing, apoptosis, or necroptosis pathways (**Figure 3C**)]. From 247 DEGs associated with stress response in general (GO declination Table S3 and Figure S4 in Supplementary Material), only 10 are connected to mechanically induced stress responses/mechanical stimulus (Figure S5 in Supplementary Material). However, when genes associated to cell junction or bicellular junction formation (GO:0030054, GO:0070830, and GO:0005911) were considered, we noticed a clear trend toward an induced gene response, including claudin-12, plakophilin 2, and FLRT3 (**Figure 4D**). This highlights an active response to promote barrier integrity of IPEC-J2 and raises the question whether *A. suum* larvae and/or their secreted products specifically target tight junction formation. Moreover, the only downregulated gene in this functional group was claudin-4 (**Figure 4D**). This is particularly interesting, because researchers suggest that claudin-4 acts to tighten the paracellular pathway (68) and downregulation of claudin-4 is observed under conditions leading to increased permeability (69). The differential regulation of claudin-12 and claudin-4 and the downregulation of IL-8 was additionally validated by quantitative PCR (Figure S7A in Supplementary Material).

Together, our results indicate that small intestinal epithelial cells show poor innate immune responses to co-incubated *A. suum* L3, reduced ribosome function and oxidative phosphorylation pathways, but specifically induce tight junction formation. Whether IPEC-J2 cells do not possess an adequate detection system or whether the parasite is inactivating the host detection systems that would otherwise raise the alarm remains unknown.

The Worm Response to the Epithelial Barrier

Ascaris suum Larvae Drive Invasion and Migration

The initial contact of *Ascaris suum* L3 with intestinal epithelial cells resulted in a transcriptomic response of 146 *A. suum* genes

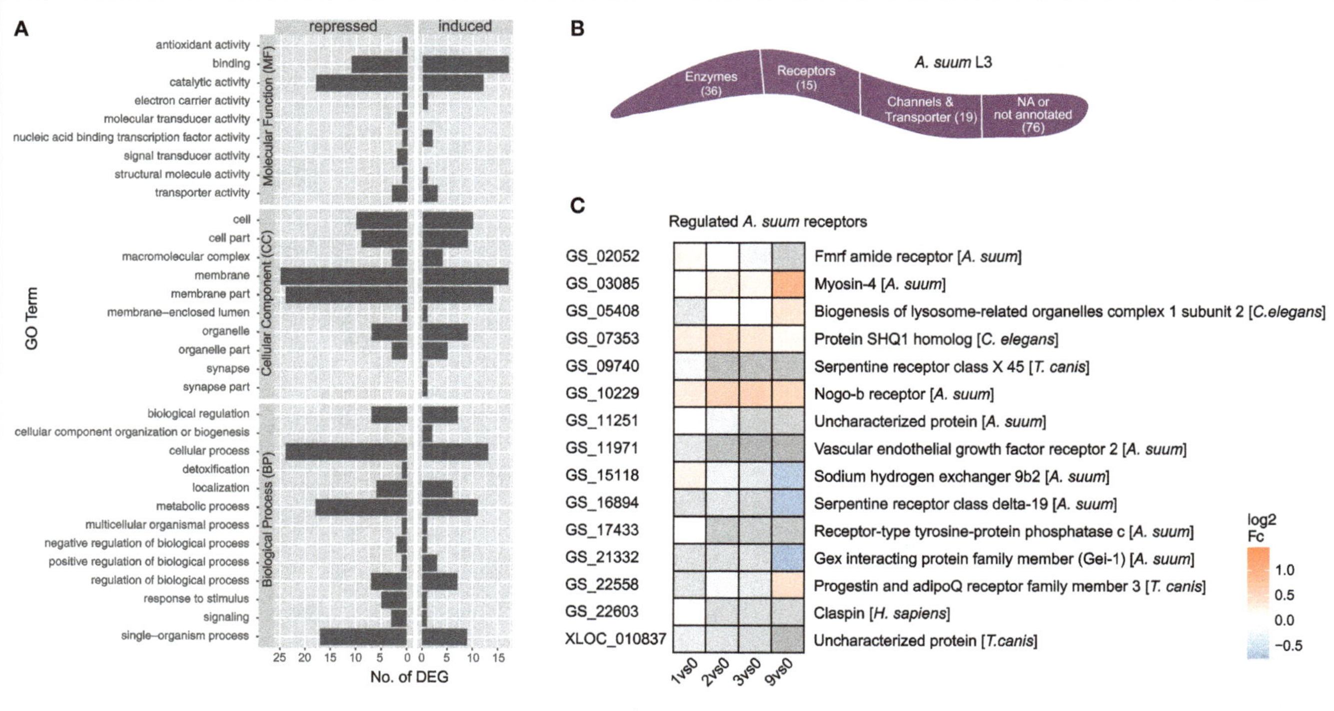

FIGURE 5 | Gene ontology (GO) profiling of *Ascaris suum* differentially expressed genes (DEGs). **(A)** Distribution of level 2 GO terms for *A. suum* L3 DEGs, categorized into molecular function, cellular component (CC), and biological process (BP). **(B)** Global classification of *A. suum* L3 DEGs into enzymes, receptors, and channels/transporter based on GO-term filter and gene description analysis (Table S3 in Supplementary Material). **(C)** Time-resolved expression of *A. suum* DEGs with GO assigned receptor function.

(68 upregulated/78 downregulated, with respect to the maximal pairwise fold-change). A total of 87 genes mapped to GO terms showed regulated functions such as *binding* and *catalytic activity* (MF), *membrane and membrane part* (CC) as well as *cellular, metabolic,* and *single-organism processes* (BP) (**Figure 5A** GO level 2). However, no significant enrichments (two-sided Fisher's Exact test in Blast2GO; adjusted $p < 0.05$) could be observed with respect to the background genome. Due to the small number of *A. suum* DEGs in general, only a few KEGG pathways could be assigned more than once, namely ABC transporters (2), cAMP signaling pathway (2, repressed), cysteine and methionine metabolism (2, repressed), glycosaminoglycan degradation (2, activated), protein digestion and absorption (3), pyrimidine metabolism (2), RNA degradation (2), and spliceosome (2) (Figure S2 in Supplementary Material). GO term filtering and gene description analysis were used to classify *A. suum* L3 DEGs into enzymes (36), receptors (15), and channels/transporters (19) (**Figure 5B**). Surprisingly, most receptor associated genes were indeed downregulated (10 out of 15, **Figure 5C**). We specifically looked for *Ascaris* C-type lectins (C-TL), a superfamily potentially involved in either site-specific tissue recognition or interference with mammalian C-TL-mediated inflammation (70), but found no C-TL within the *A. suum* DEGs of our early response experiment.

In contrast, the 20 most upregulated *A suum* L3 genes (Table S1 in Supplementary Material) included genes associated with motor activity (GS_03085 Myosin-4, GS_04138 Troponin T, GS_00138 Myoglobin) and structure (GS_04352 Cuticle collagen domain-containing protein, GS_11610 Cuticle collagen 6, GS_09547 Cuticle collagen 34, GS_00653 Protein disulfide-isomerase 2). The upregulation of genes associated with motor activity/motility driven by epithelial-contact is particularly interesting in the absence of host peristalsis, the luminal content/microbes, or mucus production and could be indicative of increased locomotion either in order to penetrate host tissue or to counteract passive movement after site-specific recognition. Increased muscular locomotor activity together with proteolytic enzymes secreted by glandular structures are thought to be essential for host tissue penetration.

The subset of upregulated genes involved in cuticle formation such as protein disulfide-isomerase 2 (PDI-2) (Table S1 in Supplementary Material and qPCR-validated in Figure S7B in Supplementary Material) suggests an epithelial trigger for driving further larval development. Nematode cuticles are formed by multiple collagenous layers that contain extensive disulfide linkages (71) and new cuticles are synthesized sequentially for each developmental stage. Cuticle biogenesis in the endoplasmic reticulum involves proline hydoxylation and disulfide bond formation by PDI (72). Mutations in the Protein disulfide-isomerase 2 (PDI-2) gene of *Caenorhabditis elegans* resulted in severe body morphology defects, uncoordinated movement, adult sterility, abnormal molting, and aberrant collagen deposition (73). The importance of PDI-2 activity for ECM formation demonstrated for *C. elegans* and more recently also for *Brugia malayi* (74) highlights its relevance as a potential anthelmintic drug target (72), including for *Ascaris* species.

At the host–parasite interface, ES proteins released by helminths play an important role in mediating host–parasite interaction, regulation, and control (75–78). To assess the transcriptional regulation of proteins potentially secreted by larval *Ascaris* parasites, we merged predicted DEGs for classical (SignalP) and non-classical (SecretomeP) secretory proteins and removed mitochondrial (TargetP) and transmembrane (TMHMM) proteins (**Figure 6A**). From the 55 ES proteins, 20 can be assigned to enzymatic activity with diverse functions including hydrolases ($n = 9$), transferases ($n = 6$), isomerases ($n = 2$), oxidoreductases ($n = 2$), and lyases ($n = 1$) as depicted in **Figure 6A**.

We hypothesized that proteolytic enzymes would be essential for parasite invasion and, therefore, upregulated by *A. suum* larvae once the epithelial barrier was detected. Within the class of proteases, nematode serine proteases have received considerable interest as they are widely distributed in parasitic nematodes with a wide variety of functions (79). Indeed, the parasite transcript with the highest maximal fold-change (comparing 0 versus 9 h time point, Table S1 in Supplementary Material) was identified as being *A. suum* aspartic protease 6 (**Figure 6B**). Aspartic proteases are a group of endopeptidases characterized by their catalytic aspartic residues that are known to drive host hemoglobin digestion by the blood-feeding nematodes *Haemonchus contortus*, *Ancylostoma caninum*, and *Necator americanus* (80, 81). Moreover, aspartic protease 1 from *N. americanus* is targeted by the bivalent human hookworm vaccine [Na-APR-1(M74), carrying a site-directed mutation abolishing its catalytic activity, and glutathione *S*-transferase (Na-GST-1)] currently being tested in clinical phase 1 studies in the US and Brazil (82–84). The Na-APR-1(M74) vaccine strategy is based on the induction of neutralizing antibodies against aspartic protease 1, thereby preventing hemoglobin degradation in the brush border membrane of the parasite's digestive tract and finally leading to diminished parasite-related blood loss and reduced numbers of hookworms [reviewed in Ref. (83, 85)]. For nematode parasites that do not feed on blood but express aspartic proteases, different functions such as skin macromolecule and epithelial degradation, aiding in tissue penetration, or host-derived nutrient digestion are suggested (86–88). Interestingly, a proteomic study on ES products of different larval stages of *A. suum* shows the presence of aspartic

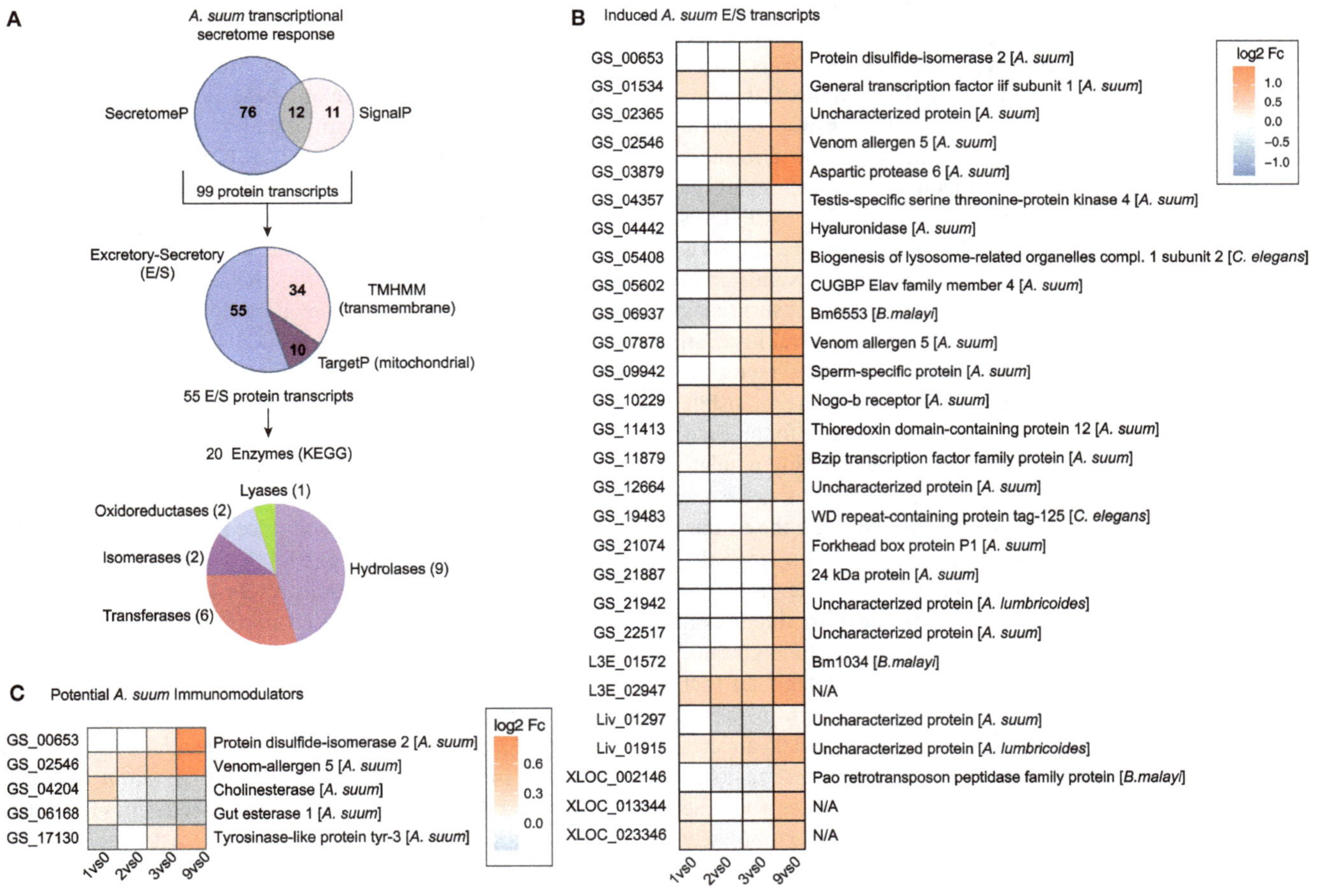

FIGURE 6 | The secretome response of *Ascaris suum*. **(A)** The pipeline to identify *A. suum* excretory-secretory (ES) transcripts used SignalP and SecretomeP to annotate classical ($n = 23$) and non-classical ($n = 88$) ES genes and excluded mitochondrial ($n = 10$; TargetP) and transmembrane ($n = 34$; TMHMM) protein transcripts. KEGG ENZYME identified enzyme classes of ES transcripts are depicted in the bottom pie chart. **(B)** Time-resolved expression of $n = 28$ induced *A. suum* ES transcripts. **(C)** Differentially expressed *A. suum* transcripts that matched to genome prediction of *A. suum* immunomodulatory ES products based on homology to other nematodes (26).

protease 6 protein in ES collected from L3-lung stage worms, but its absence in the ES of hatched L3 larvae (89), thereby directly supporting our findings on the protein level and highlighting an epithelial trigger and early role for this specific enzyme.

The same study revealed the high abundance of glycosyl hydrolases (family 31, GH31) in *A. suum* L4 ES (89) suggesting degradation of complex carbohydrates to be essential for its energy metabolism. Among the ES enzymes upregulated directly in response to epithelial cell contact, we indeed identified a hyaluronidase (**Figure 6**, GS_04442). There is evidence that some bacterial species use hyaluronidases to utilize host hyaluronic acid (HA), an essential part of the ECM of epithelial tissue, as a carbon source for their energy metabolism (90). This might indicate that *A. suum* L3 not only produce proteolytic enzymes that help in epithelial tissue invasion but that epithelial ECM components can be directly hydrolyzed to feed on. Moreover, the release of hyaluronidase by *A. suum* has been described earlier for larvae isolated from the lungs of infected pigs (91). Besides its role in facilitating larval migration, the authors added another functional point: the modulation of developmental processes by hydrolyzing HA present in extracellular cuticle during molting. The role of *A. suum* hyaluronidase in either breaking up the internal cuticle-epidermal connection critical for molting (91), larval migration (92), or larval energy metabolism, therefore, remains speculative.

A comparison of the herein identified *A. suum* DEGs with a draft genome-based list of potential *A. suum* immunomodulators (26) revealed three upregulated transcripts (**Figure 6C**, GS_00653 PDI-2, GS_02546 venom allergen-5 and GS_17130 tyrosinase like protein tyr-3). Genomic and proteomic evidence suggest the abundance of venom allergen-like (VAL) proteins (SCP/TAPs superfamily) also in the ES compartment of *A. suum*. The early upregulation of VAL genes (venom allergen-5: qPCR validated in Figure S7B in Supplementary Material) is perhaps not surprising and has been associated in previous studies with larval invasion (78, 93, 94), although there is only limited understanding on the detailed function of those proteins in the host–parasite relationship.

In summary, we provide transcriptomic evidence for an early response pattern of genes that *A. suum* L3 specifically regulate during contact with host epithelial cells. Among those genes are factors that might facilitate parasite invasion through the epithelial barrier (aspartic protease 6), migration (myosin, troponin, and myoglobin), feeding (hyaluronidase), and development (PDI2) of the parasite. However, the parasite–host interaction not only depends on proteins but might also include glycans, lipids, miRNAs, or other small molecules and metabolites that have not been studied here, but can also contribute to parasite-epithelial communication (75). Furthermore, intestinal parasites and microbes have co-evolved together in their respective hosts. For that reason, the complex interaction of parasites with the bacterial community and the microbiota–host interaction likely also contributes to the parasite–host communication.

Interspecies Interaction Is Dominated by Four *A. suum* Genes

Inference of interspecies gene co-expression networks (GENs) is an important systems biology approach to predict pathogen–host interactions. We applied established and efficient procedures to infer and analyze GENs including pairwise correlation, cluster (module) analysis, and functional enrichment (95, 96). Thereby, genes featuring a similar expression profile over time are associated by direct network links as well as gene clusters and are considered to participate in common functionality or in concurrent and thus interlinked processes. It must be noted that the recommended sample number of 20 is not met; however, our analysis compensates with distinctly higher read coverage than recommended (>10 million), an encompassing context of all samples due to the time series as well as strict GEN creation parameters ($p < 0.05$, rho > 0.95), resulting in a few but prominent and explicit signals.

Based on node degrees of the co-expression network that was reduced to interspecies nodes and interspecies edges (**Figure 7A**, GEN2), we identified four highly interacting *A. suum* genes (**Figures 7B,C**). Three of the four highly interacting *A. suum* genes could be annotated by the iterative strategy (**Figure 1B**); GS_12056 with the "elongation of very long-chain fatty acids" (UniProt:ASU_11627, GO:0016021 integral components of the membrane), GS_09942 as "sperm-specific protein" (UniProt:ASU_04668, PROSITE:PS50202) and GS_11251 as "Uncharacterized protein," or with the InterProScan classification, "rhodopsin-like G protein-coupled receptors (GPCRs)" (UniProt:ASU_01462, GO:0016021 integral components of membrane) (**Figure 7E**). The one gene lacking thorough characterization, L3E_01572, is annotated only with the associated GO-term (UniProt:Bm1034, GO:0016021 integral component of membrane). The overall gene regulation, based on maximal fold change values, of *S. scrofa* genes connected to the four *A. suum* genes was diverse as illustrated in **Figure 7D**. In addition to node degrees, the four *A. suum* genes are further emphasized by the fact that they participate in the four largest clusters of GEN1 identified by MCODE (Cluster 1, 2, 4, and 5, **Figure 7B**; Table S2 in Supplementary Material). Those four clusters are dominated by *S. scrofa* genes except for one *A. suum* gene each. The network data links the parasite's fatty acid biosynthesis with host cluster 1, which is comprised of mostly repressed genes like Cystatin E/M and macrophage inhibitory factor 1 (MIF), known to be induced by bacterial invaders (97), and ribosomal proteins (RPS21, RPS16, RPL13, RPL18, RPL8) involved in peptide and protein synthesis (Table S2 in Supplementary Material). GO profiling of *S. scrofa* DEGs per cluster revealed significantly over-represented terms (two-sided Fisher's Exact test, $p < 0.05$) in cluster 1 (**Figures 7B,C**; Figure S3 in Supplementary Material) associated with structural molecule activity (MF), cell, cell part and macromolecular complex (CC). In parallel, the sperm-specific protein of *A. suum* interacted with cluster 2 that contained mostly repressed genes for cellular and metabolic processes (BP). A dominant activation of genes was found in cluster 5 with the interspecies link to GS_11251 (*A. suum*) that shares structural similarity to known rhodopsin-like G protein-coupled receptors according to InterPro. GPCRs transduce extracellular signals through interaction with guanine nucleotide-binding (G) proteins, highlighting its potential for interspecies linkage.

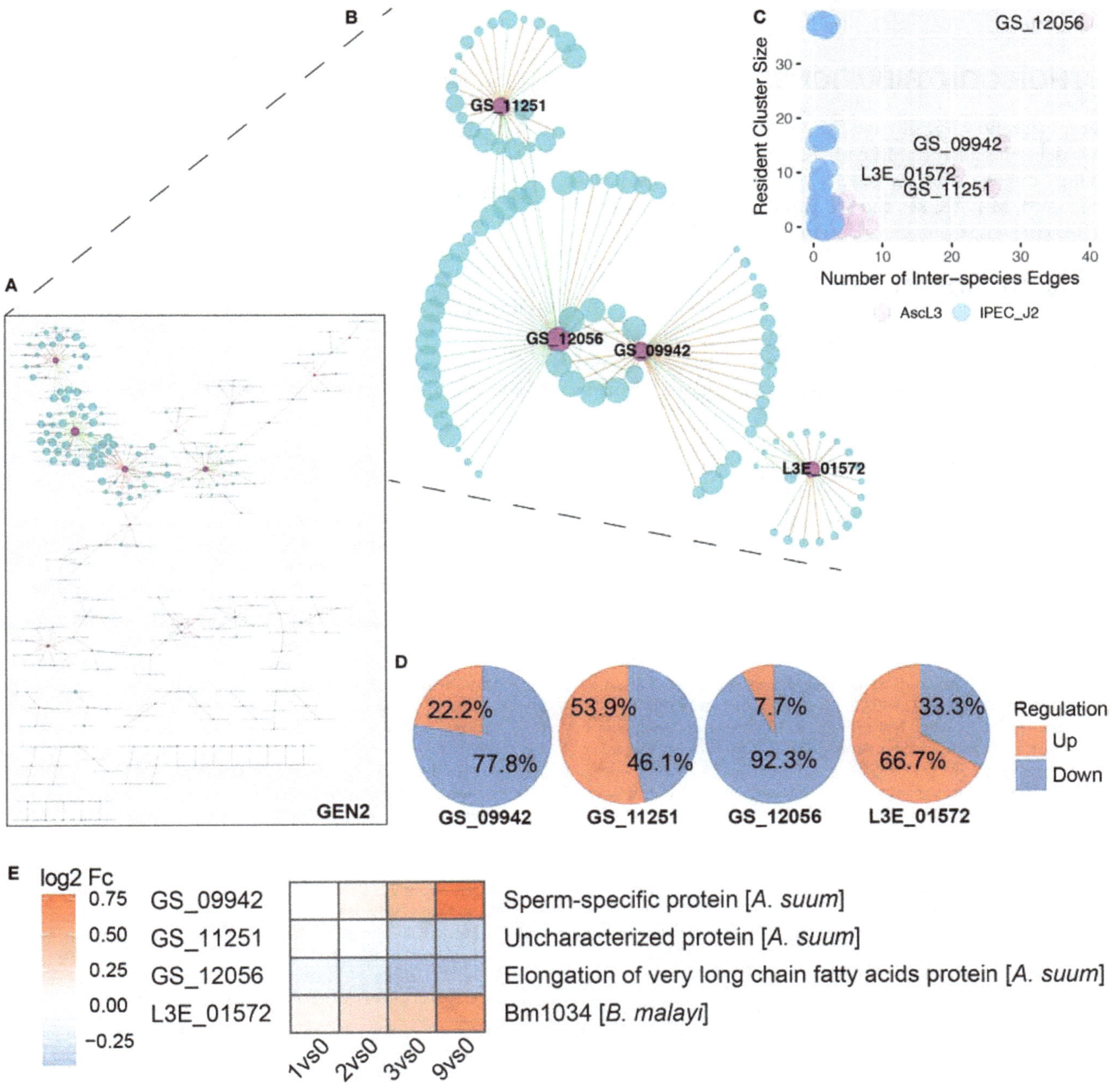

FIGURE 7 | Inferred interspecies gene co-expression network. **(A)** Gene co-expression network reduced to interspecies nodes and interspecies edges (GEN2). Nodes represent co-expressed genes of *S. scrofa* (blue) and *A. suum* (violet) with node sizes corresponding to node degree (number of node interactions in GEN1). Edges between two nodes represent correlations that are either positive (green) or negative (red) with a Spearman correlation > 0.95. **(B)** The four most prominent interspecies clusters (Cluster 1, 2, 4, and 5, Table S2 in Supplementary Material) of the interspecies network GEN1 projected to GEN2 (i.e., without intra-species edges). **(C)** Number of interspecies edges versus cluster size for *A. suum* (AscL3, violet) and *S. scrofa* (IPEC-J2, blue) nodes [differentially expressed genes (DEGs)]. **(D)** Averaged gene regulation direction (based on max Fc) for all *S. scrofa* (IPEC-J2) DEGs connected to the four indicated *A. suum* (AscL3) genes. **(E)** Annotation and gene expression of the four interspecies network dominating *A. suum* genes over time by heatmapping the log2 Fc.

Even though more extensive interpretations are limited for the DEGs that have no functional information assigned, the prominent appearance of the four *A. suum* genes in the GENs and clusters render them into attractive and suitable candidates for targeted approaches.

DATA DEPOSITION

All sequencing data generated in this project are available from the NCBI Sequence Read Archive (SRA) and collectively available *via* the BioProject: PRJNA450204.

All analysis code is provided at https://gitlab.com/mkuhring/project_asuum.

AUTHOR CONTRIBUTIONS

Conceptualization: FE, BR, and SH. Investigation: FE, MK, AR, and AM. Formal analysis: MK and BR. Visualization: FE and MK. Writing—original draft: FE and MK. Writing—review and editing: FE, AM, MK, AR, BR, and SH. Funding acquisition: SH and BR. Resources: AM and AR. Supervision: SH and BR.

ACKNOWLEDGMENTS

The authors thank Christiane Palissa, Bettina Sonnenburg, Marion Müller, Yvonne Weber, Beate Anders, and Julia Hinzmann for excellent technical support and Ulrike Lodemann and Henriette Loß for their help in RNA quality assessment. The study was supported by the Federal Ministry of Education and Research (BMBF) within the consortium "InfectControl 2020," project Art4Fun to SH and by the German Research Foundation (DFG), national research training group (GRK) 2046 to SH, and a starting grant of Freie Universität Berlin to SH and BR.

SUPPLEMENTARY MATERIAL

TABLE S1 | Differentially expressed genes pig and worm total.

TABLE S2 | Co-expression analysis: GEN nodes, GEN edges, GEN cluster

TABLE S3 | Gene ontology (GO) term declination for GO filters.

TABLE S4 | Genome of Ascaris suum L3 and IPEC-J2.

REFERENCES

1. Bethony J, Brooker S, Albonico M, Geiger SM, Loukas A, Diemert D, et al. Soil-transmitted helminth infections: ascariasis, trichuriasis, and hookworm. *Lancet* (2006) 367:1521–32. doi:10.1016/S0140-6736(06)68653-4
2. Hotez PJ, Alvarado M, Basáñez M-G, Bolliger I, Bourne R, Boussinesq M, et al. The global burden of disease study 2010: interpretation and implications for the neglected tropical diseases. *PLoS Negl Trop Dis* (2014) 8(7):e2865. doi:10.1371/journal.pntd.0002865
3. Utzinger J, Becker SL, Knopp S, Blum J, Neumayr AL, Keiser J, et al. Neglected tropical diseases: diagnosis, clinical management, treatment and control. *Swiss Med Wkly* (2012) 142:w13727. doi:10.4414/smw.2012.13727
4. Thamsborg SM, Nejsum P, Mejer H. Chapter 14 – Impact of *Ascaris suum* in livestock. In: Holland C, editor. *Ascaris: The Neglected Parasite*. Amsterdam: Elsevier (2013). p. 363–81.
5. Vlaminck J, Geldhof P. Chapter 16 – Diagnosis and control of *Ascariasis* in pigs. In: Holland C, editor. *Ascaris: The Neglected Parasite*. Amsterdam: Elsevier (2013). p. 395–425.
6. Leles D, Gardner SL, Reinhard K, Iñiguez A, Araujo A. Are *Ascaris lumbricoides* and *Ascaris suum* a single species? *Parasit Vectors* (2012) 5:42. doi:10.1186/1756-3305-5-42
7. Shao C-C, Xu M-J, Alasaad S, Song H-Q, Peng L, Tao J-P, et al. Comparative analysis of microRNA profiles between adult *Ascaris lumbricoides* and *Ascaris suum*. *BMC Vet Res* (2014) 10:99. doi:10.1186/1746-6148-10-99
8. Rosa BA, Jasmer DP, Mitreva M. Genome-wide tissue-specific gene expression, co-expression and regulation of co-expressed genes in adult nematode *Ascaris suum*. *PLoS Negl Trop Dis* (2014) 8:e2678. doi:10.1371/journal.pntd.0002678
9. Katakam KK, Thamsborg SM, Dalsgaard A, Kyvsgaard NC, Mejer H. Environmental contamination and transmission of *Ascaris suum* in Danish organic pig farms. *Parasit Vectors* (2016) 9:80. doi:10.1186/s13071-016-1349-0
10. Douvres FW, Tromba FG, Malakatis GM. Morphogenesis and migration of *Ascaris suum* larvae developing to fourth stage in swine. *J Parasitol* (1969) 55:689–712. doi:10.2307/3277198
11. Murrell KD, Eriksen L, Nansen P, Slotved HC, Rasmussen T. *Ascaris suum*: a revision of its early migratory path and implications for human ascariasis. *J Parasitol* (1997) 83:255–60. doi:10.2307/3284450
12. Fritz JH, Le Bourhis L, Magalhaes JG, Philpott DJ. Innate immune recognition at the epithelial barrier drives adaptive immunity: APCs take the back seat. *Trends Immunol* (2008) 29:41–9. doi:10.1016/j.it.2007.10.002
13. Ganz T. Epithelia: not just physical barriers. *Proc Natl Acad Sci U S A* (2002) 99:3357–8. doi:10.1073/pnas.072073199
14. Dawson H, Solano-Aguilar G, Beal M, Beshah E, Vangimalla V, Jones E, et al. Localized Th1-, Th2-, T regulatory cell-, and inflammation-associated hepatic and pulmonary immune responses in *Ascaris suum*-infected swine are increased by retinoic acid. *Infect Immun* (2009) 77:2576–87. doi:10.1128/IAI.00827-07
15. Masure D, Wang T, Vlaminck J, Claerhoudt S, Chiers K, Van den Broeck W, et al. The intestinal expulsion of the roundworm *Ascaris suum* is associated with eosinophils, intra-epithelial T cells and decreased intestinal transit time. *PLoS Negl Trop Dis* (2013) 7:e2588. doi:10.1371/journal.pntd.0002588
16. Nossol C, Barta-Böszörményi A, Kahlert S, Zuschratter W, Faber-Zuschratter H, Reinhardt N, et al. Comparing two intestinal porcine epithelial cell lines (IPECs): morphological differentiation, function and metabolism. *PLoS One* (2015) 10:e0132323. doi:10.1371/journal.pone.0132323
17. Schierack P, Nordhoff M, Pollmann M, Weyrauch KD, Amasheh S, Lodemann U, et al. Characterization of a porcine intestinal epithelial cell line for in vitro studies of microbial pathogenesis in swine. *Histochem Cell Biol* (2006) 125:293–305. doi:10.1007/s00418-005-0067-z
18. Westermann AJ, Barquist L, Vogel J. Resolving host–pathogen interactions by dual RNA-seq. *PLoS Pathog* (2017) 13(2):e1006033. doi:10.1371/journal.ppat.1006033
19. Love MI, Huber W, Anders S. Moderated estimation of fold change and dispersion for RNA-seq data with DESeq2. *Genome Biol* (2014) 15:550. doi:10.1186/s13059-014-0550-8
20. Köster J, Rahmann S. Snakemake—a scalable bioinformatics workflow engine. *Bioinformatics* (2012) 28:2520–2. doi:10.1093/bioinformatics/bts480
21. Urban JF Jr, Douvres FW, Tromba FG. A rapid method for hatching *Ascaris suum* eggs in vitro. *Proc Helminthol Soc Wash* (1981) 48(2):241–3.
22. Bolger AM, Lohse M, Usadel B. Trimmomatic: a flexible trimmer for Illumina sequence data. *Bioinformatics* (2014) 30:2114–20. doi:10.1093/bioinformatics/btu170
23. Wood DE, Salzberg SL. Kraken: ultrafast metagenomic sequence classification using exact alignments. *Genome Biol* (2014) 15:R46. doi:10.1186/gb-2014-15-3-r46
24. Kim D, Pertea G, Trapnell C, Pimentel H, Kelley R, Salzberg SL. TopHat2: accurate alignment of transcriptomes in the presence of insertions, deletions and gene fusions. *Genome Biol* (2013) 14:R36. doi:10.1186/gb-2013-14-4-r36
25. Trapnell C, Hendrickson DG, Sauvageau M, Goff L, Rinn JL, Pachter L. Differential analysis of gene regulation at transcript resolution with RNA-seq. *Nat Biotechnol* (2013) 31:46–53. doi:10.1038/nbt.2450
26. Jex AR, Liu S, Li B, Young ND, Hall RS, Li Y, et al. *Ascaris suum* draft genome. *Nature* (2011) 479:529–33. doi:10.1038/nature10553
27. Howe KL, Bolt BJ, Shafie M, Kersey P, Berriman M. WormBase ParaSite – a comprehensive resource for helminth genomics. *Mol Biochem Parasitol* (2017) 215:2–10. doi:10.1016/j.molbiopara.2016.11.005
28. Zerbino DR, Achuthan P, Akanni W, Amode MR, Barrell D, Bhai J, et al. Ensembl 2018. *Nucleic Acids Res* (2018) 46:D754–61. doi:10.1093/nar/gkx1098

29. Liao Y, Smyth GK, Shi W. featureCounts: an efficient general purpose program for assigning sequence reads to genomic features. *Bioinformatics* (2014) 30:923–30. doi:10.1093/bioinformatics/btt656
30. Ritchie ME, Phipson B, Wu D, Hu Y, Law CW, Shi W, et al. limma powers differential expression analyses for RNA-sequencing and microarray studies. *Nucleic Acids Res* (2015) 43:e47. doi:10.1093/nar/gkv007
31. Ashburner M, Ball CA, Blake JA, Botstein D, Butler H, Cherry JM, et al. Gene ontology: tool for the unification of biology. The Gene Ontology Consortium. *Nat Genet* (2000) 25:25–9. doi:10.1038/75556
32. The Gene Ontology Consortium. Expansion of the gene ontology knowledgebase and resources. *Nucleic Acids Res* (2017) 45:D331–8. doi:10.1093/nar/gkw1108
33. Rice P, Longden I, Bleasby A. EMBOSS: the European molecular biology open software suite. *Trends Genet* (2000) 16:276–7. doi:10.1016/S0168-9525(00)02024-2
34. Camacho C, Coulouris G, Avagyan V, Ma N, Papadopoulos J, Bealer K, et al. BLAST+: architecture and applications. *BMC Bioinformatics* (2009) 10:421. doi:10.1186/1471-2105-10-421
35. Conesa A, Götz S, García-Gómez JM, Terol J, Talón M, Robles M. Blast2GO: a universal tool for annotation, visualization and analysis in functional genomics research. *Bioinformatics* (2005) 21:3674–6. doi:10.1093/bioinformatics/bti610
36. Jones P, Binns D, Chang H-Y, Fraser M, Li W, McAnulla C, et al. InterProScan 5: genome-scale protein function classification. *Bioinformatics* (2014) 30:1236–40. doi:10.1093/bioinformatics/btu031
37. The UniProt Consortium. UniProt: the universal protein knowledgebase. *Nucleic Acids Res* (2017) 45:D158–69. doi:10.1093/nar/gkw1099
38. Kinsella RJ, Kähäri A, Haider S, Zamora J, Proctor G, Spudich G, et al. Ensembl BioMarts: a hub for data retrieval across taxonomic space. *Database (Oxford)* (2011) 2011:bar030. doi:10.1093/database/bar030
39. Smedley D, Haider S, Durinck S, Pandini L, Provero P, Allen J, et al. The BioMart community portal: an innovative alternative to large, centralized data repositories. *Nucleic Acids Res* (2015) 43:W589–98. doi:10.1093/nar/gkv350
40. Kanehisa M, Sato Y, Kawashima M, Furumichi M, Tanabe M. KEGG as a reference resource for gene and protein annotation. *Nucleic Acids Res* (2016) 44:D457–62. doi:10.1093/nar/gkv1070
41. Kanehisa M, Sato Y, Morishima K. BlastKOALA and GhostKOALA: KEGG tools for functional characterization of genome and metagenome sequences. *J Mol Biol* (2016) 428:726–31. doi:10.1016/j.jmb.2015.11.006
42. Durinck S, Spellman PT, Birney E, Huber W. Mapping identifiers for the integration of genomic datasets with the R/Bioconductor package biomaRt. *Nat Protoc* (2009) 4:1184–91. doi:10.1038/nprot.2009.97
43. Gomez S, Adalid-Peralta L, Palafox-Fonseca H, Cantu-Robles VA, Soberón X, Sciutto E, et al. Genome analysis of excretory/secretory proteins in *Taenia solium* reveals their abundance of antigenic regions (AAR). *Sci Rep* (2015) 5:9683. doi:10.1038/srep09683
44. Petersen TN, Brunak S, von Heijne G, Nielsen H. SignalP 4.0: discriminating signal peptides from transmembrane regions. *Nat Methods* (2011) 8:785–6. doi:10.1038/nmeth.1701
45. Bendtsen JD, Jensen LJ, Blom N, Von Heijne G, Brunak S. Feature-based prediction of non-classical and leaderless protein secretion. *Protein Eng Des Sel* (2004) 17:349–56. doi:10.1093/protein/gzh037
46. Bendtsen JD, Kiemer L, Fausbøll A, Brunak S. Non-classical protein secretion in bacteria. *BMC Microbiol* (2005) 5:58. doi:10.1186/1471-2180-5-58
47. Emanuelsson O, Nielsen H, Brunak S, von Heijne G. Predicting subcellular localization of proteins based on their N-terminal amino acid sequence. *J Mol Biol* (2000) 300:1005–16. doi:10.1006/jmbi.2000.3903
48. Krogh A, Larsson B, von Heijne G, Sonnhammer EL. Predicting transmembrane protein topology with a hidden Markov model: application to complete genomes. *J Mol Biol* (2001) 305:567–80. doi:10.1006/jmbi.2000.4315
49. Yu G, Wang L-G, Han Y, He Q-Y. clusterProfiler: an R package for comparing biological themes among gene clusters. *OMICS* (2012) 16:284–7. doi:10.1089/omi.2011.0118
50. Revelle W. *psych: Procedures for Personality and Psychological Research.* Evanston: Northwestern University (2018). Available from: https://CRAN.R-project.org/package=psych Version = 1.8.4
51. Shannon P, Markiel A, Ozier O, Baliga NS, Wang JT, Ramage D, et al. Cytoscape: a software environment for integrated models of biomolecular interaction networks. *Genome Res* (2003) 13:2498–504. doi:10.1101/gr.1239303
52. Bader GD, Hogue CWV. An automated method for finding molecular complexes in large protein interaction networks. *BMC Bioinformatics* (2003) 4:2. doi:10.1186/1471-2105-4-2
53. Okonechnikov K, Conesa A, García-Alcalde F. Qualimap 2: advanced multi-sample quality control for high-throughput sequencing data. *Bioinformatics* (2016) 32:292–4. doi:10.1093/bioinformatics/btv566
54. Zakrzewski SS, Richter JF, Krug SM, Jebautzke B, Lee I-FM, Rieger J, et al. Improved cell line IPEC-J2, characterized as a model for porcine jejunal epithelium. *PLoS One* (2013) 8:e79643. doi:10.1371/journal.pone.0079643
55. Fink C, Hoffmann J, Knop M, Li Y, Isermann K, Roeder T. Intestinal FoxO signaling is required to survive oral infection in *Drosophila*. *Mucosal Immunol* (2016) 9:927–36. doi:10.1038/mi.2015.112
56. Goodridge HS, Marshall FA, Else KJ, Houston KM, Egan C, Al-Riyami L, et al. Immunomodulation via novel use of TLR4 by the filarial nematode phosphorylcholine-containing secreted product, ES-62. *J Immunol* (2005) 174:284–93. doi:10.4049/jimmunol.174.1.284
57. Kane CM, Cervi L, Sun J, McKee AS, Masek KS, Shapira S, et al. Helminth antigens modulate TLR-initiated dendritic cell activation. *J Immunol* (2004) 173:7454–61. doi:10.4049/jimmunol.173.12.7454
58. MacDonald AS, Maizels RM. Alarming dendritic cells for Th2 induction. *J Exp Med* (2008) 205:13–7. doi:10.1084/jem.20072665
59. Perrigoue JG, Marshall F, Artis D. On the hunt for helminths: innate immune cells in the recognition and response to helminth parasites. *Cell Microbiol* (2008) 10:1757–64. doi:10.1111/j.1462-5822.2008.01174.x
60. Cohen-Kedar S, Baram L, Elad H, Brazowski E, Guzner-Gur H, Dotan I. Human intestinal epithelial cells respond to β-glucans via Dectin-1 and Syk. *Eur J Immunol* (2014) 44:3729–40. doi:10.1002/eji.201444876
61. Patel S, McCormick BA. Mucosal inflammatory response to *Salmonella typhimurium* infection. *Front Immunol* (2014) 5:311. doi:10.3389/fimmu.2014.00311
62. Aprianto R, Slager J, Holsappel S, Veening J-W. Time-resolved dual RNA-seq reveals extensive rewiring of lung epithelial and pneumococcal transcriptomes during early infection. *Genome Biol* (2016) 17:198. doi:10.1186/s13059-016-1054-5
63. Zaph C, Troy AE, Taylor BC, Berman-Booty LD, Guild KJ, Du Y, et al. Epithelial-cell-intrinsic IKK-β expression regulates intestinal immune homeostasis. *Nature* (2007) 446:552–6. doi:10.1038/nature05590
64. Gerbe F, Sidot E, Smyth DJ, Ohmoto M, Matsumoto I, Dardalhon V, et al. Intestinal epithelial tuft cells initiate type 2 mucosal immunity to helminth parasites. *Nature* (2016) 529:226–30. doi:10.1038/nature16527
65. Howitt MR, Lavoie S, Michaud M, Blum AM, Tran SV, Weinstock JV, et al. Tuft cells, taste-chemosensory cells, orchestrate parasite type 2 immunity in the gut. *Science* (2016) 351:1329–33. doi:10.1126/science.aaf1648
66. McSorley HJ, Blair NF, Smith KA, McKenzie ANJ, Maizels RM. Blockade of IL-33 release and suppression of type 2 innate lymphoid cell responses by helminth secreted products in airway allergy. *Mucosal Immunol* (2014) 7(5):1068–78. doi:10.1038/mi.2013.123
67. Kakkar R, Hei H, Dobner S, Lee RT. Interleukin 33 as a mechanically responsive cytokine secreted by living cells. *J Biol Chem* (2012) 287:6941–8. doi:10.1074/jbc.M111.298703
68. Günzel D, Yu ASL. Claudins and the modulation of tight junction permeability. *Physiol Rev* (2013) 93:525–69. doi:10.1152/physrev.00019.2012
69. Günzel D, Fromm M. Claudins and other tight junction proteins. *Compr Physiol* (2012) 2:1819–52. doi:10.1002/cphy.c110045
70. Loukas A, Maizels RM. Helminth C-type lectins and host–parasite interactions. *Parasitol Today* (2000) 16:333–9. doi:10.1016/S0169-4758(00)01704-X
71. Cox GN, Staprans S, Edgar RS. The cuticle of *Caenorhabditis elegans*: II. Stage-specific changes in ultrastructure and protein composition during postembryonic development. *Dev Biol* (1981) 86:456–70. doi:10.1016/0012-1606(81)90204-9
72. Page AP, Stepek G, Winter AD, Pertab D. Enzymology of the nematode cuticle: a potential drug target? *Int J Parasitol Drugs Drug Resist* (2014) 4:133–41. doi:10.1016/j.ijpddr.2014.05.003

73. Winter AD, McCormack G, Page AP. Protein disulfide isomerase activity is essential for viability and extracellular matrix formation in the nematode *Caenorhabditis elegans*. *Dev Biol* (2007) 308:449–61. doi:10.1016/j.ydbio.2007.05.041
74. Winter AD, McCormack G, Myllyharju J, Page AP. Prolyl 4-hydroxlase activity is essential for development and cuticle formation in the human infective parasitic nematode *Brugia malayi*. *J Biol Chem* (2013) 288:1750–61. doi:10.1074/jbc.M112.397604
75. Coakley G, Buck AH, Maizels RM. Host parasite communications – messages from helminths for the immune system. *Mol Biochem Parasitol* (2016) 208:33–40. doi:10.1016/j.molbiopara.2016.06.003
76. Cooper D, Eleftherianos I. Parasitic nematode immunomodulatory strategies: recent advances and perspectives. *Pathogens* (2016) 5(3):58. doi:10.3390/pathogens5030058
77. Ebner F, Schwiertz P, Steinfelder S, Pieper R, Zentek J, Schütze N, et al. Pathogen-reactive T helper cell analysis in the pig. *Front Immunol* (2017) 8:565. doi:10.3389/fimmu.2017.00565
78. Hewitson JP, Grainger JR, Maizels RM. Helminth immunoregulation: the role of parasite secreted proteins in modulating host immunity. *Mol Biochem Parasitol* (2009) 167:1–11. doi:10.1016/j.molbiopara.2009.04.008
79. Yang Y, Wen YJ, Cai YN, Vallée I, Boireau P, Liu MY, et al. Serine proteases of parasitic helminths. *Korean J Parasitol* (2015) 53:1–11. doi:10.3347/kjp.2015.53.1.1
80. Williamson AL, Brindley PJ, Abbenante G, Prociv P, Berry C, Girdwood K, et al. Cleavage of hemoglobin by hookworm cathepsin D aspartic proteases and its potential contribution to host specificity. *FASEB J* (2002) 16:1458–60. doi:10.1096/fj.02-0181fje
81. Yatsuda AP, Bakker N, Krijgsveld J, Knox DP, Heck AJR, de Vries E. Identification of secreted cysteine proteases from the parasitic nematode *Haemonchus contortus* detected by biotinylated inhibitors. *Infect Immun* (2006) 74:1989–93. doi:10.1128/IAI.74.3.1989-1993.2006
82. Bottazzi ME. The human hookworm vaccine: recent updates and prospects for success. *J Helminthol* (2015) 89:540–4. doi:10.1017/S0022149X15000206
83. Hotez PJ, Diemert D, Bacon KM, Beaumier C, Bethony JM, Bottazzi ME, et al. The human hookworm vaccine. *Vaccine* (2013) 31:B227–32. doi:10.1016/j.vaccine.2012.11.034
84. Seid CA, Curti E, Jones RM, Hudspeth E, Rezende W, Pollet J, et al. Expression, purification, and characterization of the *Necator americanus* aspartic protease-1 (Na-APR-1 (M74)) antigen, a component of the bivalent human hookworm vaccine. *Hum Vaccin Immunother* (2015) 11:1474–88. doi:10.1080/21645515.2015.1036207
85. Hotez PJ, Bethony JM, Diemert DJ, Pearson M, Loukas A. Developing vaccines to combat hookworm infection and intestinal schistosomiasis. *Nat Rev Microbiol* (2010) 8:814. doi:10.1038/nrmicro2438
86. Brown A, Girod N, Billett EE, Pritchard DI. *Necator americanus* (human hookworm) aspartyl proteinases and digestion of skin macromolecules during skin penetration. *Am J Trop Med Hyg* (1999) 60:840–7. doi:10.4269/ajtmh.1999.60.840
87. Jolodar A, Fischer P, Büttner DW, Miller DJ, Schmetz C, Brattig NW. Onchocerca volvulus: expression and immunolocalization of a nematode cathepsin D-like lysosomal aspartic protease. *Exp Parasitol* (2004) 107:145–56. doi:10.1016/j.exppara.2004.06.006
88. Mello LV, O'Meara H, Rigden DJ, Paterson S. Identification of novel aspartic proteases from *Strongyloides ratti* and characterisation of their evolutionary relationships, stage-specific expression and molecular structure. *BMC Genomics* (2009) 10:611. doi:10.1186/1471-2164-10-611
89. Wang T, Van Steendam K, Dhaenens M, Vlaminck J, Deforce D, Jex AR, et al. Proteomic analysis of the excretory-secretory products from larval stages of *Ascaris suum* reveals high abundance of glycosyl hydrolases. *PLoS Negl Trop Dis* (2013) 7:e2467. doi:10.1371/journal.pntd.0002467
90. Starr CR, Engleberg NC. Role of hyaluronidase in subcutaneous spread and growth of group A *Streptococcus*. *Infect Immun* (2006) 74:40–8. doi:10.1128/IAI.74.1.40-48.2006
91. Rhoads ML, Fetterer RH, Urban JF. Release of hyaluronidase during in vitro development of *Ascaris suum* from the third to fourth larval stage. *Parasitol Res* (2001) 87:693–7. doi:10.1007/s004360100410
92. Hotez PJ, Narasimhan S, Haggerty J, Milstone L, Bhopale V, Schad GA, et al. Hyaluronidase from infective *Ancylostoma* hookworm larvae and its possible function as a virulence factor in tissue invasion and in cutaneous larva migrans. *Infect Immun* (1992) 60:1018–23.
93. Bower MA, Constant SL, Mendez S. *Necator americanus*: the Na-ASP-2 protein secreted by the infective larvae induces neutrophil recruitment in vivo and in vitro. *Exp Parasitol* (2008) 118:569–75. doi:10.1016/j.exppara.2007.11.014
94. Murray J, Gregory WF, Gomez-Escobar N, Atmadja AK, Maizels RM. Expression and immune recognition of *Brugia malayi* VAL-1, a homologue of vespid venom allergens and *Ancylostoma* secreted proteins. *Mol Biochem Parasitol* (2001) 118:89–96. doi:10.1016/S0166-6851(01)00374-7
95. Ballouz S, Verleyen W, Gillis J. Guidance for RNA-seq co-expression network construction and analysis: safety in numbers. *Bioinformatics* (2015) 31:2123–30. doi:10.1093/bioinformatics/btv118
96. van Dam S, Võsa U, van der Graaf A, Franke L, de Magalhães JP. Gene co-expression analysis for functional classification and gene-disease predictions. *Brief Bioinform* (2017) 19(4):575–92. doi:10.1093/bib/bbw139
97. Beswick EJ, Reyes VE. Macrophage migration inhibitory factor and interleukin-8 produced by gastric epithelial cells during *Helicobacter pylori* exposure induce expression and activation of the epidermal growth factor receptor. *Infect Immun* (2008) 76:3233–40. doi:10.1128/IAI.01534-07

10

The Serine/Threonine-Protein Phosphatase 1 from *Haemonchus contortus* is Actively Involved in Suppressive Regulatory Roles on Immune Functions of Goat Peripheral Blood Mononuclear Cells

*Muhammad Ehsan, WenJuan Wang, Javaid Ali Gadahi, Muhammad Waqqas Hasan, MingMin Lu, YuJian Wang, XinChao Liu, Muhammad Haseeb, RuoFeng Yan, LiXin Xu, XiaoKai Song and XiangRui Li**

Department of Preventive Veterinary Medicine, College of Veterinary Medicine, Nanjing Agricultural University, Nanjing, China

***Correspondence:**
XiangRui Li
lixiangrui@njau.edu.cn

Serine/threonine-protein phosphatases (STPs), as integral constituents of parasitic excretory/secretory proteins, are assumed to be released during the host–parasite interactions. However, knowledge about these phosphatases and their immunoregulatory and immune protective efficiencies with host peripheral blood mononuclear cells (PBMCs) is scant. In this study, an open reading frame of STP from *Haemonchus contortus* designated as HcSTP-1 was amplified and cloned using reverse-transcription-polymerase chain reaction (RT-PCR) method. The 951-bp nucleotides sequence was encoded to a protein of 316 amino acid residues, conserved in characteristics motifs GDXHG, GDYVDRG, GNHE, HGG, RG, and H. The HcSTP-1 protein was detected at approximately 35 kDa as recombinant protein fused in an expression vector system and resolved on sodium dodecyl sulfate-polyacrylamide gel electrophoresis. Immunohistochemically, HcSTP-1 was found to be localized in both male and female adult worm sections. Using immunofluorescence assay, the binding activity of rHcSTP-1 was confirmed on surface of goat PBMCs, which resulted in expression of multiple cytokines and various immunoregulatory activities *in vitro*. The RT-PCR results showed that mRNA level of interleukin-2, TGF-β1, IFN-γ, and IL-17 (with 10 μg/ml) was upregulated and IL-10 was decreased. However, IL-6 showed no change after PBMCs incubated with rHcSTP-1 protein. Further functional analysis showed that migratory activity of cells, intracellular nitrite production (NO), and apoptotic efficiency of PBMCs were elevated at significant level, whereas the proliferation of goat PBMCs and monocytes-associated major histocompatibility complex (MHC)-I and MHC-II expressions were decreased significantly at concentration-dependent fashion. Our results showed that the HcSTP-1 protein engaged in vital suppressive regulatory roles on host immune cells, which might represent a potential molecular target for controlling *H. contortus* infection in future.

Keywords: *Haemonchus contortus*, serine/threonine phosphatase, peripheral blood mononuclear cells, cytokines, immune responses

INTRODUCTION

Among gastrointestinal nematodes, *Haemonchus contortus* (barber pole worm) is most important parasite, responsible for health and economic problems in livestock industry worldwide (1). In severely infected animals like sheep and goats, the adult parasite penetrates in abomasal mucosa to feed on blood, results in anemia, loss of body weight and growth, and even death of the animals (2). Existing approaches for control of nematode parasites including *H. contortus*, mainly through widespread antihelmintics have resulted in stern drug resistance in domestic livestock (3, 4). Hence, the emergence of drug resistance in *H. contortus* demands for discoveries of novel anti-parasite drugs, vaccines, and development of immunological control strategies against nematode infections. In this regard, a comprehensive insight into the developmental biology of *H. contortus* at the molecular level might pinpoint some key antigens as new drug targets for parasite control (5).

The serine/threonine-protein phosphatase 1 (STP-1) belong to phosphoprotein phosphatase (PPP) family, and protein phosphatases (PPs) is largest class which is divided functionally into two major groups: first serine/threonine phosphatases (commonly cytoplasmic structural component, concerned with transcriptional activity and signal transduction) and second tyrosine phosphatases (typically bound with membrane and implicated in receptor-arbitrated signal transduction) (6). PPs can also be divided into four subclasses, such as PP1, PP2A, PP2B, and PP2C, based on substrate and inhibitory specificities (7). Furthermore, it was reported that PPs have been implicated in range of biological functions, such as exocytosis and apoptosis, neuronal activity, ion channel electrophysiology, and cell cycle (8–12).

Previously, various STPs from number of parasites have been identified and characterized, including those of *Oesophagostomum dentatum*, *Trichostrongylus vitrinus*, *Toxoplasma gondii*, *Toxocara canis*, and *Plasmodium falciparum* (13–17), and also suggested that STP-1 from *H. contortus* play a key role in some biological processes, such as spermatogenesis (18). However, information regarding the functions of STPs in parasitic nematode *H. contortus* is scant.

In our previous comparative proteomics analysis of excretory/secretory proteins (ESPs) from *H. contortus* (HcESPs), 59 proteins were identified at early and late adult developmental stages of parasite and amongst all, serine/threonine-protein phosphatase (STPs) were recognized as vital interacting proteins bind to the goat peripheral blood mononuclear cells (PBMCs) *in vivo* (19). The main objectives of current study were to clone and characterize a stage-specific gene from *H. contortus* designated as HcSTP-1, to express its recombinant protein in an expression vector system, and to evaluate potential immune regulatory roles of this protein (rHcSTP-1) with goat PBMCs *in vitro*. Our findings will provide valuable bases to better understand the biology of this parasite and to develop effective drugs and useful vaccines, which could be helpful in the prevention and control of *H. contortus* infection.

MATERIALS AND METHODS

Ethics Statement

All animals and laboratory experiments were strictly performed in accordance with the recommendations of the Animal Ethics Committee, Nanjing Agricultural University, China. All experimental procedures used in this study were permitted by the science and Technology Agency of Jiangsu Province [ID: SYXK (SU) 2010-0005].

Animals, Parasites, and PBMC Isolation

The native crossbred goats (3–6 months old) were housed indoor, provided with hay and corn (whole shelled) and water *ad libitum*. The anti-parasitic drug, levamisole (8 mg/kg body weight) was used with 2 weeks interval to keep goats free from naturally acquired helminth infection. The fecal samples were checked twice per week, using standard parasitological techniques and goats with no sign of helminths infection were used in subsequent experiments.

Sprague-Dawley (SD) rats with average body weight of 150 g, were bought at Experimental Animal Center of Jiangsu, PR China (Certified: SCXK 2008-0004). The rats were raised in microbe free condition.

The *H. contortus* strain was maintained by serial passage in helminth-free goats, at laboratory of immunology and molecular parasitology, Nanjing Agricultural University. The parasite eggs, larvae, and adults worms were collected and preserved according to the methods stated previously (20). The blood samples were taken from jugular vein of dewormed goats and PBMCs were collected by gradient centrifugation method (21). The PBMCs were cultured as the procedure stated previously (22).

Cloning and Sequence Analysis *H. contortus* STP-1 Gene

The freshly adults *H. contortus* parasites were collected from abomasum of the infected goats and the extraction of RNA was carried out using Trizol method according to the previously described procedure (23), followed by cDNA synthesis as per the manufacturer's guidelines of cDNA synthesis Kit (TaKaRa Biotech), and was preserved at −20°C for down-stream applications.

The open reading frame of HcSTP-1 was amplified by reverse-transcription-polymerase chain reaction (RT-PCR), from conserved domain sequences of *H. contortus* STP-1 gene (GenBank: GQ280010.1). For the subsequent cloning, underlined *BamH* I and *Xho* I restriction enzyme were inserted at the 5′-end of forward primer: (5′-GGATCCATGGACCCTACTCAAT-3′), and reverse primer: (5′-CTCGAGTTATTGACAAGGTGGAGC-3′). The amplified PCR fragment was electrophoresed and eluted with Gel purification Kit (Omega, USA) in accordance with kit protocol. The eluted product was then inserted into pMD19-T cloning vector (TaKaRa Biotechnology, China). The recombinant plasmid pMD19-T/HcSTP-1 was inserted into DH5α competent strain of *Escherichia coli* and cultured in Luria–Bertini medium

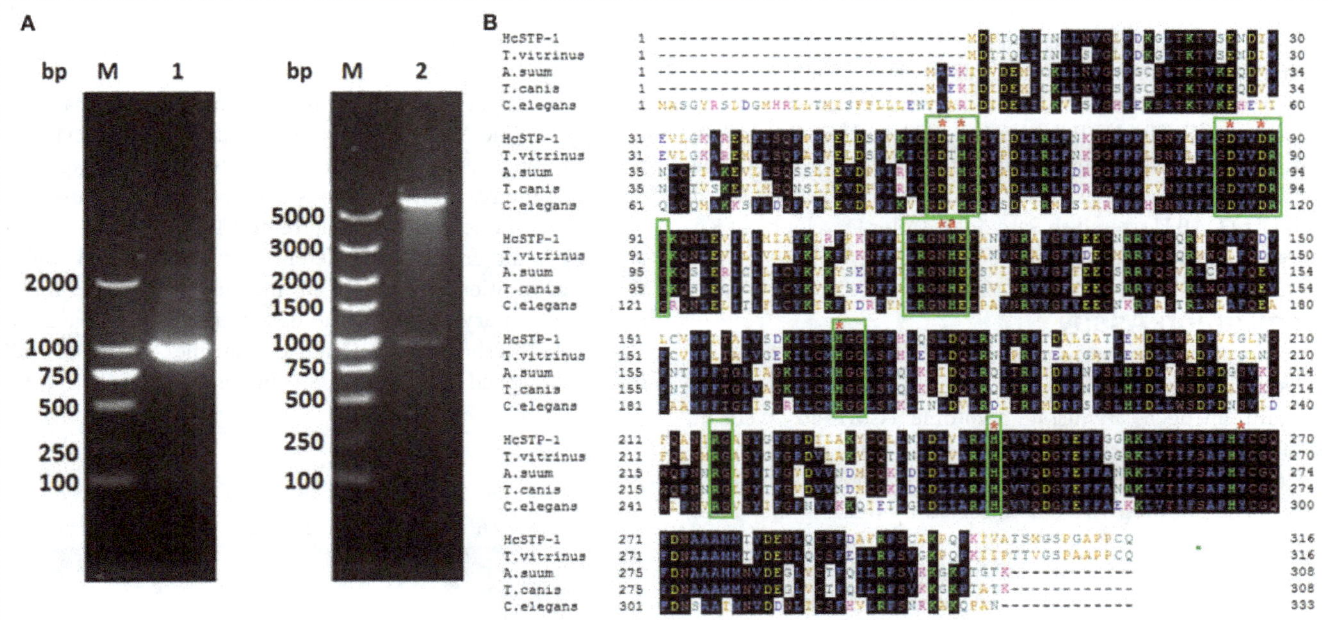

FIGURE 1 | Cloning and sequence analysis of HcSTP-1 gene. **(A)** Electrophoresis of PCR product of HcSTP-1 open reading frame (Lane 1). Restriction enzyme digestion of pET32a-HcSTP-1 with *BamH* I and *Xho* I (Lane 2) and molecular weight DNA marker (Lane M). **(B)** The comparison of amino acid sequence of *Haemonchus contortus* serine/threonine-protein phosphatase 1 (STP-1) and with predicted STPs from *Trichostrongylus vitrinus* (CAM84506.1), *A. suum* (CAJ98743.1), *Toxocara canis* (KHN86897.1), and *C. elegans* (NP_505086.2). Amino acids predicted to be involved in the catalytic metal binding are indicated by asterisks "*," and the histidine residue proposed for proton donation is indicated with "a." The conserved motifs found in all sequences including Prosite motif PS00125 (LRGNHE) are boxed in green color.

with ampicillin (100 μg/ml). The positive clones followed by sequencing (Invitrogen Biotech, Shanghai, China) were validated by sequence analysis online using Blast program.[1] The obtained nucleotide sequence was translated into amino acids sequence and aligned and compared with different nematode species using GENETYX Version 7.0.9 software. In addition, a number of online approaches/programs were used to detect N-terminal signal peptides/http://www.cbs.dtu.dk/services/SignalP/, Transmembrane protein prediction/http://www.cbs.dtu.dk/services/TMHMM/, T cell motifs/DNAstar: EditSeq, Protean, B cell epitopes/http://tools.immuneepitope.org/tools/bcell/iedb_input, and GPI modification Site Prediction/http://mendel.imp.ac.at/sat/gpi/gpi_server.html.

Expression and Purification of Recombinant HcSTP-1 Protein

The recognized recombinant pMD19-T/HcSTP-1 plasmid was digested with dual restriction enzymes *BamH* I and *Xho* I and ligated into prokaryotic expression vector pET32a (+) (Novagen, USA). Finally, the successful cloned STP-1 gene in a recombinant expression vector was sequenced to confirm its placement in the accurate reading frame. The recombinant plasmid pET32a (+)-HcSTP-1 was transferred into *E. coli* strain (BL21) and induced with 1 mM isopropyl-β-D-thiogalactopyranoside (IPTG; Sigma-Aldrich) after the OD_{600} of the culture reached 0.6 at 37°C. The cell pellet after centrifugation was lysed using 10 μg/ml of lysozyme (Sigma-Aldrich) followed by sonication, and was resolved on 12% (w/v) sodium dodecyl sulfate-polyacrylamide gel electrophoresis (SDS-PAGE). The purification of recombinant protein was carried out according to the manufacturer's instructions of Ni^{2+}-nitrilotriacetic acid (Ni-NTA) column (GE Healthcare, USA). The histidine-tagged protein (empty pET32a) used as control protein in multiple assays in this study was purified and expressed similar to the procedure described for rHcSTP-1 protein and determined at 12% SDS-PAGE after Coomassie blue staining and quantified by Bradford method (24).

Immuno-Blot Analysis

Polyclonal antibodies against recombinant protein were generated from SD rats by subcutaneous injection of 300 μg of rHcSTP-1 protein mixed equally with Freund's complete. After 2 weeks of first immunization, rats were injected three times at 1 week interval with same protein and Freund's incomplete mixture. The sera were collected after 10 days of last injection and preserved at −80°C for later use. The sera against *H. contortus* parasites were collected from naturally infected goats (25), and sera collected from normal goats or rats were used as negative control.

The SDS-PAGE products of recombinant HcSTP-1 and soluble/ES products from adult parasites, were shifted nitrocellulose membrane (Millipore, USA) for western blot analysis. After blocked with 5% (w/v) skimmed milk powder in TBST (TBS with 0.5% Tween-20) at 37°C for 2 h, the strips were incubated

[1]https://blast.ncbi.nlm.nih.gov/Blast.cgi.

with anti-*H. contortus* sera from goats or rat anti-sera against rHcSTP-1 (1:300 dilutions) as first antibody for treatment groups and normal goat serum or normal rat serum for control groups at 4°C overnight. Then, the membranes were incubated with the secondary antibody, HRP-conjugated goat anti-rat IgG (Santa Cruz, USA) in TBST (1:3,000 dilutions) at 37°C for 2 h. At end, the immunoreactions were visualized within 3–5 min, as per defined protocol of DAB Horseradish Peroxidase Color Development Kit (Beyotime Biotechnology).

Localization Assay

The mature parasites were suspended in TISSUE-TEK® O.C.T. compound (SAKURA, Torrance, CA, USA) and snap-frozen in liquid nitrogen. By using cryotome (CM1950, Wetzlar, Germany), worms were cut into sections with 10-µm thickness and fixed on poly-L-lysine hydrobromide glass slides. Non-specific bindings were confiscated by treating the slides with 10% normal goat serum, followed by incubation with rat-anti-STP-1 antiserum (1:300 dilutions) or normal rat serum as first antibody and Cy3-labeled Goat Anti-Rat IgG (1:3,000 dilutions) as second antibody (Beyotime, Shanghai, China) at 37°C for 2 h in each step. For DNA staining, the sections were marked with 1.5 µM 2-(4-amidinophenyl)-6-indolecarbamidine dihydrochloride (DAPI: Sigma, MO, USA) for 5 min. Finally, Anti-Fade Fluoromount Medium (Beyotime, Shanghai, China) was used and sections were examined under confocal microscope.

Binding of rHcSTP-1 on the Surface of Goat PBMCs

Freshly collected PBMCs, after washed with phosphate buffer saline (PBS: Ca^{2+}/Mg^{2+}-free, pH 7.4), were maintained at density of 1×10^5 cells/ml in cell culture medium (RPMI 1640), containing 10% fetal bovine serum (FBS), 100 U/ml penicillin and 100 mg/ml streptomycin (Gibco, Life Technology), and incubated with rHcSTP-1 or control protein pET32a or control buffer (PBS) at constant temperature (37°C) and humidity (5% CO_2) for 4 h. Protein binding at surface of goat PBMCs were confirmed by immunofluorescence assay (IFA). Briefly, PBMCs after being washed and stabled with 4% paraformaldehyde on poly-L-lysine-treated slides were then permeabilized using 1% TritonX-100 in PBS at normal temperature. The PBMCs were subjected to primary antibodies rat anti-rHcSTP-1-IgG (1:300 dilutions) or normal rat serum followed by Cy3-coupled goat anti-rat IgG (Beyotime, China) (1:3,000 dilutions) as second antibody for 1 h at 37°C temperature. At last, the slides were stained in darkness with DAPI (Sigma, USA) for 5 min, and subjected to Anti-Fade Fluoromount solution (Beyotime, China) before laser scanning confocal microscopic examination (LSM710, Zeiss, Jena, Germany) at 100× magnifications.

Detection of Cytokine Transcripts by RT-PCR

The PBMCs were stimulated with Concanavalin A (ConA/10 µg/ml), and treated with rHcSTP-1 (10, 20, and 40 µg/ml) or pET32a protein (10 µg/ml) and control buffer (PBS) in 24-well plate containing RPMI 1640 medium at 5% CO_2 and 37°C. The PBMCs were collected after 48 h of culture, by centrifugation and PrimeScript™ RT reagent kit (TaKaRa, CA, USA) was utilized to extract RNA from cells sediment as per the manufacturer's guidelines. The cDNA-based quantifications of cytokine transcriptions were evaluated as previously stated protocol of RT-PCR. The reaction conditions and set of primers used for cytokines [interleukin-2 (IL-2), IL-10, TGF-β1, IL-6, IFN-γ, and IL-17] and endogenous reference gene (β-actin), as well as their amplification efficiencies are mentioned in Tables S1–S3 in Supplementary Material. The data were analyzed based on Raw cycle thresholds (Ct), obtained from the ABI Prism 7500 software (Applied Biosystems, USA) by comparative Ct ($2^{-\Delta\Delta}$ Ct) method (26).

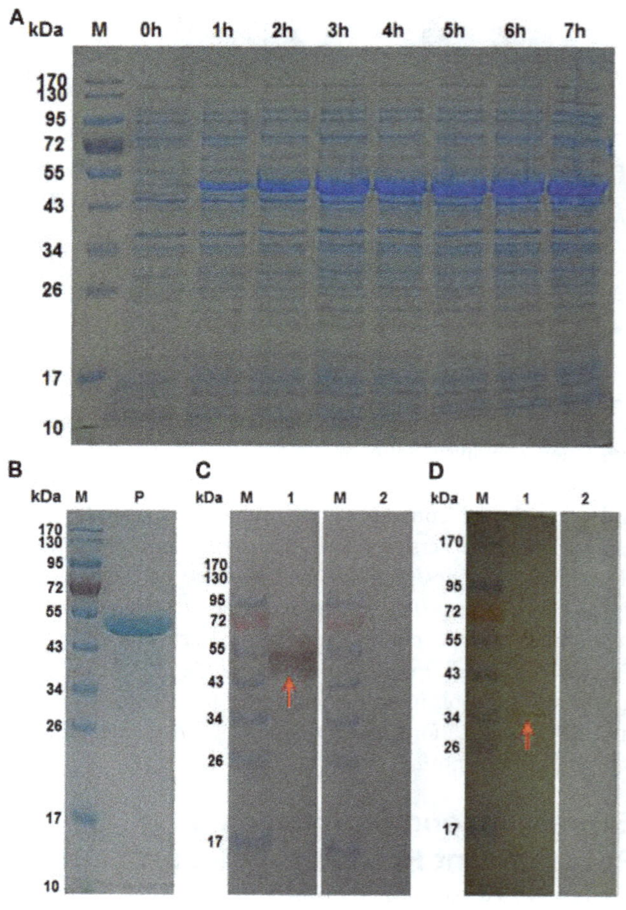

FIGURE 2 | Expression, purification and immuno reactivity of rHcSTP-1. **(A)** Recombinant expression vector before (Lane 0 h) and after 1 mM IPTG induction (Lane 1–7 h). Lane M: standard protein molecular weight marker. **(B)** Purified rHcSTP-1 protein resolved on sodium dodecyl sulfate-polyacrylamide gel electrophoresis (Lane P). **(C)** Western blot of rHcSTP-1 protein. (Lane 1) Purified recombinant protein was electrophoresed and transferred to a membrane probed with serum from goat infected with *Haemonchus contortus* and (Lane 2) with normal goat serum as negative control. **(D)** Western blot of total ES proteins of *H. contortus*. (Lane 1) ES proteins from *H. contortus* parasites were detected by rat antibodies against serine/threonine-protein phosphatase 1 (STP-1) protein and (Lane 2) with serum from normal rat as control.

Analysis of Major Histocompatibility Complex (MHC)-I and -II Molecule Expression

After separation of PBMCs by standard Ficoll-hypaque (GE Healthcare, USA) gradient centrifugation and two times washing with the PBS (Ca^{2+}/Mg^{2+}-free, pH 7.4), were poured into flat-bottom six well culture plates (Corning Inc., USA) containing RPMI 1640 medium (Invitrogen, USA) supplemented with 10% FBS and penicillin + streptomycin (Invitrogen, USA). The monocytes stick to the bottom of the plate, were collected (27) and adjusted at density of 1×10^6 cells/ml, whereas, Non-sticky cells were discarded by multiple washing steps. The purified monocytes were incubated in 24-well culture plates with different concentrations of rHcSTP-1 (treatment group) or pET32a protein and PBS (control group) at 37°C for 24 h. Subsequently, the monocytes were marked with monoclonal antibodies MHC-I (MCA2189A647, AbDserotec, Bio-Rad, USA) and MHC-II (MCA2225PE, AbDserotec), followed by flow cytometric analysis at FACS Calibur cytometer (BD Biosciences, San Jose, CA, USA) (**Figure 7A**).

Cell Proliferation Assay

The 100 µl of freshly isolated PBMCs at density of 1×10^6 cells/ml was poured into 96-well culture plate and stimulated with ConA (10 µg/ml). The PBMCs were incubated with serial concentrations of rHcSTP-1 protein (10, 20, and 40 µg/ml) in treatment group and pET32a empty protein or control vehicle (PBS) were added into control groups at 5% humidity and 37°C temperature for 72 h. Detection of PBMC proliferation was carried out according to the previously mentioned procedure of cell proliferation assay kit (28). 10 µl of CCK-8 solution (Beyotime China) was mixed in every well of plate 6 h prior to harvest and absorbance were checked by using spectrophotometer (Bio-Rad, USA) at wavelength 450 nm (OD_{450}). Result presented here are from three independent experiments.

Cell Migration Assay

The migration activity of cultured PBMCs was measured with 8.0-µm pores Millicell® insert (Merck-Millipore, USA) as stated previously. Briefly, in treatment group 200 µl of freshly separated cells were poured into the upper chamber with various concentrations of rHcSTP-1 (10, 20, and 40 µg/ml) and pET32a control protein or equal volume of control buffer (PBS) were added in control groups. Subsequently, 1,300 µl cell culture medium was filled in the lower chamber for 2 h incubation at 37°C and 5% CO_2. After that, columns were removed, and PBMC passed through polycarbonate layer were figure out by a Neubauer counting chamber. Data were resulted as percentage of seeded PBMCs. Three independent experiments were conducted.

Intracellular Nitrite Production by PBMCs

The goat PBMCs were separated and washed with Ca^{2+}/Mg^{2+}-free PBS (pH 7.4). 100 µl of cells containing DMEM medium was poured in 96-well plate with varying concentrations of rHc-STP-1 (10, 20, and 40 µg/ml), similarly the control groups were incubated with recombinant protein of pET32a or PBS (control buffer). NO production by cells was determined by Griess assay (29), by using Total Nitric Oxide Assay Kit (Beyotime, China) according to the manufacturer's instructions. The values in the

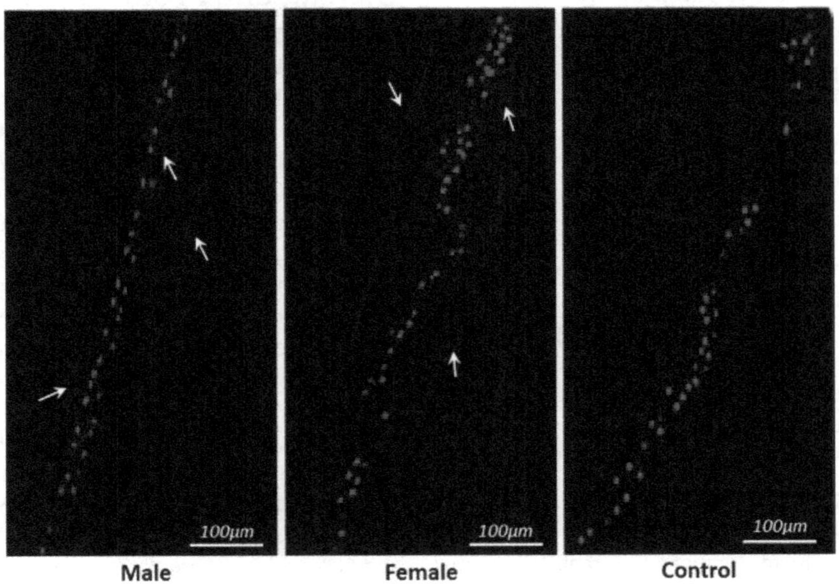

FIGURE 3 | Localization of serine/threonine-protein phosphatase 1 protein within parasite structure. Immunohistochemically STP-1 protein localizes inner and outer structure of *Haemonchus contortus* male and female adult worms. The red color indicates target protein stained with Cy3 and blue dots are localization of nuclei stained with DAPI. No red fluorescence was detected in control panel. Scale-bars: 100 µm.

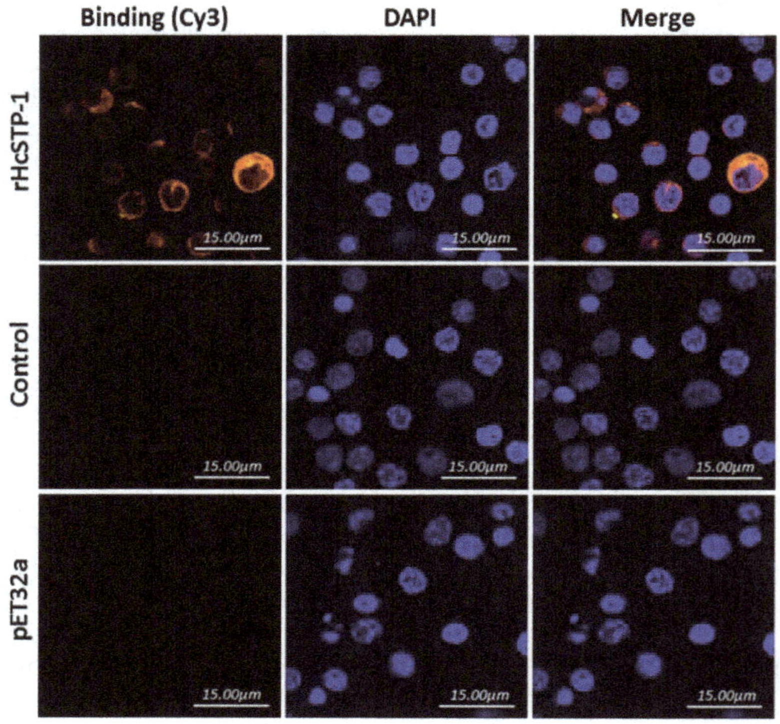

FIGURE 4 | Binding of rHcSTP-1 protein with goat peripheral blood mononuclear cells *in vitro*. The cells were incubated with rat sera anti-rHcSTP-1-O IgG, anti-HisTag protein (pET32a) or negative rat IgG as primary antibody followed by Cy3-labeled goat anti-rat IgG (red) as secondary antibody. Red fluorescence on surface of cells showed target protein staining (Cy3) and nuclei of cells were visualized by DAPI (blue). No red fluorescence was observed in control groups. The results were analyzed by using confocal laser scanning microscopy.

reaction mixture were measured at microplate spectrophotometer (Bio-Rad Laboratories, USA) at 540 nm (OD_{540}) wavelength. Data presented here are results of triplicate experiments.

Apoptotic Efficiency of rHcSTP-1 on PBMC

Efficiency of rHcSTP-1 to induce apoptosis of PBMC was assessed by flow cytometric analysis (BD Biosciences, USA). The PBMCs (1×10^7 cells/ml) treated with different rHcSTP-1 protein concentrations (5, 10, 20, and 40 µg/ml) and empty pET32a protein, were stained with Annexin V-FITC kit (Miltenyi Biotec, Germany) according to the manufacturer's protocols. The apoptosis rate was calculated by the percentage of early (Annexin V^+ PI−) and late (Annexin V^+ PI^+) PBMC apoptosis. Cells without any treatment were set as control. Data were analyzed using Flow Jo 7.6 software (Tree Star, USA).

Statistical Analysis

Data analysis regarding all experiments was performed by using the statistical package, GraphPad Premier 6.0 (GraphPad Prism, San Diego, CA, USA). Data are presented as mean ± SEM. The differences between groups were compared by one-way ANOVA, followed by a Tukey test and were considered statistically significant at $p < 0.05$.

RESULTS

Cloning and Protein Expression of *H. contortus* STP-1

The RT-PCR generated fragment of STP-1 gene with molecular size of 951 bp, was obtained from *H. contortus* cDNA and successfully cloned into an expression vector system, confirmed by enzymatic digestion with *BamH* I and *Xho* I (**Figure 1**). After that, cloned HcSTP-1 sequence was translated into 316 amino acids with predicted 35 kDa molecular mass and calculated pI of 6.328. The nucleotide and amino acid sequence identity HcSTP-1 using BLASTx and BLASTp revealed highly sequence resemblance with STPs from other parasite species, existing at NCBI database (see text footnote 1). In this study, characterization of HcSTP-1 cDNA showed 98% significant sequence identity to *H. contortus* (ADJ96628.1), 80% with *C. briggsae* (XM_002631635.1) (data not shown). Multiple sequence alignment showed that HcSTP-1 polypeptide shares a significant similarity of 91% with *T. vitrinus* (GenBank: CAM84506.1), 62% with *T. canis* (GenBank: KHN86897.1), 62% with *Ascaris suum* (GenBank: CAJ98743.1), and 58% with *Caenorhabditis elegans* (GenBank: NP_505086.2). The BLAST analysis predicted number of conserved metal ion-binding sites and histidine residue predicted to be involved in proton donation. The amino acids expressing STP protein motif LRGNHE was found during sequence analysis. The aligned STPs sequences were highly similar in central regions, particularly in term of characteristics sequence motifs, such as GDXHG, GDYVDRG, GNHE, HGG, RG, and H (30), whereas there was a higher variation occurred regarding to N- and C-terminal regions among all align sequences (**Figure 1**). Further sequence analysis indicated lack of signal peptide, transmembrane domain, and GPI anchor site, whereas T and B cell motifs were predicted in deduced protein structure (Figures S1–S4 in Supplementary Material).

The recombinant product of HcSTP-1 gene inserted into *E. coli* was expressed after IPTG induction and detected after staining with Coomassie brilliant blue R-250 on SDS-PAGE. The rHcSTP-1 protein was expressed with molecular weight of about 53 kDa (**Figure 2**, Lane P) along with 18 kDa calculated mass of vector protein (pET32a). The target protein was confirmed at its original size of 35 kDa after reduction from vector protein. Polyclonal antibodies against rHcSTP-1 were identified by immuno-blot analysis, which revealed that rHcSTP-1 could be recognized by sera from goats infected with *H. contortus* and native STP-1 protein from *H. contortus* could be recognized by antibodies generated against rHcSTP-1 protein (**Figures 2C,D**, Lane 1). However, no protein was detected with normal sera taken from un-immunized goats/rats (**Figures 2C,D**, Lane 2).

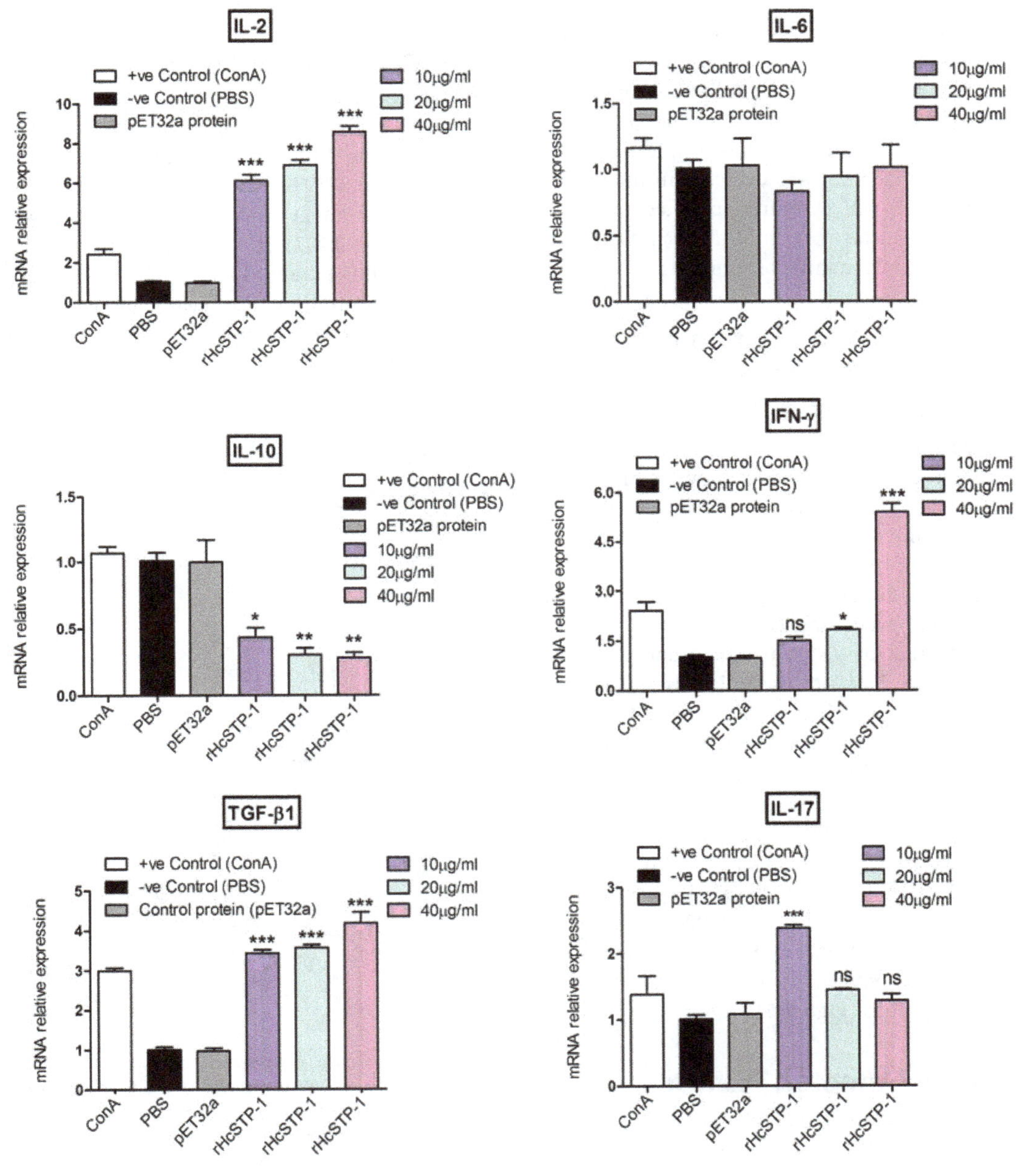

FIGURE 5 | Relative expression of multiple cytokines in goat peripheral blood mononuclear cells stimulated by the recombinant HcSTP-1. Cells were incubated with the recombinant serine/threonine-protein phosphatase 1 (STP-1) for 48 h, the mRNAs encoding interleukin-2 (IL-2), IL-6, IL-10, IFN-γ, TGF-β1, and IL-17 were quantified by reverse-transcription-polymerase chain reaction. The significant level was set at $^{*}p < 0.05$, $^{**}p < 0.01$, $^{***}p < 0.001$, and ns non-significant compared with the untreated group (control). Data are representative of three independent experiments.

HcSTP-1 Localized Outer and Inner Lining of *H. contortus* Worm Sections

The partial body sections of male and female adult worms are shown in **Figure 3**. Immunohistochemical analysis was performed to detect distribution of native STP-1 protein within the worms. The red lining at outer and inner layer of membranes and in gut region strongly indicated the presence of this protein within worms sections. However, no fluorescence was detected in the control section (**Figure 3**).

rHcSTP-1 Binding Confirmation on Surface of Goat PBMCs

The interaction of HcSTP-1 with PBMCs, which are key elements for immune responses, was investigated by using IFA. As shown in **Figure 4**, the Cy3-labeled target protein and the DAPI labeled nuclei displayed red and blue fluorescence, respectively. The red visualization on the surface of cells in treatment group (rHcSTP-1) indicated the binding of the protein whereas, no red labeling was detected in the control groups (pET32a or PBS), which clearly specified that rHcSTP-1 could bind on the surface of goat PBMCs and exerts its immune effects in a multiple manners (**Figure 4**).

rHcSTP-1 Decreased Anti-Inflammatory and Increased Pro-Inflammatory Cytokines Expression in a Balanced Th1-Th2 State *In Vitro*

The mRNA levels of cytokines produced by cultured goat immune cells (PBMCs) in response to STP-1 protein were tested at RT-PCR machine. As depicted in results of **Figure 5**, transcriptions level of IL-2 [ANOVA, $F_{(5,12)} = 198.9, p = 0.0001$] and transforming growth factor-β1 (TGF-β1) [ANOVA, $F_{(5,12)} = 108.0, p = 0.0001$] were increased significantly at dose-dependent manner to that of pET32a protein and PBS control group. However, the IL-10 transcription was decreased [ANOVA, $F_{(5,12)} = 19.04, p = 0.0001$] dose dependently to that of control groups. Here, we also noted that interferon gamma (IFN-γ) at protein concentration of 10 μg/ml showed no difference ($p = 0.337$); however, at 20 μg/ml ($p = 0.002$) and 40 μg/ml [ANOVA, $F_{(5,12)} = 105.6, p = 0.0001$] the transcription level was augmented significantly. After incubation with rHcSTP-1 protein, the expressions of IL-17 at 10 μg/ml reached at its significant level [ANOVA, $F_{(5,12)} = 11.76, p = 0.0003$], while at 20 and 40 μg/ml remained non-significant. However, IL-6 was not significantly different [ANOVA, $F_{(5,12)} = 0.604, p = 0.699$] when compared with control groups (**Figure 5**).

rHcSTP-1 Protein Affected PBMCs Proliferation

Antiproliferative effects of rHcSTP-1, compared to the negative control and control protein treated groups were evaluated by using cell counting kit (CCK8). The results demonstrated that, cells stimulated with ConA and incubated with rHcSTP-1 protein downregulated [ANOVA, $F_{(5,12)} = 67.38, p = 0.0001$] the multiplication efficiency dose dependently (**Figure 6**). However, no significant change was observed between control groups [ANOVA, $F_{(5,12)} = 67.38, p = 0.557$].

rHcSTP-1 Inhibited MHC-I and -II Expression on Goat Monocytes

In response to the rHcSTP-1, the expression of MHC-I and -II surface markers on monocytes were evaluated, and results showed that as compared to expression in control groups, rHcSTP-1 significantly decreased MHC-I (**Figures 7B,D**) molecule expression [$F_{(5,12)} = 780.3$] as well as MHC-II [$F_{(5,12)} = 157.2$] on the surface of the goat monocytes in a dose-dependent manner $p < 0.0001$ (**Figures 7C,E**).

PBMC Migration Assay

To investigate impact of the rHcSTP-1 on immune cell migration, the percentage of migrated cells through Millipore polycarbonate membrane into the lower chamber was calculated. Results showed that 16.67 ± 0.8819% cells with control and 16.33 ± 1.764% cells with control protein group (pET32a) were migrated into lower chamber ($p = 0.087$). At 10 μg/ml (27.00 ± 1.528%), 20 μg/ml (32.67 ± 2.603%), and 40 μg/ml (35.00 ± 2.309%) rHcSTP-1 protein concentrations, significant amount of cells were passed through membrane (**Figure 8**). However, no difference was found between control and 5 μg/ml (20.00 ± 1.155%) protein concentration ($p = 0.084$).

rHcSTP-1 Involved in Intra-PBMCs NO Production

Nitric oxide plays a crucial role in the host defense mechanism by preventing growth or killing the parasite directly during

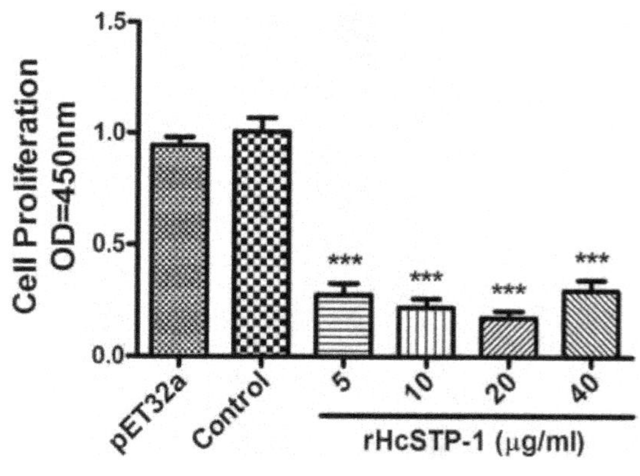

FIGURE 6 | Influences of different concentrations of rHcSTP-1 on peripheral blood mononuclear cells proliferation *in vitro*. Cells were simulated with ConA and treated with control buffer, His-Tag protein (pET32a), and various concentrations of recombinant serine/threonine-protein phosphatase 1 (STP-1) protein for 72 h. Proliferation test was conducted by CCK-8 and OD450 value was measured using microplate spectrophotometer. Cell proliferation index was calculated by considering the OD450 values in controls as 100%. The data are expressed as mean ± SEM of three independent experiments (***$p < 0.001$).

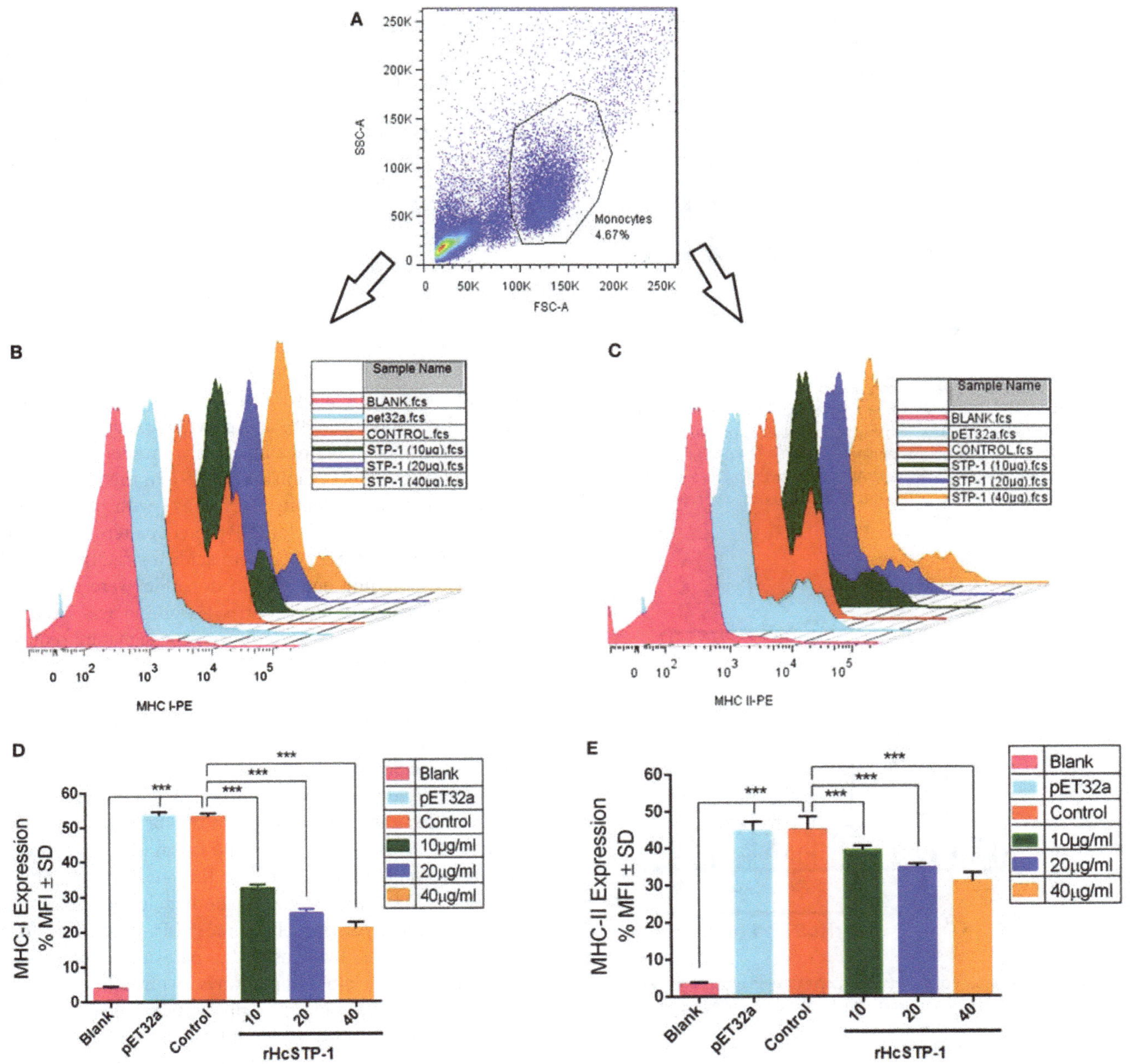

FIGURE 7 | rHcSTP-1 suppressed both major histocompatibility complex (MHC) class-I and II on goat monocytes. Monocytes were cultured in the presence of control buffer, HisTag protein (pET32a), and multiple concentrations of rHcSTP-1 for 24 h. MHC-II expression was measured by flow cytometric analysis and calculated as the percentage of mean fluorescence intensity (MFI). **(A)** Histogram corresponds to one representative of three independent experiments. **(B,C)** Stagger offset showing expression level of MHCs on monocytes. **(D,E)** Bar graphs represent the MFI ± SD of controls. The data are representative of three independent experiments (***$p < 0.001$).

infection. By using total nitric oxide kit, we found that no significant production was occurred [ANOVA, $F_{(5,12)} = 25.92$, $p = 0.504$] at 5 and 10 µg/ml compared with the groups treated as control. Here, we also observed that at 20 and 40 µg/ml, a significant level of NO was produced [ANOVA, $F_{(5,12)} = 25.92$, $p = 0.0001$]. However, production of NO between control (PBS) and pET32a group was also non-significant [ANOVA, $F_{(5,12)} = 25.92$, $p = 0.473$] (**Figure 9**).

rHcSTP-1 Dramatically Modulated Early and Late Apoptosis of PBMCs

It has been suggested that STPs obviously involved in various cellular processes including cell viability and cell death (10). The apoptotic activity of rHcSTP-1 on PBMCs was evaluated by using the externalization of membrane phospholipid phosphatidylserine (PS) as a marker of cell apoptosis. Flow cytometry assay revealed that cells incubated with different

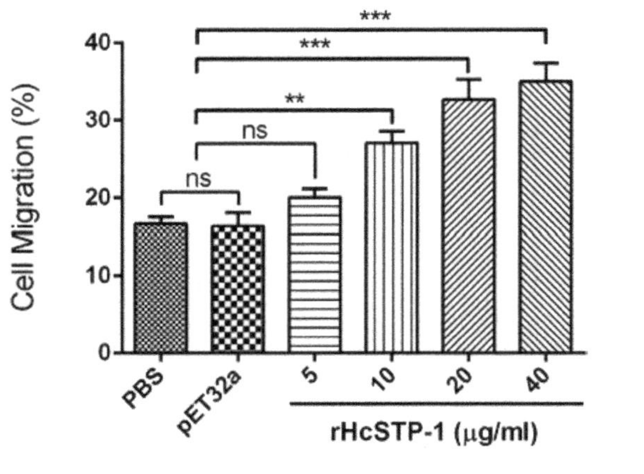

FIGURE 8 | Effects of the various concentrations of rHcSTP-1 on peripheral blood mononuclear cell migration *in vitro*. Cells were treated with control buffer, HisTag protein (pET32a), and multiple concentrations of rHcSTP-1. The migration percentage was determined randomly. The difference between the mean values was calculated using ANOVA. Data are representative of three independent experiments (**$p < 0.01$, ***$p < 0.001$, and ns non-significant versus the control).

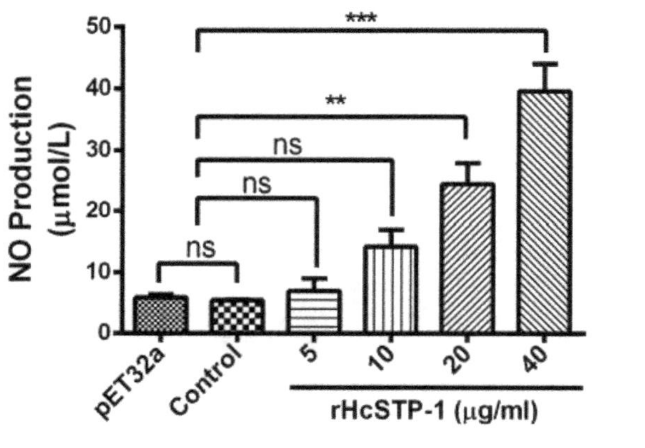

FIGURE 9 | Measurement of the intracellular nitric oxide production by goat peripheral blood mononuclear cells *in vitro*. Nitric oxide concentration in the supernatant of cell cultures was performed according to the instructions of Griess assay by Total Nitric Oxide Assay Kit. The data were presented here as mean ± SEM of three independent experiments (**$p < 0.01$ and ***$p < 0.001$).

protein concentrations (5, 10, 20, and 40 μg/ml) showed significantly increased frequency of apoptotic percentage in both early [ANOVA, $F_{(5,12)} = 69.08$, $p = 0.0001$] and late stage apoptosis [ANOVA, $F_{(5,12)} = 68.30$, $p = 0.0001$] compared with the control groups. Meanwhile, no significant change was observed [ANOVA, $F_{(5,12)} = 200.8$, $p = 0.0986$] between control and pET32a group (**Figure 10**).

DISCUSSION

Identification and development of novel drug targets are always a primacy in the biological study of socio-economically important parasites. Helminths ESPs including some antigens with unknown biological functions were characterized (31–33), and due to their sequences homology, these molecules have been proven as promising vaccine candidate against nematodes infections (34, 35). Among PPs, PP1 elaborate numerous biological activities, such as membrane receptors/channels regulations, protein synthesis, glycogen metabolism, transcription, cellular division, and apoptosis (36). In current investigation, an ES protein of *H. contortus* (STP-1) was characterized and localization of this protein through IFA confirmed its attachment with host immune cells for the first time, in shape of surface ligand complex (37), which is characteristic feature of ES proteins to suppress or modulate the immune functions of host PBMCs.

The PP1 is a major ubiquitously expressed STP, which shares a conserved catalytic domain with all other isotypes (PP2A, PP2B, PP4, PP5, PP6, and PP7) (38) and provides extensive information regarding their functions involved in numerous vital cellular mechanisms in all organisms (30, 39). In this study, highly significant amino acid identity of HcSTP-1 with presence of a conserved motif (LRGNHE) for STP protein pattern at positions 115–120 (18), involvement of amino acids for catalytic activity like metal ion-binding and proton donation were found (7). In the central regions of polypeptides, the amino acid sequences were highly conserved, particularly with the signature sequence motifs of the PPP family (GDXHG, GDXVDRG, GNHE, HGG, RG, and H) (30). However, the N- and C-terminal amino acids were variable, which suggested that it might be involved in protein binding and regulatory activity.

Previous studies suggested that STPs were associated with male reproductive processes of parasites, including sperm maturation, motility, and viability (40). In our previous proteomic analysis, STP-1 was found at adult and late adult developmental stages of *H. contortus in vivo* (19). In this study, immunohistochemically HcSTP-1 was localized in both male and female adult worms of *H. contortus*. Somehow, most PPs considered to be conserved during free-living as well as parasitic developmental stages; however, the biological pathways involved in the growth, development, survival, and/or reproduction reflects between invertebrates and vertebrates. Based on current information, a deep insight into the biochemical localization of STPs in *H. contortus* is required to understand the gender dependent immune stimulation by STPs during host–parasite interface.

The immune (Th1 and Th2) and inflammatory responses are deeply allied with secretion of various chemokines and cytokines by number of immune cell types (lymphocytes and monocytes), which perform crucial immunoregulatory functions (41), against parasitic infections like *H. contortus* (42). In this study, the levels of mRNA transcripts for IL-2, interleukin-10, transforming growth factor beta 1, interleukin-6, interferon-γ, and interleukin-17 in cultured PBMCs after treatment with rHcSTP-1 were detected for the first time. Schallig (43) suggested that sheep challenged with *H. contortus* infection responded cell mediate immune reaction (Th1), categorized by upregulation of IFN-γ and IL-2 mRNA expression. Similarly, in current research, goat PBMCs in response to rHcSTP-1 protein showed higher expression levels

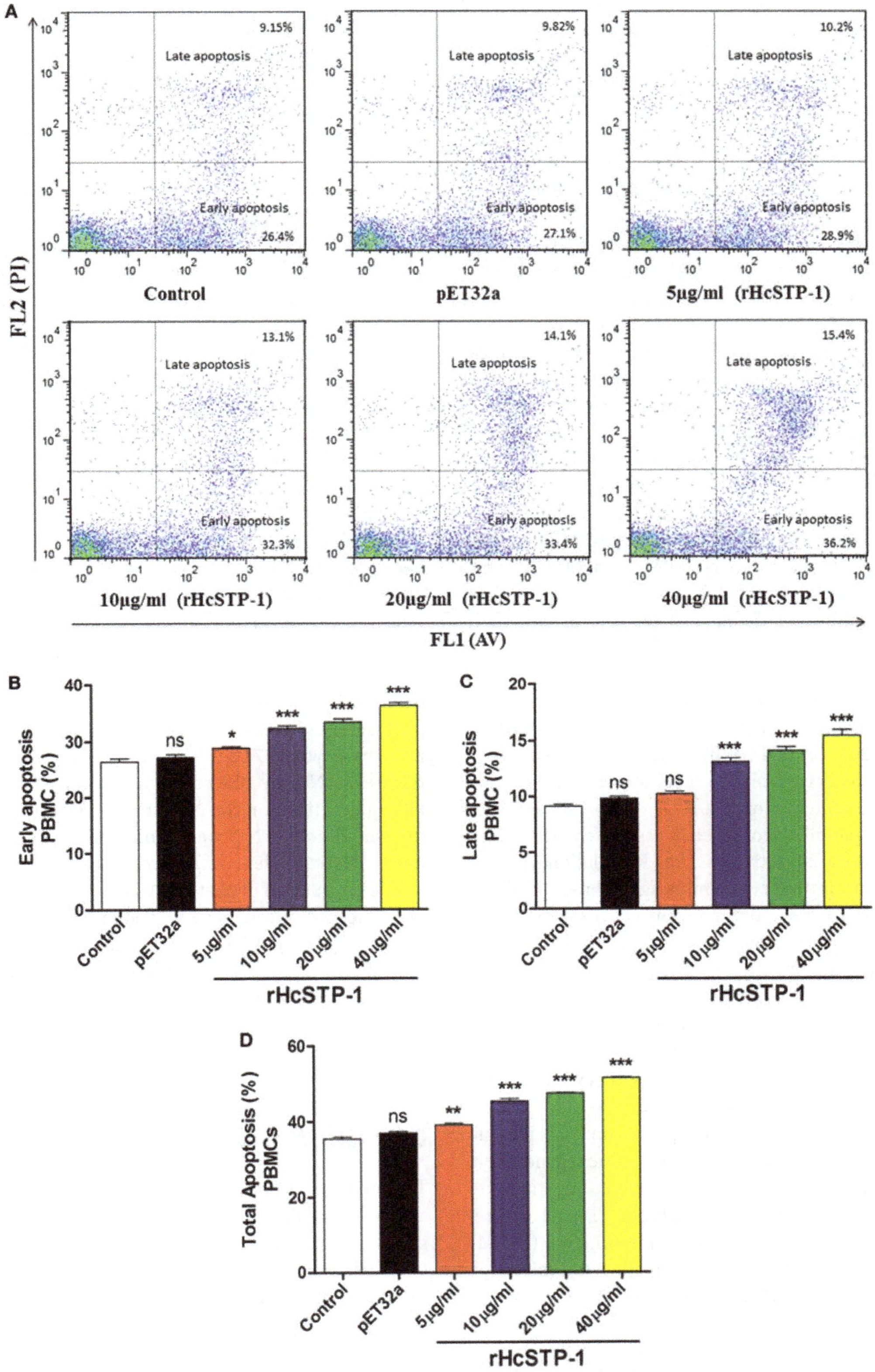

FIGURE 10 | Apoptotic analysis of peripheral blood mononuclear cells (PBMCs) by flow cytometry. **(A)** The dot plot showing percentages of PBMCs undergoing early and late stage apoptosis dually stained with Annexin V-FITC/PI. **(B)** Bar graph showing percentage of early stage apoptosis of PBMCs after rHcSTP-1 treatment. **(C)** Bar graph showing percentage of late stage apoptosis of PBMCs after rHcSTP-1 treatment. **(D)** The effect of the different protein treatments on total % (early + late) of apoptotic cells. Data are presented as the mean ± SEM (n = 3) from triplicate experiments. Asterisks designate treatment groups are significantly differ in respect to control one (*p < 0.05, **p < 0.01, ***p < 0.001, and ns non-significant).

of IL-2 and IFN-γ, suggesting that these cytokines might be in favor of non-protective Th responses against hemonchosis. The immunosuppressive cytokine IL-10 was responsible for inhibition of Th2 immune responses (44, 45). In this research, rHcSTP-1 protein showed a significant Th2 type immune response by decreased IL-10 cytokine in culture PBMCs, and thus exerts suppressive potential on differentiation of T_{reg} cells, which might be immune modulatory role of HcSTP-1 against parasite infection.

Previously, some researches demonstrated that IL-17 cytokine were involved in pathogenesis and inflammatory responses by numerous parasites (46–48). It was also elucidated that decreased level of IL-17 resulted favorable host protective responses (49). In our previous study, HcESPs were found to induce IL-17 cytokine by stimulation of the Th17 cells and resulted in inflammatory reaction favorable for worm survival in host. In this study, we found that rHcSTP-1 with concentration of 10 μg/ml significantly upregulated IL-17 cytokine. Our findings indicated that HcSTP-1 protein of *H. contortus* was adept in Th17 cells induction, which lead to inflammatory response. However, the resulted inflammatory reactions might be in favor of parasitic infection. TGF-β1 is functionally multidimensional cytokine that controls various immune system activities differentially on different cell types and potentially regulate various biological processes (50). It also plays vital roles to inhibit proliferation and to stimulate the apoptosis of various immune cells subset (51). In this investigation, the binding of recombinant protein HcSTP-1 to the goat PBMCs increased the production of TGF-β1, which could be a one of mechanism of rHcSTP-1 protein to facilitate immune evasion during host–parasite interactions.

Major histocompatibility complex is associated with many important immunological activities like: stimulation of antibody production and immune responses against microbial and parasitic pathogens (52, 53), although some cytokines especially IFN-γ and TGF-β (54) have been proven to upregulate MHC-I and -II gene expression in different immune cells. Here, we noted that STP-1 protein of *H. contortus* potentially suppress the MHC-I and -II molecules expression in goat monocytes. This indicated that STP-1 protein interferes with the MHC-I and -II antigen presentation pathway, which might be a key mechanism for evasion from the host's immune response.

The cellular processes such as cell migration part play an importance role in immune surveillance and tissue regeneration, by recruiting of immune cells into the surrounding tissue to destroy invading microorganisms. In addition, Type-1 as precise inhibitor of protein serine/threonine phosphatase (PHI-1) participated in regulatory events by modulating the migration of human endothelial and epithelial cells (55). Moreover, it was suggested that helminths actively induce migration of immune cell to infected sites (56). In this research, migration experiment concluded that rHcSTP-1 is an important binding protein to the goat PBMCs, which regulate the migration of immune cells to combat with invading *H. contortus* parasite and might be a contributor of HcESPs in the PBMCs migration.

Many proteins including ser/thr phosphatases were thought to be implicated in regulation of apoptosis (57). Till now, studies on cell death regulation by PPP subfamilies like PP2A and PP2B were well documented (10, 58); however, few studies highlighted the direct association and involvement of PP1, PP4, PP5, PP6, and PP7 members of phosphatase family in apoptosis (59–62). This study showed that rHcSTP-1 was involved in apoptosis as well as cell necrotic activity at dose-dependent manner.

In addition, cell proliferation is an indispensable process which is regulated or suppressed by both antigen-presenting cells (APCs) and T cells, thus modulate the host immune responses (63). In our earlier work, HcESPs significantly suppressed PBMCs multiplication at dose-dependent manner. In this study, PBMCs proliferation was decreased at significant level, which ultimately increased the pre- and post-apoptotic percentage in response to rHcSTP-1 treatment. Our study demonstrated that rHcSTP-1 as a constituent of HcESPs might interfere with modulatory activity on PBMCs proliferation and cell death regulation; however, the exact mechanism and pathways involved during host–parasite interaction upon HcSTP-1 protein involvement remains to be determined.

The immune cell-derived molecule, nitric oxide (NO) has been concerned with host non-specific defense against variety of infections such as hemonchosis, leishmaniasis, trypanosomiasis, malaria, toxoplasmosis, and schistosomiasis (64, 65). Previous studies provoked that PPs including P1 and P2A are involved in iNOS assertion in murine macrophages (66). Another study also witnessed that serine-threonine phosphatases post-transcriptionally regulate iNOS translation in rat hepatocytes (67). Furthermore, IFN-γ and TNF-α activated release of NO by macrophages was usually associated with killing functions on the helminths (68). In our previous study, the generation of NO was significantly suppressed by HcESPs due to decreased level of IFN-γ (69). In this study, intracellular nitrite production of goat PBMCs was significantly upregulated in a concentration-dependent fashion. These findings suggested that *H. contortus* STP-1 protein could induce the production of NO through increasing IFN-γ level which might mediate immunomodulatory functions on NO production and thus intensified the harmful effects of some chemical factors produced by the host cells on the helminths during host–parasite interface.

CONCLUSION

The current observations highlighted that *H. contortus* STP-1 as an important constituents of HcESPs localized in both gender, play pivotal stage-specific regulatory roles in interactions with host immune cells. This protein after being bind to host immune cells, regulate cytokines expression, cell proliferation, MHC expression, cell migration, NO production, and cell death regulation differentially. This study might be a powerful clue and would have major fundamental significant contribution in the discovery of novel therapeutic approaches to control hemonchosis. However, immune cells specific role of rHcSTP-1 and other related phosphatases subunits with PBMC sub-populations like T cell and B cell, NK cell, APCs, and macrophages involved in host–parasite relationship in activating immune and cellular response are worthy for future research.

AUTHOR CONTRIBUTIONS

XLi concerned with project designing, management, and coordination of this study. ME analyzed data and wrote the manuscript. WW, JG, ML, and YW provided technical support during experiments. MWH, MH, and XLiu participated in data analysis. LX, RY, and XS helped for providing all necessary materials during experiments.

REFERENCES

1. Coles GC. The future of veterinary parasitology. *Vet Parasitol* (2001) 98:31–9. doi:10.1016/S0304-4017(01)00421-6
2. Jasmer DP, Lahmers KK, Brown WC. *Haemonchus contortus* intestine: a prominent source of mucosal antigens. *Parasite Immunol* (2007) 29:139–51. doi:10.1111/j.1365-3024.2006.00928.x
3. Kaplan RM, Vidyashankar AN. An inconvenient truth: global worming and anthelmintic resistance. *Vet Parasitol* (2012) 186:70–8. doi:10.1016/j.vetpar.2011.11.048
4. Kotze AC, Hunt PW, Skuce P, Von Samson-Himmelstjerna G, Martin RJ, Sager H, et al. Recent advances in candidate-gene and whole-genome approaches to the discovery of anthelmintic resistance markers and the description of drug/receptor interactions. *Int J Parasitol Drugs Drug Resist* (2014) 4:164–84. doi:10.1016/j.ijpddr.2014.07.007
5. Britton C, Roberts B, Marks ND. Functional genomics tools for *Haemonchus contortus* and lessons from other helminths. *Adv Parasitol* (2016) 93:599–623. doi:10.1016/bs.apar.2016.02.017
6. Sarmiento M, Zhao Y, Gordon SJ, Zhang ZY. Molecular basis for substrate specificity of protein-tyrosine phosphatase 1B. *J Biol Chem* (1998) 273: 26368–74. doi:10.1074/jbc.273.41.26368
7. Barford D, Das AK, Egloff MP. The structure and mechanism of protein phosphatases: insights into catalysis and regulation. *Annu Rev Biophys Biomol Struct* (1998) 27:133–64. doi:10.1146/annurev.biophys.27.1.133
8. Cohen PT. Novel protein serine/threonine phosphatases: variety is the spice of life. *Trends Biochem Sci* (1997) 22:245–51. doi:10.1016/S0968-0004(97)01060-8
9. Herzig S, Neumann J. Effects of serine/threonine protein phosphatases on ion channels in excitable membranes. *Physiol Rev* (2000) 80:173–210. doi:10.1152/physrev.2000.80.1.173
10. Klumpp S, Krieglstein J. Serine/threonine protein phosphatases in apoptosis. *Curr Opin Pharmacol* (2002) 2:458–62. doi:10.1016/S1471-4892(02)00176-5
11. Berndt N. Roles and regulation of serine/threonine-specific protein phosphatases in the cell cycle. *Prog Cell Cycle Res* (2003) 5:497–510.
12. Sim AT, Baldwin ML, Rostas JA, Holst J, Ludowyke RI. The role of serine/threonine protein phosphatases in exocytosis. *Biochem J* (2003) 373:641–59. doi:10.1042/bj20030484
13. Delorme V, Garcia A, Cayla X, Tardieux I. A role for *Toxoplasma gondii* type 1 ser/thr protein phosphatase in host cell invasion. *Microbes Infect* (2002) 4:271–8. doi:10.1016/S1286-4579(02)01538-1
14. Boag PR, Ren P, Newton SE, Gasser RB. Molecular characterisation of a male-specific serine/threonine phosphatase from *Oesophagostomum dentatum* (Nematoda: Strongylida), and functional analysis of homologues in *Caenorhabditis elegans*. *Int J Parasitol* (2003) 33:313–25. doi:10.1016/S0020-7519(02)00263-1
15. Hu M, Abs EL-Osta YG, Campbell BE, Boag PR, Nisbet AJ, Beveridge I, et al. *Trichostrongylus vitrinus* (Nematoda: Strongylida): molecular characterization and transcriptional analysis of Tv-stp-1, a serine/threonine phosphatase gene. *Exp Parasitol* (2007) 117:22–34. doi:10.1016/j.exppara.2007.03.008
16. Kutuzov MA, Andreeva AV. Protein Ser/Thr phosphatases of parasitic protozoa. *Mol Biochem Parasitol* (2008) 161:81–90. doi:10.1016/j.molbiopara.2008.06.008
17. Ma GX, Zhou RQ, Hu SJ, Huang HC, Zhu T, Xia QY. Molecular characterization and functional analysis of serine/threonine protein phosphatase of *Toxocara canis*. *Exp Parasitol* (2014) 141:55–61. doi:10.1016/j.exppara.2014.03.019
18. Campbell BE, Rabelo EM, Hofmann A, Hu M, Gasser RB. Characterization of a *Caenorhabditis elegans* glc seven-like phosphatase (gsp) orthologue from *Haemonchus contortus* (Nematoda). *Mol Cell Probes* (2010) 24:178–89. doi:10.1016/j.mcp.2010.02.001
19. Gadahi JA, Wang S, Bo G, Ehsan M, Yan R, Song X, et al. Proteomic analysis of the excretory and secretory proteins of *Haemonchus contortus* (HcESP) binding to goat PBMCs In vivo revealed stage-specific binding profiles. *PLoS One* (2016) 11:e0159796. doi:10.1371/journal.pone.0159796
20. Ehsan M, Gao W, Gadahi JA, Lu M, Liu X, Wang Y, et al. Arginine kinase from *Haemonchus contortus* decreased the proliferation and increased the apoptosis of goat PBMCs in vitro. *Parasit Vectors* (2017) 10:311. doi:10.1186/s13071-017-2244-z
21. Nicholson IC, Mavrangelos C, Fung K, Ayhan M, Levichkin I, Johnston A, et al. Characterisation of the protein composition of peripheral blood mononuclear cell microsomes by SDS-PAGE and mass spectrometry. *J Immunol Methods* (2005) 305:84–93. doi:10.1016/j.jim.2005.07.005
22. Yuan C, Zhang H, Wang W, Li Y, Yan R, Xu L, et al. Transmembrane protein 63A is a partner protein of *Haemonchus contortus* galectin in the regulation of goat peripheral blood mononuclear cells. *Parasit Vectors* (2015) 8:211. doi:10.1186/s13071-015-0816-3
23. Gadahi JA, Ehsan M, Wang S, Zhang Z, Wang Y, Yan R, et al. Recombinant protein of *Haemonchus contortus* 14-3-3 isoform 2 (rHcftt-2) decreased the production of IL-4 and suppressed the proliferation of goat PBMCs in vitro. *Exp Parasitol* (2016) 171:57–66. doi:10.1016/j.exppara.2016.10.014
24. Bradford MM. A rapid and sensitive method for the quantitation of microgram quantities of protein utilizing the principle of protein-dye binding. *Anal Biochem* (1976) 72:248–54. doi:10.1016/0003-2697(76)90527-3
25. Yi D, Xu L, Yan R, Li X. *Haemonchus contortus*: cloning and characterization of serpin. *Exp Parasitol* (2010) 125:363–70. doi:10.1016/j.exppara.2010.03.002
26. Livak KJ, Schmittgen TD. Analysis of relative gene expression data using real-time quantitative PCR and the 2(-Delta Delta C(T)) Method. *Methods* (2001) 25:402–8. doi:10.1006/meth.2001.1262
27. Kaleab B, Ottenoff T, Converse P, Halapi E, Tadesse G, Rottenberg M, et al. Mycobacterial-induced cytotoxic T cells as well as nonspecific killer cells derived from healthy individuals and leprosy patients. *Eur J Immunol* (1990) 20:2651–9. doi:10.1002/eji.1830201219
28. Wang W, Wang S, Zhang H, Yuan C, Yan R, Song X, et al. Galectin Hco-gal-m from *Haemonchus contortus* modulates goat monocytes and T cell function in different patterns. *Parasit Vectors* (2014) 7:342. doi:10.1186/1756-3305-7-342
29. Sun J, Zhang X, Broderick M, Fein H. Measurement of nitric oxide production in biological systems by using griess reaction assay. *Sensors* (2003) 3:276. doi:10.3390/s30800276
30. Shi Y. Serine/threonine phosphatases: mechanism through structure. *Cell* (2009) 139:468–84. doi:10.1016/j.cell.2009.10.006
31. García-Coiradas L, Angulo-Cubillán F, Méndez S, Larraga V, De La Fuente C, Cuquerella M, et al. Isolation and immunolocalization of a putative protective antigen (p26/23) from adult *Haemonchus contortus*. *Parasitol Res* (2008) 104:363. doi:10.1007/s00436-008-1204-0

32. Lejambre LF, Windon RG, Smith WD. Vaccination against *Haemonchus contortus*: performance of native parasite gut membrane glycoproteins in Merino lambs grazing contaminated pasture. *Vet Parasitol* (2008) 153:302–12. doi:10.1016/j.vetpar.2008.01.032
33. García-Coiradas L, Angulo-Cubillán F, Valladares B, Martínez E, De La Fuente C, Alunda JM, et al. Immunization against lamb haemonchosis with a recombinant somatic antigen of *Haemonchus contortus* (rHcp26/23). *Vet Med Int* (2010) 2010:8. doi:10.4061/2010/852146
34. Knox DP, Redmond DL, Skuce PJ, Newlands GFJ. The contribution of molecular biology to the development of vaccines against nematode and trematode parasites of domestic ruminants. *Vet Parasitol* (2001) 101:311–35. doi:10.1016/S0304-4017(01)00558-1
35. Knox DP, Smith WD. Vaccination against gastrointestinal nematode parasites of ruminants using gut-expressed antigens. *Vet Parasitol* (2001) 100:21–32. doi:10.1016/S0304-4017(01)00480-0
36. Ceulemans H, Bollen M. Functional diversity of protein phosphatase-1, a cellular economizer and reset button. *Physiol Rev* (2004) 84:1–39. doi:10.1152/physrev.00013.2003
37. Sun Y, Yan R, Muleke CI, Zhao G, Xu L, Li X. Recombinant galectins of *Haemonchus contortus* parasite induces apoptosis in the peripheral blood lymphocytes of goat. *Int J Pept Res Ther* (2007) 13:387–92. doi:10.1007/s10989-006-9045-0
38. Li BW, Rush AC, Crosby SD, Warren WC, Williams SA, Mitreva M, et al. Profiling of gender-regulated gene transcripts in the filarial nematode Brugia malayi by cDNA oligonucleotide array analysis. *Mol Biochem Parasitol* (2005) 143:49–57. doi:10.1016/j.molbiopara.2005.05.005
39. Ingebritsen TS, Cohen P. The protein phosphatases involved in cellular regulation. 1. Classification and substrate specificities. *Eur J Biochem* (1983) 132:255–61. doi:10.1111/j.1432-1033.1983.tb07357.x
40. Smith GD, Wolf DP, Trautman KC, Da Cruz E, Silva EF, Greengard P, et al. Primate sperm contain protein phosphatase 1, a biochemical mediator of motility. *Biol Reprod* (1996) 54:719–27. doi:10.1095/biolreprod54.3.719
41. Grencis RK. Cytokine regulation of resistance and susceptibility to intestinal nematode infection – from host to parasite. *Vet Parasitol* (2001) 100:45–50. doi:10.1016/S0304-4017(01)00482-4
42. Shakya KP, Miller JE, Horohov DW. A Th2 type of immune response is associated with increased resistance to *Haemonchus contortus* in naturally infected Gulf coast native lambs. *Vet Parasitol* (2009) 163:57–66. doi:10.1016/j.vetpar.2009.03.052
43. Schallig HD. Immunological responses of sheep to *Haemonchus contortus*. *Parasitology* (2000) 120(Suppl):S63–72. doi:10.1017/S003118209900579X
44. Taylor A, Verhagen J, Blaser K, Akdis M, Akdis CA. Mechanisms of immune suppression by interleukin-10 and transforming growth factor-beta: the role of T regulatory cells. *Immunology* (2006) 117:433–42. doi:10.1111/j.1365-2567.2006.02321.x
45. Grencis RK, Humphreys NE, Bancroft AJ. Immunity to gastrointestinal nematodes: mechanisms and myths. *Immunol Rev* (2014) 260:183–205. doi:10.1111/imr.12188
46. Larkin BM, Smith PM, Ponichtera HE, Shainheit MG, Rutitzky LI, Stadecker MJ. Induction and regulation of pathogenic Th17 cell responses in schistosomiasis. *Semin Immunopathol* (2012) 34:873–88. doi:10.1007/s00281-012-0341-9
47. Song X, Gao H, Qian Y. Th17 differentiation and their pro-inflammation function. *Adv Exp Med Biol* (2014) 841:99–151. doi:10.1007/978-94-017-9487-9_5
48. Katawa G, Layland LE, Debrah AY, Von Horn C, Batsa L, Kwarteng A, et al. Hyperreactive onchocerciasis is characterized by a combination of Th17-Th2 immune responses and reduced regulatory T cells. *PLoS Negl Trop Dis* (2015) 9:e3414. doi:10.1371/journal.pntd.0003414
49. Wen X, He L, Chi Y, Zhou S, Hoellwarth J, Zhang C, et al. Dynamics of Th17 cells and their role in *Schistosoma japonicum* infection in C57BL/6 Mice. *PLoS Negl Trop Dis* (2011) 5:e1399. doi:10.1371/journal.pntd.0001399
50. Li MO, Wan YY, Sanjabi S, Robertson AK, Flavell RA. Transforming growth factor-beta regulation of immune responses. *Annu Rev Immunol* (2006) 24:99–146. doi:10.1146/annurev.immunol.24.021605.090737
51. Lebman DA, Edmiston JS. The role of TGF-beta in growth, differentiation, and maturation of B lymphocytes. *Microbes Infect* (1999) 1:1297–304. doi:10.1016/S1286-4579(99)00254-3
52. Keskinen P, Ronni T, Matikainen S, Lehtonen A, Julkunen I. Regulation of HLA class I and II expression by interferons and influenza A virus in human peripheral blood mononuclear cells. *Immunology* (1997) 91:421–9. doi:10.1046/j.1365-2567.1997.00258.x
53. Lüder CGK, Lang T, Beuerle B, Gross U. Down-regulation of MHC class II molecules and inability to up-regulate class I molecules in murine macrophages after infection with *Toxoplasma gondii*. *Clin Exp Immunol* (1998) 112:308–16. doi:10.1046/j.1365-2249.1998.00594.x
54. Panek RB, Benveniste EN. Class II MHC gene expression in microglia. Regulation by the cytokines IFN-gamma, TNF-alpha, and TGF-beta. *J Immunol* (1995) 154:2846–54.
55. Tountas NA, Brautigan DL. Migration and retraction of endothelial and epithelial cells require PHI-1, a specific protein-phosphatase-1 inhibitor protein. *J Cell Sci* (2004) 117:5905–12. doi:10.1242/jcs.01506
56. Mcgovern KE, Wilson EH. Role of chemokines and trafficking of immune cells in parasitic infections. *Curr Immunol Rev* (2013) 9:157–68. doi:10.2174/1573395509666131217000000
57. Sun H, Wang Y. Novel Ser/Thr protein phosphatases in cell death regulation. *Physiology (Bethesda)* (2012) 27:43–52. doi:10.1152/physiol.00034.2011
58. Liu Q, Wilkins BJ, Lee YJ, Ichijo H, Molkentin JD. Direct interaction and reciprocal regulation between ASK1 and calcineurin-NFAT control cardiomyocyte death and growth. *Mol Cell Biol* (2006) 26:3785–97. doi:10.1128/MCB.26.10.3785-3797.2006
59. Cohen PT, Philp A, Vazquez-Martin C. Protein phosphatase 4 – from obscurity to vital functions. *FEBS Lett* (2005) 579:3278–86. doi:10.1016/j.febslet.2005.04.070
60. Festjens N, Vanden Berghe T, Cornelis S, Vandenabeele P. RIP1, a kinase on the crossroads of a cell's decision to live or die. *Cell Death Differ* (2007) 14:400–10. doi:10.1038/sj.cdd.4402085
61. Huang H-S, Lee EYC. Protein phosphatase-1 inhibitor-3 is an in vivo target of caspase-3 and participates in the apoptotic response. *J Biol Chem* (2008) 283:18135–46. doi:10.1074/jbc.M709735200
62. Kang Y, Lee JH, Hoan NN, Sohn HM, Chang IY, You HJ. Protein phosphatase 5 regulates the function of 53BP1 after neocarzinostatin-induced DNA damage. *J Biol Chem* (2009) 284:9845–53. doi:10.1074/jbc.M809272200
63. Loke PN, Macdonald AS, Robb A, Maizels RM, Allen JE. Alternatively activated macrophages induced by nematode infection inhibit proliferation via cell-to-cell contact. *Eur J Immunol* (2000) 30:2669–78. doi:10.1002/1521-4141(200009)30:9<2669::AID-IMMU2669>3.0.CO;2-1
64. Kotze AC, Mcclure SJ. *Haemonchus contortus* utilises catalase in defence against exogenous hydrogen peroxide in vitro. *Int J Parasitol* (2001) 31:1563–71. doi:10.1016/S0020-7519(01)00303-4
65. Wandurska-Nowak E. [The role of nitric oxide (NO) in parasitic infections]. *Wiad Parazytol* (2004) 50:665–78.
66. Dong Z, Yang X, Xie K, Juang SH, Llansa N, Fidler IJ. Activation of inducible nitric oxide synthase gene in murine macrophages requires protein phosphatases 1 and 2A activities. *J Leukoc Biol* (1995) 58:725–32. doi:10.1002/jlb.58.6.725
67. Taylor BS, Liu S, Villavicencio RT, Ganster RW, Geller DA. The role of protein phosphatases in the expression of inducible nitric oxide synthase in the rat hepatocyte. *Hepatology* (1999) 29:1199–207. doi:10.1002/hep.510290419
68. Gazzinelli RT, Oswald IP, James SL, Sher A. IL-10 inhibits parasite killing and nitrogen oxide production by IFN-gamma-activated macrophages. *J Immunol* (1992) 148:1792–6.
69. Gadahi JA, Yongqian B, Ehsan M, Zhang ZC, Wang S, Yan RF, et al. *Haemonchus contortus* excretory and secretory proteins (HcESPs) suppress functions of goat PBMCs in vitro. *Oncotarget* (2016) 7:35670–9. doi:10.18632/oncotarget.13487

11

A Lactate Fermentation Mutant of *Toxoplasma* Stimulates Protective Immunity Against Acute and Chronic Toxoplaomosis

Ningbo Xia[1], Taifang Zhou[1], Xiaohan Liang[1], Shu Ye[1], Pengfei Zhao[1], Jichao Yang[1], Yanqin Zhou[1], Junlong Zhao[1,2,3] and Bang Shen[1,3]*

[1] State Key Laboratory of Agricultural Microbiology, Huazhong Agricultural University, Wuhan, China, [2] Hubei Cooperative Innovation Center for Sustainable Pig Production, Wuhan, China, [3] Key Laboratory of Preventive Medicine in Hubei Province, Wuhan, China

***Correspondence:**
Bang Shen
shenbang@mail.hzau.edu.cn

Toxoplasma gondii is an important zoonotic pathogen infecting one-third of the world's population and numerous animals, causing significant healthcare burden and socioeconomic problems. Vaccination is an efficient way to reduce global sero-prevalence, however, ideal vaccines are not yet available. We recently discovered that the *Toxoplasma* mutant lacking both lactate dehydrogenases *LDH1* and *LDH2* (*Δldh*) grew well *in vitro* but was unable to propagate in mice, making it a good live vaccine candidate. Here, we tested the protection efficacy of ME49 *Δldh* using a mouse model. Vaccinated mice were efficiently protected from the lethal challenge of a variety of wild-type strains, including type 1 strain RH, type 2 strain ME49, type 3 strain VEG, and a field isolate of Chinese 1. The protection efficacies of a single vaccination were nearly 100% for most cases and it worked well against the challenges of both tachyzoites and tissue cysts. Re-challenging parasites were unable to propagate in vaccinated mice, nor did they make tissue cysts. High levels of *Toxoplasma*-specific IgG were produced 30 days after immunization and stayed high during the whole tests (at least 125 days). However, passive immunization of naïve mice with sera from vaccinated mice did reduce parasite propagation, but the overall protection against parasite infections was rather limited. On the other hand, *Δldh* immunization evoked elevated levels of Th1 cytokines like INF-γ and IL-12, at early time points. In addition, splenocytes extracted from immunized mice were able to induce quick and robust INF-γ and other pro-inflammatory cytokine production upon *T. gondii* antigen stimulation. Together these results suggest that cellular immune responses are the main contributors to the protective immunity elicited by *Δldh* vaccination, and humoral immunity also contributes partially. We also generated uracil auxotrophic mutants in ME49 and compared their immune protection efficiencies to the *Δldh* mutants. The results showed that these two types of mutants have similar properties as live vaccine candidates. Taken together, these results suggest that mutants lacking LDH were severely attenuated in virulence but were able to induce strong anti-toxoplasma immune responses, therefore are good candidates for live vaccines.

Keywords: *Toxoplasma*, lactate dehydrogenase, live vaccine, toxoplasmosis, cellular immunity

INTRODUCTION

Toxoplasma gondii is an obligate intracellular parasite that infects all warm-blooded animals and humans (1). Generally, its infection in healthy people causes no or mild flu-like symptoms, thus most of the infections are not noticed. However, in susceptible pregnant women, *T. gondii* infection may have severe consequences such as abortion, neonatal death, congenital defects, and mental retardation of delivered babies (2, 3). In addition, it is also a high risk for individuals with compromised immune functions, such as AIDS and organ transplant patients (2). Due to the broad host range, a variety of agricultural important animals such as pigs and sheep are constantly challenged by *T. gondii*, causing substantial economic losses and public health problems (2, 4, 5). Folic acid metabolism inhibitors such as pyrimethamine and sulfadiazine are commonly used to treat toxoplasmosis but they do not work on chronic infections (6).

The control of *Toxoplasma* infection is rather difficult, one reason is that it has complex life cycle and multiple routes of transmission (7, 8). Cats are the definitive hosts of *T. gondii* and the oocysts shed by cats are thought to be a key source of human and animal infections (9). In addition, *T. gondii* can be transmitted between intermediate hosts through predation. Most of the *Toxoplasma* infection cases belong to chronic infection, where the parasites are encysted in muscles and central nerve system (called tissue cysts) of infected animals lifelong (7). Ingestion of raw or undercooked meat from such animals represents another important route of transmitting the parasites to humans and animals (2, 5). As mentioned above, encysted parasites at the chronic infection stage are resistant to most of the current therapeutics. Another challenge to the control of toxoplasmosis is the complex population structure of *T. gondii* strains. North America and Europe are dominated by three clonal strains (type I, II, and III), which display different acute virulence in mice (10, 11). However, in other parts of the world, the strains are much more diverse, particularly in South America (12, 13). A recent study demonstrated that genetically distinct strains may be able to superinfect the same host, indicating the lack of sufficient cross protection from immunization with one single strain (14). This study had important highlights for the design of *Toxoplasma* vaccines, particularly whole parasite-based vaccines.

Scientists have done tremendous amount of work to pursue an ideal vaccine against *T. gondii*. The first generation of vaccines contained killed parasites, or native antigens derived from soluble or secretory proteins of cultured tachyzoites. These vaccines only provided limited protection against further infections (15, 16). Then when the recombinant DNA technology became available, a variety of subunit vaccines were tried, mainly using surface or secretory proteins such as SAG1 and MIC2 (17–20). These recombinant protein or vector-based subunit vaccines were safer and easier to make than native antigen-based vaccines, however, they did not provide sufficient protection either [reviewed in Ref. (21, 22)]. The strategy that holds the most promise for a good *Toxoplasma* vaccine seems to be live attenuated vaccines. Currently there is one commercial vaccine (Toxovax®) available, which is derived from the S48 strain originally isolated from an aborted lamb and licensed for use to avoid congenital toxoplasmosis in ewes (23). The exact mechanisms of Toxovax® as a vaccine are not well understood, but thought to be linked to its inability to form cysts or oocysts to complete the life cycle (24). Tachyzoites can be cleared efficiently by hosts' immunity, therefore mutants defective in cyst formation have the potential to be vaccines. Encouraged by the success of Toxovax® and to design safer live vaccines, scientists turned to genetically modified parasites. Among these, uracil auxotroph mutants defective in *de novo* UMP (uridine 5′-monophosphate) synthesis are promising (25–27). Mutants with inactivated *CPSII* or *OMPDC* grew well *in vitro* in the presence of extra uracil (25–27), but were unable to establish acute infection in animals, therefore were severely attenuated. These mutants were extensively studied in mice and displayed great potential to be good vaccines, but still need to be tested in other animals like pigs, sheep, and cats.

We recently discovered that *T. gondii* mutants with both lactate dehydrogenase genes deleted (*Δldh*) grew robustly *in vitro* but failed to propagate *in vivo* (28), very similar to the uracil auxotroph mutants. The reason for this growth difference is that, under *in vivo* conditions when oxygen is limited, lactate fermentation becomes a key energy supply pathway to support parasite replication. By contrast, oxidative phosphorylation alone provides enough energy for parasite reproduction *in vitro* when oxygen is rich. As such, *Δldh* mutant was greatly attenuated *in vivo*, even in immune-deficient animals (28). In this study, we set to analyze the protective immunity of the *Δldh* mutant as a vaccine using the mouse model. The results showed that vaccination of mice with tachyzoites of this mutant induced efficient protection against the challenge of a variety of strains.

RESULTS

Tissue Cysts Derived From ME49 *Δldh* Were Severely Attenuated in Mice

Our previous study reported that the virulence of ME49 *Δldh* tachyzoites was significantly (>640-fold) reduced compared to that of the wild-type (WT) strain ME49, no mortality was detected even at the infection dose of 3.2×10^4 tachyzoites/mouse (28). However, we did observe that many of the *Δldh* tachyzoites infected mice formed brain cysts, although the amount was much less than that of WT parasites infected mice. To see whether the residual amount of cysts in *Δldh* infected mice have normal virulence, 50 cysts derived from WT or *Δldh* parasites were used to infect ICR mice by oral administration, and the survival of infected mice was monitored for 40 days. The results showed that 50 cysts of ME49 killed 80% of the mice. However, none of the *Δldh* cyst infected mice died (**Figure 1**), nor did they show any obvious clinical symptoms, suggesting that the virulence of the *Δldh* cysts was also significantly attenuated, just like the tachyzoites of this strain.

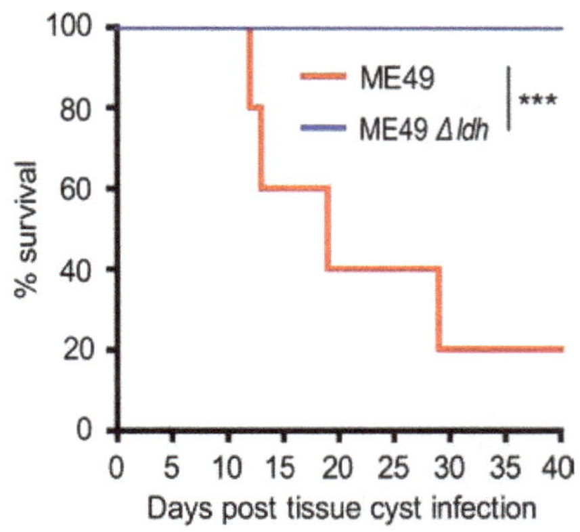

FIGURE 1 | Virulence tests of *Toxoplasma* cysts in mice. ICR mice were infected with brain cysts of ME49 or ME49 *Δldh* (50 cysts/mouse, $n = 5$ mice for ME49 strain and $n = 7$ mice for ME49 *Δldh* strain) by oral administration and their survival was monitored for 40 days. ***$p < 0.001$, Gehan–Breslow–Wilcoxon test.

Δldh Vaccination Elicited Strong Protective Immunity Against Tachyzoites Infection

The *Δldh* mutant grew robustly *in vitro* but was unable to propagate *in vivo*, this unique property makes it a good vaccine candidate (28). To check this possibility and assess the immune protection offered by *Δldh* vaccination, ICR mice were first immunized with ME49 *Δldh* by intraperitoneal injection (10^4 tachyzoites/mouse). Thirty days later, they were challenged with 10^4 tachyzoites of the type 2 strain ME49, type 3 strain VEG, or Chinese 1 strain C7719. Subsequently survival of the mice was monitored for another 30 days. The mortality rates for non-immunized mice were 100% upon the infection of ME49 and C7719, whereas VEG caused 90% mortality. However, for *Δldh*-vaccinated mice, the survival rates were 100% upon the challenge of all three strains and no obvious symptoms were observed during the 30-day infection period (**Figures 2A–C**). These results indicate that *Δldh* vaccination is able to offer efficient protection against lethal parasite infections.

The above results showed that 30 days post *Δldh* vaccination, mice were well protected. To see whether *Δldh* vaccination provides longer time protective immunity, mice were vaccinated with ME49 *Δldh* and 75 days later, they were challenged with type 1 strain RH *Δhxgprt*, type 2 strain ME49, or Chinese 1 strain C7719. The survival rates of immunized mice that were re-infected with ME49 or C7719 were 100% (**Figures 2E,F**), similar to the above infections 30 days post-vaccination. However, if challenged with the most virulent type 1 strain RH *Δhxgprt*, only 60% of the immunized mice survived (**Figure 2D**). As will be discussed below, the protection against RH infection was also 100% if the challenge occurred 20 days after immunization. To examine the efficiency of even longer time protection, ME49 *Δldh* vaccinated mice were challenged with WT parasites 125 days post-vaccination. The results showed that the immune protection against ME49 and VEG challenge was still 100% (**Figures 2G,H**). Together, these results suggest that ME49 *Δldh* immunization can provide both short- and long-term protection against strains with intermediate virulence, but the protection against strongly virulent strains is limited to a short time after vaccination and then decreased gradually.

Δldh Immunization Stimulated Protective Immunity Against Bradyzoites Infection

A significant portion of *T. gondii* infections were acquired through ingestion of tissue cysts that contain bradyzoites. In order to check whether *Δldh* vaccination provided protection against bradyzoites infection, ICR mice were first immunized with 10^4 tachyzoites of ME49 *Δldh*. Thirty days after immunization, they were orally challenged with 50 cysts of the ME49 strain. The results show that 100% of *Δldh*-immunized mice survived the cyst challenging, whereas all naïve mice died of this infection (**Figure 3**). These results suggest that *Δldh* strain also elicited protective immunity against bradyzoite infection.

Δldh Immunization Blocked Cyst Formation From New Infections

One caveat of chemotherapies against acute toxoplasmosis is that the drugs may drive the parasites to slowly replicating bradyzoites to form tissue cysts, which lead to lifelong chronic infection. To examine whether the *Δldh* mutant vaccination could provide protective immunity against chronic *T. gondii* infection, the cyst forming competent but less virulent (compared with ME49) strain TgPIG-WH1 (genotyped as ToxoDB #3) was used to challenge the vaccinated ICR mice. As shown in **Figure 4A**, at the infection dose of 10^4 tachyzoites/mouse through intraperitoneal injection, TgPIG-WH1 killed only 10% of the non-immunized mice, consistent with its reduced virulence. Thirty days post TgPIG-WH1 challenge, survived mice were sacrificed and the numbers of tissue cysts in the brains were determined by DBA-FITC staining, and compared to that of vaccinated but not re-challenged, as well as non-immunized but TgPIG-WH1 infected mice. The results in **Figure 4B** showed that infection of naïve mice by TgPIG-WH1 resulted in about 500 cysts per brain on average. However, cyst number in *Δldh* immunized and subsequently TgPIG-WH1 infected mice was reduced to around 100, which was very similar to that of vaccinated but not re-challenged mice, suggesting that they were probably derived from vaccination but not TgPIG-WH1 infection. Together, these results indicate that *Δldh* immunization also provides protective immunity against chronic toxoplasmosis.

Δldh Vaccinated Mice Were Able to Clear Challenging Parasites Rapidly

The above results demonstrated that vaccinating mice with ME49 *Δldh* provided efficient protection against both acute and chronic toxoplasmosis. To further examine the fate of challenging parasites, the propagation dynamics of a luciferase expressing strain RH-Luc in vaccinated mice were determined by bioluminescent imaging. In naïve mice, RH-Luc infection resulted in rapid replication of the parasites. At the infection dose of 10^4 tachyzoites/mouse, luminescent signals were detectable just 1 day after infection and increased over 1,000-fold 5 days post-infection

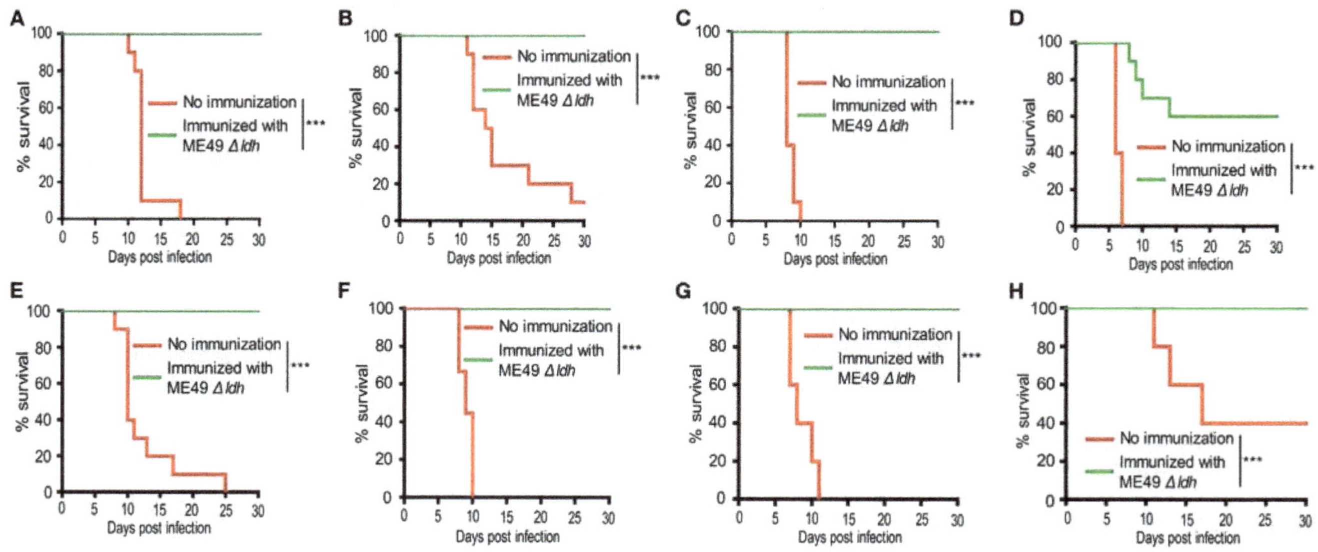

FIGURE 2 | *Δldh* parasite immunization protected mice from *Toxoplasma gondii* tachyzoites infection. ICR mice were pre-immunized with 10^4 tachyzoites of the ME49 *Δldh* mutant. **(A–C)** 30 days post-immunization, they were challenged with 10^4 tachyzoites of the ME49 **(A)**, VEG **(B)**, or C7719 **(C)** strains (10 mice for each strain) by intraperitoneal injection and their survival was monitored for another 30 days. **(D–F)** 75 days post-immunization, 10^4 tachyzoites of the RH *Δhxgprt* **(D)**, ME49 **(E)**, C7719 **(F)** strains were used to challenge the mice and their survival was monitored for another 30 days. **(G,H)** 125 days post-immunization, 10^4 tachyzoites of the ME49 **(G)**, VEG **(H)** strains were used to challenge the mice and their survival was monitored for another 30 days. Non-immunized mice were included as control. $^{***}p < 0.001$, Gehan–Breslow–Wilcoxon tests.

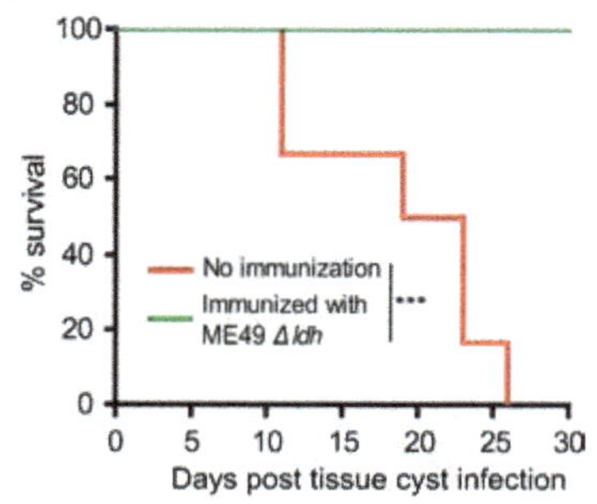

FIGURE 3 | *Δldh* mutant vaccination protected mice from *Toxoplasma gondii* cysts infection. ICR mice were pre-immunized with ME49 *Δldh* as in **Figure 2**, 30 days post-immunization they were challenged with 50 fresh brain cysts of the ME49 strain and their survival was monitored for another 30 days ($n = 10$ mice for each strain). Non-immunized mice were included as control. $^{***}p < 0.001$, Gehan–Breslow–Wilcoxon test.

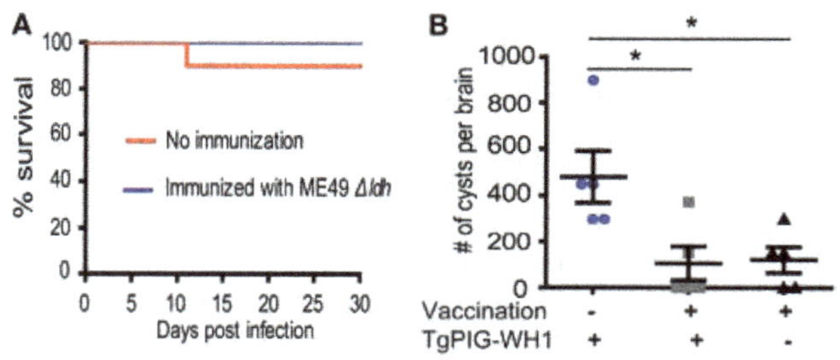

FIGURE 4 | *Δldh* mutant immunization prevented cyst formation from further infections. **(A)** ICR mice were pre-immunized with ME49 *Δldh* as in **Figure 2** and 30 days later challenged with 10^4 tachyzoites of TgPIG-WH1. Non-immunized mice were included as control and survival of mice were monitored for another 30 days ($n = 10$ mice for each strain). **(B)** Cyst loads in the brains of non-immunized but TgPIG-WH1 challenged mice, immunized and TgPIG-WH1 challenged mice, and *Δldh* immunized but not TgPIG-WH1 challenged mice [not shown in **(A)**]. The mice survived at day 30 in **(A)** were sacrificed, and the number of *Toxoplasma* cysts in the brain homogenate was determined by DBA-FITC staining and fluorescent microscopy. Data from the analysis of five mice in each group were graphed, $^{*}p < 0.05$, Student's *t*-test.

(**Figures 5A,B**). However, in the vaccinated mice, luminescent signals were not detectable at both time points, indicating little propagation and probably rapid clearance of the challenging RH-Luc (**Figures 5A,B**). It should be noted that in this experiment, RH-Luc infection was performed 30 days after *Δldh* immunization. We also followed the survival of these RH-Luc infected mice for 20 days, all naïve mice died within 8 days but all vaccinated mice survived with no symptoms (**Figure 5C**). These results suggest that, at least within a limited time period, *Δldh* immunization enables rapid clearance of the challenging parasites, which explains its efficient immune protection.

Δldh Vaccination Significantly Increased the Levels of Pro-Inflammatory Cytokines and *T. gondii* Specific IgG Antibodies

To estimate the potential mechanisms of immune protection offered by *Δldh* vaccination, we first examined the cytokine level changes upon vaccination. Sera samples obtained from vaccinated mice 30, 75, or 125 days post-vaccination were subject to ELISA analysis to check the levels of IFN-γ, IL-12,

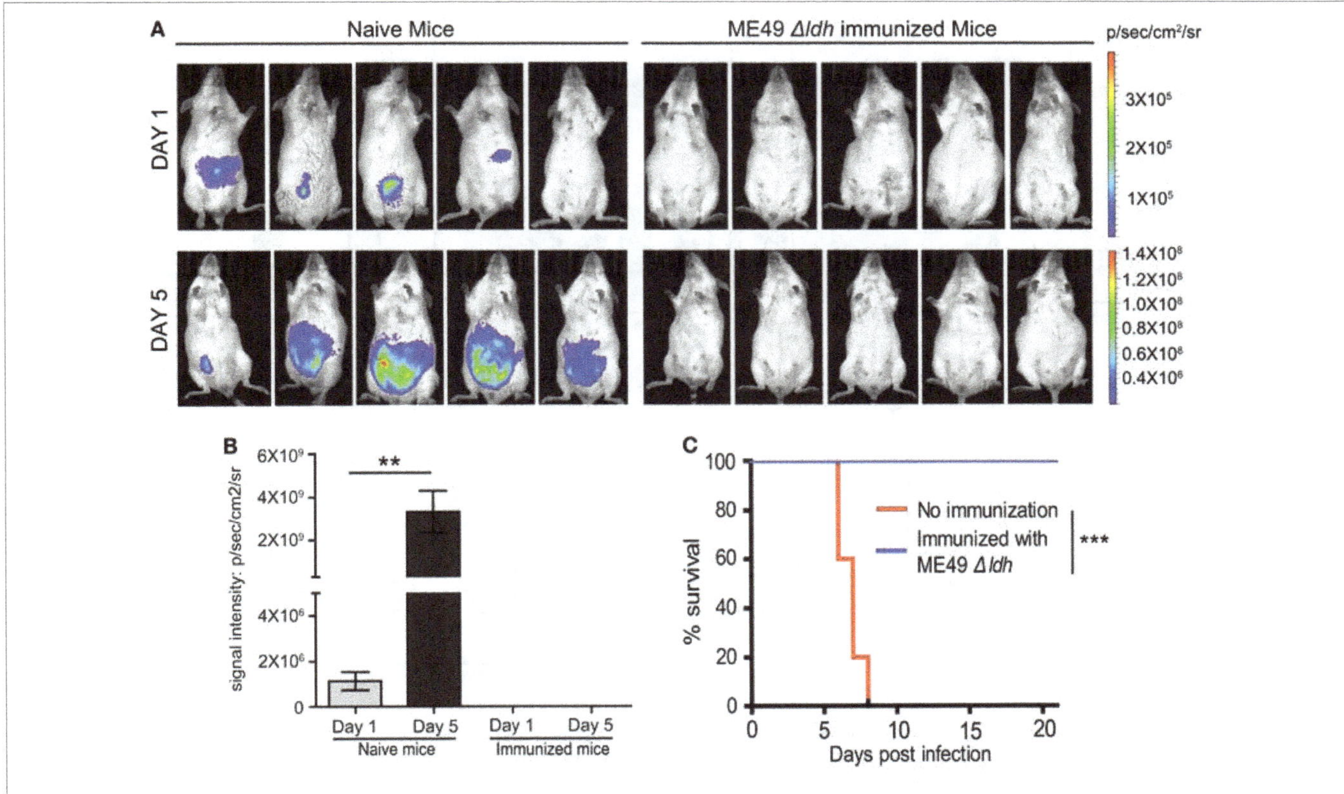

FIGURE 5 | *Δldh* parasite vaccination elicited rapid clearance of challenging parasites. **(A)** Naïve or pre-immunized mice were challenged with 10^4 tachyzoites of RH-Luc (five mice for each group). Parasite loads in mice 1 and 5 days post RH-Luc infection were analyzed by live animal imaging on the IVIS Spectra system. p/sec/cm²/sr: photons per second per cm² per steradian. **(B)** Total bioluminescent signals of mice from **(A)** were calculated and graphed, $^{**}p < 0.01$, Student's *t*-test. **(C)** Survival curves of naïve or *Δldh* immunized mice infected with RH-Luc, $^{***}p < 0.001$, Gehan–Breslow–Wilcoxon test.

IL-10, and TNF-α. The IL-12–IFN-γ axis is key to activate cellular immune clearance of *T. gondii*. Their levels, as well as the levels of another pro-inflammatory cytokine TNF-α, increased significantly both 30 and 75 days post-vaccination, compared to control mice (**Figures 6A–C**). However, the levels at day 75 were lower than that at day 30, which was likely caused by the activation of anti-inflammatory response, as evidenced by high levels of IL-10 in vaccinated mice 30 days post-infection (**Figure 6D**). At 125 days post-infection, the levels of all cytokines were back to normal as in naïve mice (**Figures 6A–D**). We also measured the *T. gondii* specific IgG levels and found that ME49 *Δldh* vaccination induced high levels of IgG 30, 75, and 125 days post-immunization (**Figure 6E**). Although it looked like there was an increase in *T. gondii* specific IgG levels over time, the differences were not statistically significant (**Figure 6E**). The relatively stable levels of parasite-specific IgG were in contrast to the changes of cytokine levels. These results, along with the above-described short- and long-term protective immunity (**Figure 2**), suggest that *Δldh* immunization probably stimulated both humoral and cell-mediated immune responses to control secondary infections.

Passive Immunization With the Sera of *Δldh*-Vaccinated Mice Provided Partial Protection Against *T. gondii* Infection

Above results demonstrated that high levels of *T. gondii* specific IgG were produced in *Δldh*-vaccinated mice. To estimate the contribution of such antisera in restricting further parasite infection, naïve mice were infected with the WT strain ME49 through intraperitoneal injection. At day 0 and day 3 after infection, sera from the ME49 *Δldh*-vaccinated mice were collected 160 days post-immunization and administered into infected mice by tail vein injection. The protection of passive immunization was estimated in two ways, parasite burden and mice survival. One week post-infection, parasite burden in peritoneal fluid was determined by quantitative PCR. The results showed that passive immunization with the sera of *Δldh*-vaccinated mice did result in significantly lower level of parasite burden compared to immunization with sera of naïve mice (**Figure 7A**). However, when the survival of mice were followed, passively immunized mice only survived for two more days, compared with the negative immunization control (**Figure 7B**). Together these results suggested that the sera of *Δldh*-vaccinated mice are able to reduce parasite propagation to some degree but do not offer full protection against lethal infections.

Robust Pro-Inflammatory Cytokine Production by Splenocytes of *Δldh*-Vaccinated Mice Upon *T. gondii* Antigen Stimulation

The above passive immunization results suggested that the contribution of humoral immunity to the protection of *Δldh*

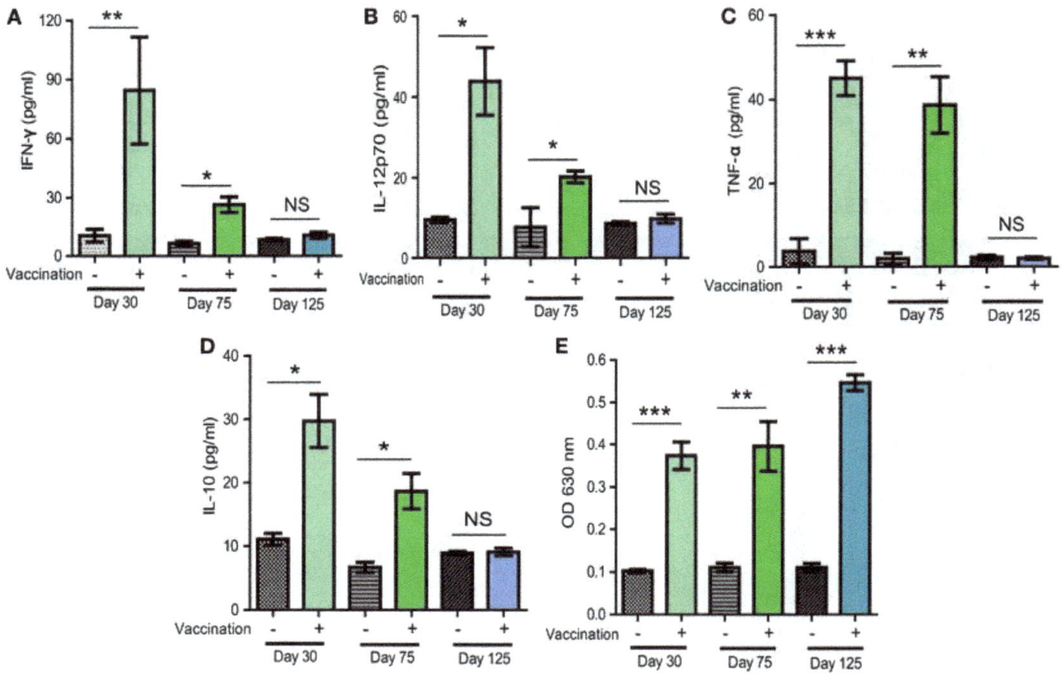

FIGURE 6 | Levels of selected cytokines and *Toxoplasma* specific IgG in sera of mice 30, 75, and 125 days after *Δldh* immunization. **(A–D)** Levels of indicated cytokines measured by ELISA. **(E)** Relative levels of *Toxoplasma* specific IgG, as determined by indirect ELISA. Sera from naïve mice were used as controls and three mice from each group were analyzed. $^{*}p < 0.05$, $^{**}p < 0.01$, $^{***}p < 0.001$, NS: not significant, Student's *t*-test.

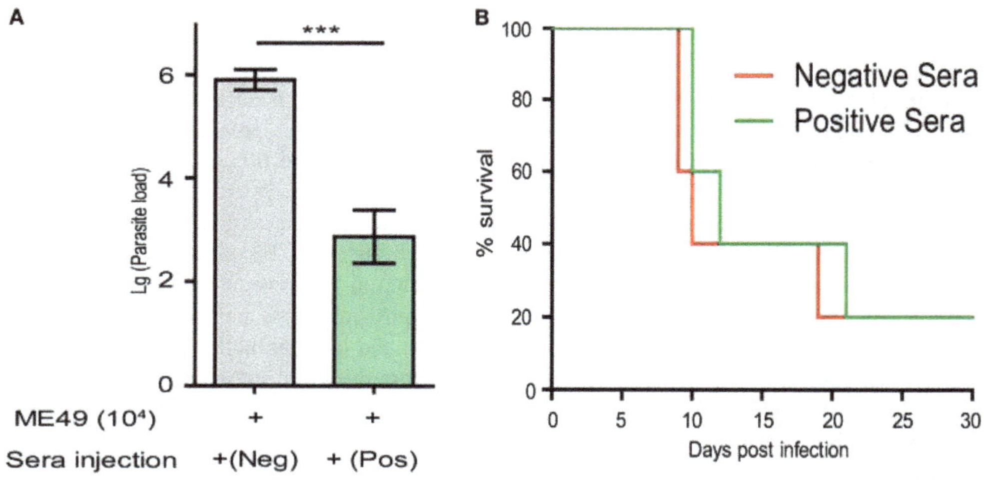

FIGURE 7 | Passive immunization using the sera from *Δldh*-vaccinated mice provided partial protection against parasite infection. **(A)** ICR mice ($n = 3$ for each group) were injected with 10^4 tachyzoites of ME49 by intraperitoneal injection. At day 0 and day 3 post-infection, mice were treated with positive sera collected from the ME49 *Δldh*-vaccinated mice (160 days post-vaccination), or negative serum from naïve mice by tail intravenous injection. Parasite loads in peritoneal fluids 7 days post-infection were estimated by quantitative PCR. $^{***}p < 0.0001$, Student's *t*-test. **(B)** Survival of passively immunized mice.

vaccination is limited. Next, we estimated cell-mediated immunity, as well as the antigen-specific memory responses by checking the antigen recall response in vaccinated mice. To do that, splenocytes from ME49 *Δldh* immunized mice were harvested 160 days post-vaccination, a time point when the cytokine levels in immunized mice was indistinguishable from that of naïve mice. These splenocytes were cultured *in vitro* and stimulated with total soluble Toxoplasma antigen (TSA) prepared from ME49 tachyzoites. Subsequently the supernatants from the cultures were collected to estimate the cytokine levels by ELISA. Compared with the no-stimulation or non-vaccinated splenocyte controls, TSA stimulated high levels of pro-inflammatory cytokines INF-γ and TNF-α (**Figures 8A,B**). Induction of IL-12 production was not as obvious (**Figure 8C**). Given that INF-γ is the key activator of

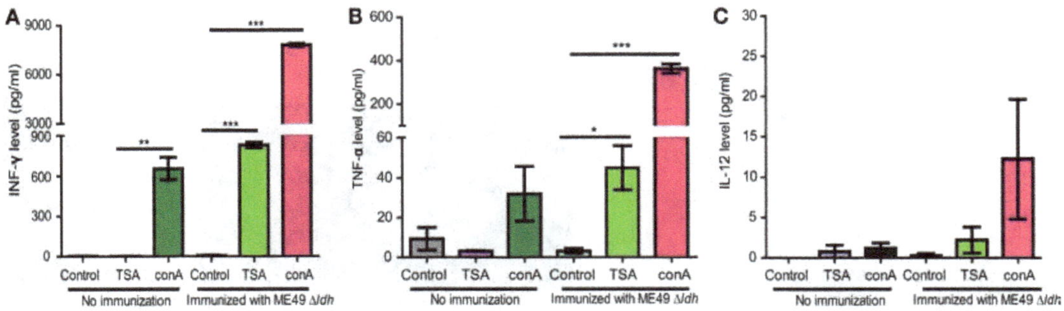

FIGURE 8 | Cytokine production by splenocytes of ME49 *Δldh*-vaccinated mice after *Toxoplasma* antigen stimulation. ICR mice were vaccinated with 10^3 tachyzoites of ME49 *Δldh* and splenocytes were harvested 160 days post-vaccination. The *in vitro* cultured splenocytes were then treated with fetal bovine serum (control), total soluble Toxoplasma antigen (TSA) or Concanavalin A (conA, positive control) for 72 h. Subsequently the levels of IFN-γ **(A)**, TNF-α **(B)** and IL-12 **(C)** in the culture supernatants were measured by ELISA. Splenocytes isolated from non-immunized naïve mice were included as controls. Three mice from each group were analyzed and each treatment condition was repeated three times, $^*p < 0.05$, $^{**}p < 0.01$, $^{***}p < 0.0001$, Student's *t*-test.

cell-mediated immunity for *T. gondii* clearance, quick and robust INF-γ production from vaccinated splenocytes upon TSA stimulation suggests that efficient cellular immune responses would be activated during secondary infections.

Compare the Protection Efficiency of *Δldh*-Based Vaccines to That of Uracil Auxotrophic Mutants

Mutants defective in *de novo* pyrimidine biosynthesis are auxotrophic to uracil, therefore they are not replicating and avirulent *in vivo* (25–27). As such, those types of mutants (such as *CPSII* and *OMPDC* deficient strains) were considered great vaccine candidates. We sought to compare the protection efficiency of our *Δldh*-based vaccines to that based on uracil auxotrophic mutants. For this purpose, we first made an *OMPDC* deletion mutant in ME49, by CRISPR/Cas9-mediated gene replacement to replace *OMPDC* by loxP sites flanked *DHFR** (**Figure 9A**). The resulted ME49 *ompdc:DHFR** (**Figure 9B**) was then transiently transfected with a Cre recombinase expressing plasmid to remove the selection marker *DHFR**, to obtain ME49 *Δompdc* (**Figure 9C**). We also generated a double knockout line (ME49 *Δompdc Δldh1*) by disrupting *LDH1* in ME49 *Δompdc* (**Figures 9D,E**).

First, the virulence of these mutants were compared in mice. With the infection dose of 10^4 tachyzoites per mouse, ME49 killed all mice within 12 days. All mice infected with *Δompdc*, *Δompdc Δldh1*, or *Δldh* mutants were survived (**Figure 10A**), indicating significant virulence attenuation of these mutants. To further check the ability of these mutants to propagate *in vivo*, mice were infected with each mutant line (10^4 tachyzoites/mouse) and a week later, the parasite burden in peritoneal fluid was examined by qPCR. ME49 displayed robust replication and high parasite burden was detected in mice with this strain (**Figure 10B**). All three mutants showed minimal replication in mice, as the parasite burden in the corresponding mutants were very low, close to (*Δldh*) or below (*Δompdc*, *Δompdc Δldh1*) the reliable detection limit of qPCR (**Figure 10B**). It seemed like there were more parasites in *Δldh*-infected mice than *Δompdc*- and *Δompdc Δldh1*-infected ones, however, because of the sensitivity of the qPCR tests, it is hard to measure the exact parasite burden differences. Next, we compared the immune protection efficiencies of these mutants. Mice were first infected with each of these mutant lines, 30 days post-infection they were challenged with the WT strain ME49 and survival of the mice was monitored. All immunized mice survived the secondary infection (**Figure 10C**), which is consistent with previous results and indicates that these mutants offered similar protection efficiencies against further infections. Together, these results suggest that the *Δldh* mutant worked comparably well as the uracil auxotrophic mutants as a vaccine candidate.

DISCUSSION

Decades of epidemiological and experimental studies have suggested that vaccination is probably the most effective way to control the ubiquitous pathogen *T. gondii*, and live attenuated vaccines hold the most promise among all vaccination strategies tried so far. Toxovax® derived from the incomplete strain S48 has been commercialized to reduce *Toxoplasma* caused abortion in sheep (23), and the uracil auxotroph mutants also look promising under experimental settings (25–27). However, these do not mean that current vaccines are ideal. In this study, we tested the possibility of using a lactate dehydrogenase null mutant (*Δldh*) as a live vaccine candidate to prevent animal toxoplasmosis, since our previous work has shown that this mutant was able to grow efficiently *in vitro* but unable to propagate *in vivo* (28). The results showed that, indeed ME49 *Δldh* immunization stimulated efficient protective immunity against the challenge of a variety of strains.

There is a long history for the search of good anti-toxoplasmic vaccines. Killed parasites, total antigens or secreted antigens extracted from cultured parasites, recombinant antigens in a variety of forms, and live attenuated parasites have all been tried over the last 60 years (16, 29–31). One important lesson from these studies is that live attenuated vaccines are the most efficient in stimulating protective immunity. The only commercially available *Toxoplasma* vaccine Toxovax® is a live vaccine derived from the S48 strain, which is used in breeding ewes to reduce

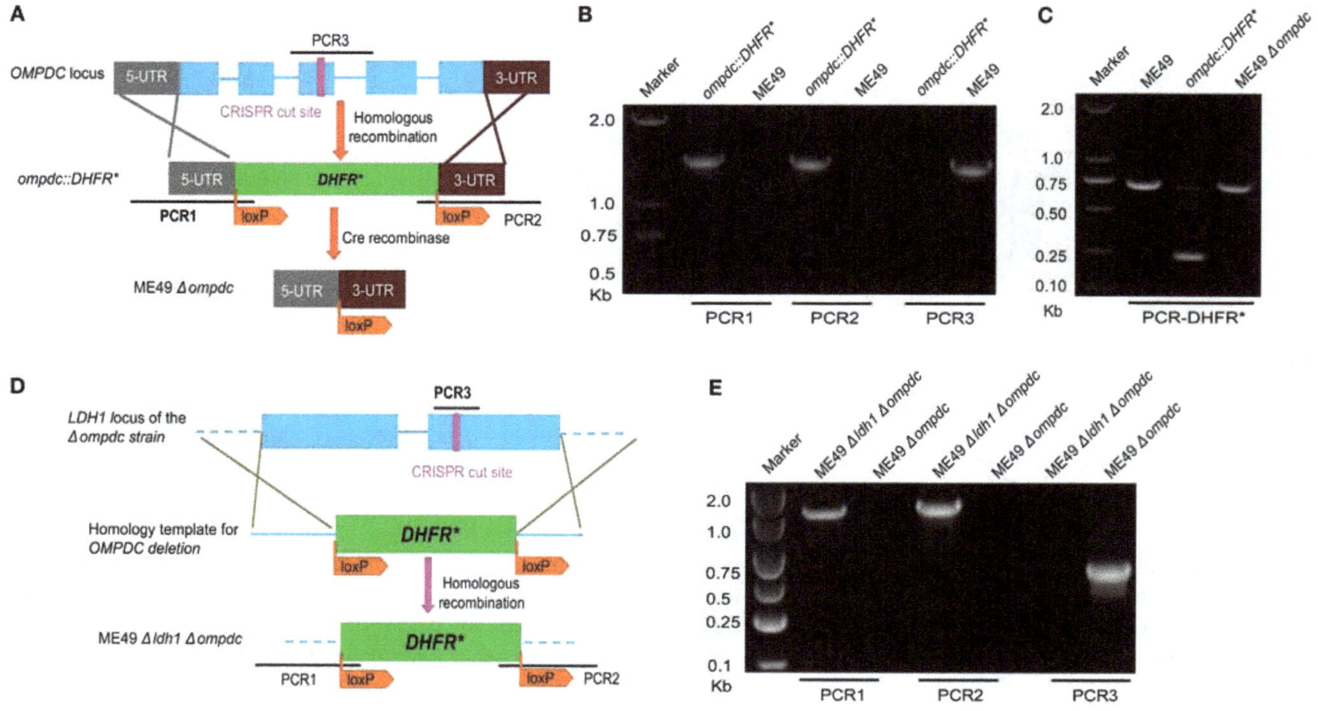

FIGURE 9 | Generation of *OMPDC* deletion mutants. **(A)** Schematic illustration of *OMPDC* replacement by the selection marker *DHFR** and subsequent removal of *DHFR** by Cre recombinase. **(B)** Diagnostic PCR on an *ompdc:DHFR** clone. PCR1 and PCR2 check the integration of *DHFR** at the 5′ and 3′ end of *OMPDC*, respectively, whereas PCR3 examines the presence of *OMPDC* sequence. **(C)** Diagnostic PCR confirming the removal of *DHFR** by Cre recombinase. This PCR generated a 700 bp product from the endogenous *DHFR* locus, and a 250 bp product from *DHFR** due to the absence of introns. Absence of the 250 bp product in *ompdc:DHFR** treated with Cre indicates removal of *DHFR**. **(D)** Diagram illustrating the deletion of *LDH1* in *Δompdc* to make the double mutant *Δompdc ldh1:DHFR**, by CRISPR/Cas9-mediated homologous gene replacement. **(E)** Diagnostic PCR on a *Δompdc ldh1:DHFR** clone.

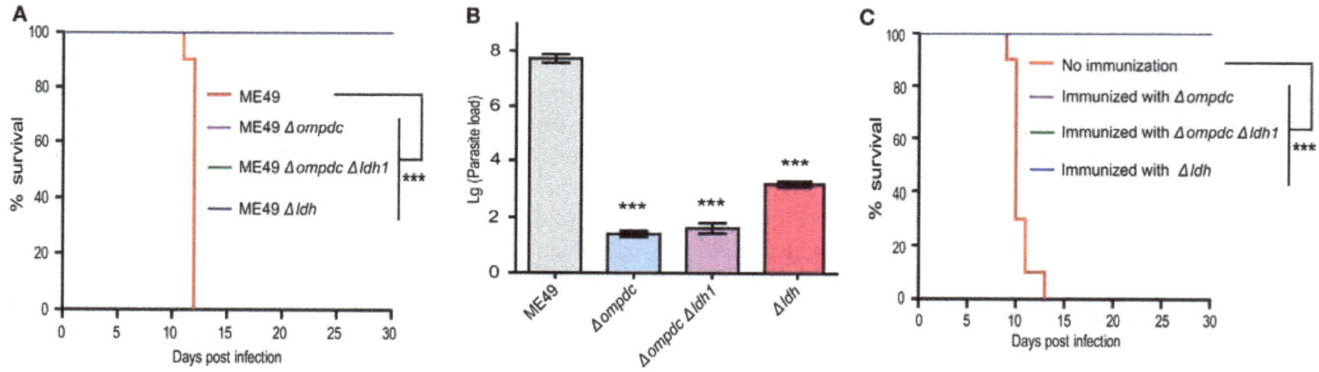

FIGURE 10 | Comparison of *Δldh* mutants-based vaccines to that based on *Δompdc* auxotrophs. **(A)** Survival curves of mice infected with indicated strains. Tachyzoites of indicated strains were used to infect ICR mice (10^4 parasites/mouse, 10 mice for each strain) by intraperitoneal injection and the survival of mice were monitored for 30 days. ***$p < 0.001$, Gehan–Breslow–Wilcoxon test. **(B)** Replication of parasites *in vivo*. ICR mice were infected with 10^4 tachyzoites of indicated strains by intraperitoneal injection and parasite loads in peritoneal fluids 7 days post-infection were determined by quantitative PCR. ***$p < 0.001$, Student's *t*-test. **(C)** Protection efficiency offered by vaccination of indicated *Toxoplasma gondii* mutants. ICR mice were immunized with indicated strains by intraperitoneal injection of 10^4 tachyzoites each. Thirty days post-immunization, they were challenged with 10^4 tachyzoites of the ME49 strain and survival of mice were monitored for another 30 days. Non-immunized mice were included as negative control. ***$p < 0.001$, Gehan–Breslow–Wilcoxon test.

incidences of dry ewes and abortion (23). Inability to complete its life cycle was thought to be why it can be used as a vaccine, since it can only grow as tachyzoites and survive in sheep for about 14 days before being cleared by sheep's immune functions (32). However, this strain is still highly virulent in mice during acute infection. It may also revert to gain cysts or oocysts formation abilities. Because of these limitations, this vaccine is not widely used. Recently the *de novo* pyrimidine synthesis pathway was found to be a good target for vaccine design, as mutants (such as *ΔcpsII* and *Δompdc*) with defective *de novo* UMP biosynthesis activity were able to grow *in vitro* in the presence of uracil but unable to propagate *in vivo* (25–27). Both *ΔcpsII* and *Δompdc* mutants were reported to induce long-term protection against both acute and chronic toxoplasmosis. Although the uracil auxotroph mutants are promising, their protection is not always 100% (25–27). The *Δldh* mutant tested in this study is similar to the uracil auxotroph mutants as a vaccine candidate, due to its drastic growth differences between *in vitro* and *in vivo* conditions.

An ideal live vaccine not only stimulates efficient protection against further infections but also leaves no parasites behind in order to prevent the risk of parasite dissemination through vaccination, particularly for meat producing animals. In the mouse model, *Δldh* vaccination induced strong protective immune responses against the challenge of a variety of strains, including type 1, 2, 3 strains and natural isolates belonging to ToxoDB #9 and ToxoDB #3. However, it should be noted that the protection to virulent type 1 strain RH-Luc is limited to short term, likely because our *Δldh* was made in the type 2 strain ME49. It was reported previously that vaccinated hosts can also be super-infected by wild strains if they contain virulent ROP5 and ROP18 alleles (14). This explains why ME49 *Δldh* vaccination only provided short-term protection against RH infection. It also suggests that using the endemic strains as starting material to design live vaccines is more likely to be successful. Nonetheless, inactivating *LDH* genes is still a feasible way of producing live attenuated vaccines. The other seemingly caveat of ME49 *Δldh* vaccination is that it still produced very small amount of tissue cysts, although we have shown that these cysts were severely attenuated and likely would not cause diseases in vaccinated animals or new hosts if transmitted to. Nevertheless, we have to admit that, ME49 *Δldh* still needs improvement in this regard, especially for meat producing animals due to the risk of transmitting the infection to humans. One strategy to improve, like we showed, is to combine *Δldh* with mutations that lead to defective *de novo* pyrimidine synthesis. The *Δompdc Δldh1* mutant is as efficient as the *Δldh* mutant in terms of stimulating protective immunity against further infections. Yet, there was little parasite replication and no cyst formation *in vivo* after vaccinating animals with this strain (**Figure 10B** and data not shown), making it safer than the *Δldh* mutant. There is another advantage to combine multiple deletions in one strain for live vaccine design. If the vaccine were to be used in cats, combination of multiple mutations reduces the chance of reversing the vaccine strain back to the virulent parental strain through sexual reproduction, which can happen when the cats are infected with other strains during the vaccination period.

In efforts to assess the potential mechanism of protective immunity from *Δldh* vaccination, we found that it was a combination of humoral and cellular immune responses, with cellular immunity being the major contributor. *Δldh* administration stimulated high levels of IL-12 and IFN-γ, two pro-inflammatory cytokines known to be crucial for activation of cell-mediated clearance of *T. gondii*. The elevated levels of IL-12 and IFN-γ did stay for a while after vaccination and then gradually decreased. They were completely back to normal levels 125 days post-vaccination. At day 160 post *Δldh* immunization, splenocytes extracted from vaccinated mice were able to respond to *T. gondii* antigen quickly and produce high levels of IFN-γ and other pro-inflammatory cytokines, which could activate cellular immune responses and clear secondary infections efficiently. On the other hand, when testing the contribution of humoral immunity by passive immunization, it was found that sera from *Δldh*-vaccinated mice was able to reduce parasite propagation but the overall protection was rather limited, since the passively immunized mice only survived 2 days longer compared to controls (**Figure 7B**). Together these results suggested that cellular immunity, instead of humoral immunity is the main source of protection from *Δldh* vaccination, similar to the uracil auxotroph mutants-based vaccines (25, 27). In our cytokine measurement studies, we noticed that *Δldh* immunization induced relatively long duration of increased IL-12 and IFN-γ levels (**Figures 6A–D**). This was somewhat unexpected, but it may be caused by the unique propagation dynamics of the *Δldh* mutants *in vivo*. As was shown, after immunization *Δldh* parasites could form very low levels of cysts in mice, which suggested that some degree of parasite replication and differentiation must have occurred. The prolonged IL-12 and IFN-γ induction might be a consequence of these parasite activities, but further work is required to completely understand this observation. In addition, it is interesting to note that *Δldh* immunization provided full protection against the challenge of type 1 virulent strain in a relatively short term (30 days). If the challenge occurred too long (>75 days) after vaccination, the protection efficiency decreased significantly. This pattern correlated well with the IL-12 and IFN-γ level changes, which may indicate that the existing of an activated cell-mediated immunity is required for full control of virulent type 1 strains. Nonetheless, even after 75 days, vaccinated mice were still partially protected against RH *Δhxgprt* infection, and fully protected from the challenge of other strain types with intermediate virulence.

In conclusion, our study demonstrated that *Δldh* mutant can potentially be used as a live attenuated vaccine. Its administration stimulated a combination of humoral and cellular immune responses that protected animals from further infections of a variety of *T. gondii* strains. We also combined a uracil auxotroph conferring mutation with *Δldh* deletion to make the double knockout *Δompdc Δldh1*, which exhibited similar protection efficiency as the *Δldh* mutant but with further reduced *in vivo* replication and cyst formation, making it safer to use as vaccines. Although the work from mice models demonstrated the great potential of these mutants as vaccine candidates, further investigations are needed to check the safety of vaccination and efficiency of protection in large animals like pigs and sheep, as well as in cats to see the protection against oocyst shedding.

MATERIALS AND METHODS

Mice and Parasite Strains

All 7-week-old ICR mice were purchased from the Hubei provincial center for disease control and prevention. All animals were maintained under standard conditions according to the regulations specified by Administration of Affairs Concerning Experimental Animals. Animal experiments were approved by the ethical committee of Huazhong Agricultural University (permit #: HZAUMO2016049).

Toxoplasma gondii type 1 strain RH *Δhxgprt* and its derivative RH-Luc that expresses a firefly luciferase, type 2 strain ME49, type 3 strain VEG, RFLP genotype ToxoDB #3 strain TgPIG-WH1, and ToxoDB #9 strain C7719 were used in this study, which were propagated with human foreskin fibroblast cells (purchased from ATCC, USA) and cultured in DMEM medium supplemented with 10% fetal bovine serum (FBS) (LifeTechnologies, Inc., Rockville, MD, USA). In addition, the *Δompdc* and *Δompdc Δldh1* mutant strains were maintained in the presence of extra 250 μM uracil (25, 27) (LifeTechnologies, Inc., Rockville, MD, USA).

Virulence Test of *Δldh* Cysts

Fresh brain cysts derived from ME49 *Δldh* or ME49 were used to infect 7-week-old female ICR mice through oral administration (50 cysts/mouse). Mice survival was monitored for 40 days and blood sample were collected afterward. MIC3-based indirect ELISA was used to check the sera to confirm infection. Sero-negative mice were not included in analysis. Cumulative mortality was graphed as Kaplan–Meier survival plots and analyzed in Prism 5 (GraphPad Software, Inc., La Jolla, CA, USA).

Immune Protection Against Acute Infection Stimulated by *T. gondii* Mutants Vaccination

ICR mice were immunized with 10^4 tachyzoites of ME49 *Δldh*, ME49 *Δompdc*, or ME49 *Δompdc Δldh1* through intraperitoneal injection. 30, 75, or 125 days post-immunization, mice were challenged with 10^4 tachyzoites of RH *Δhxgprt*, ME49, VEG, C7719, or TgPIG-WH1 by intraperitoneal injection (10 mice for each group), or 50 fresh cysts of ME49 by oral administration. Non-immunized naïve mice with the same challenging doses and routes were included as controls and subsequently these animals were monitored for another 30 days to check their clinical symptoms and survival. In addition, naïve or *Δldh* immunized mice were infected with 10^4 tachyzoites of the luciferase expressing RH-Luc strain by intraperitoneal injection (five mice/group). Propagation of RH-Luc in these mice was monitored 1 and 5 days post-infection, by bioluminescent imaging on the IVIS Spectrum imaging system (PerkinElmer, Inc., Boston, MA, USA). To do this, each mouse was injected with 200 μl of 15.4 mg/ml D-luciferin, anesthetized in a chamber containing 2% isoflurane and then imaged by IVIS Spectrum according to the manufacturer's instructions, as well as previous descriptions (33). Data acquisition and analysis were performed using the Living Image 4 software (PerkinElmer, Inc., Boston, MA, USA).

Prevention of Cyst Formation by *Δldh* Immunization

ICR mice were first immunized with ME49 *Δldh* as above and then challenged with 10^4 tachyzoites of TgPIG-WH1. Subsequently the mice were monitored for another 30 days and seropositive mice were sacrificed to harvest the brains. Immunized but not TgPIG-WH1 challenged, and non-immunized but TgPIG-WH1 challenged mice were included as controls (10 mice per group). The number of *Toxoplasma* cysts in each mouse brain was determined by DBA-FITC staining, as previously described (34).

Cytokines and *Toxoplasma*-Specific IgG Level Measurements

Sera samples were collected from mice and stored at −20°C until analysis. The levels of IL12p70, INF-γ, IL-10, and TNF-α were measured using commercial ELISA kits following the manufacturer's instructions (4A Biotech, Inc., Beijing, China). To analyze the levels of *T. gondii* specific IgG by ELISA, 96-well microtiter plates were coated with 100 μl/well 0.5 μg/ml soluble tachyzoite antigens diluted in PBS and incubated at 4°C overnight. The plates were then washed and blocked with 1% BSA. Sera samples were diluted 50-fold and added to each well to incubate for 60 min at 37°C. After extensive washing, the bound IgG antibodies were detected by HRP conjugated goat anti-mouse IgG secondary antibodies and tetramethylbenzidine as substrate. A minimum of three mice was included for each experiment and all sera samples were analyzed three times.

Cytokine Production by Splenocytes After *T. gondii* Antigen Stimulation

ICR mice were immunized with ME49 *Δldh* tachyzoites and seropositive animals were sacrificed 160 days after immunization. Subsequently the spleens were collected from the mice and homogenized in red cell lysis solution (Biosharp, Inc., Beijing, China) to obtain splenocyte suspensions. The recovered splenocytes were washed once in RPMI 1640 (LifeTechnologies, Inc., Rockville, MD, USA), resuspended and counted (35). Viability of the cells was determined by trypan blue staining. Then 3×10^5 viable splenocytes were plated in each well of 96-well plates and cultured in RPMI 1640 supplemented with 20% FBS (LifeTechnologies, Inc., Rockville, MD, USA) and 100 U/ml penicillin–streptomycin. Meanwhile the splenocytes were stimulated with total *T. gondii* soluble antigens (final concentration 50 μg/ml) isolated from tachyzoites of ME49 for 3 days. The supernatants from these cultures were harvested for cytokines level measurements, which was performed as above. *T. gondii* soluble antigens were prepared as the following: freshly egressed tachyzoites of ME49 were collected, purified by filtration, and lysed by sonication in a waterbath sonicator for 30 min. Subsequently the samples were spinned at 12,000 rcf for 10 min at 4°C and the supernatant was collected as TSA, which was subject to protein concentration determination by BCA Protein Assay Kit (Beyotime Biotechnology, Beijing, China) before use. The splenocytes were also stimulated with 5 μg/ml concanavalin A (LifeTechnologies, Inc., Rockville, MD, USA) or 20% FBS as positive and negative controls, respectively. The same experiments were also done with non-immunized naïve mice for further comparisons. Three naïve mice and three immunized mice were analyzed, and each supernatant sample was examined three times by ELISA for technical replication.

Passive Immunization With the Sera of *Δldh*-Vaccinated Mice

ICR mice (16 mice in total, two groups with 8 mice in each group) were infected with the WT strain ME49 through intraperitoneal injection (10^4 tachyzoites/mouse). At day 0 and day 3 after infection, sera from naïve mice or the ME49 *Δldh*-vaccinated mice 160 days post-immunization were collected and administered into infected mice by tail vein injection (100 µl/mouse). The protection of passive immunization was estimated in two ways. First, three mice from each group were sacrificed 7 days post-infection to measure the parasite burden in peritoneal fluids by quantitative PCR, as previously described (28). Second, the survival of the other five mice in each group was monitored daily for 30 days.

Generation of *Δompdc* and *Δompdc Δldh1* Mutants

Both *OMPDC* and *LDH1* deletions were made by CRISPR/Cas9-mediated homologous gene replacements, using the methods described previously (36, 37). All primers and plasmids used in the mutant constructions are listed in **Tables 1** and **2**, respectively. *LDH1* and *OMPDC* specific CRISPR plasmids were generated by replacing the *UPRT* targeting guide RNA (gRNA) in *pSAG1-Cas9-sgUPRT* with corresponding gRNAs, using Q5 site-directed mutagenesis (36, 37). The plasmid p*OMPDC*:loxp-*DHFR**-loxp was constructed by cloning the 5′- and 3′-homology arms (1,044 and 981 bps, respectively) of *OMPDC*, as well as the loxp-*DHFR**-loxp (3,672 bps) amplified from pDONR-G265-loxP-*DHFR**-loxp into pUC19 through Gibson assembly (New England Biolabs, Ipswich, MA, USA). It was used as the homologous template to replace *OMPDC* with the loxp-*DHFR**-loxp. The plasmid pLDH1:loxp-*DHFR**-loxp used to replace *LDH1* with loxp-*DHFR**-loxp was constructed in a similar way. All the plasmids were verified by DNA sequencing before use. To constructed the *OMPDC* knockout strain, ME49 was co-transfected with the *OMPDC* specific CRISPR plasmid and homologous template (*OMPDC*:loxp-*DHFR**-loxp), selected with 1 µM pyrimethamine and 250 µM uracil (LifeTechnologies, Inc., Rockville, MD, USA), and single cloned by limiting dilution. The resulted ME49 *ompdc:DHFR** was then transiently transfected with a Cre recombinase expressing plasmid (pmin-Cre-eGFP) (38) to remove the selection marker *DHFR**, to obtain ME49 *Δompdc*. All clones were identified by diagnostic PCRs, as demonstrated in **Figures 9A,D**. The *Δompdc Δldh1* double mutant were made by replacing *LDH1* in ME49 *Δompdc* with loxp-*DHFR**-loxp, using the same strategy as the *OMPDC* deletion.

Statistical Analysis

Statistical comparisons were performed in Prism 5 (GraphPad Software, Inc., La Jolla, CA, USA) using Student's *t*-tests,

TABLE 1 | Primers used in this study.

Primer	Sequence	Use
gRNA-LDH1-Fw	5′-GCCGGTCTGACCAAGGTGCCGTTTTAGAGCTAGAAATAGC-3′	To construct the *LDH1* specific CRISPR plasmid
gRNA-OMPDC-Fw	5′-GAGCTTGACTCCACCCTCACGTTTTAGAGCTAGAAATAGC-3′	To construct the *OMPDC* specific CRISPR plasmid
gRNA-R	5′-AACTTGACATCCCCATTTAC-3′	To construct gene specific CRISPR plasmids
pUC19-Fw	5′-GGCGTAATCATGGTCATAGC-3′	Amplification of pUC19 for Gibson assembly
pUC19-Rv	5′-CTCGAATTCACTGGCCGTCG-3′	Amplification of pUC19 for Gibson assembly
loxp-*DHFR**-loxp-Fw	5′-CAACCCGCGCAGAAGACATC-3′	Amplification of loxp-*DHFR**-loxp for Gibson assembly
loxp-*DHFR**-loxp-Rv	5′-GGACACGCTGAACTTGTGGC-3′	Amplification of loxp-*DHFR**-loxp for Gibson assembly
U5ompdc-Fw	5′-CGACGGCCAGTGAATTCGAGGTACGTTTGCGATTGTGAGC-3′	Amplification of 5′-homology of *OMPDC* for pOMPDC:loxp-*DHFR**-loxp construction
U5ompdc-Rv	5′-GATGTCTTCTGCGCGGGTTGCAGTTCTTTGGAATTGTCACGG-3′	Amplification of 5′-homology of *OMPDC* for pOMPDC:loxp-DHFR*-loxp construction
U3ompdc-Fw	5′-GCCACAAGTTCAGCGTGTCCCGTGCTGAAAGCGAAACACTATC-3′	Amplification of 3′-homology of *OMPDC* for pOMPDC:loxp-DHFR*-loxp construction
U3ompdc-Rv	5′-GCTATGACCATGATTACGCCGTCAGTTTCTCTGTGCGAGTTG-3′	Amplification of 3′-homology of *OMPDC* for pOMPDC:loxp-DHFR*-loxp construction
U5ldh1-Rv	5′-GATGTCTTCTGCGCGGGTTGTTCTCCTCTGCACAAGTGCG-3′	Amplification of *PUC19:LDH1-5UTR-3UTR* for pLDH1: loxp-*DHFR**-loxp construction
U3ldh1-Fw	5′-GCCACAAGTTCAGCGTGTCCTGGCAAAACAGGAGCGGAAT-3′	Amplification of *PUC19:LDH1-5UTR-3UTR* for pLDH1: loxp-*DHFR**-loxp construction
5′-UpU5OMPDC	5′-GACAGTTATGGCCCGTCTTC-3′	PCR1 of *Δompdc:DHFR**
3′-In*DHFR**-Fw	5′-CGTGACCACGCCAAAGTAG-3′	PCR1 of *Δompdc:DHFR**
5′-In*DHFR**-Rv	5′-GCACTTGCAGGATGAATTCC-3′	PCR2 of *Δompdc:DHFR**
3′-DnU3OMPDC	5′-GAGCATTGTGCATTTGCGTC-3′	PCR2 of *Δompdc:DHFR**
5′-UpgRNA OMPDC	5′-CGTCAGCTTCGTTAGACCAG-3′	PCR3 of *Δompdc:DHFR**
3′-DngRNA OMPDC	5′-CAGCTGTACTATGAACGGGTG-3′	PCR3 of *Δompdc:DHFR**
5′-In*DHFR*	5′-GTCCGAGTCTGTGCTTCAC-3′	To identify the deletion of loxP-*DHFR**
3′-In*DHFR*	5′-CCTGCGCAGCAGTTGATTTG-3′	To identify the deletion of loxP-*DHFR**
5′-InU5ldh1	5′-CTGTCCAGCGTAGCAATCAC-3′	PCR1 of *Δompdc Δldh1*
3′-In *DHFR**	5′-ACCACGCCAAAGTAGAAAGG-3′	PCR1 of *Δompdc Δldh1*
5′-In*DHFR**	5′-TGCTGGACTGTTGCTGTCTG-3′	PCR2 of *Δompdc Δldh1*
3′-InU3ldh1	5′-GTGGCCGACCTTTTCAGAGC-3′	PCR2 of *Δompdc Δldh1*
5′-UpgRNA ldh1	5′-GCTAGACGCGGAGAGTTGTG-3′	PCR3 of *Δompdc Δldh1*
3′-DngRNA ldh1	5′-AGCTGCTTCTCCGTGACTAC-3′	PCR3 of *Δompdc Δldh1*
RT-tubulin-F	5′-CACTGGTACACGGGTGAAGGT-3′	β-tubulin-based qPCR
RT-tubulin-R	5′-ATTCTCCCTCTTCCTCTGCG-3′	β-tubulin-based qPCR

TABLE 2 | Plasmids used in this study.

Plasmid name	Use	Source
pSAG1-Cas9-sgUPRT	Template for gene-specific CRISPR plasmid construction	Addgene plasmid #54467
pSAG1-Cas9-sgLDH1	LDH1-specific CRISPR plasmid	(28)
pSAG1-Cas9-sgOMPDC	OMPDC-specific CRISPR plasmid	This work
pOMPDC: loxp-*DHFR**-loxp	To replace OMPDC with loxp-*DHFR**-loxp	This work
pLDH1: loxp-*DHFR**-loxp	To replace LDH1 with loxp-*DHFR**-loxp	This work
pLDH1:*DHFR*	Template for *PUC19:LDH1-5UTR-3UTR* amplification	(28)
pDONR-G265-loxP-*DHFR**-loxp	Template for loxp-*DHFR**-loxp amplification	This work
pmin-Cre-eGFP	To remove the selection marker DHFR*	(38)

Gehan–Breslow–Wilcoxon test or one-way ANOVA with Bonferroni posttests as indicated in figure legends.

AUTHOR CONTRIBUTIONS

BS, NX, and TZ conceived and designed the experiments; NX, TZ, XL, SY, PZ, and JY performed the experiments; BS, NX, TZ, YZ, and JZ analyzed the data; BS and NX wrote the paper.

ACKNOWLEDGMENTS

The authors are grateful to Drs. Min Cui, Min Hu, Rui Fang, and Lan He from the college of veterinary medicine, Huazhong Agricultural University for their thoughtful suggestions during this study.

REFERENCES

1. Elmore SA, Jones JL, Conrad PA, Patton S, Lindsay DS, Dubey JP. *Toxoplasma gondii*: epidemiology, feline clinical aspects, and prevention. *Trends Parasitol* (2010) 26(4):190–6. doi:10.1016/j.pt.2010.01.009
2. Montoya JG, Liesenfeld O. Toxoplasmosis. *Lancet* (2004) 363(9425):1965–76. doi:10.1016/S0140-6736(04)16412-X
3. Petersen E, Pollak A, Reiter-Owona I. Recent trends in research on congenital toxoplasmosis. *Int J Parasitol* (2001) 31(2):115–44. doi:10.1016/S0020-7519(00)00140-5
4. Dubey JP. Toxoplasmosis in pigs – the last 20 years. *Vet Parasitol* (2009) 164(2–4):89–103. doi:10.1016/j.vetpar.2009.05.018
5. Dubey JP, Hill DE, Jones JL, Hightower AW, Kirkland E, Roberts JM, et al. Prevalence of viable *Toxoplasma gondii* in beef, chicken, and pork from retail meat stores in the United States: risk assessment to consumers. *J Parasitol* (2005) 91(5):1082–93. doi:10.1645/GE-683.1
6. Alday PH, Doggett JS. Drugs in development for toxoplasmosis: advances, challenges, and current status. *Drug Des Devel Ther* (2017) 11:273–93. doi:10.2147/DDDT.S60973
7. Dubey JP. Advances in the life cycle of *Toxoplasma gondii*. *Int J Parasitol* (1998) 28(7):1019–24. doi:10.1016/S0020-7519(98)00023-X
8. Hunter CA, Sibley LD. Modulation of innate immunity by *Toxoplasma gondii* virulence effectors. *Nat Rev Microbiol* (2012) 10(11):766–78. doi:10.1038/nrmicro2858
9. VanWormer E, Fritz H, Shapiro K, Mazet JA, Conrad PA. Molecules to modeling: *Toxoplasma gondii* oocysts at the human-animal-environment interface. *Comp Immunol Microbiol Infect Dis* (2013) 36(3):217–31. doi:10.1016/j.cimid.2012.10.006
10. Howe DK, Sibley LD. *Toxoplasma gondii* comprises three clonal lineages: correlation of parasite genotype with human disease. *J Infect Dis* (1995) 172(6):1561–6. doi:10.1093/infdis/172.6.1561
11. Khan A, Dubey JP, Su C, Ajioka JW, Rosenthal BM, Sibley LD. Genetic analyses of atypical *Toxoplasma gondii* strains reveal a fourth clonal lineage in North America. *Int J Parasitol* (2011) 41(6):645–55. doi:10.1016/j.ijpara.2011.01.005
12. Lorenzi H, Khan A, Behnke MS, Namasivayam S, Swapna LS, Hadjithomas M, et al. Local admixture of amplified and diversified secreted pathogenesis determinants shapes mosaic *Toxoplasma gondii* genomes. *Nat Commun* (2016) 7:10147. doi:10.1038/ncomms10147
13. Behnke MS, Khan A, Lauron EJ, Jimah JR, Wang Q, Tolia NH, et al. Rhoptry proteins ROP5 and ROP18 are major murine virulence factors in genetically divergent South American strains of *Toxoplasma gondii*. *PLoS Genet* (2015) 11(8):e1005434. doi:10.1371/journal.pgen.1005434
14. Jensen KD, Camejo A, Melo MB, Cordeiro C, Julien L, Grotenbreg GM, et al. *Toxoplasma gondii* superinfection and virulence during secondary infection correlate with the exact ROP5/ROP18 allelic combination. *MBio* (2015) 6(2):e02280. doi:10.1128/mBio.02280-14
15. Ezz Eldin HM, Kamel HH, Badawy AF, Shash LS. A comparative study between excretory/secretory and autoclaved vaccines against RH strain of *Toxoplasma gondii* in murine models. *J Parasit Dis* (2015) 39(3):526–35. doi:10.1007/s12639-013-0390-6
16. Waldeland H, Frenkel JK. Live and killed vaccines against toxoplasmosis in mice. *J Parasitol* (1983) 69(1):60–5. doi:10.2307/3281275
17. Darcy F, Maes P, Gras-Masse H, Auriault C, Bossus M, Deslee D, et al. Protection of mice and nude rats against toxoplasmosis by a multiple antigenic peptide construction derived from *Toxoplasma gondii* P30 antigen. *J Immunol* (1992) 149(11):3636–41.
18. Petersen E, Nielsen HV, Christiansen L, Spenter J. Immunization with *E. coli* produced recombinant *T. gondii* SAG1 with alum as adjuvant protect mice against lethal infection with *Toxoplasma gondii*. *Vaccine* (1998) 16(13):1283–9. doi:10.1016/S0264-410X(98)00039-5
19. Dautu G, Munyaka B, Carmen G, Zhang G, Omata Y, Xuenan X, et al. *Toxoplasma gondii*: DNA vaccination with genes encoding antigens MIC2, M2AP, AMA1 and BAG1 and evaluation of their immunogenic potential. *Exp Parasitol* (2007) 116(3):273–82. doi:10.1016/j.exppara.2007.01.017
20. Beghetto E, Nielsen HV, Del Porto P, Buffolano W, Guglietta S, Felici F, et al. A combination of antigenic regions of *Toxoplasma gondii* microneme proteins induces protective immunity against oral infection with parasite cysts. *J Infec Dis* (2005) 191(4):637–45. doi:10.1086/427660
21. Pan M, Lyu C, Zhao J, Shen B. Sixty years (1957–2017) of research on toxo plasmosis in China-an overview. *Front Microbiol* (2017) 8:1825. doi:10.3389/fmicb.2017.01825
22. Zhang NZ, Chen J, Wang M, Petersen E, Zhu XQ. Vaccines against *Toxoplasma gondii*: new developments and perspectives. *Expert Rev Vaccines* (2013) 12(11):1287–99. doi:10.1586/14760584.2013.844652
23. Buxton D, Innes EA. A commercial vaccine for ovine toxoplasmosis. *Parasitology* (1995) 110(Suppl):S11–6. doi:10.1017/S003118200000144X
24. Buxton D, Thomson K, Maley S, Wright S, Bos HJ. Vaccination of sheep with a live incomplete strain (S48) of *Toxoplasma gondii* and their immunity to challenge when pregnant. *Vet Rec* (1991) 129(5):89–93. doi:10.1136/vr.129.5.89
25. Fox BA, Bzik DJ. Avirulent uracil auxotrophs based on disruption of orotidine-5'*t* monophosphate decarboxylase elicit protective immunity to *Toxoplasma gondii* *Infect Immun* (2010) 78(9):3744–52. doi:10.1128/IAI.00287-10

26. Fox BA, Bzik DJ. De novo pyrimidine biosynthesis is required for virulence of *Toxoplasma gondii*. *Nature* (2002) 415(6874):926–9. doi:10.1038/415926a
27. Fox BA, Bzik DJ. Nonreplicating, cyst-defective type II *Toxoplasma gondii* vaccine strains stimulate protective immunity against acute and chronic infection. *Infect Immun* (2015) 83(5):2148–55. doi:10.1128/IAI.02756-14
28. Xia N, Yang J, Ye S, Zhang L, Zhou Y, Zhao J, et al. Functional analysis of *Toxoplasma* lactate dehydrogenases suggests critical roles of lactate fermentation for parasite growth in vivo. *Cell Microbiol* (2018) 20(1). doi:10.1111/cmi.12794
29. Cutchins EC, Warren J. Immunity patterns in the guinea pig following *Toxoplasma* infection and vaccination with killed *Toxoplasma*. *Am J Trop Med Hyg* (1956) 5(2):197–209. doi:10.4269/ajtmh.1956.5.197
30. Krahenbuhl JL, Ruskin J, Remington JS. The use of killed vaccines in immunization against an intracellular parasite: *Toxoplasma gondii*. *J Immunol* (1972) 108(2):425–31.
31. Zhang NZ, Wang M, Xu Y, Petersen E, Zhu XQ. Recent advances in developing vaccines against *Toxoplasma gondii*: an update. *Expert Rev Vaccines* (2015) 14(12):1609–21. doi:10.1586/14760584.2015.1098539
32. Innes EA, Panton WR, Thomson KM, Maley S, Buxton D. Kinetics of interferon gamma production in vivo during infection with the S48 vaccine strain of *Toxoplasma gondii*. *J Comp Pathol* (1995) 113(1):89–94. doi:10.1016/S0021-9975(05)80074-X
33. Saeij JP, Boyle JP, Grigg ME, Arrizabalaga G, Boothroyd JC. Bioluminescence imaging of *Toxoplasma gondii* infection in living mice reveals dramatic differences between strains. *Infect Immun* (2005) 73(2):695–702. doi:10.1128/IAI.73.2.695-702.2005
34. Huskinson-Mark J, Araujo FG, Remington JS. Evaluation of the effect of drugs on the cyst form of *Toxoplasma gondii*. *J Infect Dis* (1991) 164(1):170–1. doi:10.1093/infdis/164.1.170
35. Vercammen M, Scorza T, Huygen K, De Braekeleer J, Diet R, Jacobs D, et al. DNA vaccination with genes encoding *Toxoplasma gondii* antigens GRA1, GRA7, and ROP2 induces partially protective immunity against lethal challenge in mice. *Infect Immun* (2000) 68(1):38–45. doi:10.1128/IAI.68.1.38-45.2000
36. Shen B, Brown KM, Lee TD, Sibley LD. Efficient gene disruption in diverse strains of *Toxoplasma gondii* using CRISPR/CAS9. *MBio* (2014) 5(3):e1114–1114. doi:10.1128/mBio.01114-14
37. Shen B, Brown K, Long S, Sibley LD. Development of CRISPR/Cas9 for efficient genome editing in *Toxoplasma gondii*. *Methods Mol Biol* (2017) 1498:79–103. doi:10.1007/978-1-4939-6472-7_6
38. Heaslip AT, Nishi M, Stein B, Hu K. The motility of a human parasite, *Toxoplasma gondii*, is regulated by a novel lysine methyltransferase. *PLoS Pathog* (2011) 7(9):e1002201. doi:10.1371/journal.ppat.1002201

12

Allocation of Interferon Gamma mRNA Positive Cells in Caecum Hallmarks a Protective Trait Against Histomonosis

Fana Alem Kidane[1], *Taniya Mitra*[1], *Patricia Wernsdorf*[1], *Michael Hess*[1,2] *and Dieter Liebhart*[1]*

[1] *Clinic for Poultry and Fish Medicine, Department for Farm Animals and Veterinary Public Health, University of Veterinary Medicine Vienna, Vienna, Austria,* [2] *Christian Doppler Laboratory for Innovative Poultry Vaccines, University of Veterinary Medicine Vienna, Vienna, Austria*

Correspondence:
Dieter Liebhart
dieter.liebhart@vetmeduni.ac.at

Histomonosis is a parasitic disease of gallinaceous birds characterized by necrotic lesions in cacum and liver that usually turns fatal in turkeys while it is less severe in chickens. Vaccination using *in vitro* attenuated *Histomonas meleagridis* has been experimentally shown to confer protection against histomonosis. The protective mechanisms that underpin the vaccine-induced immune response are not resolved so far. Therefore, the actual study aimed to evaluate the location and quantitative distribution patterns of signature cytokines of type 1 [interferon gamma (IFN-γ)] or type 2 [interleukin (IL)-13] immune responses in vaccinated or infected hosts. An intergroup and interspecies difference in the spatial and temporal distribution patterns of cytokine mRNA positive cells was evident. Quantification of cells showed a significantly decreased percentage of IFN-γ mRNA positive cells at 4 days post-inoculation (DPI) in caeca of turkeys inoculated exclusively with the attenuated or the virulent inocula, compared to control birds. The decrement was followed by a surge of cells expressing mRNA for IFN-γ or IL-13, reaching a peak of increment at 10 DPI. By contrast, turkeys challenged following vaccination showed a slight increment of cecal IFN-γ mRNA positive cells at 4 DPI after which positive cell counts became comparable to control birds. The increase in infected birds was accompanied by an extensive distribution of positively stained cells up to the muscularis layer of cecal tissue whereas the vaccine group maintained an intact mucosal structure. In chickens, the level of changes of positive cells was generally lower compared to turkeys. However, control chickens were found with a higher percentage of IFN-γ mRNA positive cells in cecum compared to their turkey counterparts indicating a higher resistance to histomonosis, similar to the observation in immunized turkeys. In chickens, it could be shown that the changes of cytokine-positive cells were related to variations of mononuclear cells quantified by immunofluorescence. Furthermore, gene expression measured by reverse transcription quantitative real time PCR confirmed variations in organs between the different groups of both bird species. Overall, it can be concluded that a proportionally increased, yet controlled, allocation of IFN-γ mRNA positive cells in caeca hallmarks a protective trait against histomonosis.

Keywords: *Histomonas meleagridis*, histomonosis, vaccination, interferon gamma, interleukin-13, *in situ* hybridization, immunofluorescence, image analysis

INTRODUCTION

Histomonosis (syn.: blackhead disease, enzootic typhlohepatitis) is a parasitic disease of gallinaceous birds caused by the flagellate *Histomonas meleagridis* (1). The disease can cause high mortality rates in turkeys (*Meleagris gallopavo*) while in chickens (*Gallus gallus*) clinical signs are less severe, however, the infection entails an impaired performance in chickens leading to severe economic losses (2, 3). In both species, the parasite is able to infiltrate the cecum and triggers severe inflammation, thickening of the cecal wall and formation of fibrinous exudates. Histomonads can then migrate to the liver leading to multifocal areas of inflammation and necrosis, which is commonly observed in infected turkeys (4). Recently, a live vaccine prepared from an *in vitro* passaged clonal culture of *H. meleagridis* has been experimentally shown as safe and capable of providing protection from the disease (5–7). However, investigations on the immune response against histomonosis are rare and relevant protective mechanisms are so far not identified.

Only a few studies investigated the immune system of poultry in response to virulent *H. meleagridis* (8). It could be demonstrated that the level of serum antibody in turkeys may not be a key component in the protection against the parasite as passive immunization using immune sera or active immunization with killed vaccines failed to protect turkeys during challenge (5, 9, 10). However, local antibodies were measured in different parts of the intestine of infected chickens, a host species more resistant to fatal histomonosis, leading to the speculation that mucosal antibodies might be components that contribute toward protection (11). In a different study, an early onset of cytokine expression in cecal tonsils of infected chickens compared to infected turkeys was demonstrated and it was hypothesized to induce a timely immune response in order to prevent the parasite from migrating to the liver (12). Recently, flow cytometry was applied and changes in various immune cell populations in cecum, liver, spleen and blood of vaccinated and/or infected turkeys and chickens were determined showing a less pronounced changes in the frequency of immune cells in vaccinated hosts compared to an exacerbated influx in infected hosts (13).

Successful immunization depends on the ability to induce response selectively and reliably, and for this type 1/type 2 classes of immunity have been characterized in mammals in association with protection following infection or vaccination (14). Type 1/type 2 immunity has also been shown in chickens (15, 16) and can serves as a model for characterizing and optimizing immune responses in poultry for a better conferment of resistance through rational vaccine design (17). Previous studies on type 1/type 2 immunity following histomonosis, however, yielded inconclusive results. Powell et al. (12) found indications for a type 2 response with a persistently enhanced expression of interleukin (IL)-13 mRNA in infected chickens and turkeys, whereas a type 1 driven response with an augmented expression of interferon gamma (IFN-γ) mRNA was described when chickens were co-infected with histomonads and the intestinal worm *Heterakis gallinarum* (18). However, these studies utilized different infection protocols and applied undefined inocula for infection and the relevant pathway elicited during vaccination with attenuated live histomonads has never been investigated.

Moreover, in characterizing the expression patterns of cytokines of type 1/type 2 immunity, the widely utilized method has been reverse transcription quantitative real time PCR (RT-qPCR). While the technique delivered valuable information on the overall changes of transcription levels in homogenized samples, parameters such as the location and quantity of the expressing cells in tissues remained unlocked. Thus, to localize avian cells expressing T helper (Th)1/Th2 signature cytokines, respectively, INF-γ and IL-13, this study employed an *in situ* hybridization (ISH) approach to localize the cells in cecum, liver and spleen of vaccinated and/or infected turkeys and chickens. For verification of variations of the cytokines between the groups and species, RT-qPCR was employed to measure transcripts of IFN-γ and IL-13 mRNA on selected samples of turkeys and chickens, considering the different approach of both techniques. Furthermore, identification of immune cells recruited during vaccination or infection was conducted using immunofluorescence (IF) to reveal changes in populations of B cells, T cells and macrophage/monocytes in selected samples from chickens.

MATERIALS AND METHODS

Animal Trial

Inoculum for Vaccination and Infection

The inocula used for vaccination or infection originated from a clonal culture of *H. meleagridis*/Turkey/Austria/2922-C6/04, established from cecal contents of a diseased turkey (19). The clonal culture was propagated for a short period of time (21 passages) to preserve virulence, hence used for challenge, or for 295 passages to achieve attenuation, according to previous protocols (5, 20). The parasites were kept as cryopreserved cultures (stored at −150°C) were then thawing and incubated at 40°C in a culture medium consisting of Medium 199 supplemented with Earle's salts, L-glutamine, 25 mM HEPES and L-amino acids (Gibco™, Invitrogen, Lofer, Austria), 15% of fetal calf serum (Gibco™) and 0.66 mg of rice starch (Sigma–Aldrich, Vienna, Austria). Before administration, the number of viable cells was determined using a Neubauer cell counting chamber (Reichert, Buffalo, NY, USA) after staining with 0.4% trypan blue solution and adjusted to 1×10^6 histomonads per ml of medium.

Birds

A total of 60 turkeys (B.U.T. 6™; Aviagen Turkeys Ltd., Tattenhall, UK) and the same number of specific pathogen-free chickens (VALO Biomedia, Osterholz-Scharmbeck, Germany) were used. The birds were numerically labeled with a subcutaneously attached tag and housed on deep litter. Unmedicated commercial turkey, respectively, chicken starter feed and water were provided *ad libitum*, except for a 5 h abstinence from feed directly after

Abbreviations: CC, control chickens; CT, control turkeys; DIG, digoxigenin; DPI, days post-inoculation; IC, infected chickens; IF, immunofluorescence; IFN-γ, interferon gamma; IL, interleukin; ISH, *in situ* hybridization; IT, infected turkeys; MLS, mean lesion score; Th, T helper; VC, vaccinated chickens; VIC, vaccinated and infected chickens; VIT, vaccinated and infected turkeys; VT, vaccinated turkeys.

inoculation. The animal trials were approved by the institutional ethics committee and the national authority according to §26 of the Law for Animal Experiments, Tierversuchsgesetz—TVG

Experimental Design and Inoculation

In the main experiment (trial 1, **Table 1**), four groups of turkeys, as well as the same number of chicken groups, were arranged in separate groups (n = 15 per group). The groups comprised of only vaccinated turkeys or chickens (VT and VC), only IT and IC, vaccinated and infected turkeys or chickens (VIT and VIC) and control turkeys or chickens (CT and CC). Birds in group VIT and VIC were vaccinated at their first day of life. The challenge of the VIT and VIC was given on their 28th day of life, together with the infection or vaccination of the other groups.

Each bird received a dosage of 6×10^5 attenuated or virulent histomonads in 0.6 ml of medium, equally split *via* oral and cloacal application. Control birds were sham inoculated with equal volumes of pure culture media only. The oral and cloacal administration was performed using crop tubes attached to a sterile syringe, respectively, pipette tips on a 1 ml pipette. The feed was withdrawn for 5 h following inoculation to promote an adequate colonization of the parasite in the gut. To confirm successful inoculation, cloacal swabs were taken from every bird in intervals of 2–3 days and parasites were incubated for 3 days at 40°C in a culture medium mentioned above. Growth was controlled by microscopical examination of viable parasites.

In a similar setting, an additional experiment (trial 2) was conducted for generating additional cecum, liver and spleen samples for IF labeling of B cells, T cells and monocytes/macrophages in the above-described organs of chickens. For that, three groups of chickens were used: IC, VC, and control chickens (CC). Each infected, respectively, vaccinated bird received 1×10^4 histomonads orally and cloacally.

Clinical Monitoring and Postmortem Lesion Scoring

The birds were monitored daily for clinical signs of histomonosis such as ruffled feathers, depression and yellowish diarrhea. Birds showing clinical signs of the disease were euthanized.

At 4, 7, 10, 14 and 21 days post-inoculation (DPI), three predefined birds per group were killed according to their tag-numbers by bleeding after intravenous injection of sodium thiopental (Sandoz, Kundl, Austria). Postmortem examination and grading of lesions in cecum and liver were performed according to a previous scheme that used scores from 0 (no lesion) to 4 (severe lesions) (11, 21).

Histological Techniques

ISH for Localization of *H. meleagridis*

Pieces of mid-cecum, liver and spleen samples intended for ISH were fixed in 4% neutral buffered formaldehyde (SAV liquid production, Flintsbach, Germany) for at least 48 h at room temperature. The tissues were then trimmed and rinsed in running tap water for an hour before proceeding to routine histological processing. The processing involved dehydration in serially graded alcohols (80, 96 and 100%), clearing in Neo-Clear® (Merck, Darmstadt, Germany) and paraffin infiltration. Finally, the tissues were embedded in paraffin wax and stored until use. For the scheduled ISH, serial sections of 4 µm were prepared using Microme HM360 rotary microtome (Microme, Walldorf, Germany) and mounted on Superfrost Plus slides (Menzel-Gläser, Braunschweig, Germany). To further ensure adhesion of sections on the slides, an overnight treatment of the slides was allowed at 37°C. The ISH with *H. meleagridis* specific digoxigenin (DIG)-labeled oligonucleotide probes was performed according to a published protocol (22).

ISH for Localization of IFN-γ or IL-13 mRNA

Generation of RNA Probes

The use of *in vitro* transcribed DIG-labeled RNA probes for detection of chicken IFN-γ and IL-13 mRNA in liver and spleen paraffin sections has been established earlier. The same approach was followed to establish turkey's staining antisense IFN-γ or IL-13 RNA probes together with negative control sense probes as previously described (23). Briefly, gene-specific primers were designed to amplify the mRNA of turkey IFN-γ and IL-13 (**Table 2**). The targets were amplified from total RNA extracted from the spleen of a non-infected turkey by RT-PCR using QIAGEN OneStep RT-PCR kit (Qiagen, Hilden, Germany). The PCR products were then separated on 1.5% Agarose gel and purified using QIAquick® Gel Extraction Kit (Qiagen). The respective cDNAs were ligated into pCR®4-TOPO® vector for cloning in One Shot® TOP10 Chemically Competent *E. coli*, according to the manufacturer's instructions (Invitrogen, Carlsbad, CA, USA). The nucleotide

TABLE 1 | Experimental scheme and sampling strategy for different groups of turkeys and chickens inoculated with attenuated and/or virulent histomonads.

	Age of birds in days/days post-inoculation						
Group	**1**	**28**	**32/4**	**35/7**	**38/10**	**42/14**	**49/21**
Vaccinated turkeys (VT)		Vaccination	x[a]	x	X	X	x
Vaccinated chickens (VC)		Vaccination	x	x	X	X	x
Infected turkeys (IT)		Infection	x	x	X	N/A[b]	N/A
Infected chickens (IC)		Infection	x	x	X	X	x
Vaccinated and infected turkeys (VIT)	Vaccination	Infection	x	x	X	X	x
Vaccinated and infected chickens (VIC)	Vaccination	Infection	x	x	X	X	x
Control turkeys (CT)		Mock infection	x	x	X	X	x
Control chickens (CC)		Mock infection	x	x	X	X	x

[a]*Necropsy and sampling of three birds.*

[b]*Not applicable due to death caused by virulent histomonads at earlier time points.*

TABLE 2 | Primers, Genbank accession number and the size of the PCR product used for RNA probe generation for *in situ* hybridization of interferon gamma (IFN-γ) and interleukin (IL)-13 mRNA.

Target	Primer sequence	Accession number	Product size (bp)
Turkey-IFN-γ	F: CACCAAGAAGATGACTTACCAG R: TGAGGATGGCTCCTTTTCC	XM_003202048	486
Turkey-IL-13	F: GCTCCATGCCCAAGATGAAG R: AGCGTTGGCAAGAAGTTCC	AM493431	289

sequence and insertion of the cloned products were verified by sequencing (LGC Genomics, Augsburg, Germany).

Plasmids validated to contain the cDNA of the cytokines were linearized with *SpeI* or *NotI* restriction enzymes (Thermo Scientific, Dreieich, Germany). Depending on the insertion, T7 or T3 RNA polymerases were used separately to generate sense or antisense DIG-labeled RNA probes using DIG RNA Labeling Kit (SP6/T7) (Roche Diagnostics, Mannheim, Germany) according to the manufacturer's protocol. The probe yield was quantified using NanoDrop spectrophotometer (Thermo Scientific) and the size of the transcribed probes was verified by gel electrophoresis. Furthermore, the efficiency of the DIG-labeling was assessed by immunoblotting dilution series of DIG-labeled RNA probes according to the manufacturer's recommended protocol given in the DIG RNA Labeling Kit (SP6/T7) (Roche Diagnostics) with some modifications mentioned in the previous work (23).

RNA ISH

The ISH protocol for staining cytokine mRNA positive cells was described in an earlier study (23). Briefly, paraffin sections were deparaffinized with Neo-Clear® (Merck) and rehydrated in a series of graded alcohols (100, 96 and 70%) and diethyl pyrocarbonate (DEPC) treated distilled water. The sections were then digested with 2.8 μg/ml of proteinase K (Invitrogen, Carlsbad, CA, USA) in 0.05 M Tris–HCl (pH 7.5), at 40°C for 30 min. Afterwards, rinsing and dehydration were performed in DEPC-treated water and increasing concentrations of ethanol. Following a short period of air drying, the sections were covered with a hybridization mix composed of 50% formamide, 4× standard saline citrate buffer (SSC), Herring's Sperm DNA (500 ng/ml), 1× Denhardt's solution, 10% dextran sulfate, and the optimal concentration of the respective DIG-labeled RNA probe. A concentration of probes that ranged from 10 to 1,000 ng/ml of hybridization buffer was tested initially to find a defined concentration for further use. Hybridization of the probe with the target RNA was performed in a humidified chamber for overnight at 40°C.

On the next day, stringency washes were made with 2× SSC at room temperature for 30 min, followed by RNase A (20 ng/ml) (Roche Diagnostics) treatment in a solution mix of 0.5 M NaCl, 5 mM Tris–HCl (pH 7.5) and 1 mM EDTA, at 40°C for 30 min. Further washing steps were done two times in 1× and 0.1× SSC at room temperature for 10 min each.

For conjugating the DIG-labeled hybrid-complexes with an enzyme to be used for the color reaction, the sections were first incubated in a blocking solution (50% of Buffer I, 0.3% TRITON®-X and 5% normal goat serum in distilled water) for 30 min in a humidified chamber. The blocking solution was replaced by anti-DIG-AP-antibody diluted 1:100 in the blocking solution mix and incubated for 1 h at room temperature. Afterward, washing and equilibration were performed in three steps. First, unbound antibody was removed by washing the slides in a 1 to 1 dilution of Buffer I (100 mM Tris–HCl pH 7.5, 150 mM NaCl) in distilled water for 15 min. Second, the washing mentioned before was repeated and finally, equilibration in Buffer II (100 mM Tris–HCl pH 7.5, 100 mM NaCl, 50 mM $MgCl_2$, final pH 9.5) was made for 10 min.

For visualizing the target molecules, color reaction was developed using a substrate mix of an equilibration buffer (Buffer II), NBT (4-nitro blue tetrazolium chloride) (0.45 mg/ml), BCIP (5-bromo-4-chloro-3-indolyl-phosphate) (0.175 mg/ml) (Roche Diagnostics) and Levamisole (240 μg/ml) (Sigma, Deisenhofen, Germany). The color reaction was performed in a humidified chamber under dark conditions for overnight. On the next day, the reaction was terminated by immersing the sections in Tris-EDTA (pH 8.0) for at least 10 min. Finally, the sections were counterstained with Gill's hematoxylin (Merck) and mounted under coverslips (Menzel-Gläser) with Aquatex® aqueous mounting medium (Merck). For controlling the specificity of the technique, ISH was performed using the respective sense probes. Moreover, a slide from sections incubated with DEPC-water instead of the probes was used in parallel as negative control.

Immunofluorescence

Cecum, liver and spleen of one bird per group obtained from trial 2 were cryopreserved after embedding in Tissue-Tek® (Sakura Finetek Europe B.V., Flemingweg, the Netherlands) on aluminum foils. Liquid nitrogen was used to freeze the embedded tissue samples. The frozen samples were then stored at −80°C until they were cut into 5 μm slices by a cryostat (CM1800, Leica Mikrosysteme GmbH, Vienna, Austria) and directly processed for IF.

A multicolor staining protocol was employed using mouse anti-chicken Bu-1-Biotin for the detection of B cells, unlabeled mouse anti-chicken CD3 for the detection of T cells and mouse anti-chicken KUL01-PE for the detection of monocytes/macrophages (all SouthernBiotech, Birmingham, AL, USA). For labeling, the cryosections were first fixed in pre-cooled acetone at −20°C. After drying and rehydration in PBS, they were treated with blocking solution (PBS, 2% bovine serum albumin and 10% goat serum) and then incubated overnight with the CD3 antibody at 4°C in a humidified chamber.

On the next day, slides were repeatedly washed with PBS and covered with the secondary antibody goat anti-mouse Alexa 488 (Invitrogen, Vienna, Austria). Following extensive washing and treatment with the blocking solution mentioned above, the other two primary antibodies (biotin-labeled anti-chicken Bu-1 and anti-chicken KUL01 directly labeled with r-phycoerythrin) were applied on the tissues and incubated overnight in a humidified chamber in the same way as mentioned before.

On the third day, streptavidin-Alexa 647 (Life Technologies, Vienna, Austria) was used for conjugation with the Bu-1 antibody. Cell nucleus staining was performed with 4, 6-diamidine-2-phenylindole dihydrochloride (DAPI) (Boehringer Mannheim GmbH, Germany). An isotype control for IgG1k (eBioscience, Vienna, Austria) together with the goat anti-mouse Alexa 488 antibody and samples without primary antibodies were included as controls to confirm the specificity of primary antibody binding.

Microscopy and Analysis of Images for Quantification of Stained Cells

Tissue sections processed by chromogenic ISH for staining cytokine mRNA expressing cells were examined using light transmission microscopy under Zeiss Axio Imager Z1 (Carl Zeiss Microscopy GmbH, Germany). Sections were examined for the location of the stained cells in context of the histological architecture of the respective tissues. Afterward, digital images of the sections were made using a USB camera and the TissueFAXs image acquisition software (TissueGnostics GmbH, Vienna, Austria). The digital images were analyzed for quantification of cells by HistoQuest (version 4.04.0150, TissueGnostics GmbH). For cell quantification, a region of interest (ROI) was selected randomly excluding artifacts, major blood vessels and edges of the sections. The ROI for each sample was a total tissue area of 2 mm^2 divided among equal sizes of eight rectangular ROI. Then, a total number of cells within those 2 mm^2 of the ROI were counted based on their blue nuclei staining after using hematoxylin as a master channel. Valid cells were gated by hematoxylin area versus hematoxylin mean intensity. By applying the software integrated color separation method named single reference shade, a second color detection was performed to automatically separate the hematoxylin (blue) nuclei staining from NBT-BCIP (dark violet) staining based on their optical density. Cutoff values for discriminating NBT-BCIP positive cells from negative cells were set interactively based on the background signal measured in the negative controls (sections treated with sense probes or no probe). In addition, backward viewing was performed to verify the correct discrimination of NBT-BCIP stained cells from negative cells by the source image, shades and color overlay. The percentage of NBT-BCIP stained cells out of the total quantified cells in each tissue section was then exported to SPSS (SPSS 21.0, IBM, Armonk, NY, USA) for statistical analysis.

The procedure for quantification of cells in triple stained IF sections were described earlier (24). Briefly, a multichannel acquisition was made using a Zeiss Axio Imager Z1 fitted with a PCO USB camera and eight regions of interest were selected in digital images of each tissue sample covering an area of 2 mm^2. The identification of each cell was achieved by TissueQuest software using the fluorescence of DAPI (master channel). Valid cells were gated by DAPI area versus DAPI mean intensity. From this population of cells, T cells, B cells and monocytes/macrophages with their respective fluorescence signals were subsequently gated. According to the setup of the respective gates, T cells, B cells and monocytes/macrophages were quantified by the software.

RT-qPCR

Stabilization of RNA in pieces of cecum, liver and spleen samples was performed by immersing the tissues in RNAlater® solution (Qiagen) according to the manufacturer's instruction. Total RNA was then extracted using RNeasy® mini kit (Qiagen) after homogenizing the tissues with QIAshredders (Qiagen) according to manufacturer's instructions. Every RNA sample was assessed for purity, quantity and integrity by using NanoDrop 2000 (ThermoFisher Scientific, Vienna, Austria) and 4200 TapeStation (Agilent Technologies, Waldbronn, Germany), respectively. The RNA samples were stored at −80°C until used.

The expression level of IFN-γ or IL-13 mRNA was quantified by applying TaqMan one-step real-time RT-qPCR using Brilliant III Ultra-Fast QRT-PCR master mix kit (Agilent Technologies, Waldbronn, Germany). Previously published primers and probes for reference genes TFRC (transferring receptor protein 1) and RPL13 (ribosomal protein L13) for turkeys or RPL13 and TBP (TATA box binding protein) for chickens, as well as for the mentioned cytokines were applied (**Table 3**) (12, 25). Amplification of the primary transcripts and quantification of their specific products were performed using AriaMx real-time PCR system (Agilent Technologies, Waldbronn, Germany) together with the Agilent AriaMx1.0 software (Agilent Technologies, Waldbronn, Germany). The thermal cycle profile was as follows: 1 cycle of RT at 50°C for 10 min followed by 95°C for 3 min to hot start, 40 cycles of amplification at 95°C for 5 s and 60°C for 10 s. Different types of controls such as non-reverse transcriptase and non-template control were run to check for genomic DNA contamination and overall PCR contamination.

The cytokines' average cycle threshold (Ct) values for every organ were normalized using geometric mean Ct of the reference genes, to exclude technical variations during sampling and processes of RT-qPCR. Fold change of cytokines was then calculated from the normalized mean Ct value of cytokines from each group by applying the formula $2^{(-\Delta\Delta Ct)}$ (26).

TABLE 3 | Reverse transcription-qPCR primers and probes.

Target	Primer and probe sequences	Reference
Turkey IFN-γ	F: AACCTTCCTGATGGCGTGAA R: CTTGCGCTGGATTCTCAAGTC P:HEX-AAAGATATCATGGACCTGGCCAAGCTTCA-BHQ1	(12)
Turkey IL-13	F: CCTGCACGGCCAGATGA R: GGCAAGAAGTTCCGCAGGTA P: CY5-TGCCAGCTGAGCACCGACAACG-BHQ1	
Chicken IFN-γ	F: GTGAAGAAGGTGAAAGATATCATGGA R: GCTTTGCGCTGGATTCTCA P: HEX-TGGCCAAGCTCCCGATGAACGA-BHQ1	
Chicken IL-13	F: CACCCAGGGCATCCAGAA R: TCCGATCCTTGAAAGCCACTT P: CY5-CATTGCAAGGGACCTGCACTCCTCTG-BHQ1	
RPL13	F: GGAGGAGAAGAACTTCAAGGC R: CCAAAGAGACGAGCGTTTG P: HEX-CTTTGCCAGCCTGCGCATG-BHQ1	(24)
TBP	F: CTGGGATAGTGCCACAGCTA R: GCACGAAGTGCAATGGTTT P: ROX-TGCAACCAAGATTCACCGTGGA-BHQ2	
TFRC	F: AGCTGTGGGTGCTACTGAA R: GGCAGAAATCTTGACATGG P: ROX-CTCTGCCATGCTGCATGCCA-BHQ2	

Statistical Analysis

The statistical package SPSS (SPSS 21.0, IBM, Armonk, NY, USA) was used to execute the descriptive and non-descriptive statistics. Mean lesion scores of cecum or liver were calculated for each group of turkeys or chickens necropsied at the specified DPI. Similarly, total mean lesion scores (MLSs) of cecum or liver were calculated for each group of turkeys or chickens by pooling the total lesion scores of each group and divided by the total number of birds in the group. For comparing differences in the mean percentage of cytokine mRNA positive cells, first normality of the data distribution obtained from percentages of quantified ISH-positive cells for each cytokine was tested using Kolmogorov–Smirnov test according to the tissue and host species. Then, since the data generated from quantification of turkey IFN-γ and IL-13 mRNA positive cells were normally distributed, mean values obtained from the different groups necropsied at different days were compared with the control using independent samples *t*-test. By contrast, due to lack of normality of data distribution in chicken tissues, Mann–Whitney *U* test was used to test the significance of mean differences. Furthermore, *t*-test was used to compare mean of normalized Ct values of the RT-qPCR data. Mean value differences were considered significant when the *P*-value was less than 0.05 ($^{*}P < 0.05$).

RESULTS

Animal Trial

Turkeys inoculated with virulent histomonads without prior vaccination (IT) exhibited typical signs of histomonosis such as a ruffled feather, depression and sulfur-colored diarrhea starting from 7 DPI. Consequently, two birds had to be euthanized due to severe suffering at 11 DPI while the remaining animals were found dead at 12 and 13 DPI. There were not any overt clinical signs in the rest of the turkeys' as well as all of the chickens' groups until the experiment was terminated at 21 DPI. Microscopical investigation of cultured cloacal swabs, however, confirmed the presence of the flagellate in the gut of birds of every group except the controls (data not shown).

Necropsy findings are given by MLS of every group on each sampling day. Total mean lesions scores differed according to the given inoculum, respectively, were found to be reduced in birds that received the vaccination (**Figure 1**). In turkeys (**Figure 1A**), the global MLS was 0.8 in cecum and 0.5 in the liver of VT. Turkeys in group IT had a total MLS of 3.2 and 2.8 in cecum and liver, respectively. In VIT, a total MLS of 2.7 in cecum and MLS of 1.3 in liver were observed. In chickens (**Figure 1B**), the highest total MLS recorded was in cecum and liver of IC (2 and 1.6, respectively). Chickens in group VC and VIC displayed a global MLS below 0.5 in both cecum and liver. None of the control birds in group CT or CC showed lesions at any sampling day.

Localization of *H. meleagridis* in Tissue Sections

Detailed results on frequencies of *H. meleagridis* localized by ISH in cecum and liver of the birds are given in **Table 4**. In cecum, histomonads could be localized in the majority of the turkeys that were inoculated either with the attenuated and/or virulent histomonads. Groups of chickens inoculated with histomonads showed the parasite localized in the cecal sections yet with less frequency than the turkeys inoculated with the same histomonads.

The presence of histomonads was generally uncommon in livers except in IT in which the parasite was detected throughout the sampling days. The protozoa could be found in only one VT collected at 21 DPI and few liver samples (3 out of 15 birds) taken from VIT. In chickens, only three liver samples taken from IC were positive for histomonads.

The spleen of all turkey and chicken samples, independent of the group they belong to, were without parasite infestation and the control groups confirmed the status of non-inoculated birds. Localization and distribution of virulent or attenuated histomonads in cecum and liver are comparatively shown in turkeys of the respective groups (**Figure 2**).

Evaluation of IFN-γ and IL-13 RNA Probes

The DIG-labeled RNA probes generated to hybridize to turkey IFN-γ or IL-13 mRNA in paraffin sections of cecum, liver and spleen could label cells containing the mRNA of the cytokines at a probe concentration of 600 or 300 ng/ml of hybridization buffer for IFN-γ or IL-13, respectively. Similarly, probes against chicken IFN-γ or IL-13 mRNA resulted in distinct coloration of target cells at a concentration of 400 or 100 ng/ml of hybridization buffer, respectively. Positive cells could be recognized by their dark purple color developing from the enzymatic reaction of NBT-BCIP. A higher or lower concentration of probes than the ones mentioned resulted in fainting or over staining of sections, hindering identification of individual cells (data not shown).

Localization and Quantitative Distribution Patterns of IFN-γ or IL-13 mRNA Positive Cells Following Vaccination or Infection

Spatial and Temporal Distribution Differences of Quantified IFN-γ mRNA Positive Cells

The spatial distribution patterns of stained cells in cecum and liver of turkeys inoculated with the tentative vaccine or the virulent inoculum are shown in **Figure 3**. In cecum, IFN-γ mRNA positive cells in VT were exclusively localized as individual cells studded to the intraepithelial region and as small aggregates of cells in the lamina propria as seen in control birds throughout the study period. Quantification of these cells (**Figure 4A**), however, revealed a significantly lower percentage of positive cells at 4 DPI. The early decrement in VT was followed by an abrupt increment characterized by a statistically significant change at 10 DPI. Relative numbers of IFN-γ mRNA positive cells gradually decreased on 14 DPI until the experiment ended at 21 DPI, although being still higher than in the control birds. In IT, the distribution pattern of positive cells at 4 DPI was similar to VT and significantly lower compared to the control group. At 7 and 10 DPI, positive cells showed an extensive spread within the lamina propria and muscularis, along with a total loss of the mucosal structure. Coincidentally, the relative number of these cells was significantly higher at 10 DPI. There were no surviving birds left in group IT from 14 DPI onward. In VIT, the distribution

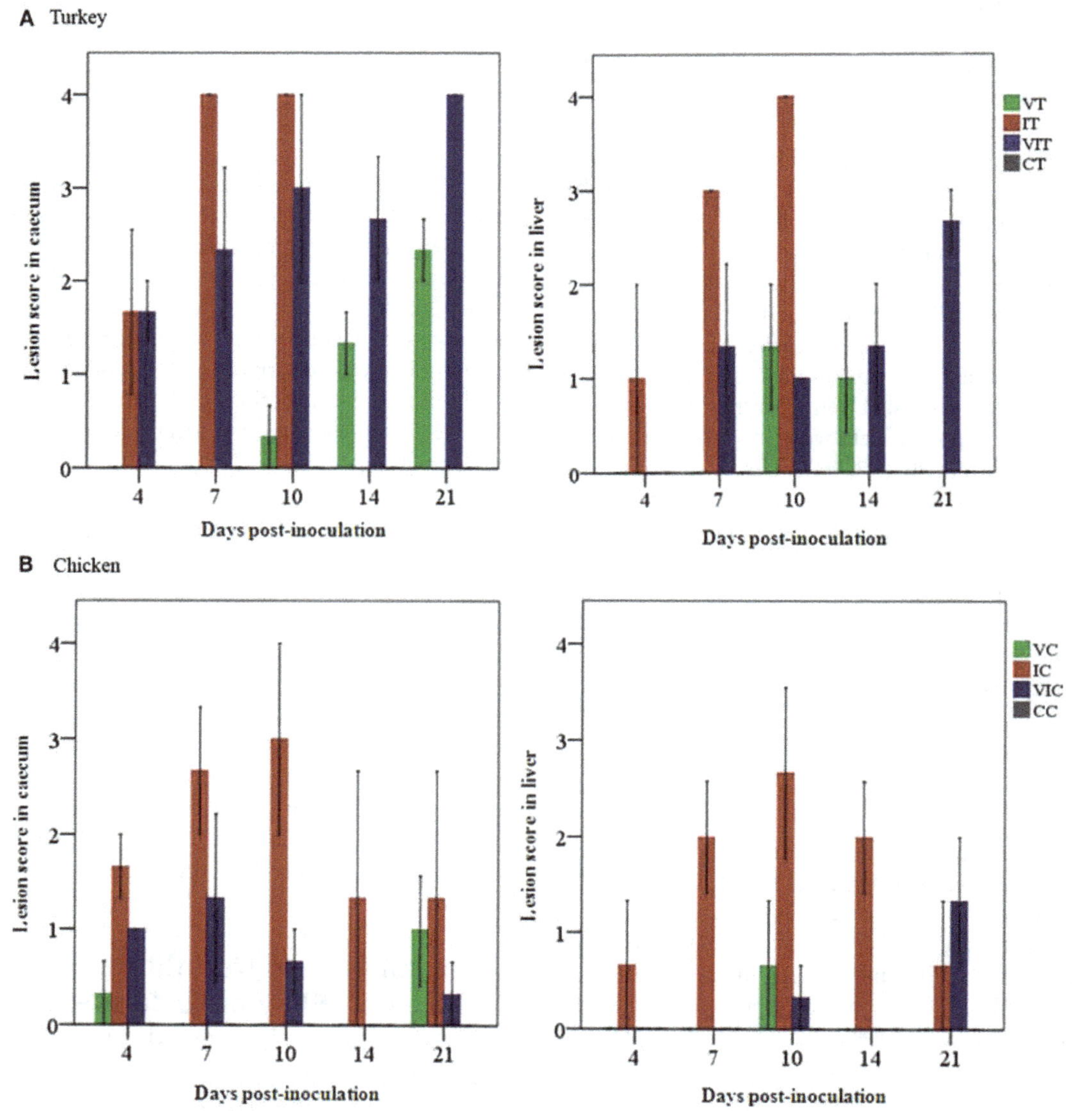

FIGURE 1 | Mean lesion scores ($n = 3$ birds/day) recorded in cecum and liver. Scores were graded from 0 to 4, indicating no lesion to severe lesion in **(A)** groups of vaccinated turkeys (VT), infected turkeys (IT) and vaccinated and infected turkeys (VIT) and in **(B)** groups of vaccinated chickens (VC), infected chickens (IC), or vaccinated and infected chickens (VIC) necropsied at different days post-inoculation. There were no lesions observed in control turkeys or chickens (CT or CC) throughout the time points.

of positive cells started out like mentioned above for the other groups. However, at 4 DPI, the percentage of cells was slightly higher than in the control, albeit statistically not significant. From 7 DPI onward, the cecal wall had infiltrated mononuclear cells with IFN-γ mRNA positive cells sporadically distributed among them. Calculation of positive cells, however, was more or less similar to birds from the control group.

In the liver of VT and CT, stained cells could be found as lymphoid aggregates and sporadically between hepatocytes. There was no change in the spatial distribution until 21 DPI when two liver samples of VT showed a restricted yet ectopic lymphoid alteration in one area with few positive cells interspersed within. Despite the similarity in the spatial distributions of stained cells in these groups, relative numbers of cells (**Figure 4A**) were higher in VT from 7 DPI onward with significant changes observed at 10 and 14 DPI. In IT, changes, both in the location and percentage of positive cells, were different at and after 7 DPI when positive cells were observed within the inflammatory infiltrates between the parenchyma and periphery of necrotized regions. The percentage of these cells was also significantly higher at 10 DPI. Positive cells in livers of VIT were similar to CT, both in location and abundance.

In spleen, positive cells had a wider spatial distribution ranging from aggregates in the periarteriolar lymphatic sheath to solitary cells in the rest of white and red pulp, regardless of the experimental treatment. Percentages of positive cells (**Figure 4A**), however, significantly decreased in VIT at 14 DPI, whereas the changes in the other groups were not statistically supported.

The location of positive cells in cecum, liver and spleen of control and affected tissues described in turkeys also applies to chickens and differences among the groups of chickens were mostly marginal. In VC, however, there was neither a location nor a percentage change in the relative numbers of positive cells in caeca throughout the experiment (**Figure 4B**). In caeca of IC, positive cells extensively spread to the lamina propria as the disease progressed at and after 7 DPI. Similarly, in VIC, a localized yet infiltrated area with positive cells was observed only at 7 DPI. Livers of VC and VIC were similar to control birds throughout the experiment, whereas positive cells were observed in infiltrates of leukocytes of affected livers of IC collected at 14 and 21 DPI. In spleen, the only noticeable changes were the significantly decreased percentage of positive cells in the spleens of IC and VIC at 21 DPI.

TABLE 4 | Number of samples positive for *Histomonas meleagridis* detected by *in situ* hybridization (n = 3 birds/day).

		Vaccinated DPI					Infected DPI					Vaccinated and infected DPI				
		4	**7**	**10**	**14**	**21**	**4**	**7**	**10**	**14**	**21**	**4**	**7**	**10**	**14**	**21**
Turkey	Cecum	0	3	3	2	2	3	3	3	N/A	N/A	3	3	3	2	2
	Liver	0	0	0	0	1	3	3	3	N/A	N/A	0	1	1	0	1
Chicken	Cecum	0	1	2	0	0	1	2	2	1	1	2	1	1	2	0
	Liver	0	0	0	0	0	0	1	2	0	0	0	0	0	0	0

DPI, days post-inoculation.

Spatial and Temporal Distribution Differences of Quantified IL-13 mRNA Positive Cells

The localization of IL-13 mRNA positive cells in turkeys and chickens was similar to the distributional localization of IFN-γ mRNA positive cells described for each group and DPI. The percentage of positive cells, however, varied at different DPI.

In turkeys (**Figure 5A**), the percentage of IL-13 mRNA positive cells increased in the cecum of VT from 7DPI onward; the only significant change, however, was the higher percentage at 10 DPI. Positive cells also increased in caeca of IT at 7 and 10 DPI; these changes nevertheless were not statistically significant. By contrast, the percentage of positive cells showed no change or was lower in VIT throughout the trial when positive cells significantly decreased at 10 and 14 DPI. In livers, the percentage of positive cells significantly increased in VT as well as IT at 10 DPI. In spleens, even though the percentages increased variably in VT and IT at and after 7 DPI, the changes were not statistically significant. By contrast, the percentage significantly decreased in spleens of VIT at 10 and 14 DPI.

In chickens, changes in the percentage of IL-13 mRNA positive cells (**Figure 5B**) were not significant, but slight changes could be noticed at 4 DPI when positive cells increased in the cecum of VC and VIC as well as in spleens of VC.

Comparison of Quantified IFN-γ or IL-13 mRNA Positive Cells

Comparison of percentages of cytokine mRNA positive cells highlighted a varying magnitude in the abundance of cells expressing

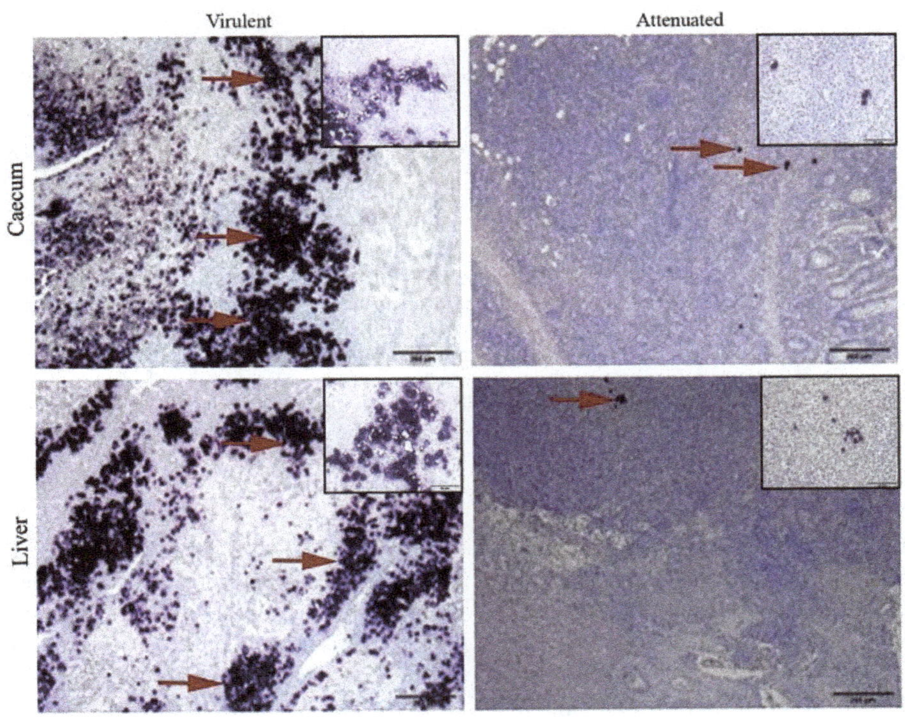

FIGURE 2 | Virulent and attenuated histomonads localized in cecum and liver by *in situ* hybridization. Stained histomonads could be seen in dark purple (examples shown in red arrow). Virulent histomonads could be seen in larger number, whereas only a few attenuated histomonads could be detected surrounded by an influx of mononuclear cells. Samples are representatives for tissues collected from turkeys inoculated with virulent histomonads (group infected turkey) necropsied on 10 days post-inoculation (DPI) and turkeys inoculated with only attenuated histomonads (group vaccinated turkeys) necropsied on 21 DPI. Insets show higher magnifications of histomonads and the surrounding cells in the respective tissue sample.

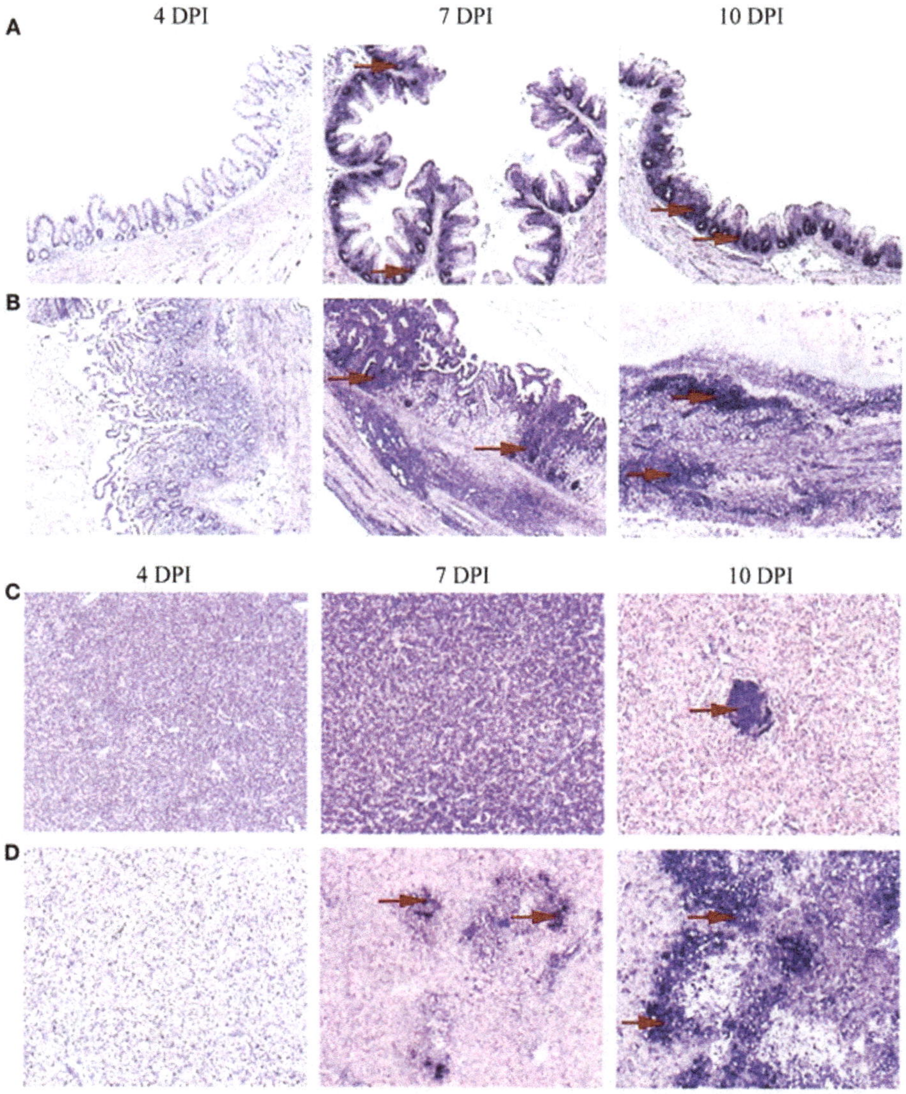

FIGURE 3 | Distribution of interferon gamma (IFN-γ) mRNA positive cells localized by *in situ* hybridization in cecum and liver. A distinct distribution pattern of cytokine mRNA positive cells in the primarily affected organs was evident between groups of turkeys that received only attenuated parasites and those inoculated with virulent *Histomonas meleagridis*. Representative distribution patterns are given using IFN-γ mRNA positive cells with areas of positive cells indicated by red arrows. At 4 days post-inoculation (DPI), positive cells were rarely distributed in caeca which then became abundant at 7 and 10 DPI with accumulation of positive cells being restricted to the lamina propria of birds that receive the attenuated culture **(A)**, whereas virulent histomonads triggered further distribution of positive cells to the muscularis layer with losing of the mucosal fold at 10 DPI **(B)**. In livers, positive cells were occasionally found as sporadic cells studded between hepatocytes and lymphoid aggregates **(C)** or in more expansive distribution comprising mononuclear infiltrates when affected by virulent histomonads **(D)**.

mRNA of IFN-γ or IL-13 pertinent to the inoculum, tissue type and host species. In turkeys (**Figure 6A**), there was a comparable level of IFN-γ and IL-13 mRNA positive cells within each type of tissue independent of the treatment group. Generally, spleen had the highest percentage of IFN-γ and IL-13 mRNA positive cells, followed by cecum whereas liver had the least percentage.

In contrast to turkeys, chicken tissues showed a divergent percentage of IFN-γ and IL-13 mRNA positive cells. Chicken IFN-γ mRNA positive cells were found to be more abundant than IL-13 mRNA positive cells in cecum and spleen of all the experimental groups (**Figure 6B**). Both tissues had more IFN-γ and IL-13 mRNA positive cells than liver. In contrast to cecum and spleen, a balanced percentage of IFN-γ and IL-13 mRNA positive cells was detected in livers of chickens, with an exception of the slight increment IFN-γ mRNA positive cells at 10 DPI in livers of VC.

Comparing percentages of cytokine mRNA positive cells between tissues of turkeys and chickens also revealed variations in the percentages of positive cells. The most obvious differences were observed in IFN-γ mRNA positive cells in the cecum and spleen of VIC and CC when compared with their counterpart turkey groups (VIT and CT).

Changes in Immune Cell Population in Chickens During Vaccination or Infection

B cells, T cells and monocytes/macrophages stained by IF in the cecum, liver and spleen cryosections of chickens from trial

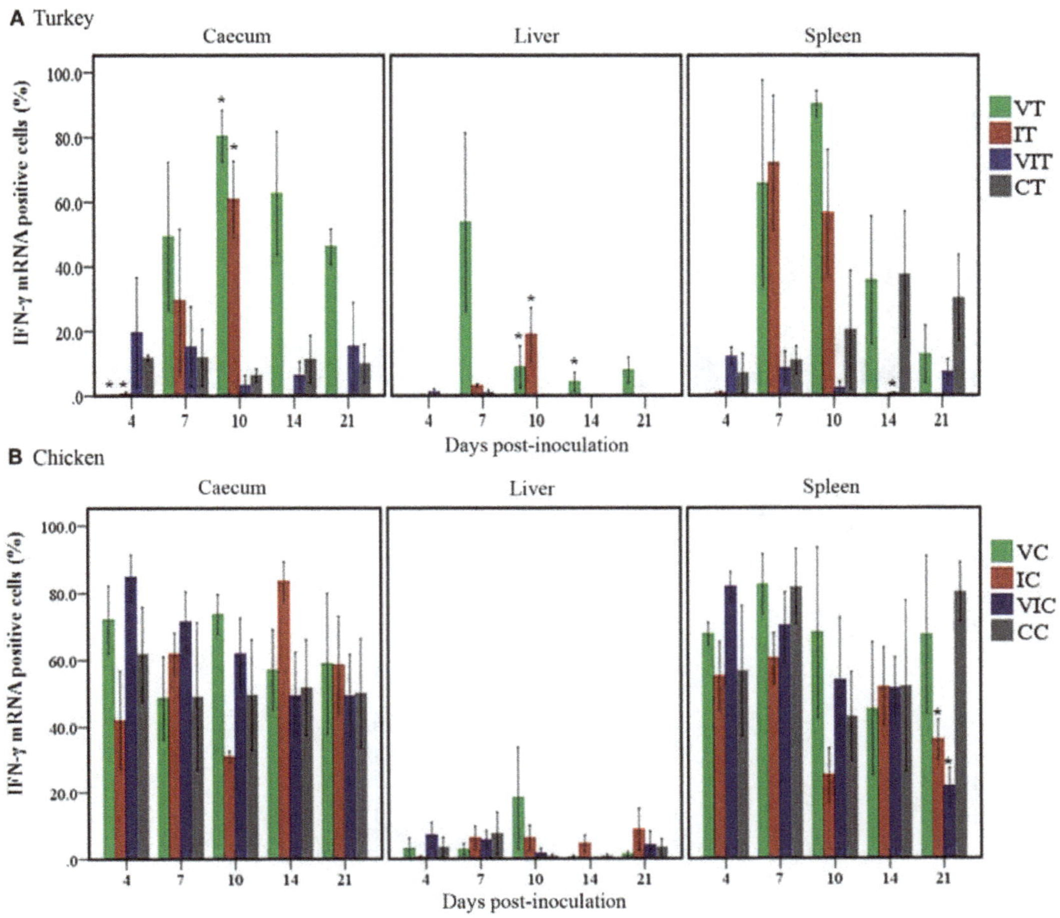

FIGURE 4 | Quantity of interferon gamma (IFN-γ) mRNA positive cells. Positive cells were quantified by TissueFAXS and its accompanying software HistoQuest in cecum, liver and spleen of turkeys **(A)** and chickens **(B)** inoculated with attenuated and/or virulent *Histomonas meleagridis*. Mean values of percentages of mRNA positive cells in each treatment group were compared with the age-matched control at the respective days post-inoculation. $n = 3$ birds/day, $^{*}P < 0.05$.

2 inoculated with either virulent or attenuated histomonads revealed changes in the population of these cells at different days post-inoculation (**Figure 7**). Quantification of the stained cells (**Figure 8**) showed distinct changes in IC which had an increased percentage of B cells, T cells and monocytes/macrophages in cecum at 4, 7 and 10 DPI as wall as in the liver at 10 and 14 DPI. By contrast, spleens of the same group showed decrement of B cells at 7 and 14 DPI and T cells from 4 DPI until 21 DPI. The levels in VCs were very similar to the control.

Fold Changes in the Expression Levels of IFN-γ and IL-13 mRNA Measured by RT-qPCR

Expression levels of IFN-γ and IL-13 mRNA were measured from samples collected at 10 and 21 DPI to supplement results obtained by quantification of the expressing cells. In most cases, results of RT-qPCR harmonized with quantification of cells.

In turkeys, cecal IFN-γ mRNA (**Figure 9A**) was upregulated in all of the inoculated groups sampled at 10 and 21 DPI although the only statistically significant change was noticed in caeca of VIT at 10 DPI. Similarly, a significant fold change was found at 10 DPI in liver and spleen of IT. By contrast, the expression was significantly downregulated at 21 DPI in spleens of VIT. In chickens (**Figure 9B**), cecal IFN-γ mRNA was significantly upregulated in IC at 10 DPI and in all groups at 21 DPI. Livers of IC also had a significantly enhanced expression at 10 DPI, whereas the changes in the other groups were lower. The expression was significantly downregulated in spleens of VC and VIC at 10 and 21 DPI.

Turkey IL-13 mRNA (**Figure 9C**) transcripts were significantly upregulated in the cecum of IT and VIT at 10 DPI. Similarly, an enhanced expression was found at 21 DPI in VT and VIT. In livers, a significant increment of expression was found in IT sampled at 10 DPI. In spleens, IL-13 transcripts showed increased fold changes at 10 DPI in IC and at 21 DPI in VT and VIT. In chickens, IL-13 expression (**Figure 9D**) was downregulated at 10 DPI in all caeca samples drawn from inoculated groups although the changes were not significant. The downregulation projected into a significant upregulation of the transcript at 21 DPI in all the groups with significant changes observed in VC and VIC. In livers, a significantly enhanced expression was observed at 10 DPI

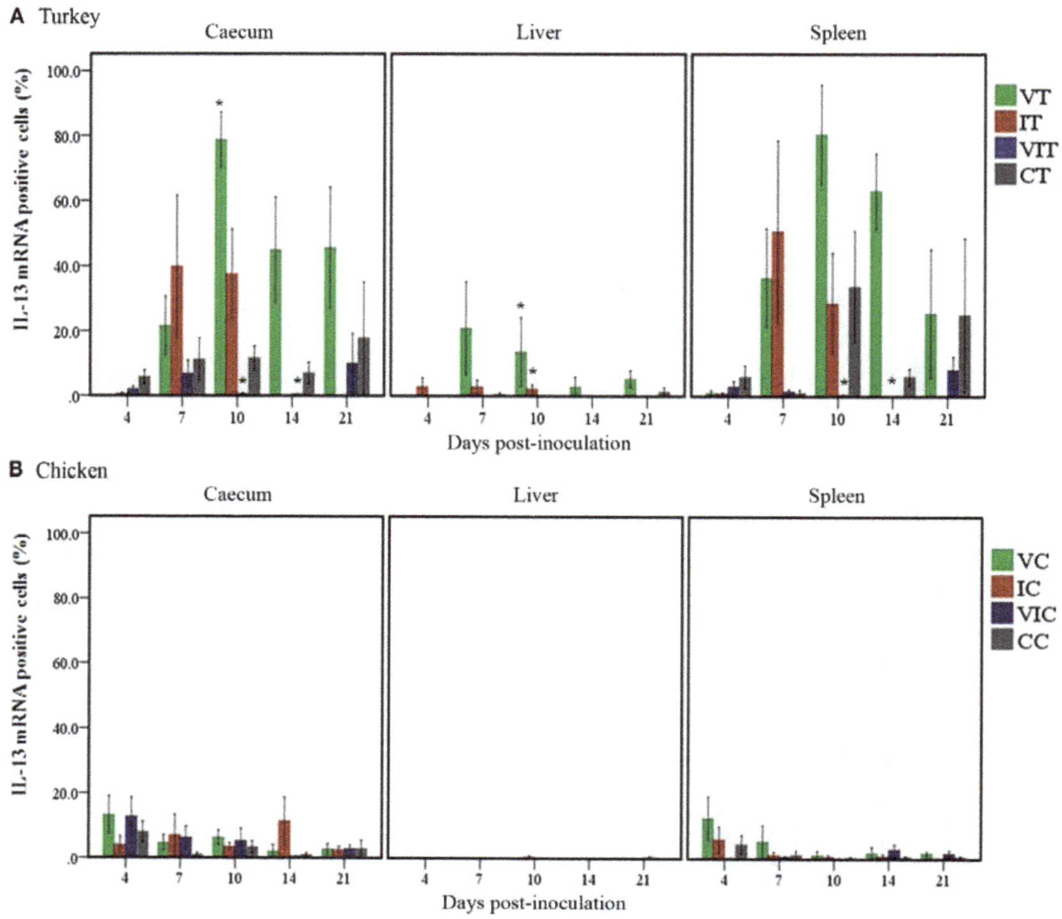

FIGURE 5 | Quantity of interleukin (IL)-13 mRNA positive cells. Positive cells were quantified in caeca, livers and spleens of groups of turkeys **(A)** and chickens **(B)** inoculated with attenuated and/or virulent *Histomonas meleagridis*. Mean percentage obtained from each treatment group was compared with the age-matched control. $n = 3$ birds/day, $^*P < 0.05$.

in VC. In spleen, the transcript was significantly downregulated in VIC at 21 DPI.

DISCUSSION

The present study quantified cells that express the mRNA of representative cytokines of type 1 and type 2 immune responses, IFN-γ, respectively, IL-13 in cecum, liver and spleen samples for elucidating cytokine expression patterns that could be attributed to vaccination or infection of turkeys and chickens with clonal cultures of *H. meleagridis*. Groups of birds were inoculated with virulent or attenuated histomonads and necropsied at different time points post-inoculation. The time points were selected based on a previous study in which cecal lesions in affected chicken reached the maximum on days 7–14 after infection and then regresses at 21 DPI (21).

Previously, the safety of the vaccine has been tested by administering 10^4 cultured histomonads exclusively *via* the oral route for turkeys and with an additional dose of 10^4 parasites cloacally to chickens. Challenges were tested in turkeys with 10^4 parasites administered by the cloaca route only (5–7). The birds in the main experiment of this study were inoculated with a 3×10^5 histomonads administrated both orally and cloacally which proved the tentative vaccine safe as noticed in vaccinated hosts together with the capability of inducing a potent immunity during challenge.

The distribution of attenuated histomonads was confined to the cecum in the majority of the samples investigated by ISH, which was in agreement with previous findings (6). On the other hand, virulent histomonads migrated further to the livers of all unprotected turkeys were a much more pronounced invasion as compared to livers of unprotected chickens. The differential kinetics in dissemination patterns of virulent histomonads in livers of turkeys and chickens was comparable to a previous study (12). However, the absence of histomonads in the spleen of all experimental birds was in contrast to a previous finding that demonstrated virulent parasites by ISH in a few spleen sections (27). This could be due to the higher dose of histomonads used in the past study which was 19 times higher per bird than in the present study.

This study employed a simultaneous assessment of localization of cytokine mRNA expressing cells and their quantitative differences in response to attenuated and virulent histomonads.

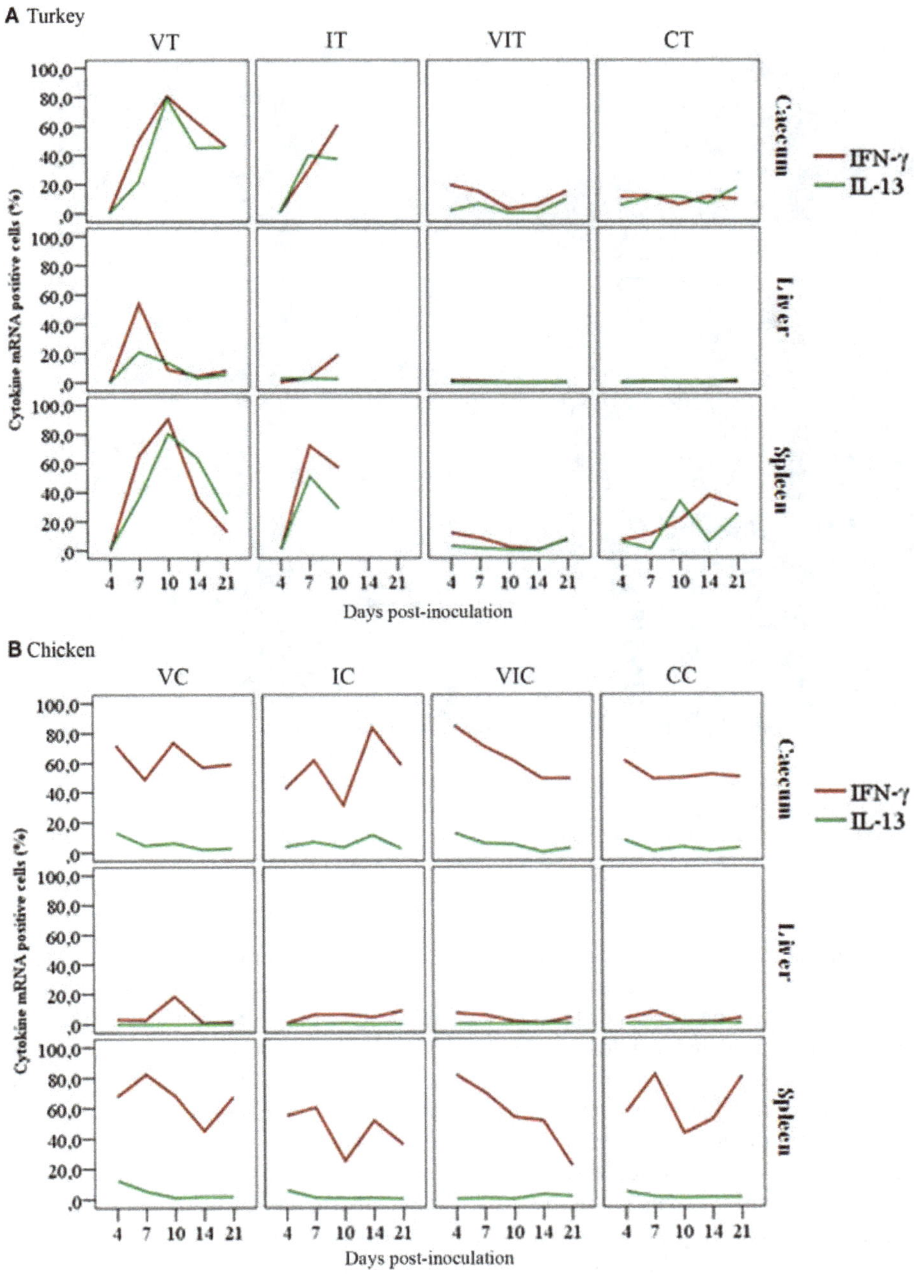

FIGURE 6 | Comparison of cytokine mRNA positive cells show a varying magnitude in the abundance of cells expressing mRNA of interferon gamma (IFN-γ) or interleukin (IL)-13. Panel **(A)** shows the percentage of turkey IFN-γ mRNA positive cells was comparable with IL-13 mRNA positive cells within the respective tissue types, regardless of their treatment condition with slight variations at different days post-inoculation. As indicated in panel **(B)**, the overall percentage of chicken IFN-γ mRNA positive cells was higher compared to the percentage of IL-13 mRNA positive cells in cecum and spleen of the respective groups throughout the trial. Remarkable differences can also be seen in the relative number of IFN-γ mRNA positive cells between cecum of control birds, turkeys (CT) and chickens (CC), with $n = 3$ birds/day.

Results showed that IFN-γ mRNA positive cells increased in the cecum of vaccinated turkeys without compromising the integrity of the tissue. By contrast, virulent histomonads caused tissue destruction along with the exacerbated increment of positive cells after a decrement of positive cells at 4 DPI. The low percentage of positive cells at this early stages in IT was in agreement with the downregulation observed by Powell et al. (12) who measured the transcript via RT-qPCR. In the present study, no data on RT-qPCR of cytokine expression were determined which limits the direct comparison. However, the authors of the last mentioned study observed a delay in cytokine response of ITs at 3 DPI which later increased to a storm of cytokines after the parasite could migrate to the liver leading to destruction of cecum and liver tissues. In concordance with this, findings of the present work showed that

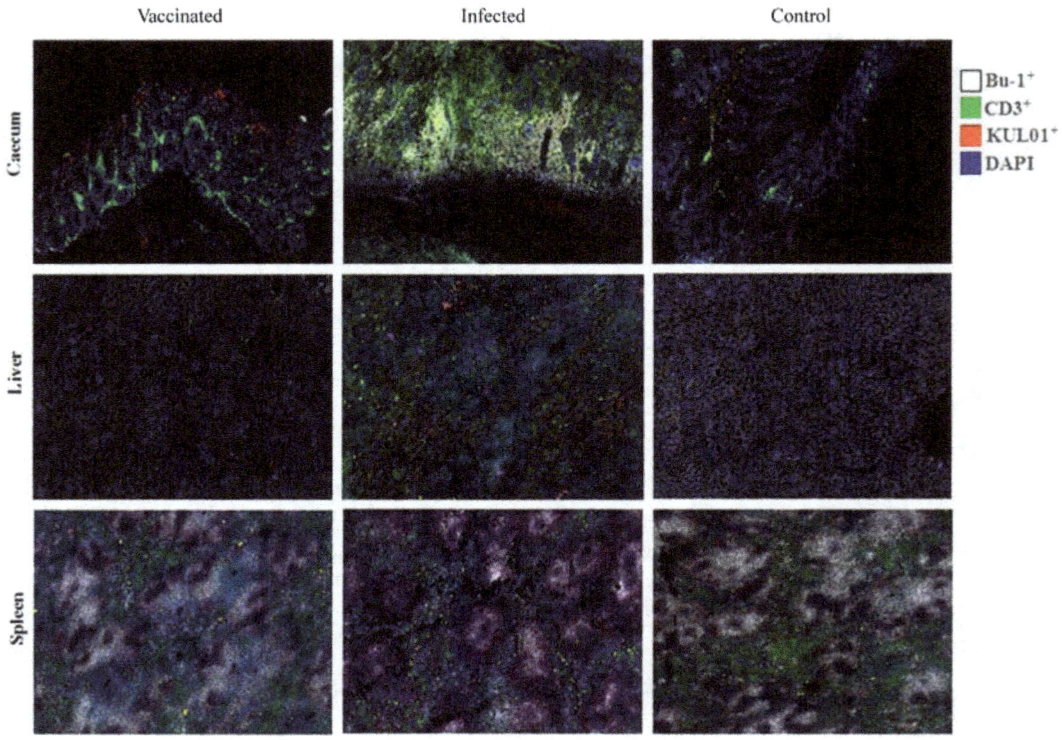

FIGURE 7 | B cells (Bu-1+), T cells (CD3+) and monocytes/macrophages (KUL01+) detected by immunofluorescence in tissues of chickens. An increase of B and T cells in the mucosa of the cecum [4 days post-inoculation (DPI)] and the liver (14 DPI) of infected chickens (inoculated with only virulent histomonads) is indicated by a higher intensity of the respective fluorochromes. By contrast, fluorescent signals of the lymphocytes in the spleen (14 DPI) are comparatively reduced in the same group.

the attenuation of the protozoa allowed the host to project the appropriate immune response without inducing tissue damage. Hence, an effective stimulation of cytokine expression that does not result in tissue damage can be considered as a desirable trait of vaccination with *in vitro* attenuated *H. meleagridis*.

In general, vaccination induces a restricted immune response to develop appropriate local and/or systemic immunity. In the present experiment, vaccinated and challenged turkeys showed a slight increment of IFN-γ mRNA positive cells in the caeca at 4 DPI. This finding indicates that the vaccine provided priming of the immune system against invading virulent histomonads. The fact that the response was shortly activated at the site of infection argues for the presence of effector memory T cells as this cell population is known to counteract re-infection by secreting antimicrobial cytokines such as IFN-γ and TNF-α (28).

The absence of any distinct separation in the relative levels of IFN-γ and IL-13 mRNA expressing cells in turkeys suggests that both type 1 and type 2 immune responses have been elicited during vaccination or infection. This could be due to the protozoa's mixed host-cellular niche. Even though it is known as an extracellular protozoan, immunohistochemical localization of the parasite in turkey liver revealed that it could occasionally be detected within host cells, mostly phagocytized by macrophages and giant cells (29). Previously, a strict intracellular pathogen (Newcastle disease virus) and extracellular helminth, *Ascaridia galli*, have been shown to cause a polarized type of cytokine expression in chickens (30).

In contrast to turkeys, a higher percentage of IFN-γ mRNA positive cells than IL-13 mRNA were noticed in chickens, regardless of the treatment conditions. Past studies on infection with virulent *H. meleagridis* or dual infection with the cecal nematode, *Heterakis gallinarum*, delivered inconclusive results in regards to type 1/type 2 responses in chicken cecal tonsils or cecum. Quantification of IFN-γ or IL-13 mRNA by RT-qPCR in cecal tonsils of turkeys and chickens infected with *H. meleagridis* inoculum prepared from an infected tissue homogenate showed a development of type 2 response with IL-13 expression although other cytokines including IFN-γ were also enhanced (12). By contrast, a dominance of type 1 response with augmented expression of IFN-γ was noticed in chicken cecum dually infected with *H. meleagridis* and *H. gallinarum* (18). Our data on the predominance of IFN-γ in chicken tissues in response to clonal cultures of histomonads was in agreement with the gene expression studies of dual infections by Schwarz et al. (18), highlighting a type 1 response in this species. Chickens probably enhance IL-13 expression only upon the encounter of the relevant pathogen. Expression of IL-13 in this species, compared to the turkeys, could be stricter, particularly in non-lymphoid tissues (31, 32). Thus, factors such as mRNA decay rate and an inter species difference in the regulation of both cytokines should be considered and explored further for defining a threshold of measurement.

In mammals, the balance between Th1/Th2 lymphocytes subsets, the main sources of signature cytokines of type 1/type 2

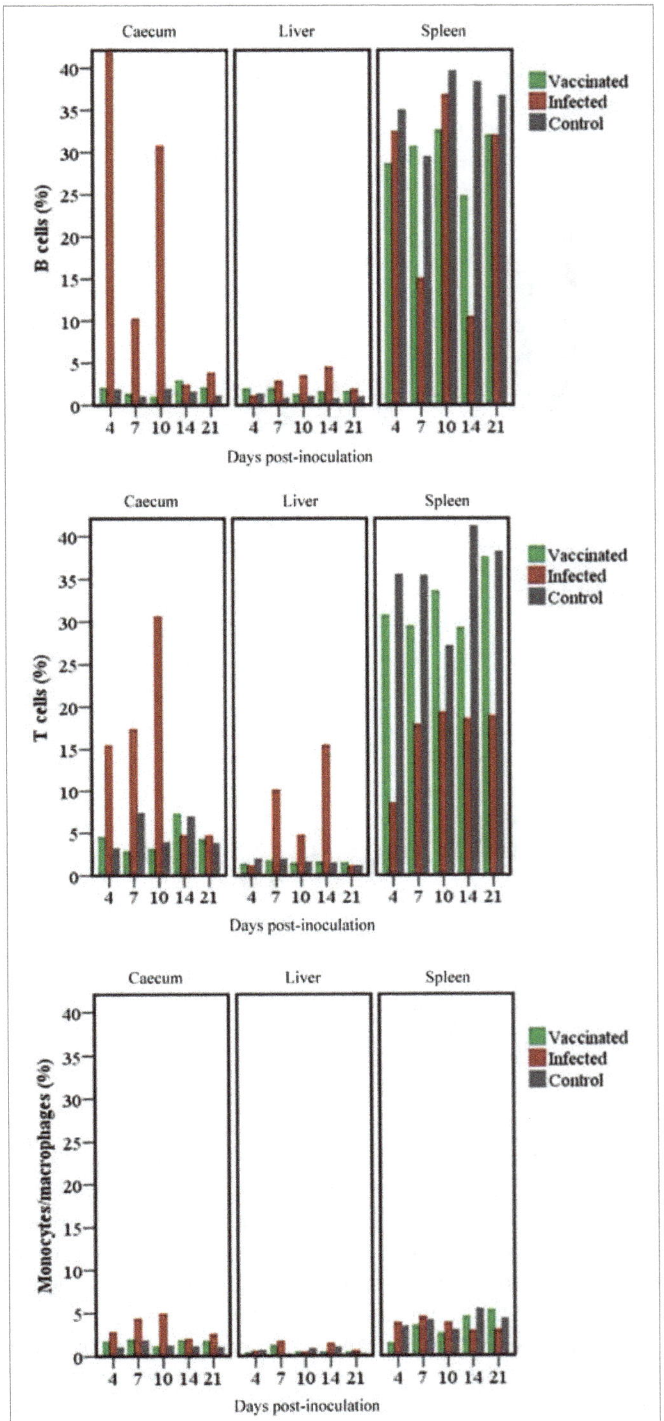

FIGURE 8 | Changes in B cells, T cells and monocytes/macrophages stained in cecum, livers and spleens of chickens. Analysis of the relative number of target cells was performed using TissueQuest after an automated image acquisition with TissueFAXS in tissues of groups of chickens inoculated with only attenuated (vaccinated) or virulent (infected) *Histomonas meleagridis*. Samples were drawn from a single chicken per group for the different days post-inoculation.

immunity, determines susceptibility to some disease states (16). In this context, the presence of a higher percentage of IFN-γ mRNA positive cells in the avian cecum seems to correlate with protection against histomonosis as noticed in chickens and vaccinated turkeys. In a study focusing on an extracellular intestinal protozoan parasite of humans, *Entameba histolytica*, it was demonstrated that asymptomatic carriers of the pathogen had higher levels of IFN-γ, reflecting a Th1 response, while patients showing disease displayed higher levels of IL-4, resembling that of a Th2 response (33). The study further revealed that re-infection in vaccinated mice was mediated by IFN-γ-producing $CD4^+$ T cells and IL-17 secreting $CD8^+$ T cells. Overall, in the mentioned study, IFN-γ was shown to enhance anti-parasitic activity in macrophages, which might be as well an important mechanism in the immune response against histomonosis of poultry. It is worth mentioning here that the mammalian key type 2 cytokine, IL-4, has been shown in the avian immune system to be less expressed compared to IL-13 in several extracellular infection models (12, 18, 23, 30, 34), hence measuring IL-13 was opted in the current study.

An important observation in the actual study was the difference in the percentage of IFN-γ mRNA positive cells in CC compared to CT. Reasons to this could be diverse and would demand research based verification. It can, however, be speculated that growth-selected turkey lines might have a trade-off between immune function and growth. Previous metanalysis on various poultry lines selected for increased growth showed a strong and significant decrease in immune function (35). In this regard, the higher surface-area abundance of these cells in the chicken cecum might be one of the reasons why this species is less susceptible to histomonosis. Their well-equipped caeca might make them immunologically competent to ward-off the protozoa at the port of entry. With this observation, it can be assumed that the presence of IFN-γ in cecum is supportive in the defense against histomonads as was shown enhancing resistance against coccidiosis (36) and *E. coli* (37) challenge. Even though further studies are needed to elucidate the specific effector function of this enhanced percentage of cells during vaccination or infection with histomonads, several effects of the cytokine might play a role in the immune response against the parasite. IFN-γ is known to promote cell-mediated immunity through activation of macrophages for phagocytosis (17). Moreover, it has been shown to stimulate secondary IgG response and enhance the expression of the genes for MHC class II in chickens (38). These traits can endow the hosts with an immune response that can better present histomonad antigens as well as efficiently fight infection.

Avian IFN-γ can be presumably be produced by macrophages, dendritic cells, $CD4^+$ and $CD8^+$ T cells, like in mammals (39–42). Recently, IFN-γ producing innate B lymphocytes have also been characterized in mice that produce high levels of IFN-γ that promotes macrophage activation, facilitating the innate immune response during early stages of infection (43). Likewise, various innate and adaptive stages of immune cells can synthesize IL-13. Hematopoietic cells of the innate immune system such as eosinophils, basophils and mast cells have been shown to produce IL-13 in mice (44). In addition, Th2 ($CD4^+$) cells are described as the main source of IL-13 during the effector phase of type 2 immune responses in worm-infested mice (45). In this study, the cellular background of the cytokine mRNAs could not be directly demonstrated due to the lack of immune cell markers for turkeys

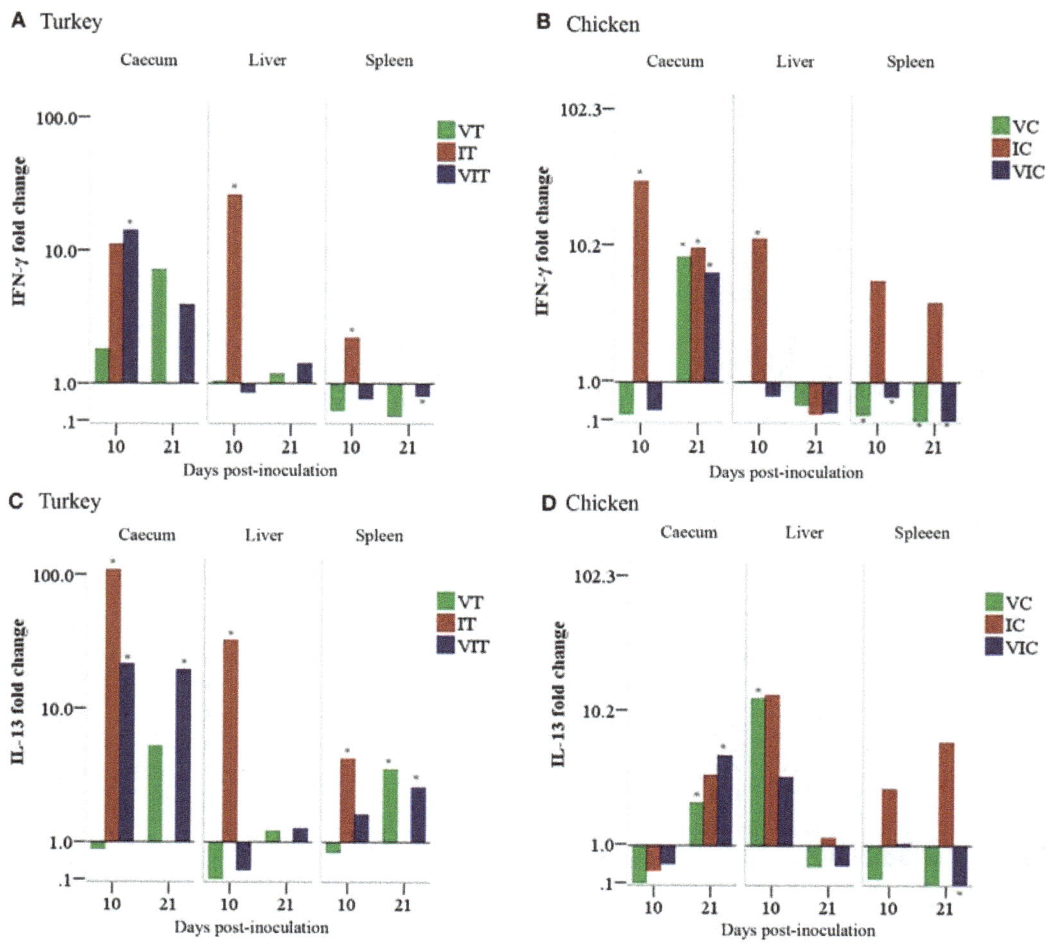

FIGURE 9 | Cytokine mRNA expression levels measured by reverse transcription-qPCR. The expression level of interferon gamma (IFN-γ) in tissues of turkeys **(A)** and chickens **(B)** as well as the expression level of interleukin (IL)-13 in tissues of turkeys **(C)** and chickens **(D)** are shown as a fold change of mRNA expression levels relative to age-matched controls. $n = 3$ birds/day, $*P < 0.05$.

and the incompatibility of the staining techniques. However, interpretation of the IF results in context of the cytokine ISH results in chickens indicate that more cell types than B cells, T cells and macrophages could be involved in producing the cytokines as the percentages of cytokine-expressing cells were higher than the immune cells quantified by IF. Nevertheless, this indication needs to be verified in prospective studies by establishing a technique enabling co-staining of cytokines and cell markers.

This study employed RT-qPCR on samples taken from selected days to observe the congruence of mRNA quantification results with that of quantification of ISH stained cells. The high percentage of IFN-γ mRNA positive cells in the cecum of VT and IT coinciding with an enhanced expression of IFN-γ mRNA at 10 DPI demonstrated the agreement of the results. By contrast, some discrepancies were observed for instance with the increased percentages of IFN-γ mRNA positive cells in liver and spleen of VT in comparison to the RT-qPCR results of both tissues at 10 DPI. The discrepancies may arise from the difference in the detection system of both techniques. ISH labels mRNA positive cells and a higher percentage indicates a wider distribution of positive cells in a given area, whereas PCR amplifies a pooled mRNA extracted from a myriad of cells which may have more or no expressed transcript. Hence, a result of a high percentage of positive cells with a low or moderate amount of the transcript might be underestimated by fewer numbers containing a higher quantity of the transcript and *vice versa* (46).

In conclusion, immunization of turkeys using *in vitro* attenuated *H. meleagridis* causes an increased percentage of IFN-γ and IL-13 mRNA positive cells in the cecum of turkeys without compromising the integrity of the tissue. Infection in non-immunized turkeys also induced an increased presence of cytokine mRNA positive cells in cecum following an early decrement but with severe destruction of the mucosa, as well as infiltration of cytokine-expressing cells up to the muscularis layer with similar destruction and cytokine distribution in livers. Overall, the cytokine expression pattern in turkeys followed both type 1 and type 2 cytokine response with attenuated and virulent histomonads. The higher percentage of IFN-γ mRNA positive cells in chicken cecum than turkeys might also be implicated in the differential survival of this species during histomonosis.

Consequently, since a higher percentage of IFN-γ mRNA positive cells have been observed in chickens as well as in immunized turkeys capable to defend histomonosis with early expression of IFN-γ mRNA, it can be concluded that increased presence of IFN-γ mRNA positive cells indicates a protective trait against histomonosis.

AUTHOR CONTRIBUTIONS

DL, MH and FK conceived and designed the work. FK, TM, DL and PW performed the animal trial and collection of samples. FK and PW performed ISH and IF experiments. FK and DL performed image acquisition and analysis. TM performed and analyzed the RT-qPCR. FK and DL interpreted the data and drafted the manuscript. MH revised the manuscript critically for important intellectual content. All authors read and approved the final manuscript.

ACKNOWLEDGMENTS

The authors are thankful to Prof. Erika Jensen-Jarolim and Sarah Meitz from Department of Comparative Medicine, Messerli Research Institute, University of Veterinary Medicine Vienna, for providing access and assistance to use their TissueFAXS platform. The authors also acknowledge the VetCore Facility for research, University of Veterinary Medicine Vienna, for providing 4200 TapeStation (Agilent) to control the quality of the RNA samples used in this study.

SUPPLEMENTARY MATERIAL

FIGURE S1 | Quantification strategy for cytokine mRNA positive cells detected by bright field microscopy and TissueFAXS image acquisition. The image is given exemplary from a single region of interest in cecum, liver and spleen tissue sections after *in situ* hybridization (ISH) staining with turkey interferon gamma antisense probe. Original bright field microscopy images **(A)**, setting a cutoff value to discriminate ISH (NBT-BCIP) positive cells **(B)** and backward viewing **(C)** to verify the correct discrimination of ISH positive (red mask) and negative cells (green mask) of the source image.

FIGURE S2 | Attenuated histomonads localized by *in situ* hybridization in the cecum of turkeys necropsied at 10 days post-inoculation showing the parasites restricted to the lumen of the cecum.

REFERENCES

1. Smith T. An infectious disease among turkeys caused by protozoa (infectious entero-hepatitis). *US Dep Agric Bur Anim Ind Bull* (1895) 8:1–38.
2. McDougald LR. Blackhead disease (histomoniasis) in poultry: a critical review. *Avian Dis* (2005) 49:462–76. doi:10.1637/7420-081005R.1
3. Hess M, Liebhart D, Bilic I, Ganas P. *Histomonas meleagridis*—new insights into an old pathogen. *Vet Parasitol* (2015) 208:67–76. doi:10.1016/j.vetpar.2014.12.018
4. Tyzzer EE. The flagellate character and reclassification of the parasite producing "blackhead" in Turkeys: *Histomonas* (Gen. nov.) *meleagridis* (Smith). *J Parasitol* (1920) 6:124. doi:10.2307/3271065
5. Hess M, Liebhart D, Grabensteiner E, Singh A. Cloned *Histomonas meleagridis* passaged *in vitro* resulted in reduced pathogenicity and is capable of protecting turkeys from histomonosis. *Vaccine* (2008) 26:4187–93. doi:10.1016/j.vaccine.2008.05.071
6. Liebhart D, Zahoor MA, Prokofieva I, Hess M. Safety of avirulent histomonads to be used as a vaccine determined in turkeys and chickens. *Poult Sci* (2011) 90:996–1003. doi:10.3382/ps.2010-01255
7. Sulejmanovic T, Liebhart D, Hess M. *In vitro* attenuated *Histomonas meleagridis* does not revert to virulence, following serial *in vivo* passages in turkeys or chickens. *Vaccine* (2013) 31:5443–50. doi:10.1016/j.vaccine.2013.08.098
8. Liebhart D, Ganas P, Sulejmanovic T, Hess M. Histomonosis in poultry: previous and current strategies for prevention and therapy. *Avian Pathol* (2017) 46:1–18. doi:10.1080/03079457.2016.1229458
9. Bleyen N, Ons E, De Gussem M, Goddeeris BM. Passive immunization against *Histomonas meleagridis* does not protect turkeys from an experimental infection. *Avian Pathol* (2009) 38:71–6. doi:10.1080/03079450802641255
10. Clarkson MJ. Immunological responses to *Histomonas meleagridis* in the Turkey and Fowl. *Immunology* (1963) 6:156–68.
11. Windisch M, Hess M. Experimental infection of chickens with *Histomonas meleagridis* confirms the presence of antibodies in different parts of the intestine. *Parasite Immunol* (2010) 32:29–35. doi:10.1111/j.1365-3024.2009.01159.x
12. Powell FL, Rothwell L, Clarkson MJ, Kaiser P. The turkey, compared to the chicken, fails to mount an effective early immune response to *Histomonas meleagridis* in the gut. *Parasite Immunol* (2009) 31:312–27. doi:10.1111/j.1365-3024.2009.01113.x
13. Mitra T, Gerner W, Kidane FA, Wernsdorf P, Hess M, Saalmüller A, et al. Vaccination against histomonosis limits pronounced changes of B cells and T-cell subsets in turkeys and chickens. *Vaccine* (2017) 35:4184–96. doi:10.1016/j.vaccine.2017.06.035
14. Yip HC, Karulin AY, Tary-Lehmann M, Hesse MD, Radeke H, Heeger PS, et al. Adjuvant-guided type-1 and type-2 immunity: infectious/noninfectious dichotomy defines the class of response Hualin. *J Immunol* (1999) 162:3942–9.
15. Kaiser P, Stäheli P. Avian cytokines and chemokines. In: Schat KA, Kaspers B, Kaiser P, editors. *Avian Immunology*. San Diego, CA: Elsevier Science Publishing (2013). p. 189–204.
16. Kidd P. Th1/Th2 balance: the hypothesis, its limitations, and implications for health and disease. *Altern Med Rev* (2003) 8:223–46.
17. Schijns VEJC, van de Zande S, Lupiani B, Reddy SM. Practical aspects of poultry vaccination. In: Schat KA, Kaspers B, Kaiser P, editors. *Avian Immunology*. San Diego, CA: Elsevier Science Publishing (2013). p. 345–62.
18. Schwarz A, Gauly M, Abel H, Daş G, Humburg J, Weiss ATA, et al. Pathobiology of *Heterakis gallinarum* mono-infection and co-infection with *Histomonas meleagridis* in layer chickens. *Avian Pathol* (2011) 40:277–87. doi:10.1080/03079457.2011.561280
19. Hess M, Kolbe T, Grabensteiner E, Prosl H. Clonal cultures of *Histomonas meleagridis*, *Tetratrichomonas gallinarum* and a *Blastocystis* sp. established through micromanipulation. *Parasitology* (2006) 133:547–54. doi:10.1017/S0031182006000758
20. Liebhart D, Grabensteiner E, Hess MA. A virulent mono-eukaryotic culture of *Histomonas meleagridis* is capable of inducing fatal histomonosis in different aged turkeys of both sexes, regardless of the infective dose. *Avian Dis* (2008) 52:168–72. doi:10.1637/8107-090707-ResNote
21. Zahoor MA, Liebhart D, Hess M. Progression of histomonosis in commercial chickens following experimental infection with an *in vitro* propagated clonal culture of *Histomonas meleagridis*. *Avian Dis* (2011) 55:29–34. doi:10.1637/9508-082110-Reg.1
22. Liebhart D, Weissenböck H, Hess M. *In-situ* hybridization for the detection and identification of *Histomonas meleagridis* in tissues. *J Comp Pathol* (2006) 135:237–42. doi:10.1016/j.jcpa.2006.08.002
23. Kidane FA, Bilic I, Mitra T, Wernsdorf P, Hess M, Liebhart D. *In situ* hybridization to detect and localize signature cytokines of T-helper (Th) 1 and Th2 immune responses in chicken tissues. *Vet Immunol Immunopathol* (2016) 175:51–6. doi:10.1016/j.vetimm.2016.05.007
24. Paudel S, Hess C, Wernsdorf P, Käser T, Meitz S, Jensen-Jarolim E, et al. The systemic multiplication of *Gallibacterium anatis* in experimentally infected chickens is promoted by immunosuppressive drugs which have a less specific

effect on the depletion of leukocytes. *Vet Immunol Immunopathol* (2015) 166:22–32. doi:10.1016/j.vetimm.2015.05.001
25. Mitra T, Bilic I, Hess M, Liebhart D. The 60S ribosomal protein L13 is the most preferable reference gene to investigate gene expression in selected organs from turkeys and chickens, in context of different infection models. *Vet Res* (2016) 47:105. doi:10.1186/s13567-016-0388-z
26. Livak KJ, Schmittgen TD. Analysis of relative gene expression data using real-time quantitative PCR and the 2(-Delta Delta C(T)) method. *Methods* (2001) 25:402–8. doi:10.1006/meth.2001.1262
27. Grabensteiner E, Liebhart D, Weissenböck H, Hess M. Broad dissemination of *Histomonas meleagridis* determined by the detection of nucleic acid in different organs after experimental infection of turkeys and specified pathogen-free chickens using a mono-eukaryotic culture of the parasite. *Parasitol Int* (2006) 55:317–22. doi:10.1016/j.parint.2006.07.004
28. Esser MT, Marchese RD, Kierstead LS, Tussey LG, Wang F, Chirmule N, et al. Memory T cells and vaccines. *Vaccine* (2003) 21:419–30. doi:10.1016/S0264-410X(02)00407-3
29. Singh A, Weissenböck H, Hess M. *Histomonas meleagridis*: immunohistochemical localization of parasitic cells in formalin-fixed, paraffin-embedded tissue sections of experimentally infected turkeys demonstrates the wide spread of the parasite in its host. *Exp Parasitol* (2008) 118:505–13. doi:10.1016/j.exppara.2007.11.004
30. Degen WGJ, Daal Nv, Rothwell L, Kaiser P, Schijns VE. Th1/Th2 polarization by viral and helminth infection in birds. *Vet Microbiol* (2005) 105:163–7. doi:10.1016/j.vetmic.2004.12.001
31. Avery S, Rothwell L, Degen WDJ, Schijns VEJC, Young J, Kaufman J, et al. Characterization of the first nonmammalian T2 cytokine gene cluster: the cluster contains functional single-copy genes for IL-3, IL-4, IL-13, and GM-CSF, a gene for IL-5 that appears to be a pseudogene, and a gene encoding another cytokinelike transcript. *J Interf Cytokine Res* (2004) 24:600–10. doi:10.1089/jir.2004.24.600
32. Powell F, Rothwell L, Clarkson M, Kaiser P. Development of reagents to study the turkey's immune response: cloning and characterisation of two turkey cytokines, interleukin (IL)-10 and IL-13. *Vet Immunol Immunopathol* (2012) 147:97–103. doi:10.1016/j.vetimm.2012.03.013
33. Quach J, St-Pierre J, Chadee K. The future for vaccine development against *Entamoeba histolytica*. *Hum Vaccin Immunother* (2014) 10:1514–21. doi:10.4161/hv.27796
34. Schwarz A, Gauly M, Abel H, Daş G, Humburg J, Rohn K, et al. Immunopathogenesis of *Ascaridia galli* infection in layer chicken. *Dev Comp Immunol* (2011) 35:774–84. doi:10.1016/j.dci.2011.02.012
35. Van Der Most PJ, De Jong B, Parmentier HK, Verhulst S. Trade-off between growth and immune function: a meta-analysis of selection experiments. *Funct Ecol* (2011) 25:74–80. doi:10.1111/j.1365-2435.2010.01800.x
36. Lowenthal JW, York JJ, O'neil TE, Rhodes S, Prowse SJ, David A, et al. In vivo effects of chicken interferon-γ during infection with *Eimeria*. *J Interf Cytokine Res* (1997) 17:551–8. doi:10.1089/jir.1997.17.551
37. Janardhana V, Ford ME, Bruce MP, Broadway MM, O'Neil TE, Karpala AJ, et al. IFN-γ enhances immune responses to *E. coli* infection in the chicken. *J Interf Cytokine Res* (2007) 27:937–46. doi:10.1089/jir.2007.0020
38. Lowenthal JW, York JJ, O'Neil TE, Steven RA, Strom DG, Digby MR. Potential use of cytokine therapy in poultry. *Vet Immunol Immunopathol* (1998) 63:191–8. doi:10.1016/S0165-2427(98)00095-6
39. Munder M, Mallo M, Eichmann K, Modolell M. Murine macrophages secrete interferon gamma upon combined stimulation with interleukin (IL)-12 and IL-18: a novel pathway of autocrine macrophage activation. *J Exp Med* (1998) 187:2103–8. doi:10.1084/jem.187.12.2103
40. Fukao T, Frucht DM, Yap G, Gadina M, O'Shea JJ, Koyasu S. Inducible expression of Stat4 in dendritic cells and macrophages and its critical role in innate and adaptive immune responses. *J Immunol* (2001) 166:4446–55. doi:10.4049/jimmunol.166.7.4446
41. Kohno K, Kataoka J, Ohtsuki T, Suemoto Y, Okamoto I, Usui M, et al. IFN-gamma-inducing factor (IGIF) is a costimulatory factor on the activation of Th1 but not Th2 cells and exerts its effect independently of IL-12. *J Immunol* (1997) 158:1541–50.
42. Tomura M, Maruo S, Mu J, Zhou XY, Ahn HJ, Hamaoka T, et al. Differential capacities of CD4+, CD8+, and CD4-CD8- T cell subsets to express IL-18 receptor and produce IFN-gamma in response to IL-18. *J Immunol* (1998) 160:3759–65.
43. Bao Y, Liu X, Han C, Xu S, Xie B, Zhang Q, et al. Identification of IFN-γ-producing innate B cells. *Cell Res* (2014) 24:161–76. doi:10.1038/cr.2013.155
44. Voehringer D, Reese TA, Huang X, Shinkai K, Locksley RM. Type 2 immunity is controlled by IL-4/IL-13 expression in hematopoietic non-eosinophil cells of the innate immune system. *J Exp Med* (2006) 203:1435–46. doi:10.1084/jem.20052448
45. Morimoto M, Morimoto M, Whitmire J, Xiao S, Anthony RM, Mirakami H, et al. Peripheral CD4 T cells rapidly accumulate at the host:parasite interface during an inflammatory Th2 memory response. *J Immunol* (2004) 172:2424–30. doi:10.4049/jimmunol.172.4.2424
46. Rosa FE, Santos RM, Rogatto SR, Domingues MAC. Chromogenic *in situ* hybridization compared with other approaches to evaluate HER2/neu status in breast carcinomas. *Braz J Med Biol Res* (2013) 46:207–16. doi:10.1590/1414-431X20132483

13

Toxoplasma Chinese 1 Strain of WH3Δ*rop16*$_{I/III}$/*gra15*$_{II}$ Genetic Background Contributes to Abnormal Pregnant Outcomes in Murine Model

Cong Wang[1†], Weisheng Cheng[2†], Qian Yu[1], Tian Xing[1], Shoubin Chen[1], Lei Liu[1], Li Yu[1], Jian Du[1], Qingli Luo[1], Jilong Shen[1,3] and Yuanhong Xu[1,3]**

[1] Department of Pathogen Biology, Provincial Laboratories of Pathogen Biology and Zoonoses, School of Basic Medicine, Anhui Medical University, Hefei, China, [2] Department of Medical Genetics, Zhongshan School of Medicine, Sun Yat-sen University, The Key Laboratory of Tropical Disease Control, Ministry of Education, Guangzhou, China, [3] Department of Clinical Laboratory, The First Affiliated Hospital of Anhui Medical University, Hefei, China

***Correspondence:**
Jilong Shen
shenjilong53@126.com;
Yuanhong Xu
xyhong1964@163.com

†These authors have contributed equally to this work.

Toxoplasma gondii infection evokes a strong Th1-type response with interleukin (IL)-12 and interferon (IFN)-γ secretion. Recent studies suggest that the infection of pregnant mice with *T. gondii* may lead to adverse pregnancy results caused by subversion of physiological immune tolerance at maternofetal interface rather than direct invasion of the parasite. Genotype-associated dense granule protein GRA15$_{II}$ tends to induce classically activated macrophage (M1) differentiation and subsequently activating NK, Th1, and Th17 cells whereas rhoptry protein ROP16$_{I/III}$ drives macrophages to alternatively activated macrophage (M2) polarization and elicits Th2 immune response. Unlike the archetypal strains of types I, II, and III, type Chinese 1 strains possess both GRA15$_{II}$ and ROP16$_{I/III}$, suggesting a distinct pathogenesis of *Toxoplasma*-involved adverse pregnancies. We constructed *T. gondii* type Chinese 1 strain of WH3Δ*rop16* based on CRISPR/Cas9 technology to explore the ROP16$_{I/III}$-deficient/GRA15$_{II}$-dominant parasites in induction of trophoblast apoptosis *in vitro* and abnormal pregnant outcomes of mice *in vivo*. Our study showed that *Toxoplasma* WH3Δ*rop16* remarkably induced apoptosis of trophoblasts. C57BL/6 pregnant mice injected with the tachyzoites of WH3Δ*rop16* presented increased absorptivity of fetuses in comparison with the mice infected with WH3 wild type (WH3 WT) parasites although no remarkable difference of virulence to mice was seen between the two strains. Additionally, the mice inoculated with WH3Δ*rop16* tachyzoites exhibited a notable expression of both IL-17A and IFN-γ, while the percentage of $CD4^+CD25^+FoxP3$ [T regulatory cells (Tregs)] were diminished in splenocytes and placenta tissues compared to those infected with WH3 WT parasites. Accordingly, expressions of IL-4, IL-10, and transforming growth factor beta 1, the pivotal cytokines of Th2 and Tregs response, were significantly dampened whereas IFN-γ and IL-12 expressions were upregulated in WH3Δ*rop16*-infected mice, which gave rise to more prominent outcomes of abnormal pregnancies. Our results indicated that the WH3Δ*rop16* parasites with *gra15*$_{II}$ background of *T. gondii* type Chinese 1 strains may cause miscarriage and stillbirth due to subversion of the maternal immune tolerance and system immunity of the animals and the GRA15$_{II}$ effector contributes to the process of adverse pregnant consequences.

Keywords: *Toxoplasma gondii*, dense granule protein GRA15, rhoptry protein ROP16, CRISPR/Cas9, adverse pregnant outcome

INTRODUCTION

During normal pregnancy, allogeneic fetal cells invading the extraembryonic trophoblasts do not impair gestation by establishing tolerance at the maternal–fetal interface (1, 2). The physiological balance of Th1/Th2 is believed to play a crucial part in maintenance of normal pregnancy of mammals including humans (3). Previous studies showed that apoptosis is a normal physiological process of trophoblasts throughout gestation and is essential to normal placental development and fetal growth (4). Thus any unfavorable impact of immunological factors on the maternal–fetal interface and/or apoptosis of trophoblasts may lead to abnormal pregnancy outcomes.

It has been elucidated that T regulatory cells (Tregs) promote immune tolerance and successful pregnancy by secreting interleukin (IL)-10 and transforming growth factor beta 1 (TGF-β1) and dampen interferon (IFN)-γ and other inflammatory cytokines to maintain the normal development of embryos (5–8). The Tregs cells have been found to be insufficient in patients who experienced recurrent spontaneous abortions (9), while excessive secretion of IFN-γ and other Th1 type cytokines may give rise to adverse pregnancies (10). Therefore, Th2-dominant response in system immunity and at maternal–fetal interface is the prerequisite for normal pregnancy (3, 11–14).

Toxoplasma gondii is an extensive intracellular protozoan parasite that is capable of affecting almost all vertebrate animals including humans and leading to reproductive failure in its hosts (15, 16). Primary infection with *Toxoplasma* during pregnancy, particularly in the first trimester, may cause stillbirths, miscarriages, or fetal abnormalities (17). The apoptosis of trophoblasts might be induced by many stimuli. For example, apoptotic process of trophoblasts is notably increased in the case of spontaneous abortion when the cells were co-cultured with inflammatory macrophages that were infected with *T. gondii* (18). Glycosyl phosphatidylinositol on the membrane of *Toxoplasma* tachyzoites, similar to LPS of bacteria, could induce oxidative stress in several tissues, and it has been found to be a key molecule which is responsible for preterm labor in mice (19, 20). Despite the fact that *Toxoplasma* infection may cause abortion or congenital fetal infection *via* direct transmission of parasite to placentas and fetuses, some studies indicate that imbalance of immune tolerance at the maternal–fetal interface, rather than a direct action of the parasite, might be attributed to the abnormal pregnancies (21, 22), resulting in apoptosis of trophoblasts in the case of abortion with *T. gondii* infection. Further researches revealed that *Toxoplasma* infection in mice lead to adverse pregnant results with a mechanism of reduction of Tregs and elevation of Th17 cells (23).

Toxoplasma gondii invasion to the host cell is actually a series of parasite protein secretions. Secretory proteins of ROPs, GRAs, MICs, RONs, and other molecules are mainly generated by the organelles of dense granules, rhoptries, and micronemes. These parasite-derived polymorphic effectors are deeply involved in dictation of virulence and modulation of host signaling pathways (24–28). For instance, Jensen et al. found that $ROP16_{I/III}$ (of types I and III strains) kinase phosphorylates Stat6/Stat3 and induces alternatively activated macrophages (M2) at early phase of infection that is associated with promoted IL-4 and IL-10 expressions and Th2-polarized response, while $GRA15_{II}$ (of type II strains) activates NF-κB and elicits classically activated macrophages (M1) that is responsible for IL-12 generation and Th1-dominant immunity, subsequently activating NK and Th17 cells (19, 28–31), resulting in oxidative stress and further activation of the pro-apoptotic pathway (28, 32).

Studies reported that type Chinese 1 (ToxoDB #9) strains dominantly prevalent in China carry both $GRA15_{II}$ and $ROP16_{I/III}$ effectors that is different from the strains of archetypical types I, II, and III of *T. gondii* in Europe and North America (33, 34). The $ROP16_{I/III}$ with $GRA15_{II}$ background in Chinese 1 strains strongly suggests the distinct pathogenesis that differs from the strains of the other continents of the world. In the current study, we explored the impact of $GRA15_{II}$ with $ROP16_{I/III}$ deletion of Chinese 1 WH3 strain parasite on adverse pregnancy outcomes in murine model by making a *T. gondii* WH3Δ*rop16* strain based on CRISPR/Cas9 technology. We hypothesize that the Toxo-WH3Δ*rop16* strain with $gra15_{II}$ background, similar to type II strains of *Toxoplasma*, might subvert the immune tolerance at the maternal–fetal interface and the systemic immunity, leading to adverse pregnancy, which is attributed to the M1/Th1/Th17 biased response. Moreover, this study would be helpful for better understanding of the genotype-associated mechanism of abnormal pregnancy caused by *Toxoplasma* predominantly circulating in China.

MATERIALS AND METHODS

Reagents

The following reagents were used in the experiment: Q5 mutagenesis kit (New England Biolabs, Ipswich, MA, USA) and ClonExpress MultiS One Step Cloning Kit (Vazyme Biotech, Nanjing, China). Phusion High-Fidelity PCR Kit (Thermo fisher, USA) was used for the PCR amplification. Percoll (GE Healthcare Life Sciences), pyrimethamine, penicillin, streptomycin, phorbol 12-myristate 13-acetate, ionomycin, HEPES, collagenase IV, and the Giemsa staining kit, were obtained from Sigma (St. Louis, MO, USA). Dulbecco's modified Eagle's medium, fetal bovine serum (FBS), and Roswell Park Memorial Institute 1640 medium (RPMI 1640) and D-Hanks solution were purchased from Wisent (Montreal, QC, Canada). Brefeldin A, FITC-labeled anti-mouse CD4, PE-labeled anti-mouse IL-17A, APC-labeled anti-mouse IL-4, Percp-cy5.5-labeled anti-mouse IFN-γ, APC-labeled anti-mouse CD25, PE-labeled anti-mouse Foxp3, FITC Annexin V Apoptosis Detection Kit, and Cytofix/Cytoperm kit were provided by BD Biosciences (New York, BD, USA). The nitrite was detected *via* Greiss Reagent System provided by Promega Biotech Company (Madison, WI, USA). The tumor necrosis factor (TNF-α), IL-17A enzyme-linked immunosorbent assay (ELISA) kit, and 1 × Fix/Perm buffer were purchased from eBioscience (San Diego CA, USA). IFN-γ, IL-12, IL-10, and TGF-β1 ELISA kit was obtained from R&D Systems (Minneapolis, MN, USA). The mouse trophoblasts (primary cells originated from C57BL/6 mice) were purchased from Wuhan Biofavor Biotechnology Company.

Propagation of *T. gondii*

Tachyzoites of *T. gondii* WH3 strain (type Chinese 1) were harvested from the continuous cell cultures in human foreskin fibroblasts (HFF, ATCC® SCRC-1041™) grown with Dulbecco's modified Eagle medium (DMEM) supplemented with 10% FBS, 100 μg/ml streptomycin, and 100 U/ml penicillin.

Generation of ROP16$_{I/III}$-Deficient Strain of Type Chinese 1

All the primers and plasmids used in the study are shown in **Table 1**. UPRT-targeting guide RNA (gRNA) in pSAG1:CAS9-U6:sgUPRT (Addgene plasmid #54467) was replaced with ROP16$_{I/III}$ targeting gRNA using Q5 mutagenesis kit. To make the homologous templates for gene replacements, homologous arms of ROP16$_{I/III}$ were amplified from the genomic DNA of type Chinese 1 WH3 WT strain as described in previous study (35). Subsequently, the homologous arms of ROP16 along with the selectable markers DHFR*-Ts were cloned into pUC19 using ClonExpress MultiS One Step Cloning Kit. The pSAG1:Cas9-U6:sgROP16$_{I/III}$ and donor DNA fragments were electroporated into *T. gondii* WH3 WT strain. After transfection, tachyzoites were immediately transferred into HFF cells. After culture for 48 h, parasites were selected with pyrimethamine for DHFR-TS. A single clone through limiting dilution in 96-well plate were seeded with HFF host cells and detected by PCR and Western blotting. Diagnostic PCRs (PCR1, PCR2, and PCR3) were used to screen individual clone. PCR reactions were performed using Taq DNA polymerase in a 25-μl reaction mixture containing 1 μl genomic DNA extracted from a single clone as templates. Subsequently, the products were examined by agarose gel electrophoresis. Rabbit polyclonal antibody against ROP18 and antibody against ROP16 was prepared in the laboratory. The invasion of WH3 WT or WH3Δ*rop16* strain in HFF cells were visualized after 48 h by Giemsa staining and the average number of tachyzoites per parasitophorous vacuole (PV) was obtained by counting 50 PVs in triplicate experiments. C57BL/6 mice were infected with 1 × 10^3 tachyzoites of WH3 WT or WH3Δ*rop16*, respectively. The animals were monitored daily for manifestations following infection and the survival rate was recorded.

Cells and Co-Culture System

Mouse peritoneal macrophages were acquired by washing the peritoneal cavity three times with ice-cold D-Hanks solution. Mouse peritoneal macrophages were cultured and suspension cells were washed off 24 h later. The transwell culture plates (Corning, Corning, NY, USA), were used to establish a co-culture system. Generally, the pore size of the bottom of the inserts is 0.4 μm, which allowed the passage of only small and soluble particles rather than cells and tachyzoites. Control macrophages (1 × 10^6) and WH3 WT (1 × 10^6) or WH3Δ*rop16* (1 × 10^6) tachyzoites infected macrophages were added to the upper well separately. The C57BL/6 primary placental trophoblasts (1 × 10^6) were co-cultured in the lower wells in 5% CO_2 at 37°C for 24 h. The co-culture system was kept in 1 ml of RPMI 1640 culture medium supplemented with 10% FBS and 1% penicillin/streptomycin. After co-culturing for 24 h, the macrophages were harvested for total RNA and culture supernatants were collected to analyze NO and TNF-α. The placental trophoblasts were collected for detection of apoptosis by flow cytometry (FCM). The apoptosis rates of trophoblasts cells were calculated as the sum of early and late apoptosis rates. The trophoblasts cells washed twice with cold PBS, and resuspended cells in 1 × binding buffer. The trophoblast cells were subjected to FITC annexin V and PI followed by gentle vortex, incubated for 15 min at 25°C in the dark and analyzed by FCM within 1 h.

Establishment of Animal Pregnant Model

The 6- to 8-week-old female and 8- to 10-week-old male C57BL/6 mice were purchased from the Animal Center of Anhui Medical University (AMU) and had free access to sterilized water and food under standard conditions, and permitted to adapt for 1 week before the experiment. The mice were treated in compliance with the Chinese National Institute of Health Guide for the Care and Use of Laboratory Animals.

TABLE 1 | Primers used in this study.

Primers	Sequence	Used for
5′-ROP16-guide RNA (gRNA) 3′-ROP16-gRNA	GTGGCAGCGCGTTTTAGAGCTAGAAATAGCAAG CGGTGCGTCCAACTTGACATCCCCATTTAC	Q5 mutagenesis changing the gRNA in pSAG1:CAS9-U6:sgUPRT to gRNA-ROP16
UpROP16 F UpROP16 R	AAAACGACGGCCAGTGAATTCAGTTTGAATCTCTGGGTAGAACAGC GGGGGTGAAAATCGAATGACACTGCCCCTGAGTCGAGCCAC	To produce UpROP16 PCR product for making pROP16:DHFR-I
DHFR-TS F DHFR-TS R	TGTCATTCGATTTTCACCCCC TCCTCCGCTCCTCTCTAGCAGGATCGATCCCCCCGGGCTGC	To produce DHFR PCR product for making pROP16:DHFR-I
DnROP16 F DnROP16 R	GCAGCCCGGGGGGATCGATCCTGCTAGAGAGGAGCGGAGGA GACCATGATTACGCCAAGCTTGCTCCGCAGTCTCTGTAAGT	To produce DnROP16 PCR product for making pROP16:DHFR-I
5′-UpROP16 5′-InDHFR	TGTGATGCTGAGTCTTGCGAGT TACCAGTCATGGACGAGATCG	PCR1
3′-InDHFR 3′-DnROP16	ACACGCATGTCTACACGAACC TGGTGGTTGCGACTGGACTA	PCR2
5′-InROP16 3′-InROP16	ATGAAAGTGACCACGAAAGG CTACATCCGATGTGAAGAAAGTT	PCR3

All procedures were followed strictly according to the ethical standards formulated by Institutional Review Board of AMU Institute of Biomedicine AMU (permit No: AMU26-081108). After 1 week of adaptation to the new environment, females were housed overnight with males (2 females for 1 male). The presence of vaginal plugs on the second day was designated day 0 of gestation (GD 0). Briefly, all pregnant mice were divided into three equal groups randomly (WH3 WT group, WH3Δ*rop16* group, and control group) with five mice in each. On gestation GD8, pregnant mice were intraperitoneally injected with 4×10^2 WH3 WT and WH3Δ*rop16* tachyzoites in 200 μl sterile PBS, and the control was exposed to only 200 μl sterile PBS at the same time. All mice were sacrificed with euthanasia on GD14, the uteruses were moved away and implantation and resorption sites were recorded. The resorption sites were defined by their small sizes, necrotic, and hemorrhagic appearance of placentas and embryos. The ratio of resorption sites to total implantation sites was calculated as the percentage of fetal loss.

The experiments that are related to using viable parasites and animal infections were performed in the AMU Biosecurity II Laboratory licensed by the local health administrative department.

Preparation of Single Cell Suspension

The placentas, uterine tissues, and spleens of experimental mice were removed aseptically. The spleen tissues were placed in a sterile nylon mesh gently. The cells were harvested after mashing through sterile nylon gauze and lysed with erythrocyte lytic buffer and cultured in RPMI 1640 supplemented with 10% FBS. At the same time, the placentas and the uterus were placed in the dish and cut into pieces followed by washing thoroughly and the shredded tissue was moved to a 50 ml centrifuge tube. The tissues digested with 2.5 mg/ml collagenase IV, 10% FBS, and 10 mM HEPES sodium salt dissolved in RPMI 1640 and then incubated at 37°C for 30 min with gentle shaking. The suspension cells were filtered through sterile nylon mesh to take away undigested tissue. The mononuclear cells were collected by discontinuous 70%/40% Percoll (GE Healthcare Life Sciences) density gradient centrifugation.

FCM Analysis of Lymphocytes

Lymphocytes from spleens, placentas, and uterine tissues were regulated to the appropriate cell number (1×10^6/ml) and cultivated in 6-well plate in 2 ml of RPMI 1640 medium supplemented with 10% FBS. For intracellular cytokine staining, ionomycin (1 mg/ml) and PMA (20 ng/ml) were used to stimulate the cells for 5 h in the presence of brefeldin A (1 mg/ml). The cells were subjected to FITC-labeled anti-mouse CD4 for 30 min at 4°C to avoid the light and were washed twice, and fixed with the Cytofix/Cytoperm kit according to manufacturer's instructions. The cells were incubated for 1 h at 4°C in the dark and were washed twice, and PE-labeled anti-mouse IL-17A, APC-labeled anti-mouse IL-4, and Percp-cy5.5-labeled anti-mouse IFN-γ were used for staining of intracellular cytokines, respectively. Tregs were marked by the FITC-labeled anti-mouse CD4 and APC-labeled anti-mouse CD25 for 30 min at 4°C in the dark and were washed twice. After surface staining, the cells were fixed and permeabilized in 1 × Fix/Perm buffer at 4°C for 1 h in the dark and washed twice, followed by PE-labeled anti-mouse Foxp3 staining at 4°C for 30 min in protection from light. After washing, the cells were analyzed on FCM.

RNA Extraction and qRT-PCR

Total RNA from the co-cultured cells, spleens, and placentas were extracted using TRIzol (Invitrogen Life Technologies, Carlsbad, CA, USA) and transcribed into cDNA using Takara Kit (Takara, Japan) following the manufacturer's instructions. The quantitative analysis was performed by testing expression of iNOS, TNF-α, IFN-γ, IL-12, IL-17A, IL-10, and TGF-β1 using SYBR Premix Ex Taq kit (Takara, Japan) by the Light Cycler 480. The glyceraldehyde-3-phosphate dehydrogenase (GAPDH) was used to normalize the results. The relative mRNA expression was counted with the comparative ΔCt method using the formula $2^{-\Delta\Delta Ct}$. The qRT-PCR was conducted in technical triplicates by using the sense and antisense primers listed in **Table 2**.

Enzyme-Linked Immunosorbent Assay

The co-cultured supernatants were obtained for TNF-α detection by ELISA. To detect cytokines in splenocyte supernatants, we used the ionomycin (1 mg/ml) and PMA (20 ng/ml) to stimulate the splenocyte cells (2×10^6) in 6-well plate in 2 ml/well of RPMI 1640 medium supplemented with 10% FBS for 5 h. Splenocyte supernatants were collected and subjected to examination for IFN-γ, IL-12, IL-17A, IL-10, and TGF-β1 by ELISA. Accurately weighed placenta tissues were homogenized with a ratio of 1 mg of placental tissues to 10 μl of PBS and centrifuged at 12,000 *g* at 4°C for 30 min. The supernatants of the tissue lysates were gathered and equal volume of the supernatants was added to each well. The cytokines of IFN-γ, IL-12, IL-17A, IL-10, and TGF-β1 were detected by ELISA according to the manufacturer's protocols. Three duplicate wells were set up for each group. The absorbance was measured at 450 nm on the ELISA plate reader (Biotek, Winooski, VT, USA).

Nitrite Detection

The co-cultured supernatant was collected for examination of nitrite oxide (NO). It was detected using the Griess Reagent

TABLE 2 | The primers used for qRT-PCR.

Primers	Forward primer (5′–3′)	Reverse primer (5′–3′)
TNF-α	ACGGCATGGATCTCAAAGAC	GTGGGTGAGGAGCACGTAGT
iNOS	CACCTTGGAGTTCACCCAGT	ACCACTCGTACTTGGGATGC
IFN-γ	AGCAAGGCGAAAAAGGATGC	TCATTGAATGCTTGGCGCTG
IL-12	GATGTCACCTGCCCAACTG	TGGTTTGATGATGTCCCTGA
IL-10	GCTCCTAGAGCTGCGGACT	TGTTGTCCAGCTGGTCCTTT
TGF-β1	CTGGATACCAACTACT GCTTCAG	TTGGTTGTAGAGGGCAAGG ACCT
IL-17A	TCTCTGATGCTGTTGCTGCT	CGTGGAACGGTTGAGGTAGT
GAPDH	CAACTTTGGCATTGTGGAAGG	ACACATTGGGGGTAGGAACAC

GAPDH, glyceraldehyde-3-phosphate dehydrogenase; IFN, interferon; IL, interleukin; iNOS, inducible nitric synthase; TNF, tumor necrosis factor; TGF-β1, transforming growth factor beta 1.

system as previously described (36) following the manufacturer's instruction. The absorbance was measured at 550 nm on an ELISA plate reader.

Statistical Analysis

The experimental data acquired were subjected to statistical analyses using one-way ANOVA and paired *t*-test after precheck of the data for homogeneity of variances. Statistical significance was defined by using GraphPad Prism Software, and $P < 0.05$ was regarded as significant. The results were presented as mean ± SD, which gives a summary of the data from at least three times experiments.

RESULTS

The WH3Δ*rop16* Strain of *T. gondii* Type Chinese 1 Was Constructed Using CRISPR/Cas9 Technology

The CRISPR/Cas9 strategy was used to inactivate ROP16 by inserting pyrimethamine-resistant DHFR (DHFR*) followed by PCR identification of a single clone (**Figure 1A**). PCR identification proved that DHFR coding sequence was successfully inserted to the target position (**Figure 1B**). Western blotting analysis showed no expression of $ROP16_{I/III}$ protein by WH3Δ*rop16* strain (**Figure 1C**). Giemsa staining results indicated that less number of parasites (13 tachyzoites vs 22 tachyzoites) per PV in WH3Δ*rop16* infected cells compared to WH3 WT-infected cells, respectively ($p < 0.05$) (**Figure 1D**). Virulence examination indicated that all animals infected by both strains died on day 12 post-infection (**Figure 1E**) and no difference of the virulence to mice was noted between WH3 WT and WH3Δ*rop16* strains.

WH3Δ*rop16* Strain Infection Drove Macrophages to M1 and Lead to Trophoblast Apoptosis

Compared to the WH3 WT group, macrophages infected with WH3Δ*rop16* strain produced a higher level of NO, iNOS, and TNF-α (**Figures 2A,B**). To elucidate the placental trophoblasts apoptosis, we detected cell apoptosis of placental tissues by fluorescein isothiocyanate/propidium iodide (FITC/PI) staining assay. Compared to the WH3 WT group, the number of total, early, and late apoptotic cells of trophoblasts was elevated when co-cultured with WH3Δ*rop16* strain-infected macrophages for 24 h (**Figure 2C**). The remarkable apoptosis of trophoblasts caused by WH3Δ*rop16* strain was observed (**Figure 2D**).

WH3Δ*rop16* Strain Infection Induced Adverse Pregnancy

Most samples of the pregnant uteruses showed significant fetal resorption and placental hemorrhage in the mice

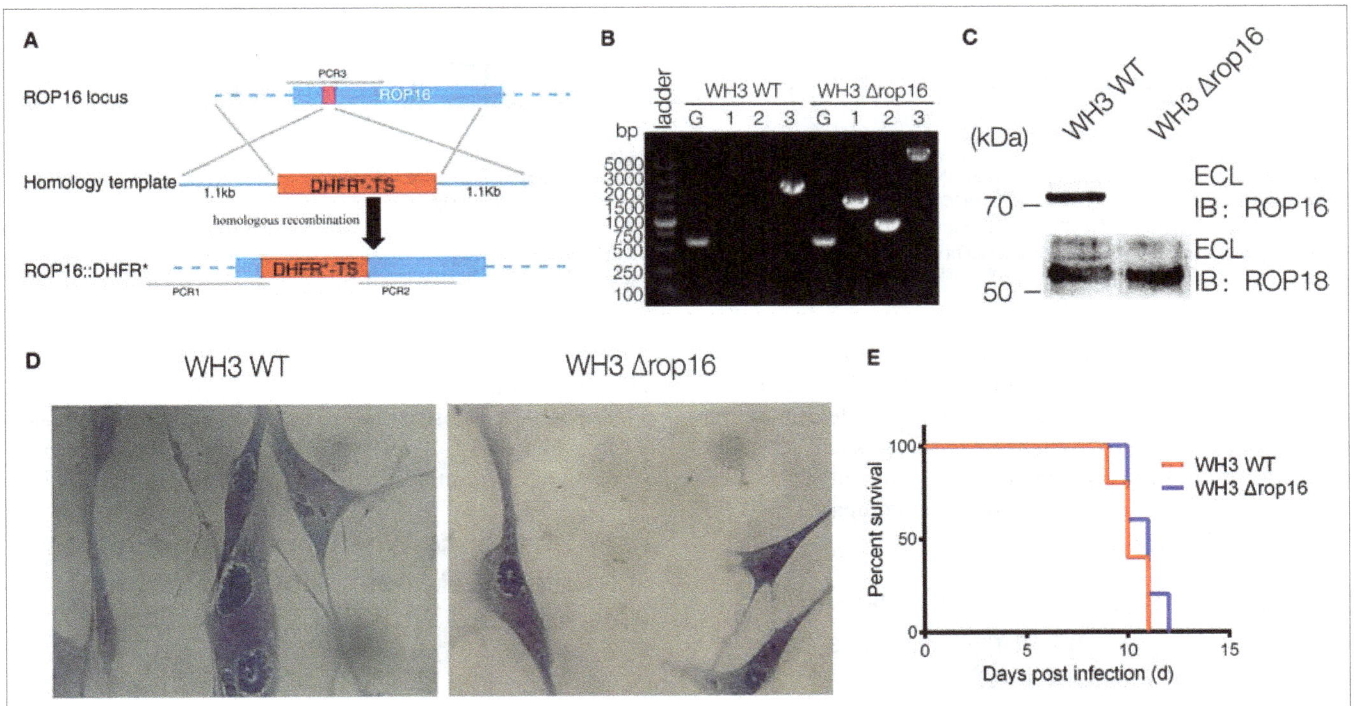

FIGURE 1 | Construction of the WH3Δ*rop16* strain of *Toxoplasma gondii* type Chinese 1 by using CRISPR-Cas9 technology. **(A)** Schematic of CRISPR/CAS9 strategy for inactivation of *rop16* by inserting pyrimethamine-resistant DHFR (DHFR*) and PCR identification of single clone. **(B)** PCR identification of WH3Δ*rop16* *T. gondii* strain. G represents the GRA1 promoter positive control, as shown in **Figure 1A**. 1: PCR1 fragment; 2: PCR2 fragment, 3: PCR3 fragment. PCR1 and PCR2 examined the integration of DHFR-TS* into corresponding genes, and PCR3 checked the deletion of ROP16 sequences. **(C)** Western blotting for detection of ROP16 expression in WH3 WT and WH3Δ*rop16*. Rabbit polyclonal antibody against ROP18 was used as the control. **(D)** The number of parasites per parasitophorous vacuole of WH3Δ*rop16* or WH3 WT. **(E)** Mouse survival after inoculation with *T. gondii* tachyzoites.

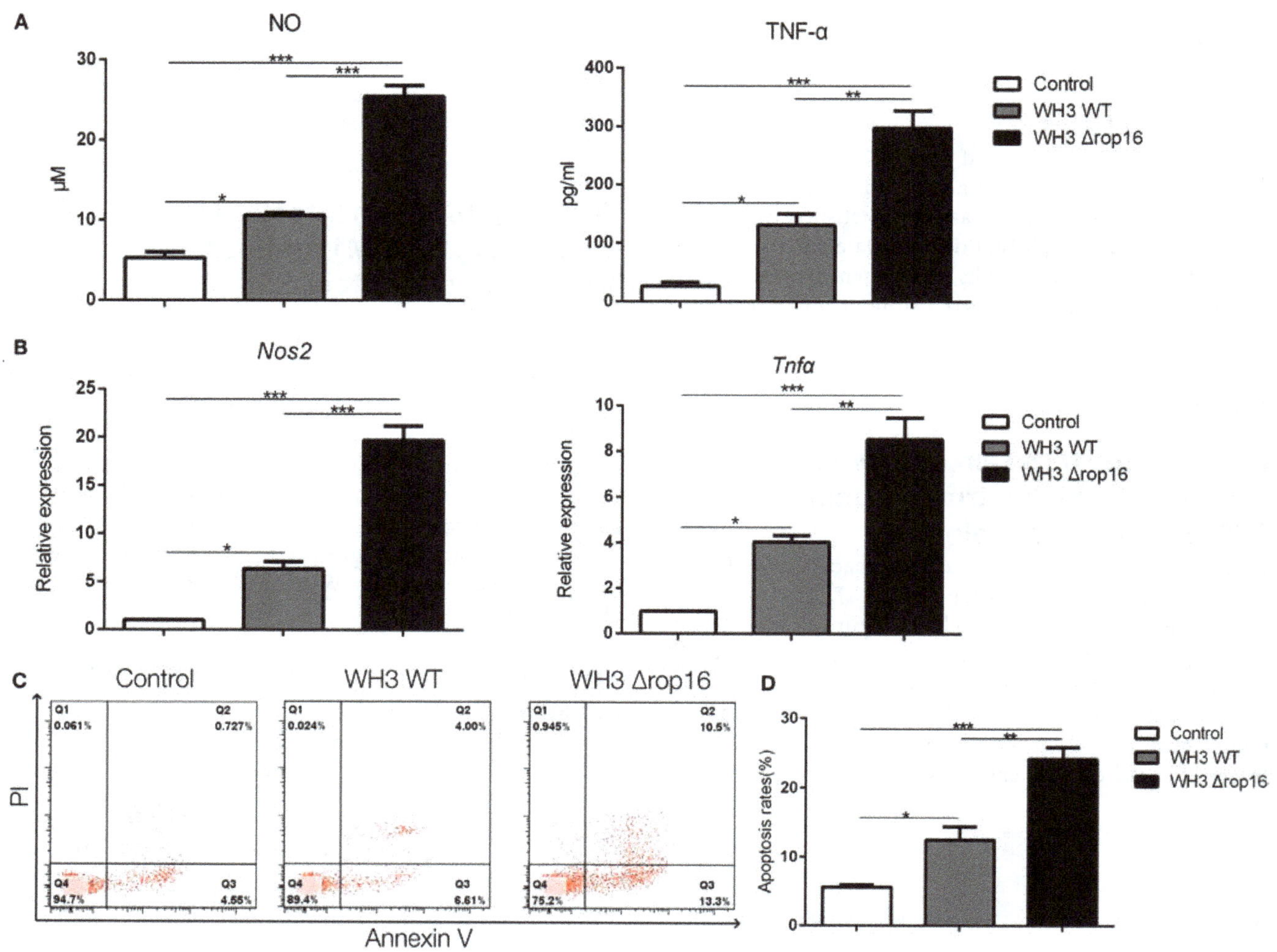

FIGURE 2 | The high production of nitrite oxide (NO), inducible nitric synthase (iNOS), and tumor necrosis factor (TNF)-α and apoptosis of trophoblasts co-cultured with macrophages infected with the WH3Δ*rop16* tachyzoites. **(A)** The culture supernatants were collected and analyzed for NO and TNF-α production. **(B)** The relative mRNA expressions of iNOS and TNF-α after co-culture. **(C)** Increased apoptosis of trophoblasts co-cultured with WH3Δ*rop16* infected macrophages. **(D)** Total, early, and late apoptosis of placental trophoblasts (**p* < 0.05, ***p* < 0.01, ****p* < 0.001).

infected with the tachyzoites of WH3Δ*rop16* in comparison with the WH3 WT group (**Figures 3A,B**). The weights of fetuses, placentas, and rate of fetal loss were determined at day 6 post infection. The weight loss of fetuses and placentas was observed and the rate of fetal loss significantly increased in mice infected with WH3Δ*rop16* strain compared to WH3 WT strain (**Figure 3C**).

WH3Δ*rop16* Strain Infection Induced Immune Bias to Th1 in the Spleens and Placentas of Pregnant Mice

We examined the IFN-γ in the lymphocytes of the spleen and placenta tissues using FCM to investigate the immune bias at maternal–fetal interface of the pregnant mice after *T. gondii* infection. The expression of IFN-γ and IL-12 were analyzed using qRT-PCR and ELISA in the spleens and placentas. Compared to WH3 WT group, Th1 subsets ($CD4^+IFN\gamma^+$) of WH3Δ*rop16* inoculated mice were remarkably elevated (**Figures 4A,B**). The data were further confirmed by using qRT-PCR and ELISA (**Figures 4C–F**). Consistent with the IFN-γ assay, the expression of IL-12 (**Figures 4C–F**) was synchronously increased in the mice of WH3Δ*rop16* infection.

Th17 Response Was Upregulated in the Spleens and Placentas of the Pregnant Mice Infected With WH3Δ*rop16* Strain

We examined the Th17 cytokine ($CD4^+IL\text{-}17A^+$) in the spleens and placentas in the three groups of mice by FCM and found that the mice infected with WH3Δ*rop16* strain exhibited a high expression of IL-17A (**Figures 5A,B**). The level of IL-17A mRNA expression in WH3Δ*rop16* group was significantly increased when compared to WH3 WT (**Figures 5C,D**), which is in parallel with the result of IL-17A detection in supernatants by ELISA (**Figures 5C,D**).

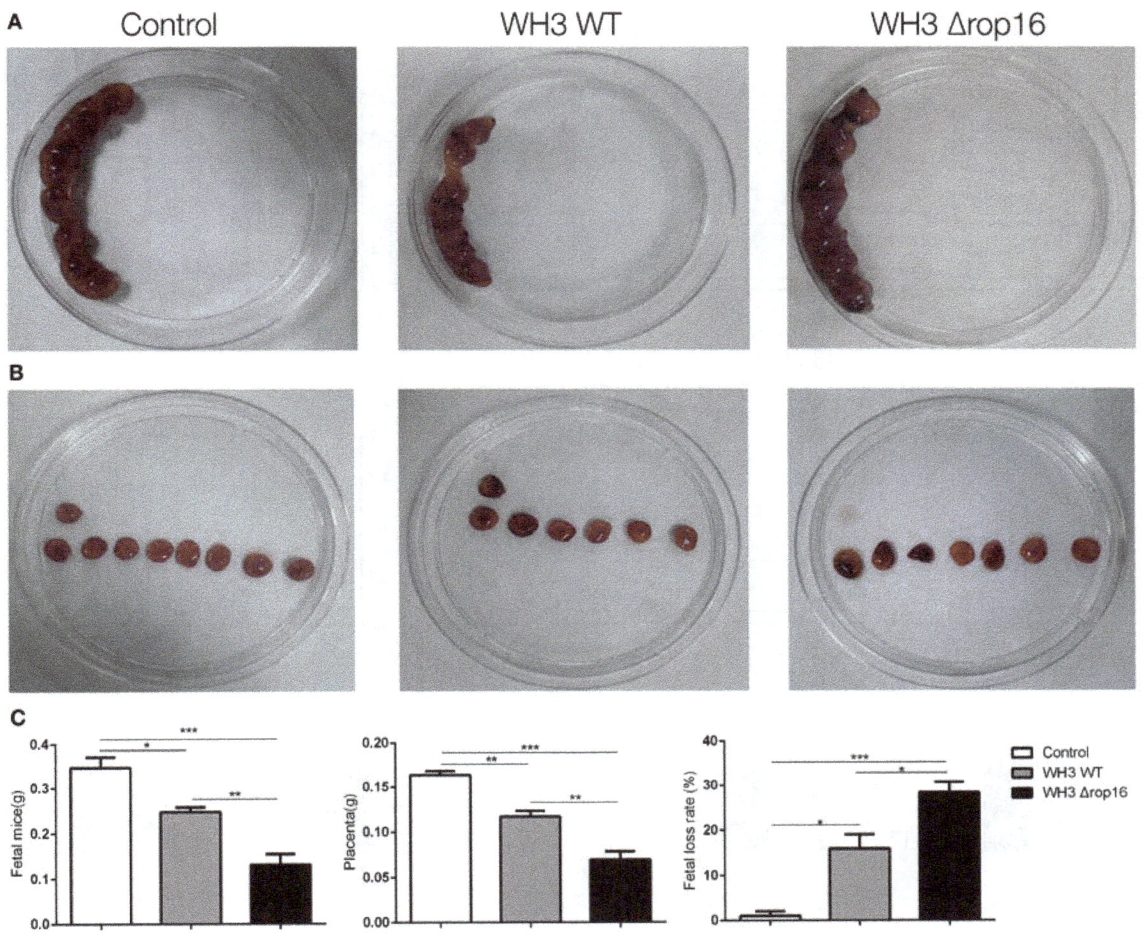

FIGURE 3 | *Toxoplasma gondii* infection induced adverse pregnancy outcomes in mice. **(A,B)** The uteruses of WH3Δ*rop16*-infected mice presented notable fetal resorption and placental bleeding in comparison with the WH3 WT group. **(C)** The weights of fetuses, placentas, and rate of fetal loss were measured at day 6 post infection. The fetal loss rate was calculated by ratio of resorption sites to the total number of implantation sites. (*$p < 0.05$, **$p < 0.01$, ***$p < 0.001$).

Percentage of Tregs Decreased in the Spleens and Placentas of the Pregnant Mice Following WH3Δ*rop16* Strain Infection

To clarify whether the mutant WH3Δ*rop16* strain infection can negatively affect the Tregs population, we detected the percentage of Tregs in the splenocytes and the cells isolated from the placentas of pregnant mice by FCM (**Figures 6A,B**). The results revealed that Tregs were significantly dampened in WH3Δ*rop16*-infected mice. Accordingly, relative mRNA expression of IL-10 and TGF-β1 in the spleens (**Figure 6C**) and placentas (**Figure 6D**) was synchronously reduced in WH3Δ*rop16* group compared to WH3 WT group. In addition, the levels of IL-10 and TGF-β1 in the spleens (**Figure 6E**) and placentas (**Figure 6F**) remarkably declined in the WH3Δ*rop16*-infected mice when compared to WH3 WT mice.

Compared to the WH3 WT-infected C57BL/6 pregnant mice, the animals inoculated with WH3Δ*rop16* tachyzoites presented a diminished expression of IL-4 determined by FCM (**Figures 7A,B**).

DISCUSSION

Toxoplasma gondii is one of the common causative agent of prenatal infections during pregnancy (15, 16). The parasite may be transmitted vertically by tachyzoites that are passed to the fetus *via* the placenta, leading to miscarriages, stillbirths, and other adverse pregnant outcomes depending on the stage of the pregnancy at which infection takes place (37). Most strains which infect humans in Europe are type II and a large proportion of cases of congenital toxoplasmosis are asymptomatic at birth if the mother acquired the infection after the second trimester of gestation (38). It has been well recognized that vertical transmission of the parasite, particularly type I virulent strain of *Toxoplasma* with superior migratory capacity, may directly cause abnormal pregnancy. However, the non-virulent strains such as PRU or ME49 may induce a decrease in the fertility if infection occurs during the later phase of gestation (39). Previous studies indicated that neither parasites nor their DNAs are detectable in the diseased tissue samples of some abnormal pregnancies and we attempted to examine the parasite by bioassay or its derived DNAs by PCR from placentas and tissues of aborted fetuses in the

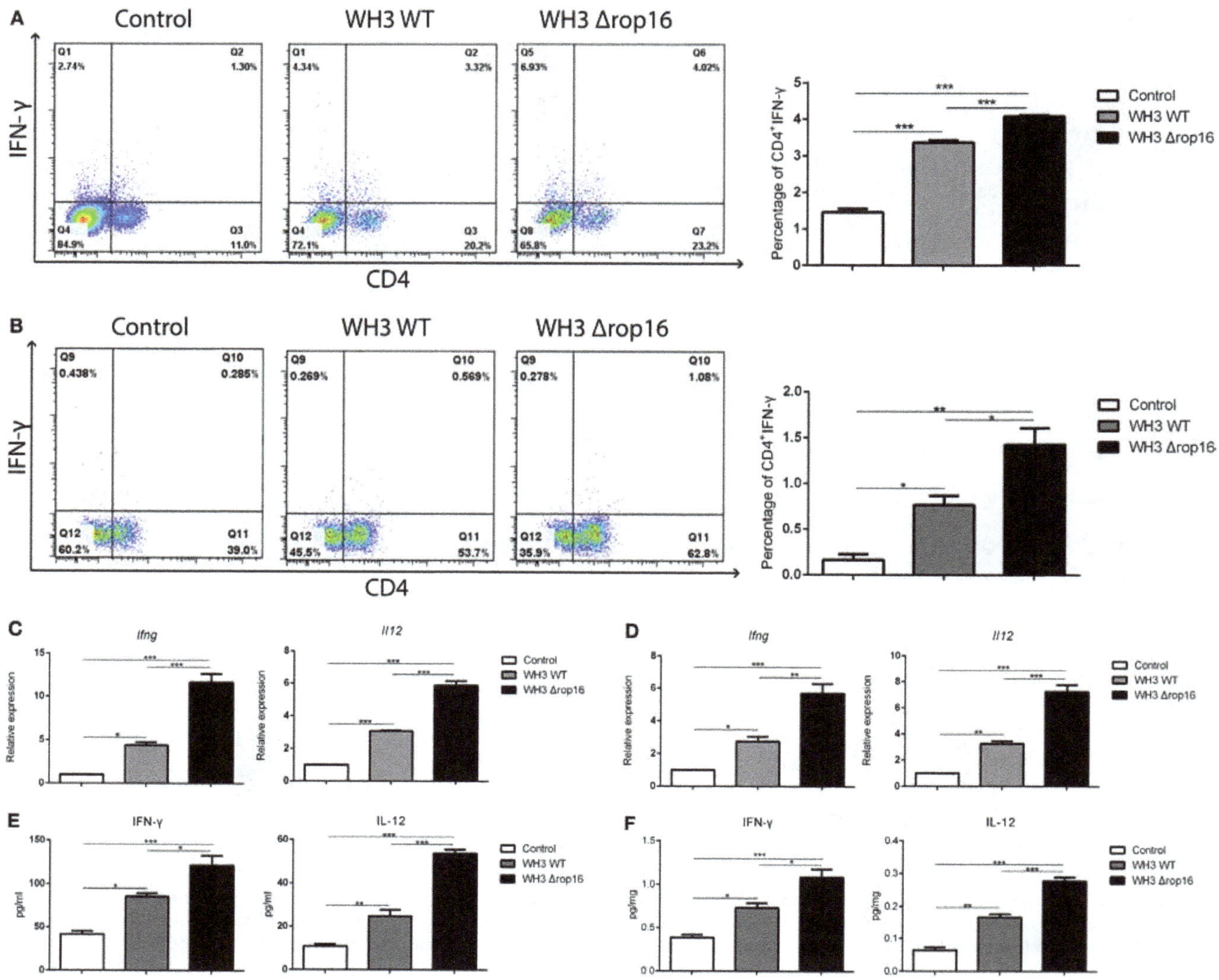

FIGURE 4 | WH3*Δrop16* strain infection upregulated Th1 response of pregnant mice. Increased percentage of Th1 (CD4⁺IFNγ⁺) cell population in the spleens **(A)** and placentas **(B)** of WH3*Δrop16* tachyzoites compared to the control. The relative mRNA expressions of interferon (IFN)-γ and interleukin (IL)-12 were sharply increased in the spleens **(C)** of WH3*Δrop16*-infected mice and placentas **(D)**. The supernatants were tested for IFN-γ and IL-12 in the spleens (pg/ml) **(E)** and placentas (pg/mg) **(F)** by enzyme-linked immunosorbent assay (**p* < 0.05, ***p* < 0.01, ****p* < 0.001).

pregnant women, some of whom showing positive IgG antibodies against *Toxoplasma*, but no positive results were obtained (data not shown). Consistent results were also reported by Senegas in murine model (40). All of these data imply that the resorption, abortion, or fetal damage might be indirectly due to lesions of the placenta induced by maternal biased immunity such as Th1/IFN-γ polarized immune response (41) and that the maternal immunity-associated but not viable parasite-generated "sterile" pathology actually takes place in abnormal pregnant consequences caused by *Toxoplasma* infection. Herein, we focused on the maternal immunity associated rather than the mother-to-child vertical transmission causative adverse outcomes of pregnancy. Our results strongly suggest that the immunity subversion-related pathogenesis is involved in early gestation induced by *T. gondii* but not due to a direct invasion of the parasite in adverse pregnancies.

It has been reported that the consequences of congenital toxoplasmosis vary in genotypes of *Toxoplasma* strain (42). Strains of *T. gondii* from Europe and North America belong to three distinct clonal lineages (type I, type II, and type III) which differ phenotypically in virulence (43, 44). Recent studies revealed that polarization of alternatively activated macrophage (M2) or classically activated macrophage (M1) of host macrophages depends on the polymorphism of ROP16 or GRA15 of *Toxoplasma* at early stage of infection. One site mutation of ROP16 at 503L/S would determine the activity or inactivity of ROP16 in phosphorylation of Stat6/Stat3. Type I and type III strains carry $ROP16_{I/III}$, which strongly drives M2 bias but $ROP16_{II}$ is negligible (30, 45, 46), while type II strains infected macrophages are classically activated through bypassing TLRs and directly activating NF-κB by the dense granule protein $GRA15_{II}$ (28, 30). Interestingly, we found that type Chinese 1 (ToxoDB #9) strains carry both $ROP16_{I/III}$

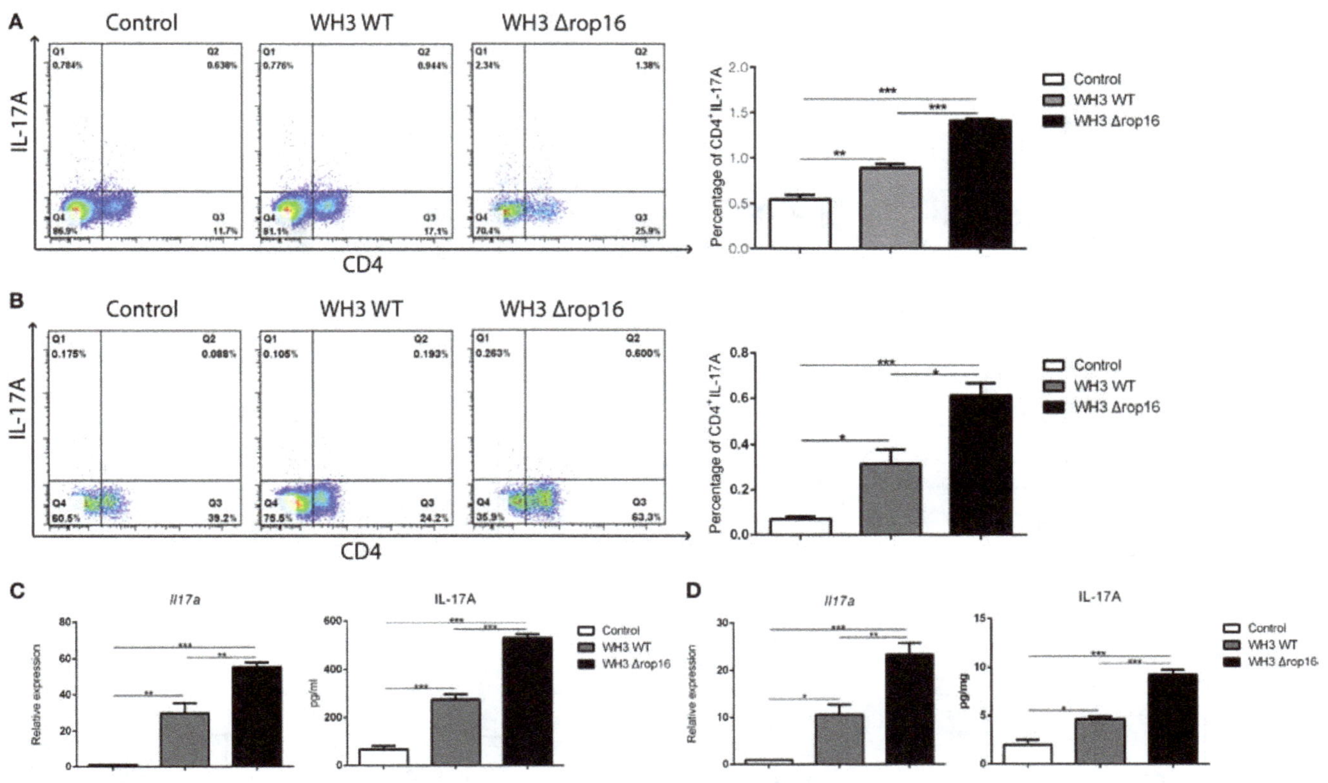

FIGURE 5 | WH3Δ*rop16* strain infection upregulated Th17 response in the spleens and placentas of the pregnant mice. The mice infected with WH3Δ*rop16* strain expressed a high level of interleukin (IL)-17A in the spleens **(A)** and placentas **(B)** determined by flow cytometry. IL-17A mRNA expression in the animals infected with WH3Δ*rop16* in the spleens **(C)** and placentas **(D)**. The IL-17A in the supernatants of spleens (pg/ml) **(C)** and placentas (pg/mg) **(D)** confirmed by enzyme-linked immunosorbent assay (*$p < 0.05$,**$p < 0.01$,***$p < 0.001$).

and GRA15$_{II}$ (33, 34). Thus, we postulated that Chinese 1 strains might have immunopathogenesis which is distinct from the archetypical strains circulating in the other parts of the world. Herewith, we constructed *T. gondii* WH3Δ*rop16* strain based on CRISPR/Cas9 strategy. The genetically manipulated parasite WH3 strain with *rop16*$_{I/III}$-deficient and *gra15*$_{II}$-dominant background (WH3Δ*rop16*/*gra15*$_{II}$), which resembles the archetypical type II of European/North American strains, may be prone to induce adverse pregnant outcomes *via* the mechanism of subverting maternal immunotolerance. We noted that WH3Δ*rop16*/*gra15*$_{II}$ efficiently *in vitro* drove macrophage polarization toward M1 cells, producing NO, TNF-α, and iNOS, and gave rise to trophoblast cells apoptosis compared to WH3 WT strain. We also found that the WH3Δ*rop16*/*gra15*$_{II}$ strain induced characteristic Th1-biased and Th17-involved inflammatory response *in vivo* at maternal–fetal interface featured by high expression of IFN-γ and IL-12, and resulted in more severe adverse pregnant consequences in murine model. These results suggest that ToxoGRA15$_{II}$ is one of the key factors involved in the imbalance of maternal immune tolerance during pregnancy which is associated with M1/Th1/Th17 skewed response. These results are in correspondence with the findings previously reported. Surely, in addition to GRA15$_{II}$, other *Toxoplasma*-derived effectors of type Chinese 1 strain may also contribute to the pathology of immunity imbalance in pregnant animals.

In the construction of the plasmids, insertion of the pyrimethamine resistance gene (dihydrofolate reductase-thymidylate synthase, DHFR-TS*) has been frequently used as the selectable marker for transformant screening of CRISPR/Cas9-based genetic deletion of *Toxoplasma* (35, 47). The DHFR-TS* is not believed to evoke the detectable phenotypical alterations in *Toxoplasma*-infected host, since it is a modified endogenous gene that exists in wild-type strains of the parasite. So far, no evidence has shown its immunogenicity which is able to induce undesirable immune response in its host cells. Moreover, we here did not use ROP16$_{II}$ insertion substituting ROP16$_{I/III}$ because, as stated above, ROP16$_{I/III}$, rather than ROP16$_{II}$, decides ROP16 kinase activity on Stat6/Stat3 and induces M2 polarization which is pivotal to M2 and subsequent Th2 response (45, 46). We deleted ROP16$_{I/III}$ in order to generate a GRA15$_{II}$ dominant transformant to explore the pathology of adverse pregnancy and the mechanisms of pathogenesis caused by the atypical strain of Chinese 1 epidemic in China.

Despite of expressing paternal antigens, the human allogenic fetus is histocompatible with the maternal immune system, presenting an immune down-modulation on CD8$^+$ T cells, Th1, and Th17 cells, which contributes to creation of an immune-privileged environment at the maternal–fetal interface. Previous investigations indicated that microbial endotoxin (LPS) administration to pregnant mice prior to delivery (16.5 day post

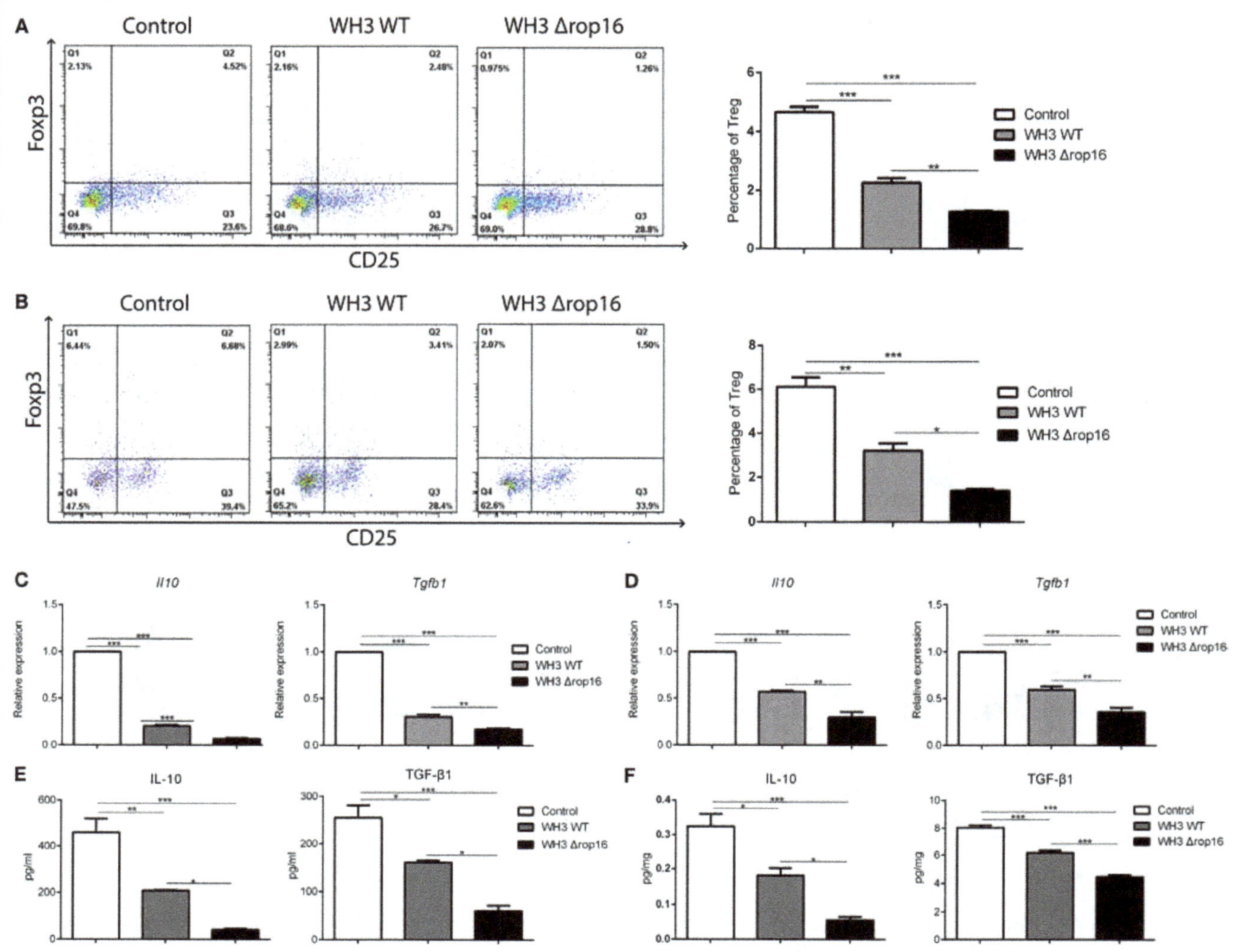

FIGURE 6 | *Toxoplasma* WH3Δ*rop16* strain infection induced impairments of T regulatory cells (Tregs). Tregs cell population in the spleens **(A)** and placentas **(B)** were detected by flow cytometry. Tregs number was significantly decreased in WH3Δ*rop16* infected group compared to control group. The relative mRNA expressions interleukin (IL)-10 and transforming growth factor beta 1 (TGF-β1) in the spleens **(C)** and placentas **(D)** were markedly reduced in WH3Δ*rop16* group. The levels of IL-10 and TGF-β1 in the spleens (pg/ml) **(E)** and placentas (pg/mg) **(F)** were significantly decreased in the group of WH3Δ*rop16* (*$p < 0.05$, **$p < 0.01$, ***$p < 0.001$).

coitum) causes a Tregs and Th17 cells involved imbalance at the maternal–fetal interface and in the spleen, inducing preterm labor (48). However, we found that mice infected with the WH3Δ*rop16/gra15II* strain at the early stage (seventh day of fertility) presented remarkable manifestations of adverse pregnant results, indicating that the mutant strain infection of *Toxoplasma* may lead to abnormal pregnant outcomes in which Tregs and Th17 cells are also involved. Various types of immune cells, such as Tregs, play a pivotal role in the maintenance of normal gestation (11, 49–52). Our study revealed that the percentage of Tregs and expression of IL-10 and TGF-β1 by Tregs as well as M2 cells were significantly diminished in the spleen and placenta tissues of early phase and metaphase of pregnancy of mice infected with the WH3Δ*rop16/gra15*$_{II}$ strain, which is consistent with the previous reports of low expression of IL-10 and TGF-β1 cytokines in mice with a high incidence of fetal rejection (53). This result demonstrates that the impairment of Tregs takes place in *T. gondii*-infected pregnant mice, particularly in mice infected with the strain of WH3 Δ*rop16/gra15*$_{II}$.

A growing body of evidence indicates that Th17 cells are involved in infiltrative inflammation in patients with recurrent spontaneous abortions (54). The imbalance of Tregs/Th17 has also been seen in human abortions (54, 55). Our previous work revealed that *T. gondii* type II strain-derived molecule of ToxoGRA15$_{II}$ is responsible for inducing M1 polarization of RAW264.7 cells *via* NF-κB activation (29, 56) eliciting host innate immunity and Th1-dominant and Th17-involved inflammatory response, and adverse pregnancy outcomes in mice (data in manuscript). Here, we also noted that expression of Th1 cytokines and IL-17A in splenocytes and placenta tissues was observably elevated in the pregnant animals infected with WH3Δ*rop16/gra15*$_{II}$ strain

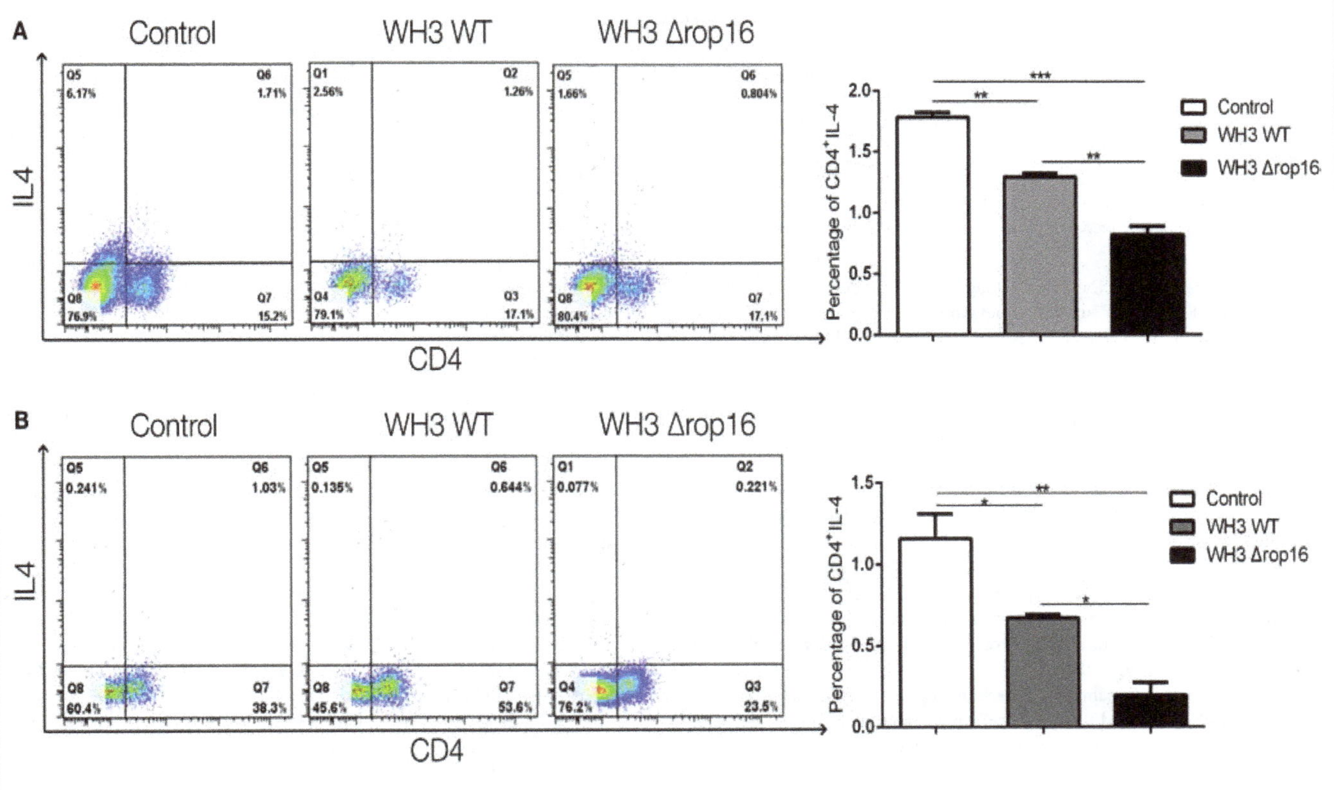

FIGURE 7 | *Toxoplasma* WH3Δ*rop16* strain infection downregulated Th2 response of pregnant mice. The expression of IL-4 in WH3Δ*rop16* group in the spleens **(A)** and placentas **(B)** compared to the control group determined with flow cytometry ($^{*}p < 0.05$, $^{**}p < 0.01$, $^{***}p < 0.001$).

of type Chinese 1 (**Figures 4** and **5**), implying a direct involvement of increased Th17 cells in fetal loss. Additional studies are on going to explore the IFN-γ/NK-involved mechanism at the maternal–fetal interface in abnormal pregnancies associated with *T. gondii* infection.

In summary, our data demonstrate that WH3Δ*rop16* strain with $GRA15_{II}$ background of *T. gondii* type Chinese 1 may cause subversion of immune tolerance at the maternal–fetus interface and in systemic immunity, leading to adverse pregnancy outcomes, which is associated with the Th1 and Th17 biased response. This study would provide an explanation for pregnancy failure caused by non/less virulent strains of type II and offer a deep insight into the pathogenesis of abnormal pregnancy caused by strains of *T. gondii* type Chinese 1 dominating in China.

AUTHOR CONTRIBUTIONS

JS and CW conceived and designed the experiments. CW, WC, QY, and TX performed the experiments. WC, CW, and JS drafted the manuscript. All authors contributed to discussion of the results followed by writing and reviewing the manuscript.

ACKNOWLEDGMENTS

The pSAG1:CAS9-U6:sgUPRT was gifted by David Sibley at Washington University School of Medicine, USA. The pDHFR-TS plasmid was a gift from Honglin Jia in Harbin Veterinary Research Institute of Chinese Academy of Agricultural Sciences, China.

REFERENCES

1. Sacks GP, Studena K, Sargent K, Redman CW. Normal pregnancy and preeclampsia both produce inflammatory changes in peripheral blood leukocytes akin to those of sepsis. *Am J Obstet Gynecol* (1998) 179(1):80–6. doi:10.1016/S0002-9378(98)70254-6
2. Trowsdale J, Betz AG. Mother's little helpers: mechanisms of maternal-fetal tolerance. *Nat Immunol* (2006) 7(3):241–6. doi:10.1038/ni1317
3. Saito S, Sakai M, Sasaki Y, Tanebe K, Tsuda H, Michimata T. Quantitative analysis of peripheral blood Th0, Th1, Th2 and the Th1: Th2 cell ratio during normal human pregnancy and preeclampsia. *Clin Exp Immunol* (1999) 117(3):550–5. doi:10.1046/j.1365-2249.1999.00997.x
4. Huppertz B, Kadyrov M, Kingdom JC. Apoptosis and its role in the trophoblast. *Am J Obstet Gynecol* (2006) 195(1):29–39. doi:10.1016/j.ajog.2005.07.039
5. Asseman C, Mauze S, Leach MW, Coffman RL, Powrie F. An essential role for interleukin 10 in the function of regulatory T cells that inhibit intes

tinal inflammation. *J Exp Med* (1999) 190(7):995–1004. doi:10.1084/jem.190.7.995
6. Santner-Nanan B, Straubinger K, Hsu P, Parnell G, Tang B, Xu B, et al. Fetal-maternal alignment of regulatory T cells correlates with IL-10 and Bcl-2 upregulation in pregnancy. *J Immunol* (2013) 191(1):145–53. doi:10.4049/jimmunol.1203165
7. Zenclussen AC, Gerlof K, Zenclussen ML, Ritschel S, Zambon Bertoja A, Fest S, et al. Regulatory T cells induce a privileged tolerant microenvironment at the fetal-maternal interface. *Eur J Immunol* (2006) 36(1):82–94. doi:10.1002/eji.200535428
8. Maloy KJ, Salaun L, Cahill R, Dougan G, Saunders NJ, Powrie F. CD4+CD25+ T(R) cells suppress innate immune pathology through cytokine-dependent mechanisms. *J Exp Med* (2003) 197(1):111–9. doi:10.1084/jem.20021345
9. Darrasse-Jeze G, Klatzmann D, Charlotte F, Salomon BL, Cohen JL. CD4+CD25+ regulatory/suppressor T cells prevent allogeneic fetus rejection in mice. *Immunol Lett* (2006) 102(1):106–9. doi:10.1016/j.imlet.2005.07.002
10. Lash GE, Otun HA, Innes BA, Kirkley M, De Oliveira L, Searle RF, et al. Interferon-gamma inhibits extravillous trophoblast cell invasion by a mechanism that involves both changes in apoptosis and protease levels. *FASEB J* (2006) 20(14):2512–8. doi:10.1096/fj.06-6616com
11. Piccinni MP, Beloni L, Livi C, Maggi E, Scarselli G, Romagnani S. Defective production of both leukemia inhibitory factor and type 2 T-helper cytokines by decidual T cells in unexplained recurrent abortions. *Nat Med* (1998) 4(9):1020–4. doi:10.1038/2006
12. Mjosberg J, Berg G, Jenmalm MC, Ernerudh J. FOXP3+ regulatory T cells and T helper 1, T helper 2, and T helper 17 cells in human early pregnancy decidua. *Biol Reprod* (2010) 82(4):698–705. doi:10.1095/biolreprod.109.081208
13. Lin H, Mosmann TR, Guilbert L, Tuntipopipat S, Wegmann TG. Synthesis of T helper 2-type cytokines at the maternal-fetal interface. *J Immunol* (1993) 151(9):4562–73.
14. Xu C, Mao D, Holers VM, Palanca B, Cheng AM, Molina H. A critical role for murine complement regulator crry in fetomaternal tolerance. *Science* (2000) 287(5452):498–501. doi:10.1126/science.287.5452.498
15. Montoya JG, Liesenfeld O. Toxoplasmosis. *Lancet* (2004) 363(9425):1965–76. doi:10.1016/S0140-6736(04)16412-X
16. Wong SY, Remington JS. Toxoplasmosis in pregnancy. *Clin Infect Dis* (1994) 18(6):853–61; quiz 862. doi:10.1093/clinids/18.6.853
17. Robbins JR, Zeldovich VB, Poukchanski A, Boothroyd JC, Bakardjiev AI. Tissue barriers of the human placenta to infection with *Toxoplasma gondii*. *Infect Immun* (2012) 80(1):418–28. doi:10.1128/IAI.05899-11
18. Xu X, He L, Zhang A, Li Q, Hu W, Chen H, et al. *Toxoplasma gondii* isolate with genotype Chinese 1 triggers trophoblast apoptosis through oxidative stress and mitochondrial dysfunction in mice. *Exp Parasitol* (2015) 154:51–61. doi:10.1016/j.exppara.2015.04.008
19. Hunter CA, Sibley LD. Modulation of innate immunity by *Toxoplasma gondii* virulence effectors. *Nat Rev Microbiol* (2012) 10(11):766–78. doi:10.1038/nrmicro2858
20. Wang H, Hirsch E. Bacterially-induced preterm labor and regulation of prostaglandin-metabolizing enzyme expression in mice: the role of toll-like receptor 4. *Biol Reprod* (2003) 69(6):1957–63. doi:10.1095/biolreprod.103.019620
21. Fu B, Li X, Sun R, Tong X, Ling B, Tian Z, et al. Natural killer cells promote immune tolerance by regulating inflammatory TH17 cells at the human maternal-fetal interface. *Proc Natl Acad Sci U S A* (2013) 110(3):E231–40. doi:10.1073/pnas.1206322110
22. Zhang H, Hu X, Liu X, Zhang R, Fu Q, Xu X. The Treg/Th17 imbalance in *Toxoplasma gondii*-infected pregnant mice. *Am J Reprod Immunol* (2012) 67(2):112–21. doi:10.1111/j.1600-0897.2011.01065.x
23. Lee SK, Kim JY, Lee M, Gilman-Sachs A, Kwak-Kim J. Th17 and regulatory T cells in women with recurrent pregnancy loss. *Am J Reprod Immunol* (2012) 67(4):311–8. doi:10.1111/j.1600-0897.2012.01116.x
24. Saeij JP, Boyle JP, Coller S, Taylor S, Sibley LD, Brooke-Powell ET, et al. Polymorphic secreted kinases are key virulence factors in toxoplasmosis. *Science* (2006) 314(5806):1780–3. doi:10.1126/science.1133690
25. Taylor S, Barragan A, Su C, Fux B, Fentress SJ, Tang K, et al. A secreted serine-threonine kinase determines virulence in the eukaryotic pathogen *Toxoplasma gondii*. *Science* (2006) 314(5806):1776–80. doi:10.1126/science.1133643
26. Saeij JP, Coller S, Boyle JP, Jerome ME, White MW, Boothroyd JC. *Toxoplasma* co-opts host gene expression by injection of a polymorphic kinase homologue. *Nature* (2007) 445(7125):324–7. doi:10.1038/nature05395
27. Reese ML, Zeiner GM, Saeij JP, Boothroyd JC, Boyle JP. Polymorphic family of injected pseudokinases is paramount in *Toxoplasma* virulence. *Proc Natl Acad Sci U S A* (2011) 108(23):9625–30. doi:10.1073/pnas.1015980108
28. Rosowski EE, Lu D, Julien L, Rodda L, Gaiser RA, Jensen KD, et al. Strain-specific activation of the NF-kappaB pathway by GRA15, a novel *Toxoplasma gondii* dense granule protein. *J Exp Med* (2011) 208(1):195–212. doi:10.1084/jem.20100717
29. Xie Y, Wen H, Yan K, Wang S, Wang X, Chen J, et al. *Toxoplasma gondii* GRA15II effector-induced M1 cells ameliorate liver fibrosis in mice infected with *Schistosomiasis japonica*. *Cell Mol Immunol* (2016) 15(2):120–34. doi:10.1038/cmi.2016.21
30. Jensen KD, Wang Y, Wojno ED, Shastri AJ, Hu K, Cornel L, et al. *Toxoplasma* polymorphic effectors determine macrophage polarization and intestinal inflammation. *Cell Host Microbe* (2011) 9(6):472–83. doi:10.1016/j.chom.2011.04.015
31. Loke P, Allison JP. PD-L1 and PD-L2 are differentially regulated by Th1 and Th2 cells. *Proc Natl Acad Sci U S A* (2003) 100(9):5336–41. doi:10.1073/pnas.0931259100
32. Melo MB, Jensen KD, Saeij JP. *Toxoplasma gondii* effectors are master regulators of the inflammatory response. *Trends Parasitol* (2011) 27(11):487–95. doi:10.1016/j.pt.2011.08.001
33. Cheng W, Liu F, Li M, Hu X, Chen H, Pappoe F, et al. Variation detection based on next-generation sequencing of type Chinese 1 strains of *Toxoplasma gondii* with different virulence from China. *BMC Genomics* (2015) 16:888. doi:10.1186/s12864-015-2106-z
34. Cai Y, Chen H, Mo X, Tang Y, Xu X, Zhang A, et al. *Toxoplasma gondii* inhibits apoptosis via a novel STAT3-miR-17-92-Bim pathway in macrophages. *Cell Signal* (2014) 26(6):1204–12. doi:10.1016/j.cellsig.2014.02.013
35. Shen B, Brown KM, Lee TD, Sibley LD. Efficient gene disruption in diverse strains of *Toxoplasma gondii* using CRISPR/CAS9. *MBio* (2014) 5(3): e01114–01114. doi:10.1128/mBio.01114-14
36. Ding AH, Nathan CF, Stuehr DJ. Release of reactive nitrogen intermediates and reactive oxygen intermediates from mouse peritoneal macrophages. Comparison of activating cytokines and evidence for independent production. *J Immunol* (1988) 141(7):2407–12.
37. Remington JS, McLeod R, Desmonts G. Toxoplasmosis. 4th ed. In: Remington JS, Klein JO, editors. *Infectious Diseases of the Fetus and Newborn Infant*. Philadelphia: WB Saunders (1995). p. 140–267.
38. Dunn D, Wallon M, Peyron F, Petersen E, Peckham C, Gilbert R. Mother-to-child transmission of toxoplasmosis: risk estimates for clinical counselling. *Lancet* (1999) 353(9167):1829–33. doi:10.1016/S0140-6736(98)08220-8
39. Vargas-Villavicencio JA, Cedillo-Pelaez C, Rico-Torres CP, Besne-Merida A, Garcia-Vazquez F, Saldana JI, et al. Mouse model of congenital infection with a non-virulent *Toxoplasma gondii* strain: vertical transmission, "sterile" fetal damage, or both? *Exp Parasitol* (2016) 166:116–23. doi:10.1016/j.exppara.2016.04.002
40. Senegas A, Villard O, Neuville A, Marcellin L, Pfaff AW, Steinmetz T, et al. *Toxoplasma gondii*-induced foetal resorption in mice involves interferon-gamma-induced apoptosis and spiral artery dilation at the maternofoetal interface. *Int J Parasitol* (2009) 39(4):481–7. doi:10.1016/j.ijpara.2008.08.009
41. Pfaff AW, Abou-Bacar A, Letscher-Bru V, Villard O, Senegas A, Mousli M, et al. Cellular and molecular physiopathology of congenital toxoplasmosis: the dual role of IFN-gamma. *Parasitology* (2007) 134(Pt 13):1895–902. doi:10.1017/S0031182007000200
42. Rico-Torres CP, Vargas-Villavicencio JA, Correa D. Is *Toxoplasma gondii* type related to clinical outcome in human congenital infection? Systematic and critical review. *Eur J Clin Microbiol Infect Dis* (2016) 35(7):1079–88. doi:10.1007/s10096-016-2656-2
43. Howe DK, Sibley LD. *Toxoplasma gondii* comprises three clonal lineages: correlation of parasite genotype with human disease. *J Infect Dis* (1995) 172(6):1561–6. doi:10.1093/infdis/172.6.1561

44. Sibley LD, Boothroyd JC. Virulent strains of *Toxoplasma gondii* comprise a single clonal lineage. *Nature* (1992) 359(6390):82–5. doi:10.1038/359082a0
45. Murray PJ. Macrophages as a battleground for *Toxoplasma* pathogenesis. *Cell Host Microbe* (2011) 9(6):445–7. doi:10.1016/j.chom.2011.05.010
46. Yamamoto M, Standley DM, Takashima S, Saiga H, Okuyama M, Kayama H, et al. A single polymorphic amino acid on *Toxoplasma gondii* kinase ROP16 determines the direct and strain-specific activation of Stat3. *J Exp Med* (2009) 206(12):2747–60. doi:10.1084/jem.20091703
47. Shen B, Brown K, Long S, Sibley LD. Chapter 6. Development of CRISPR/Cas9 for efficient genome editing in *Toxoplasma gondii*. In: Reeves A, editor. *In Vitro Mutagenesis Methods and Protocols*. Warrenville, IL: Coskata, Inc. (2017) 79–106.
48. Arenas-Hernandez M, Romero R, St Louis D, Hassan SS, Kaye EB, Gomez-Lopez N. An imbalance between innate and adaptive immune cells at the maternal-fetal interface occurs prior to endotoxin-induced preterm birth. *Cell Mol Immunol* (2016) 13(4):462–73. doi:10.1038/cmi.2015.22
49. Somerset DA, Zheng Y, Kilby MD, Sansom DM, Drayson MT. Normal human pregnancy is associated with an elevation in the immune suppressive CD25+ CD4+ regulatory T-cell subset. *Immunology* (2004) 112(1):38–43. doi:10.1111/j.1365-2567.2004.01869.x
50. Tilburgs T, Scherjon SA, van der Mast BJ, Haasnoot GW, Versteeg VDV-MM, Roelen DL, et al. Fetal-maternal HLA-C mismatch is associated with decidual T cell activation and induction of functional T regulatory cells. *J Reprod Immunol* (2009) 82(2):148–57. doi:10.1016/j.jri.2009.05.003
51. Tilburgs T, Roelen DL, van der Mast BJ, de Groot-Swings GM, Kleijburg C, Scherjon SA, et al. Evidence for a selective migration of fetus-specific CD4+CD25bright regulatory T cells from the peripheral blood to the decidua in human pregnancy. *J Immunol* (2008) 180(8):5737–45. doi:10.4049/jimmunol.180.8.5737
52. Quinn KH, Lacoursiere DY, Cui L, Bui J, Parast MM. The unique pathophysiology of early-onset severe preeclampsia: role of decidual T regulatory cells. *J Reprod Immunol* (2011) 91(1–2):76–82. doi:10.1016/j.jri.2011.05.006
53. Blois S, Tometten M, Kandil J, Hagen E, Klapp BF, Margni RA, et al. Intercellular adhesion molecule-1/LFA-1 cross talk is a proximate mediator capable of disrupting immune integration and tolerance mechanism at the feto-maternal interface in murine pregnancies. *J Immunol* (2005) 174(4):1820–9. doi:10.4049/jimmunol.174.4.1820
54. Wang WJ, Hao CF, Yi L, Yin GJ, Bao SH, Qiu LH, et al. Increased prevalence of T helper 17 (Th17) cells in peripheral blood and decidua in unexplained recurrent spontaneous abortion patients. *J Reprod Immunol* (2010) 84(2):164–70. doi:10.1016/j.jri.2009.12.003
55. Liu YS, Wu L, Tong XH, Wu LM, He GP, Zhou GX, et al. Study on the relationship between Th17 cells and unexplained recurrent spontaneous abortion. *Am J Reprod Immunol* (2011) 65(5):503–11. doi:10.1111/j.1600-0897.2010.00921.x
56. Li Y, Poppoe F, Chen J, Yu L, Deng F, Luo Q, et al. Macrophages polarized by expression of ToxoGRA15II inhibit growth of hepatic carcinoma. *Front Immunol* (2017) 8:137. doi:10.3389/fimmu.2017.00137

14

Leptin Functions in Infectious Diseases

Radheshyam Maurya [1*], Parna Bhattacharya [2], Ranadhir Dey [2] and Hira L. Nakhasi [2]

[1] Department of Animal Biology, School of Life Science, University of Hyderabad, Hyderabad, India, [2] Division of Emerging and Transfusion Transmitted Diseases, Center for Biologics Evaluation and Research, Food and Drug Administration, Silver Spring, MD, United States

Correspondence:
Radheshyam Maurya
rmusl@uohyd.ernet.in;
radhemaurya@rediifmail.com

Leptin, a pleiotropic protein has long been recognized to play an important role in the regulation of energy homeostasis, metabolism, neuroendocrine function, and other physiological functions through its effects on the central nervous system (CNS) and peripheral tissues. Leptin is secreted by adipose tissue and encoded by the obese (*ob*) gene. Leptin acts as a central mediator which regulates immunity as well as nutrition. Importantly, leptin can modulate both innate and adaptive immune responses. Leptin deficiency/resistance is associated with dysregulation of cytokine production, increased susceptibility toward infectious diseases, autoimmune disorders, malnutrition and inflammatory responses. Malnutrition induces a state of immunodeficiency and an inclination to death from communicable diseases. Infectious diseases are the disease of poor who invariably suffer from malnutrition that could result from reduced serum leptin levels. Thus, leptin has been placed at the center of many interrelated functions in various pathogenic conditions, such as bacterial, viruses and parasitic infections. We review herein, the recent advances on the role of leptin in malnutrition in pathogenesis of infectious diseases with a particular emphasis on parasitic diseases such as Leishmaniasis, Trypanosomiasis, Amoebiasis, and Malaria.

Keywords: leptin, leishmaniasis, trypanosomiasis, amoebiasis, malaria, bacteria, virus, malnutrition

INTRODUCTION

Leptin is a hormone derived from adipocytes in response to the nutritional status, and it signals to the central nervous system (CNS) and peripheral organs (1). The circulating plasma leptin concentrations are mostly influenced by the total body fat mass index, metabolic hormones, and gender. Women have higher concentrations of circulating leptin compared to men (2). The central function of leptin is metabolic homeostasis that can be attained by the delivery of information about the total body fat mass to the hypothalamus that in turn alters the CNS function and regulates glucocorticoids, insulin hormone and food intake & energy balance (3, 4). Concurrently, leptin is also a critical regulator of immunity and functions as a pro-inflammatory cytokine-like interleukin (IL)-1, IL-6, IL-8, IL-18, and tumor necrosis factor-α (TNF-α), and its deficiency increases susceptibility to infectious (5–8).

Leptin was identified as the gene defect responsible for the obesity syndrome in Leptin-deficient (*ob/ob*) mice and reported as the product of *Ob* gene (9, 10). Leptin is a 16 kDa α-helix type protein like the long-chain helical cytokine family such as IL-6, IL-2, IL-12, leukocyte inhibitory factor (LIF), Granulocyte-colony stimulating factor (G-CSF), Ciliary neurotrophic factor (CNTF), and Oncostatin M (11, 12). Most of the biological functions of leptin are exerted through leptin receptor (Ob-R) signaling via the Janus kinase/signal transducer and activator of transcription (JAK/STAT) pathway (13, 14). In general, leptin enhances the immune response via activating antigen presenting cells (APCs), Th1 cells function and proliferation, and mediating the secretion of the pro-inflammatory cytokines, such as TNF-α, IL-2, or IL-6 (7, 15, 16). Leptin-deficient (*ob/ob*; double knockout obese gene) and leptin receptor-deficient (*db/db*; double knockout obese receptor gene) mice display marked reduction in the size & thymic atrophy and exhibit defective immune responses (17, 18). Similarly, reduced leptin levels in starved and malnourished individuals is further associated with alterations of the immune response and thymic atrophy. However, these conditions can be reversed by leptin administration (19–22).

Over the past decade, the role leptin in infectious diseases was extensively explored. It has been reported that leptin deficiency is correlated with starvation or nutritional deprivation/malnutrition (23). Malnutrition affects both innate & acquired immunity of the host (24) thereby increasing the incidences of infections and mortality (25). The immune dysfunction in malnutrition or restricted calorie intake reduced the memory T cells, total CD4+ and CD8+ T cell numbers compared to well-nourished infected controls (26–29). Interestingly, leptin has a crucial role in mediating phagocytosis, T cell number, function, and metabolism in both obesity and malnutrition. The systemic circulating leptin deficiency in malnutrition is also correlated with several other bacterial, viral and parasitic infections such as tuberculosis (30), pneumonia (31), sepsis (32), colitis (33), viral infection (34, 35) leishmaniasis (36), trypanosomiasis (37), amoebiasis (38), and malaria (39) due to defective cytokine production (40–45). Hence, nutritional status is critically essential for immune cell function in both malnutrition and infection. Understanding how leptin is altered in malnutrition and infection will lead to better insight of and treatment for diseases where nutritional status determines clinical outcome. Furthermore, there has been increasing evidence that leptin is involved in the pathogenesis of various infectious diseases. In the present review, we will discuss the emerging role of leptin in different infectious diseases and will further highlight how malnutrition or starvation could play a role.

LEPTIN AND IMMUNITY

Leptin is a pleiotropic molecule, which can function as a hormone as well as cytokine (adipokine). Almost all immune cells such as neutrophils, monocytes, lymphocytes express leptin receptor and it belongs to the family of class-I cytokine receptors (46–48). Leptin regulates angiogenesis, hematopoiesis, innate & adaptive immunity and induces the Th1 response by increasing IFN-γ, IL-2, and TNF-α production, subsequently leading to the activation of monocyte/macrophages and prevents the apoptosis of various immune cells by delaying the cleavage of Bid and Bax (49–55).

In innate immunity, leptin enhances the activity and function of neutrophils by the release of oxygen free radicals, increased CD11b expression and intercellular adhesion molecule-1 (ICAM-1), which leads to migration of immune cells at the sites of inflammation (56–58). Leptin activates the monocytes and dendrite cells (DCs) that in turn leads to the production of pro-inflammatory cytokines such as TNF-α, IL-6 along with IL-12, a key cytokine that facilitates the shifting of T-cells toward the Th1 phenotype (59–62). Leptin also promotes DCs survival by triggering the activation of nuclear factor-kappa B (NF-kappa B) and up-regulates B-cell lymphoma 2 (Bcl-2) and B-cell lymphoma-extra-large (Bcl-xL) gene expression via the PI3K-Akt signaling pathway (62). Moreover, upon leptin stimulation, DCs also exhibit increased production of multiple cytokines including IL-1, IL-6, IL-12, TNF-α, MIP-1α and induces the expression of surface molecules, such as CD1a, CD80, CD83, or CD86 (63, 64). Indirectly, leptin leads to the activation of natural killer (NK) cells upon modulation of IL-1, IL-6, and TNF-α via monocytes and macrophages (61) resulting an increased IL-12 and reduced IL-15 expression in NK cells (65, 66).

In adaptive immunity, leptin induces the maturation and survival of thymic T-cells by reducing their rate of apoptosis through inhibition of FAS-directed apoptosis pathway (16, 67). Eventually, leptin has anti-apoptotic effects on mature T-cells, by up-regulating the expression of Bcl-xL (68), T-box transcription factor (T-bet) (69), and synergizes with other cytokines in lymphocyte proliferation and activation possibly via signal transducer and activator of transcription 3 (STAT3) signaling (70, 71). Leptin deficiency in both mouse and human results in severe immune defects characterized by decrease in total lymphocytes, CD4+ helper T cell number, increased thymocyte apoptosis, and a skewing away from the Th1 toward Th2 phenotype thereby resulting in increased susceptibility to intracellular infections (16, 17, 72–74). Leptin mediates T-cells polarization by inducing the cell-mediated immune response through the secretion of IL-2, IL-12, TNF-α, and IFN-γ from Th1 cells and suppresses the production of IL-10 and IL-4 from Th2 cells (13, 75–78). In facts, thymocytes treated with leptin induces CD4+CD8+ cell differentiation mainly to CD4+ mature thymocytes (79). Additionally, leptin also activates human B cells to secrete cytokines, such as IL-6, IL-10, and TNF-α, through the activation of JAK2/STAT3 and p38MAPK/ERK1/2 signaling pathways (80, 81). Leptin-STAT3 signaling also influences the production of C-X-C chemokine receptor type 3 (CXCR3) and C-C chemokine receptor type 5 (CCR5) ligands, which are preferentially expressed on Th1 cells and enhances pro-inflammatory cytokines such as IL-1β, TNF-α, and IL-6 in serum (39, 82, 83). In conclusion, leptin acts as a Th1 cytokine and regulates all immune cells through leptin receptor and affects innate & adaptive immune responses together facilitating a shift toward Th1 response. The brief role of leptin in innate & adaptive immune response was summarized in **Figure 1**.

LEPTIN IN MALNUTRITION

Nutritional deficiency impaired phagocyte function, cell-mediated immunity, cytokine production, antibody response and the complement system (24, 25, 84) and predisposed to

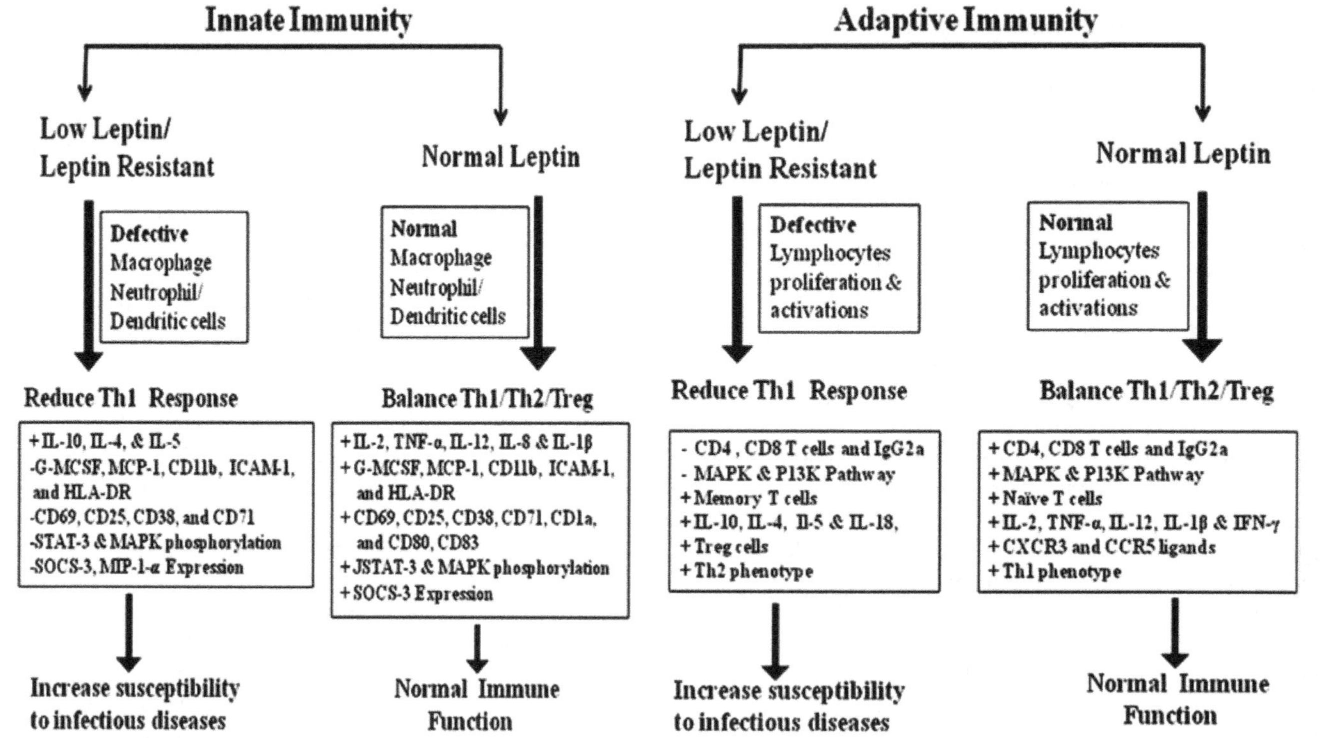

FIGURE 1 | The role of leptin in Innate and adaptive immunity: innate immunity; Leptin plays a crucial role in the activation and proliferation of macrophage, neutrophil, and dendritic cells through the up and down regulation of various cytokine/chemokines. Adaptive immunity; Leptin-induced the activation and proliferation of total lymphocytes (T and B cells), regulatory T cells and Naive T cells through the up and down regulation of pro-inflammatory and anti-inflammatory cytokines. The Innate and adaptive immune response induced by leptin signaling through the phosphorylation of MAKP/STAT-3/P13K pathways (15–18, 49–55).

death from infectious diseases (85). Concurrently, malnutrition is the most common cause of secondary immunodeficiency worldwide associated with protein-energy malnutrition (PEM) (86, 87), a nutritional deficiency in which individuals suffer from protein but not calorific malnutrition (88). Strikingly, PEM causes a drastic reduction in body fat mass and decreases the circulating concentration of leptin, which, in turn, impairs the generation of proinflammatory mediators [IFN-γ, TNF-α and (NO) nitric oxide] (89, 90), and increases the incidence of infectious diseases (72, 83). Malnutrition is a primary risk factor for many infectious diseases. From recent research, it seems that malnutrition is a predictor of tuberculosis disease and is associated with worse outcomes. Active tuberculosis is correlated with weight loss, cachexia, and low serum concentrations of leptin which in turn suppresses the lymphocyte stimulation and Th1 cytokines such as IL-2, IFN-γ, and TNF-α secretion (91–96). PEM significantly reduced the lymphocyte stimulation as well as secretion of the Th1 cytokines such as IL-2, IFN-γ, and TNF-α, in M. tuberculosis-infected guinea pig (92, 97). Furthermore, PEM also diminishes leptin concentrations and increases serum levels of stress hormones, i.e., glucocorticoids which impairs macrophage functions by limiting NF-kB translocation into the nucleus (96). Macrophages from experimental PEM mice are less sensitive to lipopolysaccharides (LPS) due to decreased NF-kB translocation resulting in impairment of active phagocytosis, cytokines response and reactive oxygen intermediates (ROIs) productions (98–101).

Serum leptin concentration decreases as malnutrition becomes more pronounced and thus serves as a biomarker of poor nutritional status in chronic cirrhosis due to viral hepatitis and candidiasis due to *Candida albicans* (102–105). Moreover, during fasting or starvation, leptin levels also fall disproportionately due to the decrease in adipose tissue fat mass (106, 107). The decrease in leptin level during starvation rendered wild-type mice susceptible to LPS and TNF-α induced lethality whereas leptin treatment restores those changes despite ongoing starvation, suggesting that the lack of leptin plays a role in the immune dysfunction during starvation (18, 108). Exogenous leptin administration modulates T cell responses in mice and prevents starvation-induced immune suppression on the development of a delay type of hypersensitivity (DTH) response and protects from starvation-induced lymphoid atrophy in mice (12, 15, 68, 109).

Taken together, Leptin is a protein hormone secreted by adipocytes, regulating body fat and food intake through neuroendocrine-signaling system. Hence, it is possible to speculate that leptin might act in the brain to directly regulate metabolic response along with peripheral immune function thereby contributing to better outcomes in various infectious diseases compared with states of relative or total leptin deficiency. Importantly, recent studies reported that serum leptin level may be used as a promising diagnostic or prognostic marker for critical illness sepsis that is triggered by an infective agent such as bacteria, viruses, fungi, or parasites (110). Therefore, from here onwards, the review focuses on the role of leptin in various infectious diseases.

LEPTIN AND BACTERIAL INFECTIONS

Leptin-deficient mice and mice rendered leptin-deficient by fasting exhibit impaired pulmonary bacterial clearance (**Table 1**) and enhanced lethality during pulmonary tuberculosis, bacterial pneumonia, and sepsis (30–32). The patients with pulmonary tuberculosis (PTB) have decreased serum leptin levels, and an increase in adiponectin may serve as a reliable biomarker for predicting the development and progression of PTB pathogenesis (111, 145, 146). Mycobacterium infection in *ob/ob* mice was hampered to produce organized granulomatous response and defective in CD4+ and CD8+ T cells functions, IFN-γ and DTH responses (30). The mechanisms underlying the defective leukocyte effector function in cells from leptin-deficient mice were associated with a reduction in leukotriene (LT) synthesis in alveolar macrophage (AMs), reduced complement receptor (CR3) expression and decreased H_2O_2 synthesis in neutrophils (PMNs) infected with *Klebsiella pneumoniae* (112–114). Restoring the level of circulating leptin to physiological levels in fasted and *ob/ob* mice significantly improved the survival and pulmonary bacterial clearance, reduced bacteraemia, reconstituted alveolar macrophage phagocytosis and increased H_2O_2 production in the PMNs resulting in increased killing of *S. pneumonia in vitro* (31, 115). Leptin binding to leptin receptor activates multiple intracellular signaling pathways, including STAT3, STAT5, and ERK1/2. STAT3 activates transcription of suppressor of cytokine signaling (SOCS)-3, a protein that inhibits JAK2 and STAT3 signaling during prolonged stimulation of the Leptin receptor long isoform (*Lep-Rb*) (147, 148). *Lep-Rb* mediated phosphorylation of Tyr^{1077} activates STAT5 signaling pathway (149). Phosphorylation of Tyr^{985} in leptin receptor recruits binding partners SH2-containing tyrosine phosphatase (SHP-2) and growth factor binding 2 (GRB2) which activate extracellular signal-regulated kinase 1 and 2 (ERK 1/2) signaling (147, 150). A mutation of the Try^{985} with L^{985} residue in the leptin receptor exhibited increased mortality and impaired pulmonary bacterial clearance following an intratracheal challenge with *K. pneumoniae* due to the disruption of ERK-dependent activation (151).

Moreover, Leptin-dependent neutrophilic phagocytosis of *L. monocytogenes* was more potent than *Escherichia coli* due to the presence of apoptotic factor Listeriolysin O, which is absent in *E. coli* (116). Exogenous leptin restored the anti-listeria resistance and monocyte chemoattractant protein-1 (MCP-1) and MIP-2 production in leptin-deficient mice (117, 152). *Clostridium difficile colitis* is a primary causative agent of nosocomial infection in humans and murine. The defective STAT3 signaling pathway leads to susceptibility to infectious colitis and bacterial peritonitis (33, 153) and leptin treatment restored the protective mucosal immune response in *C. difficile colitis* by the STAT3 inflammatory pathway (33).

In contrast to above finding, disruption of leptin receptor-mediated STAT3 signaling pathway improved AMs phagocytosis and host defense against *P. pneumonia* in ($Lepr^{s1138/s1138}$) s/s mice following an intratracheal challenge with *S. pneumonia* (154). These effects are mediated by an intracellular signaling pathway that is dependent on ERK1/2 activation in AMs resulting an increased in LT synthesis, which enhanced the phagocytosis in cells from *s/s* mice (154). Mice infected with *Helicobacter pylori*-induced pro-inflammatory cytokine response and enhanced the leptin secretion from gastric mucosa which may be playing a role in weight gain after eradication of *H pylori* infection (118–120) suggesting that leptin has a local effect rather than systemic action in patients with gastritis (121, 155). These findings reveal the existence of a relevant neuroendocrine control of leptin in systemic immune defense in various bacterial diseases thereby highlighting the possible therapeutic potential of leptin analogous to control infectious diseases.

LEPTIN AND VIRAL INFECTIONS

Mice deficient in the leptin receptor or malnourished leads to impaired viral clearance (**Table 1**), diminished lung IFNγ level and reduced survival during influenza-A pneumonia infections (156). The mice lacking functional leptin receptor in T cells ($LepR^{T-/-}$) limits pH1N1 influenza mortality and infection severity in obese mice suggesting that leptin signaling in T cells may be a critical mediator of pH1N1 severity in obese mice (122, 123). Moreover, Leptin resistant obese mice or decreased leptin level in obese individuals may increase the susceptibility to influenza virus infection by suppressing the memory T-cell function and IFN-α, IFN-β, and IFN-γ mRNA expression which leads to an increase in viral titer and infiltration (124). Furthermore, mice lacking functional leptin receptor in tissue-specific lung epithelial and macrophage cells have improved viral clearance and reduced lung injury following influenza-A infection suggesting that leptin signaling is also associated with non-myeloid cells such as natural killer cells and T cells (125). Leptin significantly upregulated the Th17 subset but suppressed Th2 subset differentiation possibly via regulating ERK1/2 phosphorylation in human bronchial epithelial cells (hBECs) infected with the respiratory syncytial virus (RSV) (126). Human immunodeficiency virus (HIV)-infected patients have an exaggerated expression of leptin receptor on their blood mononuclear cells while low leptin levels in their serum leads to an immune deficiency in these patients (127, 128). Importantly, leptin therapy, a novel strategy now in clinical trials, and its beneficial positive role in HIV patients in correction of metabolic complications related to HIV-associated lipodystrophy syndrome (HALS) has been reported recently (129). Leptin also diminishes the oxidative status of monocytes suggesting that leptin can alter the redox status of monocytes, which leads to immunological alterations in HIV infection (35). Therefore, taken together these findings reveal that leptin could control the systemic immune defense failure in viral specific immune cells dysfunction and

TABLE 1 | The distinctive immune responses in various infectious diseases upon leptin treatment were summarized.

Infectious group	Infectious species	Effect of leptin on the Immune response	Model used (*in-vitro* & *in-vivo*)	References
Bacterial disease	*Mycobacterium tuberculosis*	Increase IFNγ & TNF-α levels and PMN cells & functions. Increase T helper CD4 T cells & CD8 T cells activity. Improve Ag- specific antibody response. Restored DTH response and Granuloma formation. Reduced IL-6 cytokine and bacterial load.	Mice and human	(30, 95, 111)
	Klebsiella pneumonia	Increase phagocytosis index and Leukotriene synthesis. Improve defective alveolar macrophage phagocytosis. Restored CD11b expression level. Decrease bacterial load and reduce mortality.	Mice	(112, 113)
	Pneumococcal pneumonia	Restored defective alveolar macrophage phagocytosis activity. Increase PMN H_2O_2 production. Reduced TNF-α, MIP-2, PGE2 in the lung. Improves pulmonary bacterial clearance and survival.	Mice	(31, 114)
	Clostridium difficile	Leptin receptor Q223R mutation leads to defective STAT3 signaling pathway and associated with an increased risk of colitis. Mutation of tyrosine 1,138 in the intracellular domain of LepRb decreased mucosal chemokine and cell recruitment. Increases inflammation, colonic chemokine expression, and cellular recruitment. Improve the bacterial clearance.	Mice	(33)
	Sepsis	Improve the Neutrophil function. Increase the phosphorylation of p38 MAP kinase. Control sepsis-induced organ damage Supresses IL-6 and MCP-1 level. Control the bacteraemia.	Mice and rat	(32, 110, 115)
	Listeria monocytogenes	Induce CD11b expression on neutrophils and lower the apoptosis. Induce effective bacterial phagocytosis and lymphocytic apoptosis in sever immune-deficiency. Improvement of anti-listerial resistance and the MCP-1 mRNA expression. Decrease defective MCP-1 expression in the liver. Control the bacteraemia.	Mice	(116, 117)
	Helicobactor pylori	Increase mucosal leptin in the infected patients compare to uninfected patients. Amount of gastric leptin correlated positively with the mucosal levels of IL-1β and IL-6, but not IL-8 cytokine. Increase of gastric leptin expression during infection may have a local rather than systemic action. Increase in serum leptin concentration. Circulating leptin correlated with body mass index, but not with bacterial load. There was no change in plasma leptin levels following cure of the infection.	Mice and human	(118–121)
Viral disease	Influenza A/H1N1 pneumonia	Global deficiency of leptin receptor (db/db) have worsened survival following influenza A infection. Leptin receptor deficiency impaired viral clearance & diminished the IFN-γ levels. Loss of leptin receptor within lung epithelium or within macrophages is not associated with worsened lung injury or mortality following infection. Decrease proinflammatory cytokines IL-6 and IL-1β level and increase survival. Disruption of leptin signaling in T cells limits worsened the pH1N1 dependent mortality and infection severity.	Human and mice	(34, 122–125)
	Respiratory Syncytial Virus	Promoted Th17 subset differentiation. Suppressed Th2 subset differentiation. Increased phosphorylation of ERK1/2 in peripheral Lymphocytes.	Human	(126)
	HIV	Leptin inhibits ROS and control oxidative burst mechanism in HIV+ monocyte patients. Leptin receptor (ob-R) expression increased in HIV+ PBMCs than control. Serum leptin level positively correlated with CD4+ T lymphocyte during antiviral therapy in HIV patients. Supresses SOCS3 & mTOR expression and Th2 subset differentiation. Reduced viral load.	Human and mice (*in-vitro* & *in-vivo*)	(35, 127–129)

(Continued)

TABLE 1 | Continued

Infectious group	Infectious species	Effect of leptin on the Immune response	Model used (*in-vitro* & *in-vivo*)	References
Parasitic disease	*Leishmania major/Leishmania donovani*	Activates macrophage phagocytosis and ROS induction. Enhances the phosphorylation of Erk1/2 & Akt in macrophages. Increases IFN-γ, IL12, IL-1β secretion in macrophage. Improve IFN-γ/IL-10 ratio, GrzA and Th1 cytokine response. Activate CD8+ T-cell compartment and reduces PD-1 & CTLA-4 expression. Increase IgG2a levels and improve IgG2a/IgG1 ratio. Improve granuloma formation and repaired tissue degeneration. Reduced parasite load in visceral organs.	Human (THP-1 and PBMCs) Mice (*in-vitro* & *in-vivo*)	(36, 49, 130–132)
	Trypanosoma cruzi	Defective leptin receptors or reduction in leptin level increase parasitemia and mortality rate. Reconstitution of central leptin signaling in brain reduces tissue parasitism and mortality rates. Improve plasma cytokines and chemokine's.	Mice	(37, 133–136)
	Entamoeba histolytica	Mutation in leptin receptor (LEPR Q223R). Substitution of arginine (223R) in the cytokine receptor homology domain 1 of LEPR are more susceptible than those have glutamine (223Q) amino acid. Q223R polymorphism also decreased leptin-dependent STAT3 activation and defective STAT3 signaling and increase susceptibility to liver & intestinal abscess. Q223R leptin receptor mutation results in defective neutrophil infiltration to the site of infection. Mutation of tyrosine 985 or 1138 in leptin receptor results in defective SHP2/ERK and STAT3 signaling. Leptin-mediated resistance to amebiasis requires leptin receptor signaling through both the STAT3 and SHP2/ERK pathways. Leptin promotes regeneration & mucin secretion by epithelial cell and control apoptosis & integrity in intestinal epithelium lining. Low serum leptin increase liver and intestinal abscess. Intestinal parasites deregulate the secretion of leptin and adiponectin and play a role in enteric parasitosis by modulating body immunity, food intake and blood chemistry.	Human and mice	(38, 137–142)
	Plasmodium berghei ANKA parasite	Higher serum leptin levels. Increase mTORC1 (Mechanistic target of rapamycin complex 1) activity in CD4+ and CD8+ T cells in a dose dependent manner. Leptin act as downstream target for mTORC1 activity in T cells during ECM. The *leptin* gene mutation in *ob/ob* is associated with observed CM resistance phenotype. CM resistance phenotype is due to involvement of Th1 cytokines TNF-α and INF-γ in the regulatory cascade controlling inflammatory responses after malarial infections.	Mice	(39, 143, 144)

further suggests the possible healing potential for leptin analogs in infectious disease.

LEPTIN AND PARASITIC INFECTIONS

Parasitic infections contribute significantly to the burden of communicable diseases worldwide. Reportedly, much of infections and mortality from parasitic illnesses are restricted mainly in developing countries (157). Malnutrition or loss of appetite is a common characteristic of many infectious diseases including parasitic infections which result in reduced serum leptin levels (158). Since, leptin has been reported to induce pro-inflammatory cytokines & chemokines, neutrophil chemotaxis, NK cell cytotoxicity, and T cell functions, therefore its deficiency leads to an increase in susceptibility to infectious diseases (64, 65, 159, 160). Furthermore, leptin exerts central effects on hypothalamic-pituitary function and disruption of these effects have been implicated into severe parasitic diseases due to immune dysfunction in host (35–38).

Moreover, very little is known about the role of leptin in pathogenesis of parasitic infections. There is a need for studying the role of leptin in controlling parasitic infections since preponderance of such infections is associated with malnutrition which goes hand in hand in developing countries. As a first step, we have highlighted some of these studies to generate interest in initiating such studies (**Table 1**).

Leishmaniasis

Leishmaniasis is a vector-borne protozoan disease caused by Leishmania parasites. Leishmaniasis is commonly prevalent in tropical and subtropical regions of the world with different immunopathology and varying degrees of morbidity and mortality. Among which, Visceral Leushmaniasis (VL) is the deadliest form of the diseases, marked by uncontrolled parasitemia in the spleen, liver, and bone marrow (161, 162).

VL is an endemic disease found mostly in economically poor societies, who invariably suffer from malnutrition. Malnutrition is characterized by the lower serum leptin level which in turn adversely alters the development of innate and adaptive immune responses during VL in both mice and children living in endemic areas (163–165). Hence, malnutrition and low serum leptin level are playing a critical role in *Leishmania* infection and its pathogenesis. Leptin improved cytokine production and phagocytosis of *Leishmania donovani* by murine and human macrophages by increasing the phagolysosome formation and oxidative killing of the parasite via intracellular reactive oxygen species (ROS) generation (36). Leptin in combination with miltefosine, the conventional antileishmanial drug, augments the protective immunity in mouse macrophage during *L. donovani* infection *in vitro* (130). Similarly, it enhances the host protective Th1 cytokine responses in THP-1, and human PMBCs derived macrophages by inducing Erk1/2 and Akt phosphorylation, which is usually dephosphorylated in *L. donovani* infection (36). It can also maintain the protective environment against *L. donovani* infection through the classical macrophage activation (36). Recently we demonstrated that leptin induces the innate immune response in bone marrow-derived antigen presenting dendritic cells, and causes heightened nitric oxide, proinflammatory cytokines (IFN-γ, IL-12, and IL1β) in the splenocytes stimulated with soluble Leishmania antigen. Besides this, leptin-induced IFN-γ production from both CD4+ and CD8+ T cells compared with untreated infected normal mice, indicates that leptin-induced heightened Th1 response (131). Alternatively, leptin deficient *ob/ob* mice had higher splenic and liver parasite burden compared with the normal infected mice. Nevertheless, leptin treatment of *ob/ob* mice failed to reduce the splenic parasite burden and host-protective cytokine response. Moreover, in contrast to DCs from a normal mouse, *ob/ob* mouse-derived DCs showed limitation in the initiation of innate immune response during *Leishmania* infection that could not be restored by leptin treatment suggesting that leptin signaling was differentially regulated in *ob/ob* mice compared with normal mice fed with healthy diet (131, 166). Interestingly, very recently we demonstrated that leptin also induces a protective CD8+ T-cell dependent immune response in malnutrition coupled with *L. donovani* infection through up-regulation of Granzyme A (GrzA) and down-regulation of cytotoxic T-lymphocyte-associated protein 4 (CTLA-4) and Programmed death-1 (PD-1) markers (132). The PD-1 ligand plays a significant role in CD8+ T cell exhaustion during the chronic infections of various infectious diseases including VL (167). It is worth mentioning here that in contrast to the above reports an increased expression or activity of leptin, has been reported in blood samples of dogs with canine leishmaniasis (CanL) and suggested possible use of leptin as a biomarker for CanL (168). In conclusion, leptin treatment may improve parasite clearance in malnourished VL condition through restoration of normal immune cell function via leptin signaling.

Trypanosomiasis

Chagas disease is caused by a protozoan parasite *Trypanosoma cruzi*. The parasite is transmitted to humans and other hosts mainly by feces of infected blood-feeding triatomines, blood transfusion, or by ingestion of contaminated food (169). Chagas disease remains a serious health problem in Central and South America and a major cause of morbidity and mortality (135, 170). *T. cruzi* uses adipocytes as a reservoir for chronic infection and displays a pro-inflammatory phenotype by upregulating cytokines such as IL-1β, IFN-γ, TNF-α, and chemokines such as CCL2, CXCL10, and CCL5 along with innate immune receptors such as Toll-like receptor (TLR)-2 and 9 (171–173). Other pathways, such as ERK and PI3K pathways were also activated upon *T. cruzi* infection (174, 175). Additionally, Adipose tissue profoundly expressed Peroxisome proliferator-activated receptor (PPAR-γ) along with adiponectin, which exerts an anti-inflammatory effect. The levels of PPAR-γ were also decreased in *T. cruzi* infected cells, which leads to the reduced secretion of adiponectin and increased inflammatory reactions (176).

Since parasite infects many organs including adipose tissue which is a source to a variety of adipokines, including leptin and could have significant role in pathogenesis of Trypanosomiasis (133, 134). Mice infected with *T. cruzi* showed significant reduction in leptin levels, possibly due to adipocyte involvement in disease progression (133, 135). It was also reported that chemically induced diabetic mice and genetically susceptible *db/db* diabetic mice with defective leptin receptors had higher parasitemia and mortality after *T. cruzi* infection, which suggests that the dysregulation of host metabolism may be beneficial to parasitic survival in the host (136). Moreover, mice with defective leptin receptor are metabolically challenged and upon infection with *T. cruzi* suffer high mortality (37). In NSE-Rb *db/db* mice, a genetically modified *db/db* mouse, central leptin signaling is reconstituted only in the brain which is sufficient to correct the metabolic defects and when infected with *T. cruzi* showed reduced parasitemia, mortality rates, and tissue parasitism as compared to normal *db/db* mice. The plasma levels of several cytokines and chemokines were also significantly increased in infected *db/db* mice compared with NSE-Rb *db/db* mice (37). In summary, the normalization of the metabolic dysfunction in NSE-Rb *db/db* mice through the restoration of leptin receptor signaling in brain reconstitute the normal immune response against *T. cruzi* infection, but not peripheral restoration, highlighting that leptin may play a role as a central regulator for both metabolic function and immune response.

Amoebiasis

Amoebiasis is the disease caused by an enteric protozoan parasite *Entamoeba histolytica*. Infection results from ingestion of the parasite cyst from feces-contaminated food or water (177). *E. histolytica* primarily lives in the intestinal mucosa and mainly restricted in colon infection causing devastating dysentery, colitis, and liver abscess by producing tissue damages (178, 179) while many deaths are associated with extraintestinal invasive disease (180, 181). Amoebiasis occurs when trophozoites disrupt the mucosal barrier and penetrate the underlying tissue and break down extracellular matrix, destroy cells, and phagocytose cellular

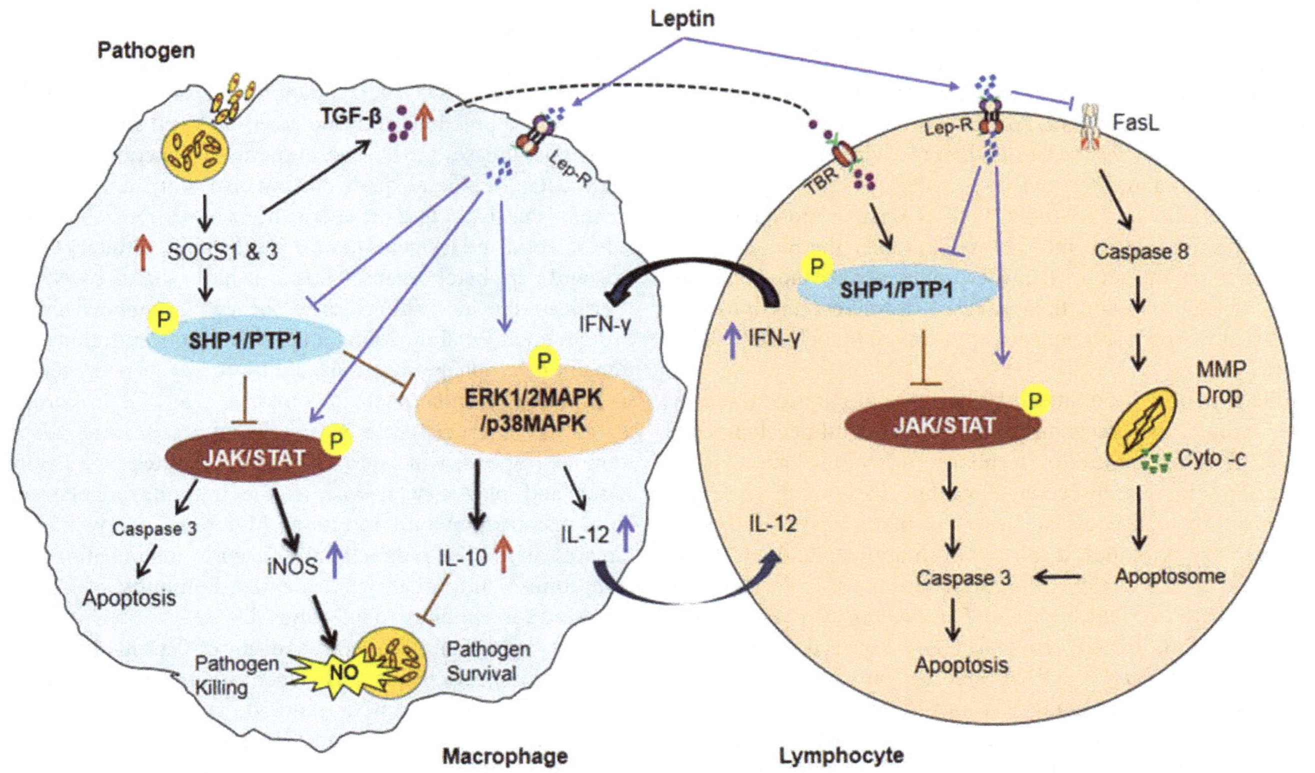

FIGURE 2 | The possible model of Leptin and Immune response in malnutrition coupled infectious diseases. In malnutrition, low adipocyte mass causes a reduction of serum leptin level resultant impairment of normal macrophages and lymphocytes activities. Infected macrophages induce the SOCS1 & 3 proteins expression subsequently upregulates ROS scavenging enzyme Thioredoxin which leads to activates SHP1/PTPase molecules. SHP1/PTP1 negatively regulates the JAK/STAT, and MAP-Kinase pathways thus inhibiting IFN–inducible macrophage functions (increased IL-10 and TGF-β level and decreased the IL-12 cytokines in infected macrophage). IL-10 suppresses the NO activity and improves the parasite survival. TGF-β activates SHP1/PTPase activity in lymphocytes through TGF-β receptor (TBR) which leads to lymphocytes apoptosis. In contrast, Leptin treatment inactivated SHP1/PTPase directed pathways and reversed the macrophage activities by up-regulating the pro-inflammatory cytokines (IFNγ, TNF-α, and IL-12) secretion and NO expression. IL-12 cytokine released from activated macrophage upon leptin treatment inhibits the SHP1/PTPase dependent T lymphocytes apoptosis by activation of JAK/STAT pathway. Moreover, Leptin directly inhibits the FasL-dependent T lymphocytes apoptosis by the inhibition of the caspase 8 activity. Caspase-8 then promotes mitochondrial outer membrane permeabilization (MOMP) by diminishing the inhibitory effect of various antiapoptotic and proapoptotic molecules. MOMP results in cytochrome-c release from the mitochondria, enabling activation of a supramolecular complex, the apoptosome that activates caspase-3 to undertake apoptotic cell death (Suppressors of cytokine signaling: SOCS1 & 3; Protein tyrosine phosphatases: SHP1/PTP1, Mitochondrial membrane potential drop: MMP drop, and P: phosphorylation) (192–206).

debris (182). Studies on amoebic liver abscess (ALA) carried out in Indian subcontinent suggest that malnutrition is associated with ALA outcome (183, 184).

Moreover, malnutrition and serum leptin levels are directly proportional to the pathogenesis of amoebiasis, and low serum leptin plays a critical role in *E. histolytica*- associated diarrheal illness and extent of liver injury (137, 185). The mucosal immune response can be suppressed by a mutation in leptin receptor and defective STAT3 signaling pathways, resulting in susceptibility to intestinal abscess due to *E. histolytica* infections (38, 138). The mechanism of mucosal immune suppression depends on homozygous allelic mutation in leptin receptor Q223R (rs1137101) that ablates STAT3 signaling, results in decreased mucosal chemokine's LIF, CXCL9, CXCL10, CCL3, and CCL4 secretion (68, 69). A mutation or polymorphism in leptin receptor at 233 (from glutamine to arginine) is liable to enhance 4 times more susceptibility to *E. histolytica* infection in children irrespective of nutritional status (139). The leptin-deficient (*ob/ob*) and LepRb-deficient (*db/db*) mice were highly susceptible to infection with *E. histolytica*, whereas wild-type C57BL/6 mice were resistant. Moreover, mice either homozygous or heterozygous for the 223R allele of leptin receptor were significantly more prone to amoebic infection. Both types of mice ceca were shown to have profound epithelial denudation because of trophozoites invasion. Leptin signaling in the intestinal epithelium and downstream STAT3 and SHP2 (Src homology phosphatase 2) signaling was required for protection in the murine model of amoebic colitis (140). Leptin-mediated specific activation of STAT3 and ERK or Akt signaling pathways in gut mucosal epithelial cells offers more resistance against amoebiasis caused by *E. histolytica* infection (141, 142). In conclusion, leptin may control the amoebic infections by the activation of leptin signaling pathway in gut mucosal epithelial cells via up-regulation of various signaling pathway.

Malaria

Malaria is caused by *Plasmodium* species, an intracellular parasite transmitted by the bite of an infected female Anopheles mosquito. It is endemic in most of the tropical countries such as sub-tropical regions of Asia, Africa, South and Central America (186). *Plasmodium falciparum* is the most virulent form of the human malaria parasites and responsible for 90% of malaria-related morbidity and mortality (187). During a mosquito bite, sporozoites are injected into host's skin, enter the bloodstream and reach to the liver. Parasites differentiate and replicate inside hepatocytes, and then released as merozoites into the bloodstream, which subsequently invades red blood cells (RBCs) (186).

Inflection of diet can affect the outcome of parasitic diseases either through the effects on parasite growth and development, or via the host immune response, or both. Leptin is a cytokine predominantly secreted by adipocytes that increases in proportion to total body fat mass, and upon exposure to pro-inflammatory cytokines, it inhibits both appetite and adiposity in malaria infection (39). Moreover, serum leptin levels were approximately five-fold higher in *Plasmodium berghei*-infected mice than in non-infected controls (188). Leptin-deficient mice infected with *P. berghei* ANKA were shown to be resistant to the development of cerebral malaria whereas the normal mice developed signs of cerebral malaria. Dietary restriction prevented severe experimental cerebral malaria (ECM) symptoms and death in mice through modulation of leptin levels and mechanistic target of rapamycin complex 1 (mTORC1) activity in T cells (143). Pharmacological inhibition of either leptin signaling with a mutant peptide, or downstream mTORC1 signaling with rapamycin, blocked ECM symptoms and reduced mortality (39). Furthermore, leptin exerts central effects on hypothalamic-pituitary function and these outcomes might affect the severity of malaria disease. Disturbance in hypothalamic-pituitary-adrenal axis during *P. falciparum* infection have been involved in the pathogenic mechanism of severe malaria (144). Importantly, the level of leptin in serum of malaria patients has been recently reported to be used as prognostic markers of treatment outcomes and pathogenesis of malaria patients (144). In conclusion, leptin could play an important role to control the immuno-compromised malarial infections by the activation of immune cells through leptin signaling pathway.

CONCLUSION AND SUMMARY

Many studies have been conducted in recent past to understand the role of leptin in immune modulation such as activation of phagocytosis, cytokine polarization and cell-mediated immunity in infectious diseases. Both obesity and malnutrition are pandemics associated with immune-deficiencies that lead to increased vulnerability to infectious disease. Interestingly, both obesity and malnutrition are related to aberrant leptin levels, obesity due to chronically elevated leptin levels, whereas malnutrition results in significantly diminished leptin levels. Emerging data from animal models and human indicates that immune dysfunction underlies the etiology of malnutrition and reduced immune-mediated protection from infections, which interplay between nutrition, leptin levels and immune responses (86, 189, 190). Malnutrition is characterized by immune suppression and increased risk of mortality from infectious diseases (191). The immune dysfunction is not only a consequence of inadequate diet but also contributes in various mechanisms, including the energy homeostasis, metabolism, the role of leptin and it signals to the hypothalamic-pituitary-adrenal axis and peripheral organs. Thus, it is likely that the CNS plays a critical role in malnutrition associated immune deficiency. Protein-energy malnutrition reduces leptin concentrations which impairs macrophage functions, ability to engulf pathogens and to produce proinflammatory cytokines (25, 27). Importantly, leptin has a crucial role in mediating innate and adaptive immune response which are significantly affected by nutritional status and play a vital role in the immune adaptation in both malnutrition and infection. Moreover, many infectious diseases directly or indirectly are linked to malnutrition which compromises the innate and adaptive immunity of host and increased susceptibility to infectious disease.

More importantly the mechanism of leptin signaling in various infectious diseases is depends on SOCS3 expression as describes in NF-κB dependent pathway. The SOCS3 expression attenuates the macrophage's response to IFN-γ at both proximal level activation and downstream expression. Hence, taken together above-mentioned observations indicate that the potential role of leptin signaling in various pathogens has been summarized in a schematic diagram (**Figure 2**) (192–205). Therefore, understanding the link between nutrition, leptin, and immune dysfunction in murine and human infectious diseases will inform targeted interventions for a vulnerable population with undernutrition, which is a crucial need for new approaches to reduce global mortality from infectious diseases. Present review provides a rationale for future studies to explore role of leptin as therapeutics to host immune dysfunction in infectious diseases during malnutrition.

AUTHOR CONTRIBUTIONS

RM conceived and conducted literature reviews, figure, and table construction and contributed to the writing of the manuscript. PB, RD, and HN critically edited and reviewed the complete manuscript, tables and figures. All authors approved the final manuscript for submission.

ACKNOWLEDGMENTS

We sincerely thank University Grant Commission (UGC), DST-SERB, DST-FIST, DST-Purse and University of Hyderabad for providing the lab infrastructure and subscription of many scientific journal and books to compile the review. FDA authors' contributions represent their best judgment and do not bind or obligate the FDA.

REFERENCES

1. La Cava A, Matarese G. The weight of leptin in autoimmunity. *Nat Rev Immunol.* (2004) 4:371–9. doi: 10.1038/nri1350
2. Grinspoon S, Gulick T, Askari H, Landt M, Lee K, Anderson E, et al. Serum leptin levels in women with anorexia nervosa. *J Clin Endocrinol Metab.* (1996) 81:3861–3.
3. Mantzoros CS, Magkos F, Brinkoetter M, Sienkiewicz E, Dardeno TA, Kim SY, et al. Leptin in human physiology and pathophysiology. *Am J Physiol Endocrinol Metab.* (2011) 301:E567–84. doi: 10.1152/ajpendo.00315.2011
4. Dardeno TA, Chou SH, Moon HS, Chamberland JP, Fiorenza CG, Mantzoros CS. Leptin in human physiology and therapeutics. *Front Neuroendocrinol.* (2010) 31:377–93. doi: 10.1016/j.yfrne.2010.06.002
5. Faggioni R, Jones-Carson J, Reed DA, Dinarello CA, Feingold KR, Grunfeld C, et al. Leptin-deficient (*ob/ob*) mice are protected from T cell-mediated hepatotoxicity: role of tumor necrosis factor α and IL-18. *Proc Natl Acad Sci USA.* (2000) 97:2367–72. doi: 10.1073/pnas.040561297
6. Procaccini C, Jirillo E, Matarese G. Leptin as an immunomodulator. *Mol Aspects Med.* (2012) 33:35–45. doi: 10.1016/j.mam.2011.10.012
7. Fernandez-Riejos P, Najib S, Santos-Alvarez J, Martín-Romero C, Pérez-Pérez A, González-Yanes C, et al. Role of leptin in the activation of immune cells. *Media Inflamm.* (2010) 2010:568343. doi: 10.1155/2010/568343
8. Sharma A, Satyam A, Sharma JB. Leptin, IL-10 and inflammatory markers (TNF-alpha, IL-6 and IL-8) in pre-eclamptic, normotensive pregnant and healthy non-pregnant women. *Am J Reprod Immunol.* (2007) 58:21–30. doi: 10.1111/j.1600-0897.2007.00486.x
9. Zhang Y, Proenca R, Maffei M, Barone M, Leopold L, Friedman JM. Positional cloning of the mouse obese gene and its human homologue. *Nature* (1994) 372:425–32. doi: 10.1038/372425a0
10. Coleman DL. Obese and diabetes: two mutant genes causing diabetes-obesity syndromes in mice. *Diabetologia* (1978) 14:141–8. doi: 10.1007/BF00429772
11. Madej T, Boguski MS, Bryant SH, Threading analysis suggests that the obese gene product may be a helical cytokine. *FEBS Lett.* (1995) 373:13–8. doi: 10.1016/0014-5793(95)00977-H
12. Tartaglia LA, Dembski M, Weng X, Deng N, Culpepper J, Devos R, et al. Identification and expression cloning of a leptin receptor, OB-R. *Cell* (1995) 83:1263–71. doi: 10.1016/0092-8674(95)90151-5
13. Licinio J, Mantzoros C, Negrão AB, Cizza G, Wong ML, Bongiorno PB, et al. Human leptin levels are pulsatile and inversely related to pituitary-adrenal function. *Nat Med.* (1997) 3:575–9. doi: 10.1038/nm0597-575
14. Mansour E, Pereira FG, Araujo EP, Amaral MEC, Morari J, Ferraroni NR, et al. Leptin inhibits apoptosis in thymus through a janus kinase-2-independent, insulin receptor substrate-1/phosphatidylinositol-3 kinase-dependent pathway. *Endocrinology* (2006) 147:5470–9. doi: 10.1210/en.2006-0223
15. Martin-Romero C, Santos-Alvarez J, Governa R, Sanchez-Margalet V. Human leptin enhances activation and proliferation of human circulating T lymphocytes. *Cell Immunol.* (2000) 199:15–24. doi: 10.1006/cimm.1999.1594
16. Matarese G, Moschos S, Mantzoros CS. Leptin in immunology. *J Immunol.* (2005) 174:3137–42. doi: 10.4049/jimmunol.174.6.3137
17. Lord GM, Matarese G, Howard JK, Baker RJ, Bloom SR, Lechler RI. Leptin modulates the T-cell immune response and reverses starvation-induced immunosuppression. *Nature* (1998) 394:897–901. doi: 10.1038/29795
18. Howard JK, Lord GM, Mataresse G, Vendetti S, Ghatei MA, Ritter MA, et al. Leptin protects mice from starvation-induced lymphoid atrophy and increases thymic cellularity in *ob/ob* mice. *J Clin Invest.* (1999) 104:1051–9. doi: 10.1172/JCI6762
19. Saucillo DC, Gerriets VA, Sheng J, Rathmell JC, Maciver NJ. Leptin metabolically licenses T cells for activation to link nutrition and immunity. *J Immunol.* (2014) 192:136–44. doi: 10.4049/jimmunol.1301158
20. Faggioni R, Feingold KR, Grunfeld C. Leptin regulation of the immune response and the immunodeficiency of malnutrition. *FASEB J.* (2001) 15:2565–71. doi: 10.1096/fj.01-0431rev
21. Paz-Filho GJ, Delibasi T, Erol HK, Wong ML, Licinio J. Cellular immunity before and after leptin replacement therapy. *J Pediatr Endocrinol Metab.* (2009) 22:1069–74. doi: 10.1515/JPEM.2009.22.11.1069
22. Farooqi IS, Matarese G, Lord GM. Beneficial effects of leptin on obesity, T cell hyporesponsiveness, and neuroendocrine/metabolic dysfunction of human congenital leptin deficiency. *J Clin Invest.* (2002) 110:1093–103. doi: 10.1172/JCI0215693
23. Moore S, Morgan G, Collinson A, Swain J, O'Connell M, Prentice A. Leptin, malnutrition, and immune response in rural Gambian children. *Arch Dis Child.* (2002) 87:192–7. doi: 10.1136/adc.87.3.192
24. Woodward B. Protein, calories, and immune defenses. *Nutr Rev.* (1998) 56:S84–92. doi: 10.1111/j.1753-4887.1998.tb01649.x
25. Schaible UE, Kaufmann SH. Malnutrition and infection: complex mechanisms and global impacts. *PLoS Med.* (2007) 4:e115. doi: 10.1371/journal.pmed.0040115
26. Najera O, Gonzalez C, Toledo G, López L, Cortés E, Betancourt M, et al. CD45RA and CD45RO isoforms in infected malnourished and infected well-nourished children. *Clin Exp Immunol.* (2001) 126:461–5. doi: 10.1046/j.1365-2249.2001.01694.x
27. Iyer SS, Chatraw JH, Tan WG, Wherry EJ, Becker TC, Ahmed R, et al. Protein-energy malnutrition impairs homeostatic proliferation of memory CD8 T cells. *J Immunol.* (2012) 188:77–84. doi: 10.4049/jimmunol.1004027
28. Chatraw JH, Wherry EJ, Ahmed R, Kapasi ZF. Diminished primary CD8 T cell response to viral infection during protein-energy malnutrition in mice is due to changes in microenvironment and low numbers of viral-specific CD8 T cell precursors. *J Nutr.* (2008) 138:806–12. doi: 10.1093/jn/138.4.806
29. Nájera O, González C, Toledo G, López L, Ortiz R. Flow cytometry study of lymphocyte subsets in malnourished and well-nourished children with bacterial infections. *Clin Diagn Lab Immunol.* (2004) 11:577–80. doi: 10.1128/CDLI.11.3.577-580.2004
30. Wieland CW, Florquin S, Chan ED, Leemans JC, Weijer S, Verbon A, et al. Pulmonary *Mycobacterium tuberculosis* infection in leptin-deficient *ob/ob* mice. *Int Immunol.* (2005) 17:1399–408. doi: 10.1093/intimm/dxh317
31. Hsu A, Aronoff DM, Phipps J, Goel D, Mancuso P. Leptin improves pulmonary bacterial clearance and survival in *ob/ob* mice during *Pneumococcal pneumonia*. *Clin Exp Immunol.* (2007) 150:332–9. doi: 10.1111/j.1365-2249.2007.03491.x
32. Tschöp J, Nogueiras R, Haas-Lockie S, Kasten KR, Castañeda TR, Huber N, et al. CNS leptin action modulates immune response and survival in sepsis. *J Neurosci.* (2010) 30:6036–47. doi: 10.1523/JNEUROSCI.4875-09.2010
33. Madan R, Guo X, Naylor C, Buonomo EL, Mackay D, Noor Z, et al. Role of leptin-mediated colonic inflammation in defense against Clostridium difficile Colitis. *Infect Immun.* (2014) 82:341–9. doi: 10.1128/IAI.00972-13
34. Zhang AJ, To KK, Li C, Lau CC, Poon VK, Chan CC, et al. Leptin mediates the pathogenesis of severe 2009 pandemic influenza a (h1n1) infection associated with cytokine dysregulation in mice with diet-induced obesity. *J Infect Dis.* (2013) 207:1270–80. doi: 10.1093/infdis/jit031
35. Sánchez-Pozo C, Rodriguez-baño J, Domínguez-Castellano A, Muniain MA, Goberna R, Sánchez-Margalet V. Leptin stimulates the oxidative burst in control monocytes but attenuates the oxidative burst in monocytes from HIV-infected patients. *Clin Exp Immunol.* (2003) 134:464–9. doi: 10.1111/j.1365-2249.2003.02321.x
36. Dayakar A, Chandrasekaran S, Veronica J, Maurya R. Leptin induces the phagocytosis and protective immune response in *Leishmania donovani* infected THP-1 cell line and human PBMCs. *Exp Parasitol.* (2016) 160:54–9. doi: 10.1016/j.exppara.2015.12.002
37. Nagajyothi F, Zhao D, Machado FS, Weiss, LM Schwartz GJ, Desruisseaux MS, et al. Crucial role of the central leptin receptor in murine *Trypanosoma cruzi* infection. *J Infect Dis.* (2010) 202:1104–13. doi: 10.1086/656189
38. Vedantama G, Viswanathan VK. Leptin signaling protects the gut from *Entamoeba histolytica* infection. *Gut Microb.* (2012) 3:2–3. doi: 10.4161/gmic.19424
39. Pulido-Mendez M, De Sanctis J, Rodriguez-Acosta A. Leptin and leptin receptors during malaria infection in mice. *Folia Parasitol.* (2002) 49:249–51. doi: 10.14411/fp.2002.046
40. Chan J, Tian Y, Tanaka KE, Tsang MS, Yu K, Salgame P, et al. Effects of protein-calorie malnutrition on tuberculosis in mice. *Proc Natl Acad Sci USA.* (1996) 93:14857–61. doi: 10.1073/pnas.93.25.14857
41. Pena-Cruz V, Reiss CS, McIntosh K. Sendai virus infection of mice with protein malnutrition. *J Virol.* (1989) 63:3541–4.
42. Ritz BW, Aktan I, Nogusa S, Gardner EM. Energy restriction impairs natural killer cell function and increases the severity of influenza

infection in young adult male C57BL/6 mice. *J Nutr.* (2008) 138:2269–75. doi: 10.3945/jn.108.093633
43. Goldberg EL, Romero-Aleshire MJ, Renkema KR, Ventevogel MS, Chew WM, Uhrlaub JL, et al. Lifespan-extending caloric restriction or mTOR inhibition impair adaptive immunity of old mice by distinct mechanisms. *Aging Cell* (2015) 14:130–8. doi: 10.1111/acel.12280
44. Kristan DM. Chronic calorie restriction increases susceptibility of laboratory mice (Mus musculus) to a primary intestinal parasite infection. *Aging Cell* (2007) 6:817–25. doi: 10.1111/j.1474-9726.2007.00345.x
45. Rodríguez L, Graniel J, Ortiz R. Effect of leptin on activation and cytokine synthesis in peripheral blood lymphocytes of malnourished infected children. *Clin Exp Immunol.* (2007) 148:478–85. doi: 10.1111/j.1365-2249.2007.03361.x
46. Procaccini C, Lourenco EV, Matarese G, La Cava A. Leptin signaling: a key pathway in immune responses. *Curr Signal Transduct Ther.* (2009) 4:22–30. doi: 10.2174/157436209787048711
47. Fantuzzi G. Three questions about leptin and immunity. *Brain Behav Immun.* (2009) 23:405–10. doi: 10.1016/j.bbi.2008.10.007
48. Sánchez-Margalet V, Martín-Romero C, Santos-Alvarez J, Goberna R, Najib S, Gonzalez-Yanes C. Role of leptin as an immunomodulator of blood mononuclear cells: mechanisms of action. *Clin Exp Immunol.* (2003) 133:11–9. doi: 10.1046/j.1365-2249.2003.02190.x
49. Gainsford T, Willson TA, Metcalf D. Leptin can induce proliferation, differentiation, and functional activation of hemopoietic cells. *Proc Natl Acad Sci USA.* (1996) 93:14564–8. doi: 10.1073/pnas.93.25.14564
50. Raso GM, Pacilio M, Esposito E, Coppola A, Di Carlo R, Meli R. Leptin potentiates IFN-gamma induced expression of nitric oxide synthase and cyclo-oxygenase-2 in murine macrophage J774A. 1. *Br J Pharmacol.* (2002) 137:799–804. doi: 10.1038/sj.bjp.0704903
51. Santos-Alvarez J, Goberna R, Sanchez-Margalet V. Human leptin stimulates proliferation and activation of human circulating monocytes. *Cell Immunol.* (1999) 194:6–11. doi: 10.1006/cimm.1999.1490
52. Bennett BD, Solar GP, Yuan JQ, Mathias J, Thomas GR, Matthews W. A role for leptin and its cognate receptor in hematopoiesis. *Curr Biol.* (1996) 6:1170–80. doi: 10.1016/S0960-9822(02)70684-2
53. Najib S, Sanchez-Margalet V. Human leptin promotes survival of human circulating blood monocytes prone to apoptosis by activation of p42/44 MAPK pathway. *Cell Immunol.* (2002) 220:43–149. doi: 10.1016/S0008-8749(03)00027-3
54. Loffreda S, Yang SQ, Lin HZ, Karp CL, Brengman ML, Wang DJ, et al. Leptin regulates proinflammatory immune responses. *FASEB J.* (1998) 12:57–65. doi: 10.1096/fasebj.12.1.57
55. Oral EA, Javor ED, Ding L, Uzel G, Cochran EK, Young JR, et al. Leptin replacement therapy modulates circulating lymphocyte subsets and cytokine responsiveness in severe lipodystrophy. *J Clin Endocrinol Metab.* (2006) 91:621–8. doi: 10.1210/jc.2005-1220
56. Bruno A, Conus S, Schmid I, Simon H-U. Apoptotic pathways are inhibited by leptin receptor activation in neutrophils. *J Immunol.* (2005) 174:8090–6. doi: 10.4049/jimmunol.174.12.8090
57. Zarkesh-Esfahani H, Pockley AG, Wu Z, Hellewell PG, Weetman AP, Ross RJ, et al. Leptin indirectly activates human Neutrophils via induction of TNF-α. *J Immunol.* (2004) 172:1809–14. doi: 10.4049/jimmunol.172.3.1809
58. Brake DK, Smith EB, Mersmann H, Smith CW, Robker RL. ICAM-1 expression in adipose tissue: effects of diet-induced obesity in mice. *Am J Physiol Cell Physiol.* (2006) 291:C1232–9. doi: 10.1152/ajpcell.00008.2006
59. Kiguchi N, Maeda T, Kobayashi Y, Fukazawa Y, Kishioka S. Leptin enhances CC-chemokine ligand expression in cultured murine macrophage. *Biochem Biophys Res Commun.* (2009) 384:311–5. doi: 10.1016/j.bbrc.2009.04.121
60. Gruen ML, Hao M, Piston DW, Hasty AH. Leptin requires canonical migratory signaling pathways for induction of monocyte and macrophage chemotaxis. *Am J Physiol Cell Physiol.* (2007) 293:C1481–8. doi: 10.1152/ajpcell.00062.2007
61. Rafail S, Ritis K, Schaefer K, Kourtzelis I, Speletas M, Doumas M, et al. Leptin induces the expression of functional tissue factor in human neutrophils and peripheral blood mononuclear cells through JAK2-dependent mechanisms and TNF-α involvement. *Thromb Res.* (2008) 122:366–75. doi: 10.1016/j.thromres.2007.12.018
62. Mattioli B, Straface E, Quaranta MG, Giordani L, Viora M. Leptin promotes differentiation and survival of human dendritic cells and licenses them for Th1 priming. *J Immunol.* (2005) 174:6820–8. doi: 10.4049/jimmunol.174.11.6820
63. Mattioli B, Giordani L, Quaranta MG, Viora M. Leptin exerts an anti-apoptotic effect on human dendritic cells via the PI3K-Akt signalling pathway. *FEBS Lett.* (2009) 583:1102–6. doi: 10.1016/j.febslet.2009.02.029
64. Lam QL, Liu S, Cao X, Lu L. Involvement of leptin signalling in the survival and maturation of bone marrow-derived dendritic cells. *Eur J Immunol.* (2006) 36:3118–30. doi: 10.1002/eji.200636602
65. Tian Z, Sun R, Wei H, Gao B. Impaired natural killer (NK) cell activity in leptin receptor deficient mice: leptin as a critical regulator in NK cell development and activation. *Biochem Biophys Res Commun.* (2002) 298:297–302. doi: 10.1016/S0006-291X(02)02462-2
66. Zhao Y, Sun R, You L, Gao C, Tian Z. Expression of leptin receptors and response to leptin stimulation of human natural killer cell lines. *Biochem Biophys Res Commun.* (2003) 300:247–52. doi: 10.1016/S0006-291X(02)02838-3
67. Velloso LA, Savino W, Mansour E. Leptin action in the thymus. *Ann N Y Acad Sci.* (2009) 1153:29–34. doi: 10.1111/j.1749-6632.2008.03973.x
68. Da Silva SV, Salama C, Renovato-Martins M, Helal-Neto, E, Citelli, M, Savino, W, et al. Increased leptin response and inhibition of apoptosis in thymocytes of young rats offspring from protein deprived dams during lactation. *PLoS ONE* (2013) 8:e64220. doi: 10.1371/journal.pone.0064220
69. Merrick JC, Edelson BT, Bhardwaj V, Swanson PE, Unanue ER. Lymphocyte apoptosis during early phase of Listeria infection in mice. *Am J Pathol.* (1997) 151:785–92.
70. Papathanassoglou E, El-Haschimi K, Li XC, Matarese G, Strom T, Mantzoros C. Leptin receptor expression and signaling in lymphocytes: kinetics during lymphocyte activation, role in lymphocyte survival, and response to high-fat diet in mice. *J Immunol.* (2006) 176:7745–52. doi: 10.4049/jimmunol.176.12.7745
71. Fujita Y, Murakami M, Ogawa Y, Masuzaki H, Tanaka M, Ozaki S, et al. Leptin inhibits stress-induced apoptosis of T lymphocytes. *Clin Ex Immunol.* (2002) 128:21–6. doi: 10.1046/j.1365-2249.2002.01797.x
72. Lord GM, Matarese G, Howard JK, Bloom SR, Lechler RI. Leptin inhibits the anti-CD3-driven proliferation of peripheral blood T cells but enhances the production of proinflammatory cytokines. *J Leukoc Biol.* (2002) 72:330–8. doi: 10.1189/jlb.72.2.330
73. Farooqi IS, Wangensteen T, Collins S, Kimber W, Matarese G, Keogh JM, et al. Clinical and molecular genetic spectrum of congenital deficiency of the leptin receptor. *N Engl J Med.* (2007) 356:237–47. doi: 10.1056/NEJMoa063988
74. Ozata M, Ozdemir IC, Licinio J. Human leptin deficiency caused by a missense mutation: multiple endocrine defects, decreased sympathetic tone, and immune system dysfunction indicates new targets for leptin action, greater central than peripheral resistance to the effects of leptin, and spontaneous correction of leptin-mediated defects. *J Clin Endocrinol Metab.* (1999) 84:3686–95. doi: 10.1210/jcem.84.10.5999
75. Chandra RK. Cell-mediated immunity in genetically obese C57BL/6J (ob/ob) mice. *Am J Clin Nutr.* (1980) 33:13–6. doi: 10.1093/ajcn/33.1.13
76. Banks AS, Davis SM, Bates SH, Myers MG Jr. Activation of downstream signals by the long form of the leptin receptor. *J Biol Chem.* (2000) 275:14563–72. doi: 10.1074/jbc.275.19.14563
77. Dunn SL, Bjornholm M, Bates SH, Chen Z, Seifert M, Myers MG Jr, et al. Feedback inhibition of leptin receptor/Jak2 signaling via Tyr1138 of the leptin receptor and suppressor of cytokine signaling 3. *Mol Endocrinol.* (2005) 19:925–38. doi: 10.1210/me.2004-0353
78. Kim SY, Lim JH, Choi SW, Kim M, Kim ST, Kim MS, et al. Preferential effects of leptin on CD4 T cells in central and peripheral immune system are critically linked to the expression of leptin receptor. *Biochem Biophys Res Commun.* (2010) 394:562–8. doi: 10.1016/j.bbrc.2010.03.019
79. De Rosa V, Procaccini C, Calì G, Pirozzi G, Fontana S, Zappacosta S, et al. A key role of leptin in the control of regulatory T cell proliferation. *Immunity* (2007) 26:241–55. doi: 10.1016/j.immuni.2007.01.011
80. Sanchez-Margalet V, Martin-Romero C. Human leptin signaling in human peripheral blood mononuclear cells: activation of the JAK-STAT pathway. *Cell Immunol.* (2001) 211:30–6. doi: 10.1006/cimm.2001.1815

81. Agrawal S, Gollapudi S, Su H, Gupta S. Leptin activates human B cells to secrete TNF-alpha, IL-6, and IL-10 via JAK2/STAT3 and p38MAPK/ERK1/2 signaling pathway. *J Clin Immunol.* (2011) 31:472–8. doi: 10.1007/s10875-010-9507-1
82. Groom JR, Luster AD. CXCR3 in T cell function. *Exp Cell Res.* (2011) 315:620–31. doi: 10.1016/j.yexcr.2010.12.017
83. Biesiada G, Czepiel J, Ptak-Belowska A, Targosz A, Krzysiek-Maczka G, Strzalka M, et al. Expression and release of leptin and proinflammatory cytokines in patients with ulcerative colitis and infectious diarrhea. *J Physiol Pharmacol.* (2012) 63:471–81.
84. Chandra RK. Nutrition, immunity and infection: from basic knowledge of dietary manipulation of immune responses to practical application of ameliorating suffering and improving survival. *Proc Natl Acad Sci USA.* (1996) 93:14304–7. doi: 10.1073/pnas.93.25.14304
85. Matarese G. Leptin and the immune system: how nutritional status influences the immune response. *Eur Cytokine Netw.* (2000) 11:7–14.
86. Gerriets VA, MacIver NJ. Role of T cells in malnutrition and obesity. *Front Immunol.* (2014) 5:379. doi: 10.3389/fimmu.2014.00379
87. Chandra R. Nutrition, and immunology: from the clinic to cellular biology and back again. *Proc Nutr Soc.* (1999) 58:681–3. doi: 10.1017/S0029665199000890
88. Cederholm T, Arner P, Palmblad J. Low circulating leptin levels in protein-energy malnourished chronically ill elderly patients. *J Intern Med.* (1997) 242:377–82. doi: 10.1046/j.1365-2796.1997.00216.x
89. Soliman AT, Zalabany El, Salama MM, Ansari BM. Serum leptin concentrations during protein-energy malnutrition: correlation with growth parameters and endocrine function. *Metabolism* (2000) 49:819–25. doi: 10.1053/meta.2000.6745
90. Blackburn GL. Pasteur's quadrant and malnutrition. *Nature* (2001) 409:397–401. doi: 10.1038/35053187
91. Dai G, McMurray DN. Altered cytokine production and impaired antimycobacterial immunity in protein-malnourished guinea pigs. *Infect Immun.* (1998) 66:3562–8.
92. Cegielski JP, McMurray DN. The relationship between malnutrition and tuberculosis: evidence from studies in humans and experimental animals. *Int J Tuberc Lung Dis.* (2004) 8:286–98.
93. Cakir B, Yonem A, Guler S, Odabasi E, Demirbas B, Gürsoy G, et al. Relation of leptin and tumor necrosis factor alpha to body weight changes in patients with pulmonary tuberculosis. *Horm Res.* (1999) 52:279–83.
94. Schwenk A, Hodgson L, Rayner CF, Griffin GE, Macallan DC. Leptin and energy metabolism in pulmonary tuberculosis. *Am J Clin Nutr.* (2003) 77:392–8. doi: 10.1093/ajcn/77.2.392
95. van Crevel R, Karyadi E, Netea MG, Verhoef H, Nelwan RH, West CE, et al. Decreased plasma leptin concentrations in tuberculosis patients are associated with wasting and inflammation. *J Clin Endocrinol Metab.* (2002) 87:758–63. doi: 10.1210/jcem.87.2.8228
96. van Lettow M, van der Meer JW, West CE, van Crevel R, Semba RD. Interleukin- 6 and human immunodeficiency virus load, but not plasma leptin concentration, predict anorexia and wasting in adults with pulmonary tuberculosis in Malawi. *J Clin Endocrinol Metab.* (2005) 90:4771–6. doi: 10.1210/jc.2004-2539
97. Hoang T, Agger EM, Cassidy JP, Christensen JP, Andersen P. Protein energy malnutrition during vaccination has limited influence on vaccine efficacy but abolishes immunity if administered during *Mycobacterium tuberculosis* infection. *Infect Immun.* (2015) 83:2118–26. doi: 10.1128/IAI.03030-14
98. Auphan N, Didonato JA, Helmberg A, Rosette C, Karin M. Immunoregulatory genes and immunosuppression by glucocorticoids. *Arch Toxicol Suppl.* (1997) 19:87–95. doi: 10.1007/978-3-642-60682-3_8
99. McCarter MD, Naama HA, Shou J, Kwi LX, Evoy DA, Calvano SE, et al. Altered macrophage intracellular signaling induced by protein-calorie malnutrition. *Cell Immunol.* (1998) 183:131–6. doi: 10.1006/cimm.1998.1241
100. Redmond HP, Gallagher HJ, Shou J, Daly JM. Antigen presentation in protein-energy malnutrition. *Cell Immunol.* (1995) 163:80–7. doi: 10.1006/cimm.1995.1101
101. Redmond HP, Leon P, Lieberman MD, Hofmann K, Shou J, Reynolds JV, et al. Impaired macrophage function in severe protein-energy malnutrition. *Arch Surg.* (1991) 126:192–6. doi: 10.1001/archsurg.1991.01410260080011
102. Palacio A, Lopez M, Perez-Bravo F, Monkeberg F, Schlesinger L. Leptin levels are associated with immune response in malnourished infants. *J Clin Endocrinol Metab.* (2002) 87:3040–6. doi: 10.1210/jcem.87.7.8636
103. Bartz S, Mody A, Hornik C, Bain J, Muehlbauer M, Kiyimba T, et al. Severe acute malnutrition in childhood: hormonal and metabolic status at presentation, response to treatment, and predictors of mortality. *J Clin Endocrinol Metab.* (2014) 99:2128–37. doi: 10.1210/jc.2013-4018
104. Testa R, Franceschini R, Giannini E, Cataldi A, Botta F, Fasoli A, et al. Serum leptin levels in patients with viral chronic hepatitis or liver cirrhosis. *J Hepatol.* (2000) 33:33–7. doi: 10.1016/S0168-8278(00)80156-7
105. Redmond HP, Shou J, Kelly CJ, Leon P, Daly JM. Protein-calorie malnutrition impairs host defense against *Candida albicans. J Surg Res.* (1991) 50:552–9. doi: 10.1016/0022-4804(91)90040-S
106. Cason J, Ainley CC, Wolstencroft RA, Norton KR, Thompson RP. Cell-mediated immunity in anorexia nervosa. *Clin Exp Immunol.* (1986) 64:370–5.
107. Ahima RS, Prabakaran D, Mantzoros C, Qu D, Lowell B, Maratos-Flier E, et al. Role of leptin in the neuroendocrine response to fasting. *Nature* (1996) 382:250–2. doi: 10.1038/382250a0
108. Faggioni R, Moser A, Feingold KR, Grunfeld C. Reduced leptin levels in starvation increase susceptibility to endotoxic shock. *Am J Pathol.* (2000) 156:1781–7. doi: 10.1016/S0002-9440(10)65049-3
109. Faggioni R, Fantuzzi G, Gabay C, Moser A, Dinarello CA, Feingold KR, et al. Leptin deficiency enhances sensitivity to endotoxin-induced lethality. *Am J Physiol.* (1999) 276:R136–42.
110. Chen M, Wang B, Xu Y, Deng Z, Xue H, Wang L, et al. Diagnostic value of serum leptin and a promising novel diagnostic model for sepsis. *Exp Therapeutic Med.* (2014) 7:881–6. doi: 10.3892/etm.2014.1506
111. Ye M, Bian L-F. Association of serum leptin levels and pulmonary tuberculosis: a meta-analysis. *J Thorac Dis.* (2018)10:1027–36. doi: 10.21037/jtd.2018.01.70
112. Mancuso P, Gottschalk A, Phare SM, Peters-Golden M, Lukacs NW, Huffnagle GB. Leptin-deficient mice exhibit impaired host defense in Gram-negative pneumonia. *J Immunol.* (2002) 168:4018–24. doi: 10.4049/jimmunol.168.8.4018
113. Moore SI, Huffnagle GB, Chen GH, White ES, Mancuso P. Leptin modulates neutrophil phagocytosis of *Klebsiella pneumoniae. Infect Immun.* (2003) 71:4182–5. doi: 10.1128/IAI.71.7.4182-4185.2003
114. Mancuso P, Huffnagle GB, Olszewski MA, Phipps J, Peters-Golden M. Leptin corrects host defense defects after acute starvation in murine *Pneumococcal pneumonia. Am J Respir Crit Care Med.* (2006) 173:212–8. doi: 10.1164/rccm.200506-909OC
115. Koca C, Kavakli HS, Alici O. Immunomodulatory role of leptin treatment in experimental sepsis caused by gram negative bacteria. *Turk J Med Sci.* (2011) 41:251–8. doi: 10.3906/sag-1009-1109
116. Morshedi A, Zarkesh-Esfahani HS, Behjati M. Effect of leptin on neutrophils phagocytosis and lymphocytes apoptosis challenge by *Listeria monocytogenes* and *Escherichia coli. Jundishapur J Microbiol.* (2013) 6:e6389. doi: 10.5812/jjm.6389
117. Ikejima S, Sasaki S, Sashinami H, Mori F, Ogawa Y, Nakamura T, et al. Impairment of host resistance to *Listeria monocytogenes* infection in the liver of *db/db* and *ob/ob* mice. *Diabetes* (2005) 54:182–9. doi: 10.2337/diabetes.54.1.182
118. Nishi Y, Isomoto H, Uotani S, Wen CY, Shikuwa S, Ohnita K, et al. Enhanced production of leptin in gastric fundic mucosa with *Helicobacter pylori* infection. *World J Gastroenterol.* (2005) 11:695–9. doi: 10.3748/wjg.v11.i5.695
119. Khosravi Y, Seow SW, Amoyo AA, Chiow KH, Tan TL, Wong WY, et al. *Helicobacter pylori* infection can affect energy modulating hormones and body weight in germ free mice. *Sci Rep.* (2015) 5:8731. doi: 10.1038/srep08731
120. Azuma T, Suto H, Ito Y, Ohtani M, Dojo M, Kuriyama M, et al. Gastric leptin and *Helicobacter pylori* infection. *Gut* (2001) 49:324–9. doi: 10.1136/gut.49.3.324
121. Khudhur S, Jameel D, Karhoot J, AL-Khafaji J, Mohsin J. Increase serum leptin level in *Helicobacter pylori* infection in Iraqi gastritis patients. *Al-Kindy Col Med J.* (2011) 7:74–7.

122. Milner J, Meyers M, Sheridan P, Mancuso P, Beck M. The role of T cell leptin signaling in 2009 pandemic *H1N1* influenza infection mortality in obese mice (VIR2P.1013). *J Immunol.* (2014) 192(Suppl. 1):75.2.
123. Milner JJ, Rebeles J, Dhungana S, Stewart DA, Sumner SC, Meyers MH, et al. Obesity increases mortality and modulates the lung metabolome during pandemic *H1N1* influenza virus infection in mice. *J Immunol.* (2015) 194:4846–59. doi: 10.4049/jimmunol.1402295
124. Hur SJ, Kim DH, Chun SC, Lee SK. Effect of adenovirus and influenza virus infection on obesity. *Life Sci.* (2013) 93:531–5. doi: 10.1016/j.lfs.2013.08.016
125. Radigan KA, Morales-Nebreda L, Soberanes S, Nicholson T, Nigdelioglu R, Cho T, et al. Impaired clearance of influenza a virus in obese, leptin receptor-deficient mice is independent of leptin signaling in the lung epithelium and macrophages. *PLoS ONE* (2014) 9:e108138. doi: 10.1371/journal.pone.0108138
126. Qin L, Tan YR, Hu CP, Liu XA, He RX. Leptin is over-secreted by respiratory syncytial virus-infected bronchial epithelial cells and regulates th2 and th17 cell differentiation. *Int Arch Allergy Immunol.* (2015) 167:65–71. doi: 10.1159/000436966
127. Sánchez-Margalet V, Martín-Romero C, González-Yanes C, Goberna R, Rodríguez-Baños J, Muniain MA. Leptin receptor expression is induced in activated mononuclear cells *in vitro* and *in vivo* in HIV-infected patients. *Clin Exp Immunol.* (2002)129:119–24. doi: 10.1046/j.1365-2249.2002.01900.x
128. Azzoni L, Crowther NJ, Firnhaber C, Foulkes AS, Yin X, Glencross D, et al. Association between HIV replication and serum leptin levels: an observational study of a cohort of HIV-1-infected South African women. *J Int AIDS Soc.* (2010) 13:33. doi: 10.1186/1758-2652-13-33
129. Sinha U, Sinharay K, Sengupta N, Mukhopadhyay P. Benefits of leptin therapy in HIV patients. *Ind J Endocrinol Metab.* (2012) 16(Suppl. 3):S637–43. doi: 10.4103/2230-8210.105583
130. Shivahare R, Ali W, Vishwakarma P, Natu SM, Puri SK, Gupta S. Leptin augments protective immune responses in murine macrophages and enhances the potential of miltefosine against experimental visceral leishmaniasis. *Acta Trop.* (2015) 150:35–41. doi: 10.1016/j.actatropica.2015.06.024
131. Maurya R, Bhattacharya P, Ismail N, Dagur PK, Joshi AB, Razdan K, et al. Differential role of leptin as an immunomodulator in controlling visceral leishmaniasis in normal and leptin-deficient mice. *Am J Trop Med Hyg.* (2016) 95:109–19. doi: 10.4269/ajtmh.15-0804
132. Dayakar A, Chandrasekaran S, Veronica J, Bharadwaja V, Maurya R. Leptin regulates Granzyme-A, PD-1 and CTLA-4 expression in T cell to control visceral leishmaniasis in BALB/c Mice. *Sci Rep.* (2017) 7:14664. doi: 10.1038/s41598-017-15288-7
133. Combs TP, Nagajyothi, Mukherjee S, de Almeida CJ, Jelicks LA, Schubert W, et al. The adipocyte as an important target cell for *Trypanosoma cruzi* infection. *J Biol Chem.* (2005) 280:24085–94. doi: 10.1074/jbc.M412802200
134. Gutierrez FR, Guedes PM, Gazzinelli RT, Silva JS. The role of parasite persistence in the pathogenesis of Chagas heart disease. *Parasite Immunol.* (2009) 31:673–85. doi: 10.1111/j.1365-3024.2009.01108.x
135. Matos Ferreira AV, Segatto M, Menezes Z, Macedo AM, Gelape C, de Oliveira Andrade L, et al. Evidence for *Trypanosoma cruzi* in adipose tissue in human chronic Chagas disease. *Microb Infect.* (2011) 13:1002–5. doi: 10.1016/j.micinf.2011.06.002
136. Tanowitz HB, Amole B, Hewlett D, Wittner M. *Trypanosoma cruzi* infection in diabetic mice. *Trans R Soc Tropic Med Hyg.* (1988) 82:90–3. doi: 10.1016/0035-9203(88)90272-6
137. Alam F, Salam A, Mahmood I, Kabir M, Chowdhury S, Haque R. Amebic liver abscess is associated with malnutrition and low serum leptin level. *J Infect Dis Ther.* (2016) 4:298. doi: 10.4172/2332-0877.1000298
138. Duggal P, Guo X, Haque R, Peterson KM, Ricklefs S, Mondal D, et al. A mutation in the leptin receptor is associated with *Entamoeba histolytica* infection in children. *J Clin Invest.* (2011) 121:1191–8. doi: 10.1172/JCI45294
139. Naylor C, Burgess S, Madan R, Buonomo E, Razzaq K, Ralston K et al. Leptin receptor mutation results in defective neutrophil recruitment to the colon during *Entamoeba histolytica* infection. *MBio* (2014) 5:e02046-14. doi: 10.1128/mBio.02046-14
140. Guo X, Roberts MR, Becker SM, Podd B, Zhang Y, Chua SC Jr, et al. Leptin signaling in intestinal epithelium mediates resistance to enteric infection by *Entamoeba histolytica. Mucosal Immunol.* (2011) 4:294–303. doi: 10.1038/mi.2010.76
141. Marie CS, Verkerke HP, Paul SN, Mackey AJ, Petri WA Jr. Leptin protects host cells from *Entamoeba histolytica* cytotoxicity by a STAT-3 dependent mechanism. *Infect Immun.* (2012) 226:2123–30.
142. Mackey-Lawrence NM, Petri WA Jr. Leptin and mucosal immunity. *Mucosal Immunol.* (2012) 5:472–9. doi: 10.1038/mi.2012.40
143. Mejia P, Treviño-Villarreal JH, Hine C, Harputlugil E, Lang S, Calay E, et al. Dietary restriction protects against experimental cerebral malaria via leptin modulation and T cell mTORC1 suppression. *Nat Commun.* (2015) 6:6050. doi: 10.1038/ncomms7050
144. Al-Fadhli MA, Saraya MA, Qasem JA. Evaluation of leptin, interleukin-1 beta and tumor necrosis factor alpha in the serum of malaria patients as prognostic markers of treatment outcome. *Asian Pac J Trop Biomed.* (2014) 4:441–5. doi: 10.12980/APJTB.4.201414B11
145. Elnemr GM, Elnashar MA, Elmargoushy NM, Elnashar NA, Elnashar MA. Adiponectin levels as a marker of inflammation in pulmonary tuberculosis. *Egypt J Hosp Med.* (2015) 59:208–14. doi: 10.12816/0012177
146. Neeraj Indora N, Sharma K, Karunanand B, Sudan DPS, Shah AK. Assessment of metabolic (Adiponectin, Leptin) and inflammatory markers (TNF-α, hs-CRP & IFN-γ) in pulmonary tuberculosis: prospective Study. *Int J Clin Biochem Res.* (2017) 4:216–9. doi: 10.18231/2394-6377.2017.0051
147. Shirshev SV, Orlova EG. Molecular mechanisms of regulation of the functional activity of mononuclear phagocytes by leptin. *Biochemistry* (2005) 70:841–7. doi: 10.1007/s10541-005-0193-1
148. Bates SH, Stearns WH, Dundon TA, Schubert M, Tso AW, Wang Y, et al. STAT3 signalling is required for leptin regulation of energy balance but not reproduction. *Nature* (2003) 421:856–9. doi: 10.1038/nature 01388
149. Gong Y, Ishida-Takahashi R, Villanueva EC, Fingar DC, Münzberg H, Myers MG Jr. The long form of the leptin receptor regulates STAT5 and ribosomal protein S6 via alternate mechanisms. *J Biol Chem.* (2007) 282:31019–27. doi: 10.1074/jbc.M702838200
150. Bjørbaek C, Buchholz RM, Davis SM, Bates SH, Pierroz DD, Gu H, et al. Divergent roles of SHP-2 in ERK activation by leptin receptors. *J Biol Chem.* (2001) 276:4747–55. doi: 10.1074/jbc.M007439200
151. Mancuso P, Myers MG, Goel D, Serezani CH, O'Brien E, Goldberg J, et al. Ablation of leptin receptor-mediated ERK activation impairs host defense against gram-negative pneumonia. *J Immunol.* (2012) 189:867–75. doi: 10.4049/jimmunol.1200465
152. Caldefie-Chezet F, Poulin A, Tridon A, Sion B, Vasson MP. Leptin: a potential regulator of polymorphonuclear neutrophil bactericidal action? *J Leukoc Biol.* (2001) 69:414–8.
153. Moshyedi AK, Josephs MD, Abdalla EK, Mackay SLD, Edwards CK, Copeland EM, et al. Increased leptin expression in mice with bacterial peritonitis is partially regulated by tumor necrosis factor alpha. *Infect Immun.* (1998) 66:1800–2.
154. Mancuso P, Peters-Golden M, Goel D. Disruption of leptin receptor-stat3 signaling enhances leukotriene production and pulmonary host defense against *Pneumococcal pneumonia. J Immunol.* (2011) 186:1081–90. doi: 10.4049/jimmunol.1001470
155. Breideri M, Miehlike S, Glasou A, Orban Z, Stolte M, Ehninger G, et al. Leptin and its receptor in normal human gastric mucosa and in *H pylori*-associated gastritis. *Scand J Gastroenterol.* (1999) 34:954–61. doi: 10.1080/003655299750025039
156. Taylor AK, Cao W, Vora KP, De La Cruz J, Shieh WJ, Zaki SR, et al. Protein-energy malnutrition decreases immunity and increases susceptibility to influenza infection in mice. *J Infect Dis.* (2013) 207:501–10. doi: 10.1093/infdis/jis527
157. Ortega YR, Eberhard ML, Kris H. Protozoan diseases: cryptosporidiosis, giardiasis and other intestinal protozoan diseases. *International Encyclopedia of Public Health.* Oxford: Academic Press (2008) p. 354–66.
158. Lõhmus M, Moalem S, Björklund M. Leptin, a tool of parasites? *Biol Lett.* (2012) 8:849–52. doi: 10.1098/rsbl.2012.0385
159. Caldefie-Chezet F, Poulin A, Vasson MP. Leptin regulates functional capacities of polymorphonuclear neutrophils. *Free Radic Res.* (2003) 37:809–14. doi: 10.1080/1071576031000097526

160. Naylor C, Petri WA Jr. Leptin regulation of immune responses. *Trends Mol Med.* (2016) 22:88–98. doi: 10.1016/j.molmed.2015.12.001
161. WHO. Control of the leishmaniasis: report of a meeting of the WHO Expert Committee on the Control of Leishmaniases, Geneva, March 22–26, 2010. *World Health Organ Tech Rep Ser.* (2010) 949:1–186.
162. Desjeux P. Leishmaniasis: current situation and new perspectives. *Comp Immunol Microbiol Infect Dis.* (2004). 27:305–18. doi: 10.1016/j.cimid.2004.03.004
163. Pearson RD, Cox G, Jeronimo SM, Castracane J, Drew JS, Evans T, et al. Visceral leishmaniasis: a model for infection-induced cachexia. *Am J Trop Med Hyg.* (1992) 47(1 Pt 2):8–15. doi: 10.4269/ajtmh.1992.47.8
164. Anstead GM, Chandrasekar B, Zhao W, Yang J, Perez LE, Melby PC. Lalnutrition alters the innate immune response and increases early visceralization following *Leishmania donovani* infection. *Infect Immun.* (2001) 69:4709–18. doi: 10.1128/IAI.69.8.4709-4718.2001
165. Ibrahim MK, Barnes JL, Anstead GM, Jimenez F, Travi BL, Peniche AG, et al. The malnutrition-related increase in early visceralization of *Leishmania donovani* is associated with a reduced number of lymph node phagocytes and altered conduit system flow. *PLoS Negl Tropic Dis.* (2013) 7:e2329. doi: 10.1371/journal.pntd.0002329
166. Macia L, Delacre M, Abboud G, Ouk TS, Delanoye A, Verwaerde C, et al. Impairment of dendritic cell functionality and steady-state number in obese mice. *J Immunol.* (2006) 177:5997. doi: 10.4049/jimmunol.177.9.5997
167. Jin HT, Anderson AC, Tan WG, West EE, Ha SJ, Araki K, et al. Cooperation of Tim-3 and PD-1 in CD8 T-cell exhaustion during chronic viral infection. *Proc Natl Acad Sci USA.* (2010) 107:14733–8. doi: 10.1073/pnas.1009731107
168. Di Loria A, Squillacioti C, De Luca A, Veneziano V, Mirabella N, Guccione J, et al. Increased leptin mRNA expression in the blood of dogs naturally infected by *Leishmania infantum. Vet J.* (2014) 202:634–6. doi: 10.1016/j.tvjl.2014.10.010
169. WHO. *Global Plan to Combat Neglected Diseases 2008–2015.* WHO/CDS/NTD/2007. Geneva: WHO (2007).
170. Machado FS, Mukherjee S, Weiss LM, Tanowitz HB, Ashton AW. Bioactive lipids in *Trypanosoma cruzi* infection. *Adv Parasitol.* (2011) 76:1–31. doi: 10.1016/B978-0-12-385895-5.00001-3
171. Miao Q, Ndao M. *Trypanosoma cruzi* infection and host lipid metabolism. *Mediators Inflamm.* (2014) 2014:902038. doi: 10.1155/2014/902038
172. Nagajyothi F, Desruisseaux MS, Thiruvur N, Weiss LM, Braunstein VL, Albanese C, et al. *Trypanosoma cruzi* infection of cultured adipocytes results in an inflammatory phenotype. *Obesity* (2008) 16:1992–7. doi: 10.1038/oby.2008.331
173. Rodrigues CM, Valadares HM, Francisco AF, Arantes JM, Campos CF, Teixeira-Carvalho A, et al. Coinfection with different *Trypanosoma cruzi* strains interferes with the host immune response to infection. *PLoS Negl Trop Dis.* (2010) 4:e846. doi: 10.1371/journal.pntd.0000846
174. Mukherjee S, Huang H, Petkova SB, Albanese C, Pestell RG, Braunstein VL, et al. *Trypanosoma cruizi* infection activates extracellular signal-regulated kinase in cultured endothelial and smooth muscle cells. *Infect Immun.* (2004) 72:5274–82. doi: 10.1128/IAI.72.9.5274-5282.2004
175. Wilkowsky SE, Barbieri MA, Stahl P, Isola ELD. *Trypanosoma cruzi*: phosphatidylinositol 3-kinase and protein kinase B activation is associated with parasite invasion. *Exp Cell Res.* (2001) 264:211–8. doi: 10.1006/excr.2000.5123
176. Hovsepian E, Penas F, Mirkin GA, Goren NB. Role of PPARs in *Trypanosoma cruzi* infection: implications for chagas disease therapy. *PPAR Res.* (2011) 2012:528435. doi: 10.1155/2012/528435
177. Stanley SL Jr. Amoebiasis. *Lancet* (2003) 361:1025–34. doi: 10.1016/S0140-6736(03)12830-9
178. Baxt LA, Singh U. New insights into *Entamoeba histolytica* pathogenesis. *Curr Opin Infect Dis.* (2008) 21:489–94. doi: 10.1097/QCO.0b013e32830ce75f
179. Mortimer L, Chadee K. The immunopathogenesis of *Entamoeba histolytica. Exp Parasitol.* (2010) 126:366–80. doi: 10.1016/j.exppara.2010.03.005
180. Petri WA Jr, Mondal D, Peterson KM, Duggal P, Haque R. Association of malnutrition with amebiasis. *Nutr Rev.* (2009) 67 (Suppl. 2):S207–15. doi: 10.1111/j.1753-4887.2009.00242.x
181. Ali IK, Clark CG, Petri WA Jr. Molecular epidemiology of amebiasis. *Infect Genet Evol.* (2008) 8:698–707. doi: 10.1016/j.meegid.2008.05.004
182. Haque R, Mondal D, Duggal P, Kabir M, Roy S, Farr BM, et al. *Entamoeba histolytica* infection in children and protection from subsequent amebiasis. *Infect Immun.* (2006) 74:904–9. doi: 10.1128/IAI.74.2.904-909.2006
183. Blessman J, Van LP, Tanich E. Epidemiology of amebiasis in a region of high incidence of amebic liver abscess in central Vietnam. *Am J Trop Med Hyg.* (2002) 66:578–83. doi: 10.4269/ajtmh.2002.66.578
184. Siddiqui MA, Ekram ARSM, Islam QT, Hoque MA, Masum QAAI. Clinico-pathological profile of liver abscess in a teaching hospital. *Teachers Assoc J Rajshahi* (2008) 21:46–8.
185. Mondal D, Haque R, Sack RB, Kirkpatrick BD, Petri WA. Attribution of malnutrition to cause-specific diarrheal illness: evidence from a prospective study of preschool children in Mirpur, Dhaka, Bangladesh. *Am J Trop Med Hyg.* (2009) 80:824–6. doi: 10.4269/ajtmh.2009.80.824
186. World Health Organization. *World Malaria Report.* Geneva: WHO (2015).
187. Bousema T, Drakeley C. Epidemiology and infectivity of *Plasmodium falciparum* and *Plasmodium vivax* gametocytes in relation to malaria control and elimination. *Clin Microbiol Rev.* (2011) 24:377–410. doi: 10.1128/CMR.00051-10
188. Robert V, Bourgouin C, Depoix D, Thouvenot C, Lombard MN, Grellier P. Malaria and obesity: obese mice are resistant to cerebral malaria. *Malaria J.* (2008) 7:81. doi: 10.1186/1475-2875-7-81
189. Finlay D, Cantrell DA. Metabolism, migration and memory in cytotoxic T cells. *Nat Rev Immunol.* (2011) 11:109–17. doi: 10.1038/nri2888
190. Hughes SM, Amadi B, Mwiya M, Nkamba H, Tomkins A, Goldblatt D. Dendritic cell anergy results from endotoxemia in severe malnutrition. *J Immunol.* (2009) 183:2818–26. doi: 10.4049/jimmunol.0803518
191. Bourke CD, Berkley JA, Prendergast AJ. Immune dysfunction as a cause and consequence of malnutrition. *Trends Immunol.* (2016) 37:386–98. doi: 10.1016/j.it.2016.04.003
192. Lam QL, Lu L. Role of leptin in immunity. *Cel Mol Immunol.* (2007) 4:1–13.
193. Vernooy JHJ, Ubags NDJ, Brusselle GG, Tavernier J, Suratt BT, Joos GF, et al. Leptin as regulator of pulmonary immune responses: involvement in respiratory diseases. *Pulmon Pharmacol Therapeut.* (2013) 26:464–72. doi: 10.1016/j.pupt.2013.03.016
194. Duncan SA, Baganizi DR, Sahu R, Singh SR, Dennis VA. SOCS proteins as regulators of inflammatory responses induced by bacterial infections: a review. *Front Microbiol.* (2017) 8:2431. doi: 10.3389/fmicb.2017.02431
195. Paracha RZ, Ahmad J, Ali A, Hussain R, Niazi U, Tareen SHK, et al. Formal modelling of toll like receptor 4 and JAK/STAT signalling pathways: insight into the roles of SOCS-1, interferon-β and proinflammatory cytokines in sepsis. *PLoS ONE* (2014) 9:e108466. doi: 10.1371/journal.pone.0108466
196. Akhtar LN, Qin H, Muldowney MT, Yanagisawa LL, Kutsch O, Clements J E, et al. Suppressor of cytokine signaling 3 inhibits antiviral IFN- β signaling to enhance HIV-1 replication in macrophages. *J Immunol.* (2010) 185:2393–404. doi: 10.4049/jimmunol.0903563
197. Wei H, Wang S, Chen Q, Chen Y, Chi X, Zhang L, et al. Suppression of interferon lambda signaling by SOCS-1 results in their excessive production during influenza virus infection. *PLoS Pathog.* (2014) 10:e1003845. doi: 10.1371/journal.ppat.1003845
198. Michaud F, Coulombe F, Gaudreault E, Paquet-Bouchard C, Rola-Pleszczynski M, Gosselin J. Epstein-Barr virus interferes with the amplification of IFN-α secretion by activating suppressor of cytokine signaling 3 in primary human monocytes. *PLoS ONE* (2010) 5:e11908. doi: 10.1371/journal.pone.0011908
199. Srivastav S, Basu Ball W, Gupta P, Giri J, Ukil A, Das PK. *Leishmania donovani* prevents oxidative burst-mediated apoptosis of host macrophages through selective induction of suppressors of cytokine signaling (SOCS) proteins. *J Biol Chem.* (2014) 289:1092–105. doi: 10.1074/jbc.M113.496323
200. Banerjee R, Kumar S, Sen A, Mookerjee A, Roy S, Pal S, et al. TGF-β-regulated tyrosine phosphatases induce lymphocyte apoptosis in *Leishmania donovani*-infected hamsters. *Immunol Cell Biol.* (2011) 89:466–74. doi: 10.1038/icb.2010.108
201. Bertholet S, Dickensheets H L, Sheikh F, Gam AA, Donnelly R P, Kenney RT. *Leishmania donovani*-induced expression of suppressor of cytokine signaling 3 in human macrophages: a novel mechanism for intracellular

parasite suppression of activation. *Infect Immun.* (2003) 71:2095–101. doi: 10.1128/IAI.71.4.2095-2101.2003

202. Blanchette J, Racette N, Faure R, Siminovitch KA, Olivier M. *Leishmania*-induced increases in activation of macrophage SHP-1 tyrosine phosphatase are associated with impaired IFN-gamma-triggered JAK2 activation. *Eur J Immunol.* (1999) 29:3737–44. doi: 10.1002/(SICI)1521-4141(199911)29:11<3737::AID-IMMU3737>3.0.CO;2-S
203. Forget G, Gregory DJ, Whitcombe LA, Olivier M. Role of host protein tyrosine phosphatase SHP-1 in *Leishmania donovani*-induced inhibition of nitric oxide production. *Infect Immun.* (2006) 74:6272–79. doi: 10.1128/IAI.00853-05
204. Alti D, Sambamurthy C, Kalangi SK. Emergence of leptin in infection and immunity: scope and challenges in vaccines formulation. *Front Cell Infect Microbiol.* (2018) 8:147. doi: 10.3389/fcimb.2018.00147
205. Stahl P, Schwarz RT, Debierre-Grockiego F, Meyer T. *Trypanosoma cruzi* parasites fight for control of the JAK-STAT pathway by disarming their host. *JAKSTAT* (2015) 3:e1012964. doi: 10.1080/21623996.2015.1012964
206. Hovsepian E, Penas F, Siffo S, Mirkin GA, Goren NB. IL-10 inhibits the NF-κB and ERK/MAPK-mediated production of pro-inflammatory mediators by up-regulation of SOCS-3 in *Trypanosoma cruzi*-infected Cardiomyocytes. *PLoS ONE* (2013) 8:e79445. doi: 10.1371/journal.pone.0079445

15

Elevated Systemic Levels of Eosinophil, Neutrophil and Mast Cell Granular Proteins in *Strongyloides Stercoralis* Infection that Diminish following Treatment

Anuradha Rajamanickam[1]*, Saravanan Munisankar[1], Yukthi Bhootra[1], Chandra Kumar Dolla[2], Thomas B. Nutman[3] and Subash Babu[1,3]

[1] National Institutes of Health – National Institute of Research in Tuberculosis (ICMR) – International Center for Excellence in Research, Chennai, India, [2] National Institute of Research in Tuberculosis (ICMR), Chennai, India, [3] Laboratory of Parasitic Diseases, National Institute of Allergy and Infectious Diseases, National Institutes of Health, Bethesda, MD, United States

****Correspondence:***
Anuradha Rajamanickam
anuradha@nirt.res.in

Infection with the helminth parasite *Strongyloides stercoralis* (*Ss*) is commonly clinically asymptomatic that is often accompanied by peripheral eosinophilia. Granulocytes are activated during helminth infection and can act as immune effector cells. Plasma levels of eosinophil and neutrophil granular proteins convey an indirect measure of granulocyte degranulation and are prominently augmented in numerous helminth-infected patients. In this study, we sought to examine the levels of eosinophil, neutrophil, and mast cell activation-associated granule proteins in asymptomatic *Ss* infection and to understand their kinetics following anthelmintic therapy. To this end, we measured the plasma levels of eosinophil cationic protein, eosinophil-derived neurotoxin, eosinophil peroxidase, eosinophil major basic protein, neutrophil elastase, myeloperoxidase, neutrophil proteinase-3, mast cell tryptase, leukotriene C4, and mast cell carboxypeptidase-A3 in individuals with asymptomatic *Ss* infection or without *Ss* infection [uninfected (UN)]. We also estimated the levels of all of these analytes in infected individuals following definitive treatment of *Ss* infection. We demonstrated that those infected individuals have significantly enhanced plasma levels of eosinophil cationic protein, eosinophil-derived neurotoxin, eosinophil peroxidase, eosinophil major basic protein, elastase, myeloperoxidase, mast cell tryptase, leukotriene C4, and carboxypeptidase-A3 compared to UN individuals. Following the treatment of *Ss* infection, each of these granulocyte-associated proteins drops significantly. Our data suggest that eosinophil, neutrophil, and mast cell activation may play a role in the response to *Ss* infection.

Keywords: eosinophils, neutrophils, mast cells, granular proteins, helminths, *Strongyloides stercoralis*

INTRODUCTION

Strongyloides stercoralis (Ss), an intestinal parasitic nematode, infects 30–100 million people worldwide (1). The clinical manifestation of *Ss* can range from clinically asymptomatic to, at its most severe, a potentially fatal disseminated infection. Granulocytes are activated during helminth infection and act as immune effector cells. *In vitro* granulocyte mediated immunity against helminths can be attained through antibody-dependent cell-mediated cytotoxicity, and antibody attaches to the parasite's cell surface and triggers degranulation and extrusion of toxic granule contents against the parasite (2).

In healthy people, eosinophils normally constitute only 2–5% of peripheral leukocytes. However, during active helminth infection, the eosinophils fraction in the blood can increase to more than 40% (3). Eosinophils have eosinophil-specific toxic proteins stored in their secondary granules. These include eosinophil cationic protein (ECP), eosinophil peroxidase (EPX), eosinophil-derived neurotoxin (EDN), and eosinophil major basic protein (MBP). ECP, EPX, and MBP are potent helminth toxins (4). MBP can provoke histamine release from mast cells; however, EDN and ECP can act as ribonucleases (4, 5). Experimental helminth infection studies revealed that eosinophils accumulate in the gastrointestinal tract, where it is believed that they assist to eliminate parasites (6). Interestingly, evidence suggests that there could be dissimilarities in the mechanisms of eosinophil-mediated killing among different life cycle stages of the same parasite (7).

Among granulocytes, neutrophils are effective at phagocytosis, and they can engulf and execute microorganisms by producing reactive oxygen intermediates in phagolysosomes. Conversely, helminths are very large to be phagocytosed, and as a outcome, the function of neutrophils in helminth-driven effector responses has been ignored till now (2). Neutrophils can be defensive against nematode parasites, and this has been exhibited conclusively in the *Strongyloides sp.* model (8). Like neutrophils, granulocytes are also critical in controlling *Streptococcus ratti* in mice (9). Myeloperoxidase (MPO) purified from human neutrophils is toxic to *Trichinella spiralis* and *Schistosoma mansoni* (10, 11) and functions in killing *S. stercoralis* larvae (12). Neutrophil elastase (NE) secreted following contact with *S. mansoni* is potentially toxic to a number of stages of this parasite (13).

Mast cells also play an important role in parasitic infections and have been implicated in the regulation of innate and adaptive immune responses following infection (14). Helminth infections are associated with elevations in tissue mast cell numbers (15). In the presence of helminth antigens, FcεRI receptor provokes mast cell degranulation, which results in the release of mast cell tryptase (MCT), carboxypeptidase-A3 (CPA-3), and leukotriene C4 (LTC4), which has direct cytotoxic effect on helminths (15, 16). During helminth infection, studies have revealed that mast cells are crucial in the expulsion of several helminth species from the gastrointestinal tract (17) including *T. spiralis*, *Nippostrongylus brasiliensis*, and *S. ratti* in rodent models (18, 19).

In this study, we wanted to characterize the presence and persistence of eosinophil, neutrophil, and mast cell degranulation proteins in *Ss* infection before and after treatment. We hypothesized that the plasma levels of granular proteins would reflect the activation profile of these important granulocyte subsets and its association to *Ss* infection. To this end, we measured the plasma levels of eosinophil granular proteins (ECP, EDN, EPX, and MBP), neutrophil granular proteins [NE, MPO, and proteinase-3 (PTN-3)], and mast cell granular proteins and mediators (MCT, LTC4, and CPA-3) in *Ss*-infected (INF) and *Ss*-uninfected (UN) individuals. Plasma levels of ECP, EPX, EDN, MBP, NE, MPO, MCT, LTC4, and CPA-3 levels were all significantly increased in *Ss* infection compared to those without *Ss* infection. These levels decreased significantly after anthelmintic treatment.

MATERIALS AND METHODS

Ethics Statement

All participants were examined as a part of a natural history study protocol (12-I-073) approved by Institutional Review Boards of the National Institute of Allergy and Infectious Diseases (USA) and the National Institute for Research in Tuberculosis (India), and informed written consent was obtained from all participants.

Study Population

We studied a total of 118 individuals including of 60 clinically asymptomatic, INF individuals and 58 UNF, endemic healthy individuals in Tamil Nadu, South India (**Table 1**). These individuals were all enrolled from a rural population. None had previous anthelmintic treatment, a history of helminth infections, or HIV. The INF individuals were followed up after 6 months of anthelmintic treatment.

Strongyloides stercoralis infection was detected by measuring IgG antibodies to the recombinant NIE antigen, as explained elsewhere (20, 21). Further confirmation was done using specialized stool examination with nutrient agar plate cultures (22). None of the study population had lymphatic filariasis (based on ELISA) or other intestinal helminths (based on the stool microscopy). All INF individuals were treated with single doses of ivermectin and albendazole, and follow-up blood draws were collected after 6 months. Treated individuals were *Ss* infection negative by stool microscopy at 6 months posttreatment (post-T). All UN individuals were negative for anti-*Ss*-NIE and for filarial and other intestinal helminths.

Measurement of Hematological Parameters

Hematological parameters were measured from fresh venous EDTA blood samples on all individuals using an ACT 5 Diff. hematology analyzer (Beckman Coulter, Brea, CA, USA).

Measurement of Eosinophils, Neutrophils, and Mast Cell Granular Proteins

Plasma levels of ECP, EDN, EPX, MBP (MyBiosource, Inc., San Diego, CA, USA), MPO, PTN-3 (R&D Systems, Minneapolis, MN, USA), NE (Cell Sciences Hycult Biotech, Canton, MA, USA), MCT, LTC4, and CPA-3 were measured using the Mybiosource ELISA kits (MyBiosource, Inc., San Diego, CA, USA), followed

TABLE 1 | Baseline demographics of the study population.

Study demographics	*Ss* infected (INF)	*Ss* uninfected (UN)
Number	60	58
Gender (male/female)	33/27	35/23
Median age (range)	36 (20–65)	39 (20–60)
NIE ELISA	Positive	Negative

the manufacturer's protocol. The detection limits were as follows: ECP, 1.56–100 ng/ml; EDN, 0.625–40 ng/ml; EPX, 78–5,000 pg/ml; MBP, 0.468–30 ng/ml; MPO, 62.50–4,000 pg/ml; PTN-3, 15.6–1,000 pg/ml; NE, 0.4–25 ng/ml; MCT, 3.12–100 ng/ml; LTC4, 78–5,000 pg/ml; and CPA-3, 0.78–50 ng/ml. We have assigned the lowest standard value to the samples that were below the threshold of detection.

Statistical Analysis

Data analyses were done using GraphPad PRISM 7 (GraphPad Software, Inc., San Diego, CA, USA). Central tendency was calculated using geometric mean (GM). Nonparametric Mann–Whitney *U* test and Wilcoxon matched pair test were used to calculate the statistical significant difference. Multiple comparisons were corrected using the Holm's correction. JMP 13 (SAS) software was used to perform Spearman rank correlation matrix.

RESULTS

Ss Infection Is Associated with Elevated Absolute Neutrophil and Eosinophil Counts and Reversal following Treatment

As shown in **Table 1**, there was no significant difference in age or gender between the two groups. We measured the hematological parameters in the two groups. As shown in **Figure 1A**, INF had significantly enhanced levels of neutrophils (GM of 6,566/μl in INF Vs GM of 4,848/μl in UN; $p = 0.0001$) and eosinophils (GM of 550/μl in INF vs GM of 281/μl in UN; $p < 0.0001$) in comparison with UN individuals. The other hematological parameters did not show any significant difference between the two groups. Upon anthelminthic treatment, the absolute numbers were significantly reversed. As shown in **Figure 1B**, absolute counts of neutrophils [GM of 6,566/μl in pretreatment (pre-T) vs GM of 6,000/μl in post-T; $p < 0.0001$] and eosinophils (GM of 550/μl in pre-T Vs GM of 483/μl in post-T; $p < 0.0001$) were significantly decreased. Other hematological parameters did not show any significant changes following treatment.

Ss Infection Is Associated with Elevated Levels of Eosinophils, Neutrophils, and Mast Cell Granular Proteins

To characterize the role of eosinophils, neutrophils, mast cell granular proteins, and lipid mediators in *Ss* infection, we measured the plasma levels of eosinophil granular proteins (ECP, EDN, EPX, and MBP), neutrophil granular proteins (NE, MPO, and PTN-3), mast cell granular proteins, and lipid mediator (MCT, LTC4, and CPA-3) in INF and UN individuals. As shown in **Figure 2A**, INF had significantly higher levels of ECP (GM of 71.18 ng/ml in INF vs. 48.59 ng/ml in UN; $p = 0.0007$), EDN (GM of 1.811 ng/ml in INF vs. 1.014 ng/ml in UN; $p = 0.0072$), EPX (GM of 1,1945 ng/ml in INF vs. 7,407 ng/ml in UN; $p = 0.0065$), and MBP (GM of 288.4 ng/ml in INF vs. 223.7 ng/ml in UN; $p = 0.0464$) in comparison to UN individuals. As shown in **Figure 2B**, INF had significantly enhanced levels of NE (GM of 8,456 ng/ml in INF vs. 6,422 ng/ml in UN; $p = 0.0363$) and MPO (GM of 45.12 pg/ml in INF vs. 37.26 pg/ml in UN; $p = 0.0340$) in comparison to UN individuals. As shown in **Figure 2C**, INF had significantly increased levels of MCT (GM of 8,456 ng/ml in INF vs. 6,422 ng/ml in UN; $p = 0.0363$), LTC4 (GM of 45.12 pg/ml in INF vs. 37.26 pg/ml in UN; $p = 0.0340$), and CPA-3 (GM of

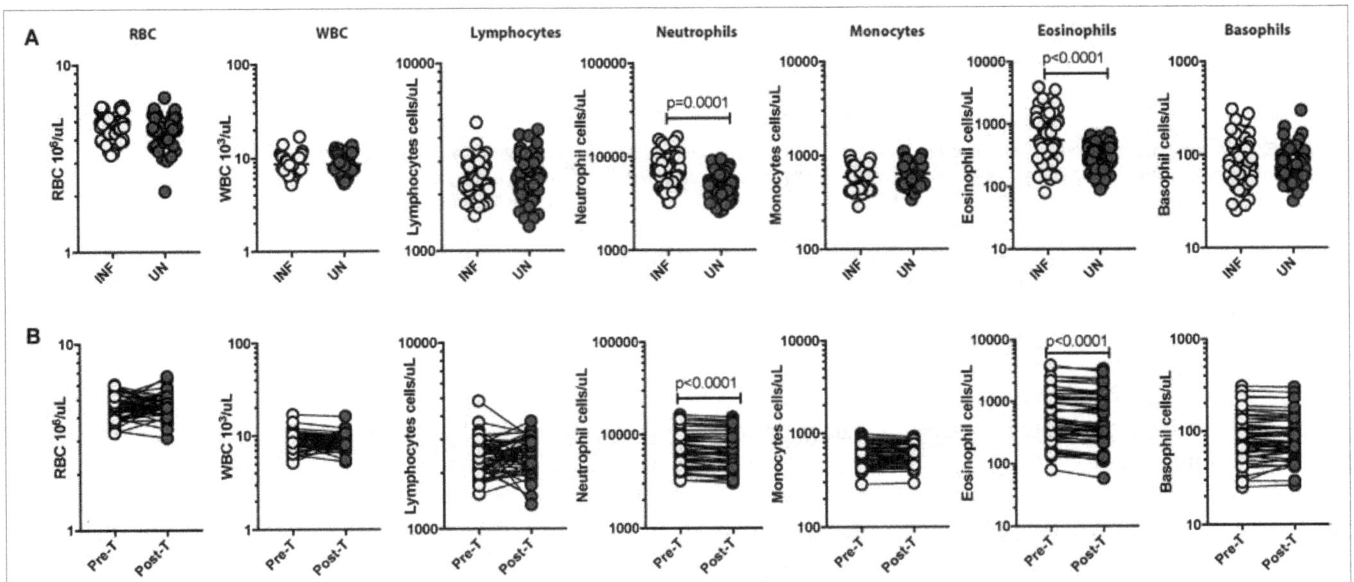

FIGURE 1 | *Strongyloides stercoralis* (Ss) infection is associated with elevated absolute neutrophil and eosinophil counts and reversal following treatment. **(A)** Absolute counts of hematological parameters from Ss-infected (INF; $n = 60$) or uninfected (UN; $n = 58$) individuals were measured. Data are shown as scatter plots with the bar representing the geometric mean. *p* Values were calculated using the Mann–Whitney test with Holm's correction for multiple comparisons. **(B)** Absolute counts of hematological parameters from Ss-infected pretreatment (pre-T; $n = 60$) and 6 months after treatment posttreatment (post-T) individuals were measured. *p* Values were calculated using the Wilcoxon matched pair test with Holm's correction for multiple comparisons.

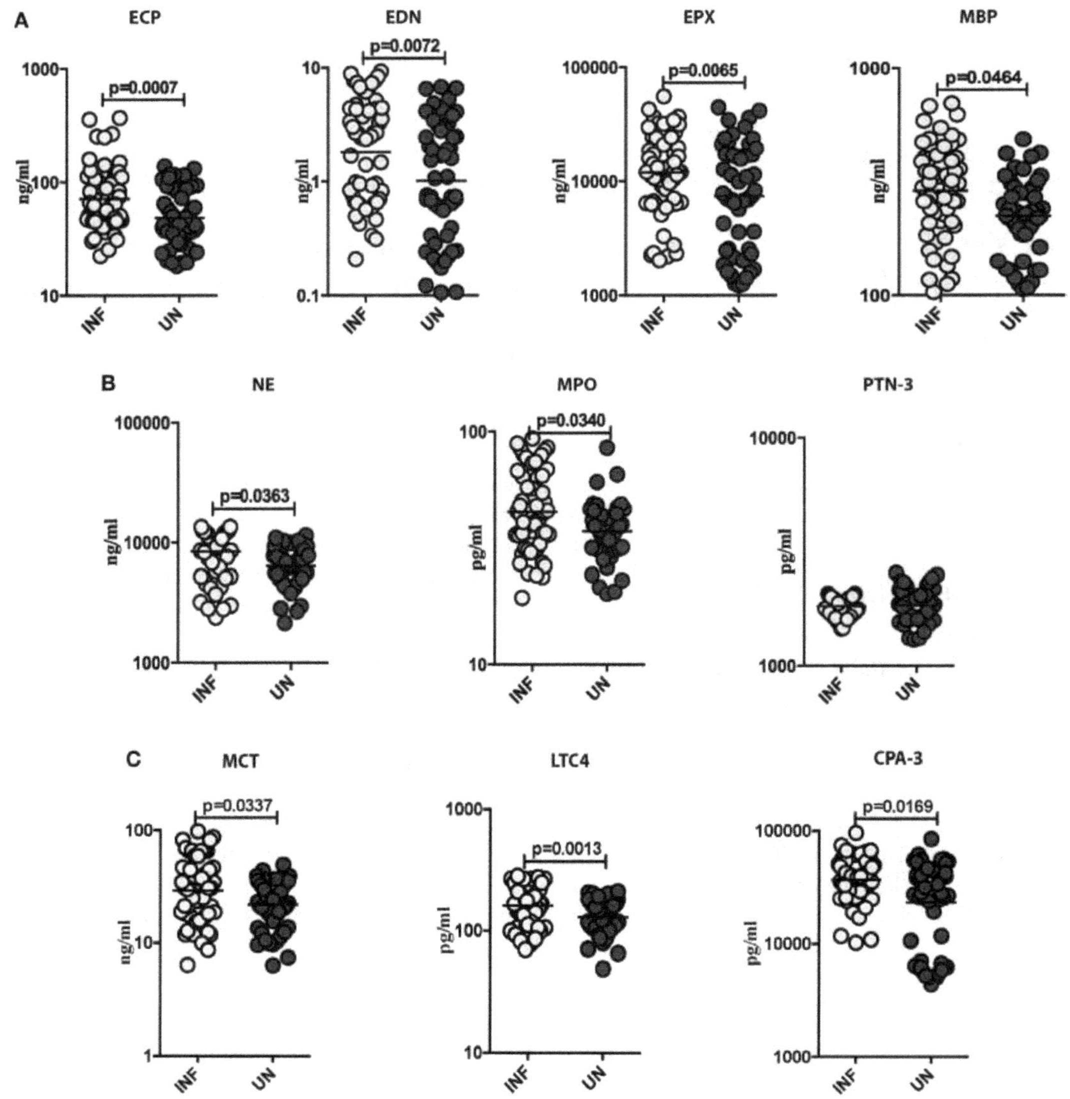

FIGURE 2 | *Strongyloides stercoralis* (*Ss*) infection is associated with elevated levels of eosinophils, neutrophils, and mast cell granular proteins. **(A)** Plasma levels of eosinophil cationic protein (ECP), eosinophil-derived neurotoxin (EDN), eosinophil peroxidase (EPX), and major basic protein (MBP), from *Ss*-infected (INF; $n = 60$) or *Ss*-uninfected (UN; $n = 58$) individuals were measured by ELISA. Data are shown as scatter plots with the bar representing the geometric mean. *p* Values were calculated using the Mann–Whitney test. **(B)** Plasma levels of plasma levels of neutrophil elastase (NE), myeloperoxidase (MPO), and proteinase-3 (PTN-3) from (INF; $n = 60$) or (UN; $n = 58$) individuals were measured by ELISA. Data are shown as scatter plots with the bar representing the geometric mean. *p* Values were calculated using the Mann–Whitney test. **(C)** Plasma levels of plasma levels of mast cell tryptase (MCT), leukotriene C4 (LTC4), and carboxypeptidase A-3 (CPA-3) from INF ($n = 60$) or UN ($n = 58$) individuals were measured by ELISA. Data are shown as scatter plots with the bar representing the geometric mean. *p* Values were calculated using the Mann–Whitney test with Holm's correction for multiple comparisons.

45.12 pg/ml in INF vs. 37.26 pg/ml in UN; $p = 0.0340$) in comparison to UN individuals.

Ss Infection Is Associated with Decreased Levels of Eosinophils, Neutrophils, and Mast Cell Granular Proteins following Anthelminthic Treatment

To determine the outcome of treatment on the levels of these granulocyte-associated proteins in those with *Ss* infection, all INF individuals were treated, and the levels of eosinophil granular proteins (ECP, EDN, EPX, and MBP), neutrophil granular proteins (NE, MPO, and PTN-3), and mast cell products (MCT, LTC4, and CPA-3) were measured in INF individuals before and after anthelminthic treatment. As shown in **Figure 3A**, the systemic levels of ECP (GM of 71.18 ng/ml in pre-T vs. 57.78 ng/ml in post-T; $p = 0.0007$), EDN (GM of 1.811 ng/ml in pre-T vs. 1.365 ng/ml in post-T; $p = 0.0006$), EPX (GM of 1,1945 ng/ml in pre-T vs. 1,1146 ng/ml in post-T; $p = 0.0005$), and MBP (GM of 288.4 ng/ml in pre-T vs. 167 ng/ml in post-T; $p = 0.0084$) were significantly decreased in INF individuals following anthelmintic treatment. For the neutrophil-associated

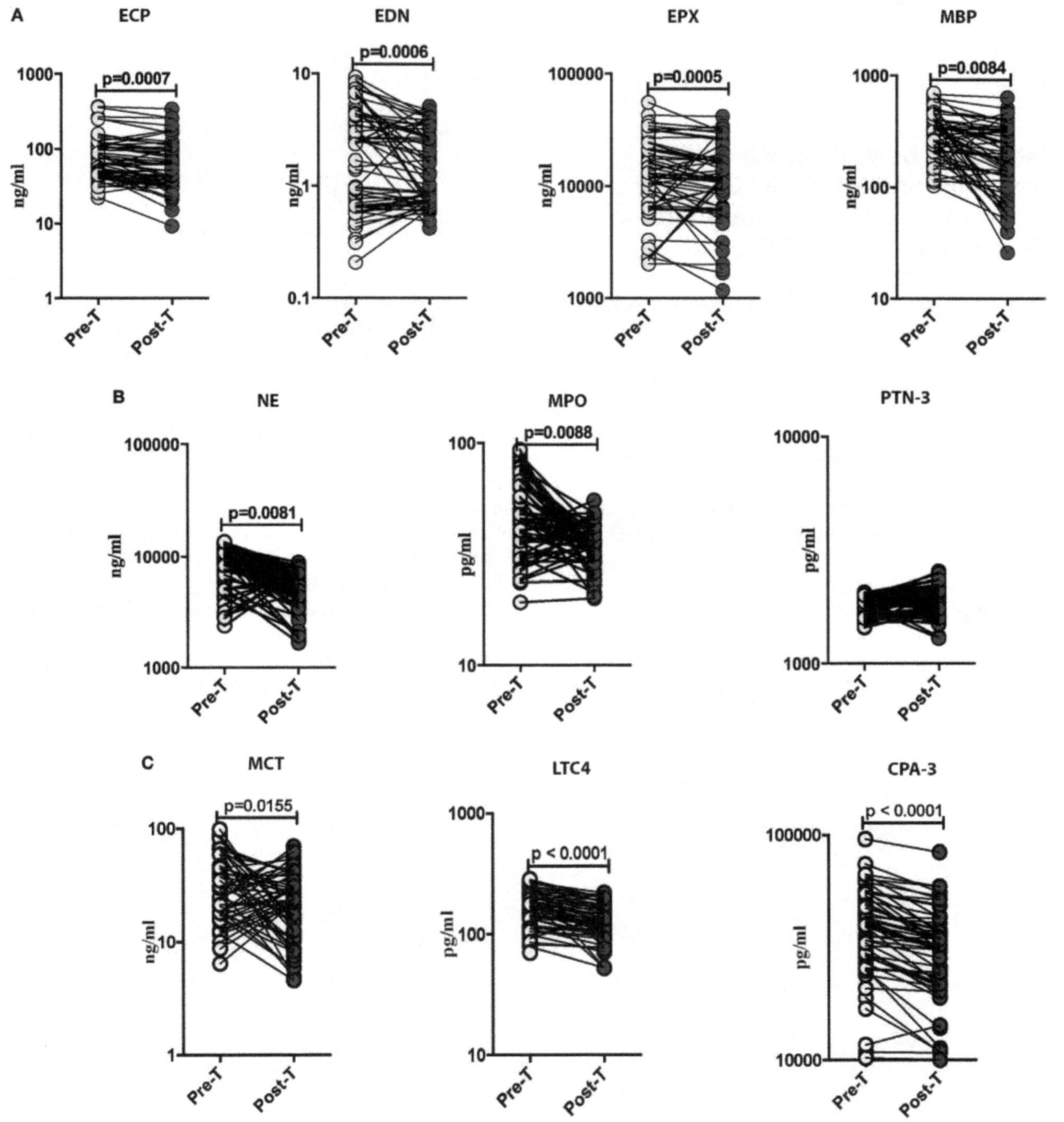

FIGURE 3 | *Strongyloides stercoralis* (*Ss*) infection is associated with decreased levels of eosinophils, neutrophils, and mast cell granular proteins following anthelminthic treatment. **(A)** Plasma levels of eosinophil cationic protein (ECP), eosinophil-derived neurotoxin (EDN), eosinophil peroxidase (EPX), and major basic protein (MBP), from *Ss*-infected pre treatment (pre-T; $n = 60$) and 6 months following treatment from posttreatment (post-T) individuals were measured by ELISA. *p* Values were calculated using the Wilcoxon matched pair test. **(B)** Plasma levels of neutrophil elastase (NE), myeloperoxidase (MPO), and proteinase-3 (PTN-3) from *Ss* infected (pre-T; $n = 60$) and 6 months following treatment from post-T individuals were measured by ELISA. *p* Values were calculated using the Wilcoxon matched pair test. **(C)** Plasma levels of mast cell tryptase (MCT), leukotriene C4 (LTC4), and carboxypeptidase A3 (CPA-3) from *Ss*-infected (pre-T; $n = 60$) and 6 months following treatment from post-T individuals were measured by ELISA. *p* Values were calculated using the Wilcoxon matched pair test with Holm's correction for multiple comparisons.

proteins, as shown in **Figure 3B**, the systemic levels of NE (GM of 8,456 ng/ml in pre-T vs. 4,491 ng/ml in post-T; $p = 0.0081$) and MPO (GM of 45.12 pg/ml in pre-T vs. 36.58 pg/ml in post-T; $p = 0.0088$) were significantly decreased in INF individuals following anthelmintic treatment. Furthermore, the systemic levels of MCT (GM of 8,456 ng/ml in pre-T vs. 4,491 ng/ml in post-T;

$p = 0.0081$), LTC4 (GM of 45.12 pg/ml in pre-T vs. 36.58 pg/ml in post-T; $p = 0.0088$), and CPA-3 (GM of 45.12 pg/ml in pre-T vs. 36.58 pg/ml in post-T; $p = 0.0088$) were also significantly diminished in INF individuals following anthelmintic treatment (**Figure 3C**).

Relationship between Eosinophils, Neutrophils, and Mast Cell Granular Protein Levels and Absolute Numbers of Eosinophils, Neutrophils, and Basophils in INF Individuals

The relationships between the levels of eosinophils, neutrophils, and mast cell granular proteins and the absolute numbers of eosinophils, neutrophils, and basophils were next assessed (**Figure 4A**). There was a significant positive correlation between absolute eosinophil count (AEC) and the levels of ECP ($r = 0.2413$; $p = 0.0085$), EPX ($r = 0.2196$; $p = 0.0169$), and MBP ($r = 0.1918$; $p = 0.0375$). There was also a significant positive correlation between levels of NE ($r = 0.2637$; $p = 0.0039$) and MPO ($r = 0.2006$; $p = 0.0294$) and the absolute neutrophil count (ANC). Finally, there was also a significant positive correlation between the levels of MCT ($r = 0.2637$; $p = 0.0039$) and the absolute basophil count. Next, we assessed the correlation between the post anthelmintic treatment levels of eosinophils, neutrophils, and mast cell granular proteins and the absolute numbers of eosinophils, neutrophils, and basophils. We did not find any significant correlation between granular proteins and the absolute numbers of eosinophils, neutrophils, and basophils at the post-T time point (**Figure 4B**).

DISCUSSION

Eosinophils are one of the foremost components of the immune system, which play a prominent role in parasitic infections. Eosinophilia is a hallmark of helminth infections, and in some host–parasite interactions, eosinophils have been witnessed to kill worms and mediate protective immunity (6, 23, 24). Eosinophils are also presumed to play a role as APCs for the initiation of the primary and secondary Th2 immune responses to *S. stercoralis* (25), indicating an elemental role for eosinophils at the boundary between innate and adaptive immune responses. Eosinophils have secondary granules, which contain MBP, ECP, EDN, and EPO, and which are directly toxic to the larvae of *S. stercoralis* (26, 27).

Eosinophils and antibodies play a crucial function in defense mechanisms against *S. stercoralis* larvae in innate (28) and adaptive immune responses (29). Previous studies have shown that mice deficient in MBP and (30) and EPO (31) are more susceptible to Strongyloides infection. O'Connell et al. have shown that MBP involved in eosinophil-mediated larval killing (12). ECP and EDN possess ribonuclease activity that form pores into the membrane of target cells, facilitating the entry of other toxic molecules into the cells with subsequent degeneration (26). Plasma levels of eosinophil granule proteins deliver an indirect measure of degranulation in the tissues and

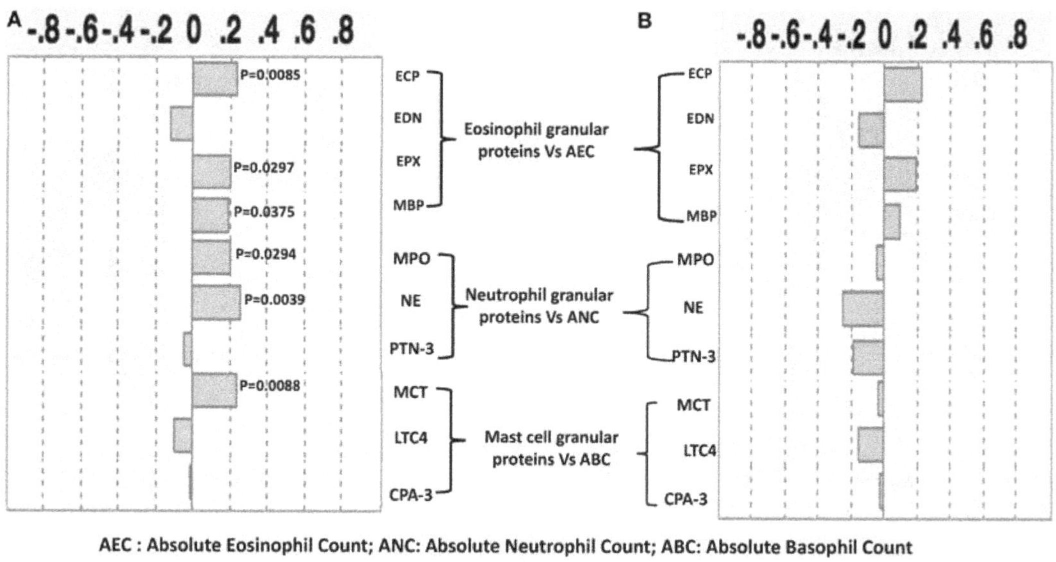

FIGURE 4 | Relationship between eosinophil, neutrophil, and mast cell granular protein levels and absolute numbers of eosinophils, neutrophils, and basophils in *Strongyloides stercoralis* (*Ss*)-infected individuals and following anthelminthic treatment. **(A)** The absolute count of eosinophils was correlated with plasma levels of eosinophil cationic protein (ECP), eosinophil-derived neurotoxin (EDN), eosinophil peroxidase (EPX), and major basic protein (MBP); the absolute count of neutrophils was correlated with plasma levels of neutrophil elastase (NE), myeloperoxidase (MPO), and proteinase-3 (PTN-3), and the absolute count of neutrophils were correlated with plasma levels of mast cell tryptase (MCT), leukotriene C4 (LTC4), and carboxypeptidase A-3 in *Ss*-infected individuals ($n = 60$). **(B)** The absolute count of eosinophils correlation with plasma levels of ECP, EDN, EPX, and MBP; the absolute count of neutrophils correlation with plasma levels of NE, MPO, and PTN-3; and the absolute count of neutrophils correlation with plasma levels of MCT, LTC4, and carboxypeptidase A-3 (CPA-3) in *Ss*-infected following anthelmintic treated individuals ($n = 60$). *p* and *r* values were calculated using the Spearman rank correlation test using JMP software.

are prominently augmented in many helminth-infected patients (32). Our data also show that eosinophil granular protein levels were increased in INF individuals. Earlier studies on onchocerciasis, lymphatic filarisis, schistosomiasis, and loiasis showed that ECP and EDN/EPX levels were elevated (32, 33). The serum concentrations of these proteins emerge consequently to reflect the functional activity of the corresponding granulocyte effector system in the host. In our study, we observed that there was a positive correlation between plasma levels of ECP, EPX and MBP, and the AEC, a finding similar to that seen in loiasis (32, 33). Thus, eosinophil granular proteins appear to reflect eosinophil activation.

Neutrophils are involved in the activation, regulation, and effector functions of innate and adaptive immune cells (34). NE and PTN-3 are directly involved in intracellular killing of phagocytosed bacteria in phagolysosomes, in conjunction with MPO and reactive oxygen species (35). During certain helminth infections, as with non-helminth induced inflammation, neutrophils are often the first cells to be recruited; these can mediate a degree of protective immunity against nematode parasites, as has been revealed most conclusively in the *Strongyloides sp.* model (9, 36, 37). Maximum killing happened by neutrophils when EPO from eosinophils attached to the surface of *S. mansoni* (38). In other mouse models, purified neutrophils have been shown to independently kill Strongyloides larvae (39). In addition, neutrophils are known to mediate adult worm killing through an MPO-dependent mechanism (12, 40). In our study, NE and MPO levels were significantly increased in INF individuals, and the levels were significantly associated with ANCs. This is similar to an earlier study on *Onchocerca volvulus* infection that showed that the plasma level of MPO was correlated with ANC (32, 41). Changes in the PTN-3 levels may be due to increased production during inflammatory activity and neutrophil or mononuclear cell leakage/degranulation. PTN-3 has antimicrobial properties and is known to efficiently kill bacteria (41). However, in our study, PTN-3 did not show any significant alterations in Ss infection. Thus, neutrophil granular proteins, similar to their eosinophil counterparts, appear to reflect neutrophil-mediated activation in *Ss* infection.

Mast cell tryptase, CPA-3, and arachidonic acid-derived lipid mediators such as LTC4 are produced during mast cell activation (42, 43). MCT is a major protein product of human mast cells (44). During the activation of mast cells, MCT levels have been shown to be elevated in anaphylaxis (45) and systemic mastocytosis (46). Infection with *T. spiralis* has shown increased numbers of gastrointestinal tract mast cells and associated levels of LTC4, that was felt to be involved in rapid worm expulsion (47). In line with these data, INF individuals showed significantly increased levels of MCT, CPA-3, and LTC4 when compared with UN individuals.

Earlier studies have demonstrated that eosinophils and neutrophils are the key players mediating microfilarial killing following anthelmintic treatment (48). Destruction of parasites occurs through eosinophil degranulation after anthelmintic treatment with DEC or ivermectin (49, 50). Cooper et al. showed that plasma levels of MCT increased following treatment for onchocerciasis (51). In this study, we show that the augmented levels of eosinophils, neutrophils, and mast cell granular proteins are significantly diminished at 6 months following treatment. This indicates that the release of these granular proteins is intimately related to the presence of active helminth infection and that elimination of the parasite removes the stimulus for increased release of these factors.

Our study adds to the growing body of literature showing the importance of granulocytes and their activation in helminth infections. While the roles of neutrophils in animal models of helminth infections are well studied (36), very scant data exist on the role of these important innate mediators in human helminth infection. Thus, our study derives strength from the fairly large sample size and the homogeneity of the population studied. Further studies exploring the exact role of these granular proteins should provide valuable insight into the regulation of the protective or pathogenic immune response in helminth infections at large.

AUTHOR CONTRIBUTIONS

Conceived and designed the experiments: AR and SB. Performed the experiments: AR, SM, and YB. Analyzed the data: AR and SB. Contributed reagents/materials/analysis tools: CD and TN. Wrote the paper: AR, TN, and SB.

ACKNOWLEDGMENTS

We thank Dr. M. Satiswaran and Prabbu Balakrishnan for valuable assistance in collecting the clinical data for this study. We thank the staff of the Department of Epidemiology, NIRT, for valuable assistance in recruiting the patients for this study.

REFERENCES

1. Puthiyakunnon S, Boddu S, Li Y, Zhou X, Wang C, Li J, et al. Strongyloidiasis – an insight into its global prevalence and management. *PLoS Negl Trop Dis* (2014) 8:e3018. doi:10.1371/journal.pntd.0003018
2. Oppenheim JJ, Yang D. Alarmins: chemotactic activators of immune responses. *Curr Opin Immunol* (2005) 17:359–65. doi:10.1016/j.coi.2005.06.002
3. Reimert CM, Fitzsimmons CM, Joseph S, Mwatha JK, Jones FM, Kimani G, et al. Eosinophil activity in *Schistosoma mansoni* infections in vivo and in vitro in relation to plasma cytokine profile pre- and posttreatment with praziquantel. *Clin Vaccine Immunol* (2006) 13:584–93. doi:10.1128/CVI.13.5.584-593.2006
4. Gessner A, Mohrs K, Mohrs M. Mast cells, basophils, and eosinophils acquire constitutive IL-4 and IL-13 transcripts during lineage differentiation that are sufficient for rapid cytokine production. *J Immunol* (2005) 174:1063–72. doi:10.4049/jimmunol.174.2.1063
5. Walsh GM. Eosinophil granule proteins and their role in disease. *Curr Opin Hematol* (2001) 8:28–33. doi:10.1097/00062752-200101000-00006
6. Klion AD, Nutman TB. The role of eosinophils in host defense against helminth parasites. *J Allergy Clin Immunol* (2004) 113:30–7. doi:10.1016/j.jaci.2003.10.050

7. Brattig NW, Tischendorf FW, Strote G, Medina-De La Garza CE. Eosinophil-larval-interaction in onchocerciasis: heterogeneity of in vitro adherence of eosinophils to infective third and fourth stage larvae and microfilariae of *Onchocerca volvulus*. *Parasite Immunol* (1991) 13:13–22. doi:10.1111/j.1365-3024.1991.tb00259.x
8. Herbert DR, Nolan TJ, Schad GA, Abraham D. The role of B cells in immunity against larval *Strongyloides stercoralis* in mice. *Parasite Immunol* (2002) 24:95–101. doi:10.1046/j.0141-9838.2001.00441.x
9. Watanabe K, Noda K, Hamano S, Koga M, Kishihara K, Nomoto K, et al. The crucial role of granulocytes in the early host defense against *Strongyloides ratti* infection in mice. *Parasitol Res* (2000) 86:188–93. doi:10.1007/s004360050030
10. Jong EC, Mahmoud AA, Klebanoff SJ. Peroxidase-mediated toxicity to schistosomula of *Schistosoma mansoni*. *J Immunol* (1981) 126:468–71.
11. Buys J, Wever R, Ruitenberg EJ. Myeloperoxidase is more efficient than eosinophil peroxidase in the in vitro killing of newborn larvae of *Trichinella spiralis*. *Immunology* (1984) 51:601–7.
12. O'Connell AE, Hess JA, Santiago GA, Nolan TJ, Lok JB, Lee JJ, et al. Major basic protein from eosinophils and myeloperoxidase from neutrophils are required for protective immunity to *Strongyloides stercoralis* in mice. *Infect Immun* (2011) 79:2770–8. doi:10.1128/IAI.00931-10
13. Freudenstein-Dan A, Gold D, Fishelson Z. Killing of schistosomes by elastase and hydrogen peroxide: implications for leukocyte-mediated schistosome killing. *J Parasitol* (2003) 89:1129–35. doi:10.1645/GE-96R
14. Bulfone-Paus S, Bahri R. Mast cells as regulators of T cell responses. *Front Immunol* (2015) 6:394. doi:10.3389/fimmu.2015.00394
15. Weller CL, Collington SJ, Williams T, Lamb JR. Mast cells in health and disease. *Clin Sci (Lond)* (2011) 120:473–84. doi:10.1042/CS20100459
16. Melendez AJ, Harnett MM, Pushparaj PN, Wong WS, Tay HK, Mcsharry CP, et al. Inhibition of Fc epsilon RI-mediated mast cell responses by ES-62, a product of parasitic filarial nematodes. *Nat Med* (2007) 13:1375–81. doi:10.1038/nm1654
17. Pennock JL, Grencis RK. The mast cell and gut nematodes: damage and defence. *Chem Immunol Allergy* (2006) 90:128–40. doi:10.1159/000088885
18. Abe T, Nawa Y. Worm expulsion and mucosal mast cell response induced by repetitive IL-3 administration in *Strongyloides ratti*-infected nude mice. *Immunology* (1988) 63:181–5.
19. Marshall JS. Mast-cell responses to pathogens. *Nat Rev Immunol* (2004) 4:787–99. doi:10.1038/nri1460
20. Bisoffi Z, Buonfrate D, Sequi M, Mejia R, Cimino RO, Krolewiecki AJ, et al. Diagnostic accuracy of five serologic tests for *Strongyloides stercoralis* infection. *PLoS Negl Trop Dis* (2014) 8:e2640. doi:10.1371/journal.pntd.0002640
21. Buonfrate D, Sequi M, Mejia R, Cimino RO, Krolewiecki AJ, Albonico M, et al. Accuracy of five serologic tests for the follow up of *Strongyloides stercoralis* infection. *PLoS Negl Trop Dis* (2015) 9:e0003491. doi:10.1371/journal.pntd.0003491
22. Sato Y, Kobayashi J, Toma H, Shiroma Y. Efficacy of stool examination for detection of *Strongyloides* infection. *Am J Trop Med Hyg* (1995) 53:248–50. doi:10.4269/ajtmh.1995.53.248
23. Huang L, Appleton JA. Eosinophils in helminth infection: defenders and dupes. *Trends Parasitol* (2016) 32:798–807. doi:10.1016/j.pt.2016.05.004
24. Huang L, Gebreselassie NG, Gagliardo LF, Ruyechan MC, Luber KL, Lee NA, et al. Eosinophils mediate protective immunity against secondary nematode infection. *J Immunol* (2015) 194:283–90. doi:10.4049/jimmunol.1402219
25. Padigel UM, Lee JJ, Nolan TJ, Schad GA, Abraham D. Eosinophils can function as antigen-presenting cells to induce primary and secondary immune responses to *Strongyloides stercoralis*. *Infect Immun* (2006) 74:3232–8. doi:10.1128/IAI.02067-05
26. Weller PF. The immunobiology of eosinophils. *N Engl J Med* (1991) 324:1110–8. doi:10.1056/NEJM199104183241607
27. Zuo L, Rothenberg ME. Gastrointestinal eosinophilia. *Immunol Allergy Clin North Am* (2007) 27:443–55. doi:10.1016/j.iac.2007.06.002
28. Satoh M, Toma H, Sato Y, Kikuchi M, Takara M, Shiroma Y, et al. Production of a high level of specific IgG4 antibody associated with resistance to albendazole treatment in HLA-DRB1*0901-positive patients with strongyloidiasis. *Am J Trop Med Hyg* (1999) 61:668–71. doi:10.4269/ajtmh.1999.61.668
29. Mir A, Benahmed D, Igual R, Borras R, O'Connor JE, Moreno MJ, et al. Eosinophil-selective mediators in human strongyloidiasis. *Parasite Immunol* (2006) 28:397–400. doi:10.1111/j.1365-3024.2006.00826.x
30. Denzler KL, Farmer SC, Crosby JR, Borchers M, Cieslewicz G, Larson KA, et al. Eosinophil major basic protein-1 does not contribute to allergen-induced airway pathologies in mouse models of asthma. *J Immunol* (2000) 165:5509–17. doi:10.4049/jimmunol.165.10.5509
31. Denzler KL, Borchers MT, Crosby JR, Cieslewicz G, Hines EM, Justice JP, et al. Extensive eosinophil degranulation and peroxidase-mediated oxidation of airway proteins do not occur in a mouse ovalbumin-challenge model of pulmonary inflammation. *J Immunol* (2001) 167:1672–82. doi:10.4049/jimmunol.167.3.1672
32. Tischendorf FW, Brattig NW, Burchard GD, Kubica T, Kreuzpaintner G, Lintzel M. Eosinophils, eosinophil cationic protein and eosinophil-derived neurotoxin in serum and urine of patients with onchocerciasis coinfected with intestinal nematodes and in urinary schistosomiasis. *Acta Trop* (1999) 72:157–73. doi:10.1016/S0001-706X(98)00088-6
33. Herrick JA, Metenou S, Makiya MA, Taylar-Williams CA, Law MA, Klion AD, et al. Eosinophil-associated processes underlie differences in clinical presentation of loiasis between temporary residents and those indigenous to Loa-endemic areas. *Clin Infect Dis* (2015) 60:55–63. doi:10.1093/cid/ciu723
34. Mantovani A, Cassatella MA, Costantini C, Jaillon S. Neutrophils in the activation and regulation of innate and adaptive immunity. *Nat Rev Immunol* (2011) 11:519–31. doi:10.1038/nri3024
35. Kobayashi SD, Voyich JM, Burlak C, DeLeo FR. Neutrophils in the innate immune response. *Arch Immunol Ther Exp (Warsz)* (2005) 53(6):505–17.
36. Bonne-Annee S, Kerepesi LA, Hess JA, O'Connell AE, Lok JB, Nolan TJ, et al. Human and mouse macrophages collaborate with neutrophils to kill larval *Strongyloides stercoralis*. *Infect Immun* (2013) 81:3346–55. doi:10.1128/IAI.00625-13
37. Bonne-Annee S, Hess JA, Abraham D. Innate and adaptive immunity to the nematode *Strongyloides stercoralis* in a mouse model. *Immunol Res* (2011) 51:205–14. doi:10.1007/s12026-011-8258-2
38. Jong EC, Chi EY, Klebanoff SJ. Human neutrophil-mediated killing of schistosomula of *Schistosoma mansoni*: augmentation by schistosomal binding of eosinophil peroxidase. *Am J Trop Med Hyg* (1984) 33:104–15. doi:10.4269/ajtmh.1984.33.104
39. Galioto AM, Hess JA, Nolan TJ, Schad GA, Lee JJ, Abraham D. Role of eosinophils and neutrophils in innate and adaptive protective immunity to larval *Strongyloides stercoralis* in mice. *Infect Immun* (2006) 74:5730–8. doi:10.1128/IAI.01958-05
40. Doyle AD, Jacobsen EA, Ochkur SI, Mcgarry MP, Shim KG, Nguyen DT, et al. Expression of the secondary granule proteins major basic protein 1 (MBP-1) and eosinophil peroxidase (EPX) is required for eosinophilopoiesis in mice. *Blood* (2013) 122:781–90. doi:10.1182/blood-2013-01-473405
41. Sørensen OE, Follin P, Johnsen AH, Calafat J, Tjabringa GS, Hiemstra PS, et al. Human cathelicidin, hCAP-18, is processed to the antimicrobial peptide LL-37 by extracellular cleavage with proteinase 3. *Blood* (2001) 97:3951–9. doi:10.1182/blood.V97.12.3951.
42. Goldstein SM, Kaempfer CE, Proud D, Schwartz LB, Irani AM, Wintroub BU. Detection and partial characterization of a human mast cell carboxypeptidase. *J Immunol* (1987) 139:2724–9.
43. Schechter NM, Irani AM, Sprows JL, Abernethy J, Wintroub B, Schwartz LB. Identification of a cathepsin G-like proteinase in the MCTC type of human mast cell. *J Immunol* (1990) 145:2652–61.
44. Schwartz LB. Diagnostic value of tryptase in anaphylaxis and mastocytosis. *Immunol Allergy Clin North Am* (2006) 26:451–63. doi:10.1016/j.iac.2006.05.010
45. Vliagoftis H, Lacy P, Luy B, Adamko D, Hollenberg M, Befus D, et al. Mast cell tryptase activates peripheral blood eosinophils to release granule-associated enzymes. *Int Arch Allergy Immunol* (2004) 135:196–204. doi:10.1159/000081304
46. Stone KD, Prussin C, Metcalfe DD. IgE, mast cells, basophils, and eosinophils. *J Allergy Clin Immunol* (2010) 125:S73–80. doi:10.1016/j.jaci.2009.11.017
47. Knight PA, Brown JK, Pemberton AD. Innate immune response mechanisms in the intestinal epithelium: potential roles for mast cells and goblet cells in the expulsion of adult *Trichinella spiralis*. *Parasitology* (2008) 135:655–70. doi:10.1017/S0031182008004319
48. Tischendorf FW, Brattig NW, Hoyer A, Medina-De La Garza CE, Geisinger F. Modulatory effects of antifilarial drugs ivermectin, CGP 6140 and CGP 20376 on the oxidative burst of eosinophilic granulocytes. *Acta Trop* (1993) 53:27–37. doi:10.1016/0001-706X(93)90003-T

49. Racz P, Tenner-Racz K, Luther B, Buttner DW, Albiez EJ. Immunopathologic aspects in human onchocercal lymphadenitis. *Bull Soc Pathol Exot Filiales* (1983) 76:676–80.
50. Wildenburg G, Darge K, Knab J, Tischendorf FW, Bonow I, Buttner DW. Lymph nodes of onchocerciasis patients after treatment with ivermectin: reaction of eosinophil granulocytes and their cationic granule proteins. *Trop Med Parasitol* (1994) 45:87–96.
51. Cooper PJ, Schwartz LB, Irani AM, Awadzi K, Guderian RH, Nutman TB. Association of transient dermal mastocytosis and elevated plasma tryptase levels with development of adverse reactions after treatment of onchocerciasis with ivermectin. *J Infect Dis* (2002) 186:1307–13. doi:10.1086/344318

16

A Role for Epitope Networking in Immunomodulation by Helminths

E. Jane Homan and Robert D. Bremel*

EigenBio LLC, Madison, WI, United States

***Correspondence:**
E. Jane Homan
jane_homan@eigenbio.com

Helminth infections, by nematodes, trematodes, or cestodes, can lead to the modulation of host immune responses. This allows long-duration parasite infections and also impacts responses to co-infections. Surface, secreted, excreted, and shed proteins are thought to play a major role in modulation. A commonly reported feature of such immune modulation is the role of T regulatory (Treg) cells and IL-10. Efforts to identify helminth proteins, which cause immunomodulation, have identified candidates but not provided clarity as to a uniform mechanism driving modulation. In this study, we applied a bioinformatics systems approach, allowing us to analyze predicted T-cell epitopes of 17 helminth species and the responses to their surface proteins. In addition to major histocompatibility complex (MHC) binding, we analyzed amino acid motifs that would be recognized by T-cell receptors [T-cell-exposed motifs (TCEMs)]. All the helminth species examined have, within their surface proteins, peptides, which combine very common TCEMs with predicted high affinity binding to many human MHC alleles. This combination of features would result in large cognate T cell and a high probability of eliciting Treg responses. The TCEMs, which determine recognition by responding T-cell clones, are shared to a high degree between helminth species and with *Plasmodium falciparum* and *Mycobacterium tuberculosis*, both common co-infecting organisms. The implication of our observations is not only that Treg cells play a significant role in helminth-induced immune modulation but also that the epitope specificities of Treg responses are shared across species and genera of helminth. Hence, the immune response to a given helminth cannot be considered in isolation but rather forms part of an epitope ecosystem, or microenvironment, in which potentially immunosuppressive peptides in the helminth network via their common T-cell receptor recognition signals with T-cell epitopes in self proteins, microbiome, other helminths, and taxonomically unrelated pathogens. Such a systems approach provides a high-level view of the antigen-immune system signaling dynamics that may bias a host's immune response to helminth infections toward immune modulation. It may indicate how helminths have evolved to select for peptides that favor long-term parasite host coexistence.

Keywords: helminth, immunomodulation, bioinformatics, T regulatory, networking, T-cell-exposed motifs

INTRODUCTION

Parasitic helminth infections affect over 2 billion people, mostly in tropical and subtropical countries, causing a vast burden of clinical and subclinical disease (1–3). To allow them to infect their hosts for extended periods, sometimes over decades, helminths have evolved to modulate their host's immune responses (4–6). Down-regulation of the immune response results in many

---

Abbreviations: APC, antigen-presenting cell; FC, frequency category; GEM, groove-exposed motif; HLA, human leucocyte allele; MHC, major histocompatibility complex; pMHC, peptide MHC; sORF, small open reading frame; TCEM, T-cell-exposed motif; TMH, transmembrane helix.

infected individuals being asymptomatic carriers and thus ensures perpetuation of the parasite life cycle.

Immune modulation by helminths extends to other immune stimulants; in infected individuals the immune response to secondary parasite infections, to other pathogens, and to vaccines is also down-regulated (7–11). While epidemiologic and socioeconomic factors also contribute to the prevalence of co-infections, helminth-induced immune modulation may predispose to infection by *Mycobacterium tuberculosis* or malaria (7, 12–14). A number of helminth infections have been associated with increased risks of cancer. The oriental liver flukes, *Clonorchis sinensis* and *Opisthorchis viverrini*, are risk factors for development of cholangiocarcinoma, typically many decades after initial infection (15). Infection with *Schistosoma haematobium* is associated with an increased risk of bladder carcinoma (16). Intestinal helminths have been thought to reduce risk of *Helicobacter pylori* associated adenocarcinoma (17), but *Opisthorchis* flukes may serve as risk factor by vectoring *H. pylori* and thus increasing associated cancers (18).

Helminth immune modulation has some beneficial effects as allergies, and inflammatory and autoimmune diseases are less common in populations infected with helminths (11, 19–21). Treatment with anthelminthics removes this effect and is reported to increase the incidence of inflammatory, autoimmune and allergic diseases (22, 23). The observation that helminth infection modulates inflammation and allergic responses has raised interest in the use of helminth infections, helminth extracts, or recombinant helminth-derived proteins as therapeutic interventions (24–27).

The mechanisms of immunomodulation arising from helminth infections have been extensively researched and are the subject of a large body of literature and many authoritative reviews (4, 11, 27–29). Among the many reports of possible modes of action (30, 31), two common themes emerge. First, certain groups of proteins appear to play a key role in bringing about changes in the host immune response. This includes proteins, which are secreted or excreted (32–34), proteins that are present in outer surface tegument or gastrointestinal surfaces, or proteins that are continually shed into the environs of the worm, either in isolation or as components of extracellular vesicles (35, 36). Extracts of secreted and surface proteins have been shown experimentally to elicit some of the immunomodulatory effects (32, 34). This has been extended to testing a number of individual proteins and identifying several proteins that can affect immune function (24, 28, 31, 37). The second unifying theme is that T regulatory (Treg) cells, and induction of IL-10, play a central role in helminth-induced host immune modulation (38–44), whether by classical Foxp3+ CD4 cells or other IL-10 secreting populations of CD4+ or CD8+ cells (45–50).

Helminth infections are not uniformly immunosuppressive. Protective immunity does emerge over time and provides the impetus for research toward vaccines (1, 51, 52), although reinfection may follow anthelmintic treatment (53, 54). Allergic responses to some helminths also occur and may also predispose to asthma (55, 56).

Studies of helminth immune modulation have largely focused on how cytokine-mediated effector mechanisms may impact the immune response. However, they have not addressed the question of whether the initial signaling in immune recognition of the parasite causes components of the immune response to be biased toward a suppressive or regulatory pathway.

In this study, we use a computational systems approach to evaluate the initial signal recognition patterns between helminth and host T cells. We evaluate the complete proteomes of 17 representative helminths and three reported co-infections based on the pattern of amino acids that would be exposed to T cells, which determine the interaction of parasite antigen and T cells. Essentially, we are attempting to see the helminth antigens as a T-cell receptor would see them, based on the minimal differentiating signal patterns from major histocompatibility complex (MHC)-bound helminth peptides that would be exposed from the MHC histotope. We have previously examined such interactions between T-cell receptor and amino acid motifs in a variety of bacterial pathogens and commensals and found distinct patterns that appear to relate to the pathogenesis of the organisms (57).

A single T-cell does not recognize, or respond to, a whole helminth; it instead engages with the few amino acids in a bound peptide MHC (pMHC) protruding from a MHC histotope, which is determined by the host human leucocyte allele (HLA) genotype. Protein antigens are processed by antigen-presenting cells (APCs) and presented to T cells as peptides bound in the groove of MHC molecules. The bound peptides (8–11 amino acids for MHC I and 13–22 amino acids for MHC II) comprise inward facing amino acids which determine peptide binding in the groove pockets [the groove-exposed motif (GEM) or pocket positions]. The intervening amino acids protrude outwards from the MHC surface or histotope and are thus exposed to the T-cell receptor, determining binding to that cognate receptor (58, 59). We refer to these amino acid motifs as the T-cell-exposed motif (TCEM). In MHC I-bound peptides, the TCEM comprises a continuous pentamer comprising positions 4, 5, 6, 7, and 8 of a nonamer, whereas in MHC II-bound peptides, the TCEM is a discontinuous pentamer in two possible recognition patterns, denoted here as TCEM IIA and IIB and comprised amino acid positions ~2,3~5~7,8~ or −1~~3~5~7,8~, respectively (where ~ is the intervening positions), relative to the central nonamer core of a longer bound peptide (60, 61). Hence, the signal that determines the outcome of the interaction with the cognate T cell is determined by the pentameric TCEM motif. This enables T cells to be polyspecific, responding to the same TCEM recognition signal, even though the MHC-bound peptide may be derived from antigens of different sources (62). The duration of TCEM signaling is determined by the stability of the pMHC complex and thus the dwell time of the peptide in the MHC groove, a function of the amino acids making up the MHC GEM. The frequency of signaling is determined by the size of the cognate T-cell population encountering the signal, which in turn is influenced by the frequency of occurrence of that TCEM in self proteins, commensal microbiome, and other pathogens.

The proteins of the human microbiome, especially the gastrointestinal microbiome, the human proteome, and the immunoglobulin repertoire are also continually processed by APCs and presented to T cells (63, 64). In examining the immunoglobulinome, it emerged that there is a frequency hierarchy of

TCEM. This includes, at one extreme, common motifs found in most immunoglobulin variable regions. These are not limited to motifs encoded by the germline but also include motifs produced by somatic mutation. At the other extreme, very rare motifs are encountered only once in several million B-cell clones (65, 66). This frequency distribution is representative of that in the rest of the human proteome and gastrointestinal microbiome (57). The frequency of appearance of a TCEM determines the frequency of stimulation of a clone or clones of cognate T cells. Hence, more common motifs would be expected to beget larger cognate T-cell populations than rare motifs. A highly bound peptide that recruits a large T-cell population and a high frequency of signal is more likely to generate a suppressive or Treg response (67–72). The human immunoglobulinome comprises the greatest diversity of motifs relative to the rest of the human proteome and microbiome and undergoes considerably more turnover. We use the immunoglobulinome variable regions as a reference scale of TCEM motif frequency (65). Here, we show that a feature of helminths is their content of common TCEM that, when in the context of a binding GEM, is potentially immunosuppressive and to which the infected host is chronically exposed.

Helminth parasites have large genomes and complex life cycles (73, 74). Considerable progress has been made in helminth genome sequencing, but many proteins remain unannotated, and transcriptomic studies that relate proteins to life stage, while more advanced for a few helminths (75–79) are mostly incomplete. With these limitations, we cannot define an exact combination of T-cell epitope modulation signals functioning within the human host, but the results we present are indicative of the complexity of potential T-cell epitope interactions within and among helminth species and with potential co-infections. Such a systems approach provides a high-level view of the antigen-immune system signaling dynamics that may bias a host immune response to helminth infections toward immune modulation and may suggest approaches to develop a further understanding of the host:parasite interrelationship.

MATERIALS AND METHODS

Helminth Proteomes

Protein FASTA files for 17 complete helminth proteomes were downloaded from Wormbase (www.wormbase.org) (80) as shown in **Table 1**. All infect humans; most have human as their primary definitive host; some (e.g., *Echinococcus granulosus*, *Trichinella spiralis*, *Fasciola hepatica*, and *Loa loa* infect humans as an accidental zoonotic host). Proteomes identified and curated by different originating laboratories varied in the size criteria applied for inclusion as did criteria for inclusion of multiple splice variants. Proteins under 50 amino acids were excluded from our analysis as end effects of the sliding analysis windows preclude making meaningful comparisons to larger proteins.

Comparative Proteomes

The proteins of the human immunoglobulinome, comprising the variable region sequences of 40 million distinct immunoglobulins, were assembled as previously described, supplemented with sequences from clinical samples and other published immunoglobulin sequences, and the TCEM frequency distributions were precomputed as previously described (61, 66, 93). Examination of the frequency of occurrence of TCEM in the large immunoglobulin dataset allows us to assign a frequency category (FC) to each TCEM motif as it occurs in the immunoglobulinome clonotypes. Each motif in each recognition pattern (TCEM I for MHC I and TCEM IIA and IIB for MHC II) is assigned a log base 2 FC based on whether it occurs in half (FC1), 1 in 4 (FC2), and 1 in 8 (FC3)

TABLE 1 | Helminth proteomes analyzed.

Class	Parasite evaluated	Proteome size[a]	15-mer peptides	Secreted and surface proteins selected for complete analysis[b]	Secreted and surface proteins selected as percentage of proteome	Project number on http://parasite.wormbase.org	Reference
Nematodes	*Ancylostoma ceylanicum*	36,687	9,508,454	3,266	8.9	prjna231479	(75)
	Ancylostoma duodenale	27,485	5,447,645	713	2.6	prjna72581	
	Necator americanus	19,153	4,868,515	737	3.8	prjna72135	(81)
	Ascaris lumbricoides	23,604	6,833,958	1,064	4.5	prjeb4950	
	Brugia malayi	11,021	6,125,076	853	7.7	prjna10729	(82)
	Loa loa	12,473	4,931,854	606	4.9	prjna246086	(83)
	Onchocerca volvulus	12,117	4,873,818	736	6.1	prjeb513	(84)
	Wucheria bancrofti	13,058	4,140,788	589	4.5	prjeb536	
	Trichinella spiralis	14,737	8,879,076	1,567	10.6	prjna257433	(85)
	Trichuris trichuria	9,650	4,050,951	522	5.4	prjeb535	(86)
Trematodes	*Clonorchis sinensis*	13,634	7,029,209	933	6.8	prjda72781	(87)
	Opisthorchis viverrini	16,356	6,848,490	874	5.3	prjna222628	(88)
	Fasciola hepatica	22,676	5,851,887	670	3.0	prjeb6687	(89)
	Schistosoma mansoni	10,772	5,443,618	629	5.8	prjea36577	(90, 91)
Cestodes	*Diphylobothrium latum*	19,966	3,872,702	529	2.6	prjeb1206	
	Echinococcus granulosus	10,245	4,932,446	804	7.8	prjeb121	(92)
	Taenia solium	12,481	4,992,618	724	5.8	prjna170813	(92)

[a]*T-cell-exposed motif (TCEM) extraction and ranking were completed on the whole proteome.*

[b]*Proteins for detailed analysis were selected from the proteome based on the presence of a transmembrane domain and/or signal peptide, which are in the top 5% of content of high frequency TCEM (those motifs more common than 1 in 1,024 clones), or which contain TCEM in any pattern (TCEM I, IIA, or IIB).*

immunoglobulin variable regions, up to FC23, which represents 1 in 8.39 million (2^{23}) clonotypes, or approximately one T-cell clone in the entire repertoire that a single human carries. A further category of FC24 designates those motifs not yet encountered in immunoglobulin variable regions analyzed to date. The mean frequency in the human immunoglobulinome is FC10, a motif which is found in 1 in 1,024 (2^{10}) variable regions. Motifs of FC1-3 are referred to as very high frequency and those of FC10 or less as high frequency.

The human proteome, including all known isoforms of each protein (totaling 88,000 proteins), but excluding immunoglobulin sequences, was assembled from Uniprot (www.uniprot.org) and its TCEMs precomputed. The proteomes of constituents of the GI microbiome were assembled and precomputed as previously described (57). This database comprised 67 bacterial species.

Proteomes of reference sequences of *Plasmodium falciparum* (3D7), *M. tuberculosis* (H37Rv), and *H. pylori* (26695) were downloaded from EupathDb (http://eupathdb.org) and Patric (https://www.patricbrc.org/) (94, 95). These proteomes were screened in their entirety for high frequency TCEM and not filtered by SP and transmembrane helix (TMH) proteins.

Determination of TCEMs and Predicted MHC Binding

T-cell-exposed motif patterns were extracted from the complete proteomes and ranked as previously described for each of three recognition patterns (61, 65). Frequencies of motif occurrence were determined with respect to the immunoglobulinome, the human proteome, and the gastrointestinal microbiome (57). MHC binding was predicted using neural network ensembles trained to the LN ic50 (96) for approximately 230,000 binding reactions using the neural platform of JMP® (SAS Institute). This is an updated version of a system described previously (61). Predicted MHC binding was computed for each sequential 9-mer and 15-mer peptides in selected protein sets, wherein the predicted binding affinity to 37 MHC I and 28 MHC II alleles was determined. To estimate population behavior comprising multiple alleles with varying affinities for any peptide, the LN ic50 binding data estimates were transformed and standardized to a zero mean unit variance within each protein using a Johnson Sb distribution (97). This transformation enables the combination of binding results from different alleles, which is akin to using the principle of the additivity of variance commonly used in quantitative genetics (98, 99). The probability of cleavage of each protein by human cathepsin B, L, or S was determined. Both binding affinity and cleavage predictions were accomplished using previously described methods by neural network predictors based on principal component analysis of amino acid physical properties (100).

Suppressive Indices

To derive an indicator of the probability of a particular peptide generating a Treg response, we combined the prediction of standardized MHC binding and the frequency of occurrence of the TCEM. The combination of these two parameters provides a metric that is directly related to the probability that a collision between a cognate T cell and a pMHC on the surface of an APC will occur. For each peptide, where the standardized predicted binding affinity is greater than the mean for the protein and allele combination, the predicted standardized affinity of each allele (A) is weighted by its cognate encounter number ($nA \times FC^{16\text{-}FC}$) and the sum that product provides the suppressive index. Thus, the final suppressive index is a composite metric of affinity and how often cognate T-cell encounters will occur in the human population (Figure S1 in Supplementary Material).

The suppressive index is therefore an indicator of the predicted response of the human population of diverse immunogenetics; the response of any particular HLA allele will vary around this mean index. Hence the suppressive index, as computed here, does not distinguish the differences in modulation, which may arise between different ethnic or immunogenetic population subsets or between individual immunogenetically distinct hosts.

Bacteria and viruses, with small proteomes, typically comprise peptides with suppressive indices of up to a few hundred and usually under about 8,000, rare motifs have indices of 20,000–50,000 (data not shown). Only exceptional proteins in bacteria and viruses have motifs with indices >200,000. A peptide scoring a suppressive index over 1 million is thus extremely rare and would only be possible with an extremely common motif (FC1-3) that binds to almost all human alleles (in either frames IIA and IIB or MHC I A and B).

Selection of Proteins Comprising Potential Suppressor Motifs

Given the large size of each helminth proteome, we focused attention particularly on proteins of the secreted and surface proteins and on those most likely to elicit a suppressive response. To this end, all proteins with signal peptides and/or transmembrane helices in an organism proteome were selected. To identify transmembrane regions and signal peptides in the primary amino acid sequence of proteins, the online resource Phobius http://phobius.sbc.su.se/was used. This combines the two types of domain identification tools generally used in genome annotation in one resource (101). Signal peptides were predicted for eukaryotic organisms.

From these, in order to focus on the likely immunomodulatory protein candidates, two subsets of proteins were then compiled from each species based on the following criteria: the proteins having the highest content of common TCEM (less than or equal to FC 10) per 100 amino acid length were selected; and those proteins having any TCEM (TCEM I, IIA, or IIB) of FC1-3 (motifs occurring at least as frequently as in one in eight immunoglobulin variable regions). These subsets were combined, duplicates were eliminated, and a full computation of predicted MHC binding and cathepsin excision sites was completed. This comprised from 2.5 to 10% of each proteome. All peptides for each protein in each species set (15-mer for MHC II and 9-mer for MHC I) were ranked by suppressive index. Any peptide having a suppressive index over 300,000 and its source protein were identified.

Proteins Reported to Be Associated With Immunomodulation

A set of sequences for proteins previously reported to be associated with immunomodulation (24, 28, 37) was assembled, using Reference sequences from GenBank. These proteins are listed in Table S1 in Supplementary Material.

Statistical Analysis

All data processing, pattern analysis, and statistical analysis were done with JMP® v13 from SAS Institute (Cary, NC, USA).

RESULTS

Analyses were conducted for all three TCEM recognition patterns in the complete proteomes. To conserve space, in some cases, we show data for TCEM IIA in the body of the paper and provide corresponding TCEM I and TCEM IIB data in Supplementary Tables. Very similar results are seen for each of the TCEM patterns.

TCEM Characteristics of the Entire Organism Proteome

Sharing of TCEMs Is Common

For each TCEM pentameric motif pattern, the maximum possible configurations of the 20 amino acid is 3.2 million (20^5). All possible motifs are found in the immunoglobulinome. The human proteome and GI microbiome comprise approximately 75 and 91%, respectively, of the possible motifs in each recognition pattern.

Table 2 shows the content the TCEM IIA motifs in the helminth species studied and the degree of sharing of motifs (Table S2 in Supplementary Material shows additional motif patterns TCEM I and IIB). The repertoire of each helminth comprises from approximately 53 to 71% of the total possible motifs in each TCEM pattern, indicating the overlap of repertoire with the immunoglobulinome. Among all 17 species of helminth, >96% of all possible TCEMs are collectively represented.

Sharing Between Helminth Species

Given the breadth of the TCEM repertoires of each species of helminth there is inevitably overlap in repertoires between the species. Overall ~415,000 TCEM motifs of each pattern are present in all of the 17 species analyzed. The remaining ~2.6 million motifs are shared in varying combinations among the species. **Figure 1** shows the motif sharing patterns. Each tile represents a unique combination of sharing of the 3.2 million TCEM IIA motifs among the 17 species, in all comprising 112,225 different motif sharing combinations. This indicates the complexity of the potential T-cell epitope sharing and cross-reactivities between species.

Each helminth species has a small set of motifs, less than 0.6%, that are unique to that species relative to the other 16 species (last column **Table 2**). The exact number of these motifs is unlikely to be significant given the different approaches to sequencing and curation adopted for each species, but it is notable that each species does have a unique signature. However, it must be recognized that such unique motifs are overlapped with amino acids comprising non-unique motifs, so their utility in directing a unique immune response is limited.

TABLE 2 | Sharing of total T-cell-exposed motif (TCEM) IIA between helminths, gastrointestinal microbiome, and human proteome.

	Total TCEM IIA	TCEM IIA as percentage of 3.2 million	TCEM IIA shared with GI microbiome	Percentage of TCEM IIA shared with GI microbiome	TCEM IIA shared with human proteome	Percentage of TCEM IIA shared with human proteome	TCEM IIA unique to helminth species	Unique TCEM IIA as percentage of species total
Immunoglobulinome	3,200,000	100.00						
GI microbiome	2,921,445	91.30						
Human proteome #1	2,412,699	75.40						
Total motifs in 17 helminths	3,101,990	96.94						
TCEM IIA common to all 17 species	418,120							
Ancylostoma ceylanicum	2,281,190	71.29	2,193,019	96.13	1,931,093	84.65	13,051	0.57
Ancylostoma duodenale	1,844,757	57.65	1,790,685	97.07	1,609,132	87.23	4,032	0.22
Necator americanus	1,845,715	57.68	1,792,570	97.12	1,611,216	87.29	5,294	0.29
Ascaris lumbricoides	2,075,222	64.85	2,005,287	96.63	1,783,734	85.95	13,400	0.65
Brugia malayi	1,835,074	57.35	1,780,913	97.05	1,595,941	86.97	2,370	0.13
Loa loa	1,796,988	56.16	1,746,152	97.17	1,569,747	87.35	3,397	0.19
Onchocerca volvulus	1,855,127	57.97	1,800,210	97.04	1,610,305	86.80	5,015	0.27
Wucheria bancrofti	1,737,656	54.30	1,689,344	97.22	1,519,185	87.43	1,925	0.11
Trichinella spiralis	1,873,959	58.56	1,811,550	96.67	1,622,466	86.58	12,512	0.67
Trichuris trichura	1,716,725	53.65	1,669,456	97.25	1,507,130	87.79	9,275	0.54
Clonorchis sinensis	2,079,755	64.99	2,006,177	96.46	1,792,125	86.17	7,740	0.37
Opisthorchis viverrini	2,032,485	63.52	1,962,333	96.55	1,758,940	86.54	6,589	0.32
Fasciola hepatica	1,918,592	59.96	1,855,938	96.73	1,670,778	87.08	10,851	0.57
Schistosoma mansoni	1,822,979	56.97	1,767,657	96.97	1,586,723	87.04	9,105	0.50
Diphyllobothrium latum	1,592,066	49.75	1,551,677	97.46	1,417,136	89.01	6,647	0.42
Echinococcus granulosus	1,788,474	55.89	1,735,938	97.06	1,575,786	88.11	4,636	0.26
Taenia solium	1,801,611	56.30	1,748,550	97.05	1,585,759	88.02	5,002	0.28

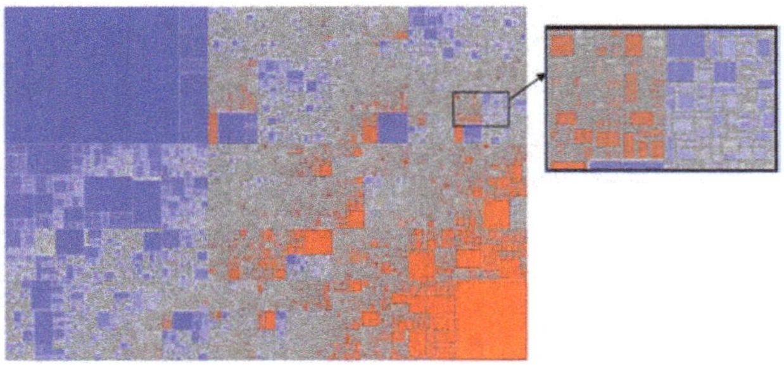

FIGURE 1 | Treemap showing the complexity of sharing patterns of T-cell-exposed motifs (TCEMs) (shown for TCEM IIA) among the 17 helminth species analyzed. A total of 112,225 unique sharing patterns were identified. The sharing pattern refers to the combination of the 17 species of helminths that carries that motif. Some sharing patterns comprised a single TCEM motif represented by a very small tile; other sharing patterns comprise large groups of shared motifs and are shown by large tiles. The tiles are colored from highly shared motif groups (blue) to minimally shared motif groups (red). The large blue box at top left represents the TCEM IIA common to all 17 species; the red box at bottom right represents the TCEM IIA absent from all species. The intervening tiles each have a unique combination of motifs and species sharing pattern. The expanded high resolution cutout provides an appreciation of the number and complexity of different patterns embedded in the lower resolution picture.

Sharing of TCEM Between Helminths and Co-Infecting Pathogens

Three unrelated pathogens cited as common co-infections with heminthiases were selected for comparison. The extent of TCEM IIA sharing with *P. falciparum*, *M. tuberculosis*, and *H. pylori* is shown in Table S3 in Supplementary Material. Across all species of helminth, approximately 50% of TCEM have matches in *P. falciparum*, 28% have matches in *M. tuberculosis*, and 16% have matches in *H. pylori*.

Distribution of High-Frequency TCEMs Within the Helminth Proteome

The frequency of occurrence of TCEMs in each helminth proteome was compared to their frequency in the immunoglobulinome. There is no significant difference in the distribution of motifs found in helminths among the frequency categories observed in the immunoglobulinome (correlation coefficients all >0.9); those motifs that are common in immunoglobulins are commonly found in helminths and rare immunoglobulin motifs are also rare in helminths.

We then examined the distribution of high frequency TCEM in the proteins of each helminth proteome to evaluate whether particular proteins might be contributing more to an immunosuppressive response. **Figure 2** shows examples of the distribution of proteins based on their content of TCEM of FC10 or lower, i.e., those motifs more common than the mean frequency in the immunoglobulin reference database. Each protein is plotted according to its size and the number of the frequent motifs. Comparable plots for the other helminths, and the three comparative co-infections, are provided in Figure S2 in Supplementary Material. While the distribution is not dissimilar from that seen in many other pathogens (57), the scatter

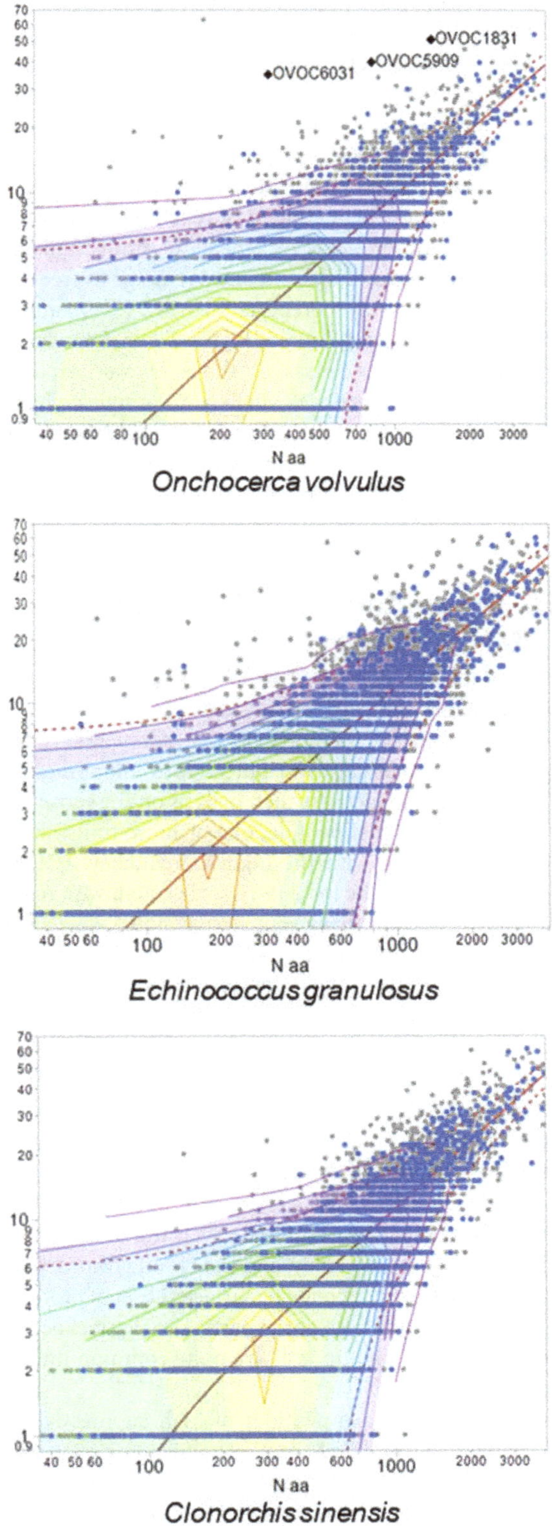

FIGURE 2 | Proteins with high content of common T-cell-exposed motif (TCEM). Each dot represents one protein of the species indicated. *X*-axis shows size of the protein ($\log_{10}$ amino acid number). *Y*-axis shows number of TCEM IIA motifs of higher than FC10, i.e., occurring more often than the mean in an immunoglobulinome reference database. Proteins shown in blue are secreted and surface proteins. Three example *Onchocerca volvulus* proteins are labeled, and sequences for these provided in Figure S3 in Supplementary Material.

of outlier proteins with a high content of frequent or rare TCEM is distinctive. As shown in **Figure 2**, the outliers are not proteins with signal peptides or transmembrane domains. Having a high content of high frequency TCEM motifs would be an indicator that a protein may have more immunosuppressive peptides, if such peptides are appropriately processed in APC and bind to MHC. On closer examination, the outliers were found to be proteins which have a high content of repetitive residues, either homorepeats of amino acids or repeats of simple amino acid motifs. Homorepeats of L, S, G, T, and Y emerge as frequent FC categories while those homorepeats of M, C, H, Q, and W are rare motifs in immunoglobulins. Figure S3 in Supplementary Material shows the sequences of those *Onchocerca volvulus* examples labeled in **Figure 2**, which are examples of proteins comprising amino acid repeats. *L. loa* is particularly striking with respect to the number of proteins with extended homorepeats that show as having a high content of common TCEM (Figure S1 in Supplementary Material).

TCEM Characteristics of Surface and TMH Proteins

Sharing of TCEM Associated With High Suppressive Index Between Helminth Species

Given the focus in the literature on the secreted, surface, and shed proteins as potential contributors to immunomodulation (32–35), we elected to focus further analysis on the subset of proteins which have a signal peptide, one or more transmembrane helices or both, along with the highest frequency TCEM. For each helminth species, the top 2.5–10% of protein with respect to their likelihood of comprising suppressive motifs were analyzed, comprising 15,816 proteins overall (**Table 1**). The number of peptides with extremely high suppressive indices over 300,000 was determined and included 903 peptides with high MHC I suppressive indices, of which 627 were unique, and 1,377 peptides with high MHC II suppressive indices, of which 977 were unique. Such highly suppressive index peptides were found in all the helminth species examined. **Table 3** shows the counts by species and suppressive index groupings. Among these, 70 proteins were identified containing more than one high suppressive index peptide at separate positions. Given the differing criteria in helminth proteome assembly, and the criteria imposed for the selection of analysis of a secreted or surface subset of proteins, the absolute numbers shown are not of particular significance except to indicate that such high indices are quite common findings in helminths.

Several helminths have peptides of high suppressive index, which comprise shared TCEM motifs, but in association with the same or different flanking peptides. Not surprisingly, the same flanking sequences are found in closely related helminths, such as *Clonorchis* and *Opisthorchis* as well as in proteins with multiple different transcripts, as shown for *Ancylostoma ceylanicum*. It should also be noted however that the same TCEM motifs may occur in the same parasites in the context of flanking peptides which are not high affinity binders. Depending on their binding affinity, these would have a shorter or even a transitory dwell time within the MHC groove. However, to the degree they may attract cognate Treg cells whose phenotype has already been determined, they may reinforce Treg signaling. **Figure 3** shows an example of peptides from *O. viverrini* and *A. lumbricoides* each comprising the same FC3 TCEM IIA motif SL~L~LV but within an array of peptides, which show different predicted MHC II binding affinities. It also indicates how binding may vary between alleles to generate different outcomes in different hosts.

TABLE 3 | Content of extremely high suppressive index peptides in secreted and surface proteins, showing peptides with suppressive index over 300,000.

	Major histocompatibility complex (MHC) I	MHC II
Ancylostoma ceylanicum	196	322
Ancylostoma duodenale	36	72
Necator americanus	32	63
Ascaris lumbricoides	81	83
Brugia malayi	56	72
Loa loa	32	56
Onchocerca volvulus	46	65
Wucheria bancrofti	34	48
Trichinella spiralis	71	150
Trichuris trichuria	20	64
Clonorchis sinensis	70	85
Opisthorchis viverrini	61	101
Fasciola hepatica	8	17
Schistosoma mansoni	30	58
Diphylobothrium latum	1	6
Echinococcus granulosus	68	62
Taenia solium	61	53
Total	903	1,377

Sharing of TCEM Associated With High Suppressive Index Between Helminths and Co-Infections

High-frequency TCEM associated with high suppressive indices was also shared between helminths and the three co-infecting pathogens examined. **Table 4** shows the count of shared motifs and the TCEM associated with highest suppressive indices in helminths and their matches in the three co-infecting agents. Shared highly suppressive motifs were found particularly for *M. tuberculosis* and *P. falciparum*. We have focused on those with suppressive indices over 300,000. **Figure 4** shows a conceptual model for how such T-cell networking among multiple helminths and co-infections may occur, based on a small illustrative group of five TCEM IIA motifs, which would each engage a finite number of T-cell clonotypes.

Proteins Previously Reported to Be Associated With Immunomodulation

Analysis of suppressive indices in 21 proteins reported to be associated with immunomodulation (Table S1 in Supplementary Material) identified only one, *T. spiralis* p53 with a peptide having a suppressive index over 300,000; the 15-mer at index position 456 has a suppressive index of 305,422, driven by the motif AV~Y~AR, which is found in 25% of all immunoglobulin variable regions. Suppressive indices of the other proteins are noted in Table S1 in Supplementary Material. Several proteins have suppressive indices in the range of 20,000–80,000.

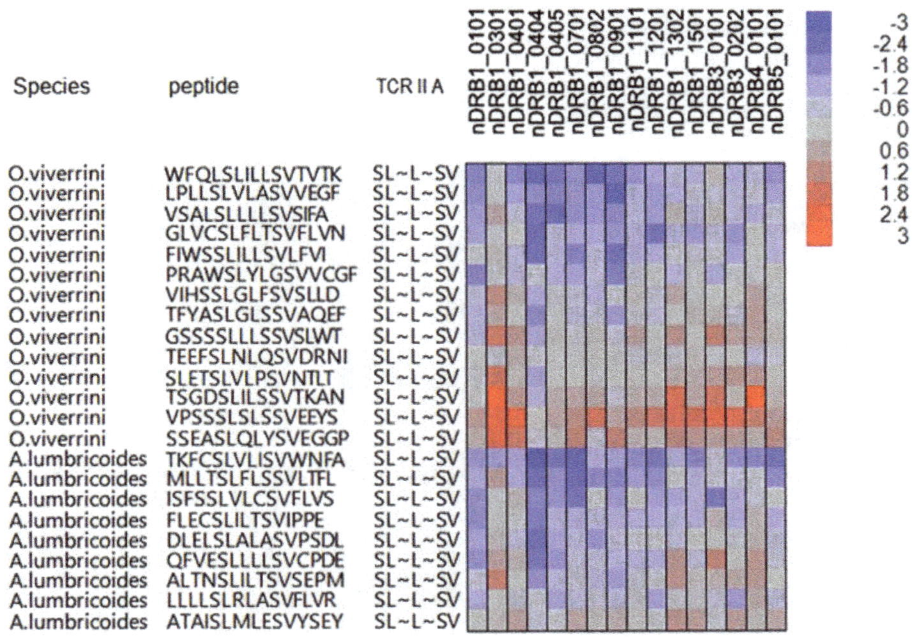

FIGURE 3 | Example of peptides of *Opisthorchis viverrini* and *Ascaris lumbricoides*, which have shared T-cell-exposed motifs (TCEMs) but in the context of differing groove-exposed motifs. *X*-axis of cell plot indicates multiple different major histocompatibility complex (MHC) II DRB alleles. Coloration of the cell plot indicates predicted binding affinity in standard deviation units below the mean for that protein. Blue indicates high binding affinity; red indicates low affinity. The peptides represent a range of suppressive indices: *O. viverrini* ranges from 621,829 to 20,788 and *A. lumbricoides* from 371,273 to 36,698 based on binding to all MHC II alleles evaluated. As the TCEM motif SL~L~LV is a common motif (FC3), these are all relatively high indices.

TABLE 4 | Sharing of helminth T-cell-exposed motifs (TCEMs) associated with extremely high suppressive index motifs with selected co-infections.

	Suppressive indices >300,000								
	***Mycobacterium tuberculosis* motifs shared**			***Plasmodium falciparum* motifs shared**			***Helicobacter pylori* motifs shared**		
	TCEM I	**TCEM IIA**	**TCEM IIB**	**TCEM I**	**TCEM IIA**	**TCEM IIB**	**TCEM I**	**TCEM IIA**	**TCEM IIB**
Ancylostoma ceylanicum	69	51	49	90	47	57	0	0	2
Ancylostoma duodenale	15	10	13	21	12	15	0	1	0
Necator americanus	9	14	8	20	14	14	0	0	1
Ascaris lumbricoides	21	24	6	41	26	14	0	2	1
Brugia malayi	16	13	5	29	16	14	0	1	1
Loa loa	8	7	9	18	9	8	0	1	1
Onchocerca volvulus	14	10	4	24	9	12	0	1	0
Wucheria bancrofti	9	6	7	17	7	11	0	1	0
Trichinella spiralis	15	17	12	32	40	34	0	10	0
Trichuris trichuria	6	11	10	5	11	18	0	1	0
Clonorchis sinensis	24	14	8	37	12	22	0	0	1
Opisthorchis viverrini	20	22	10	35	21	28	0	1	3
Fasciola hepatica	4	8	4	7	5	3	0	0	0
Schistosoma mansoni	7	8	6	17	13	8	0	2	1
Diphyllobothrium latum	0	0	2	0	0	4	0	0	0
Echinococcus granulosus	25	10	13	34	5	18	0	0	3
Taenia solium	26	9	7	33	9	13	0	0	1

DISCUSSION

Reports of immunomodulation by helminths have led to a search for individual proteins, which may cause this effect. A comprehensive explanation of helminth associated immunomodulation has been elusive, but a recurring theme is that Treg cells play a central role (38, 40). In the present analysis, we apply a systems approach examining the potential magnitude of networking of T-cell responses between parasites, host, and co-infecting microrganisms and offering

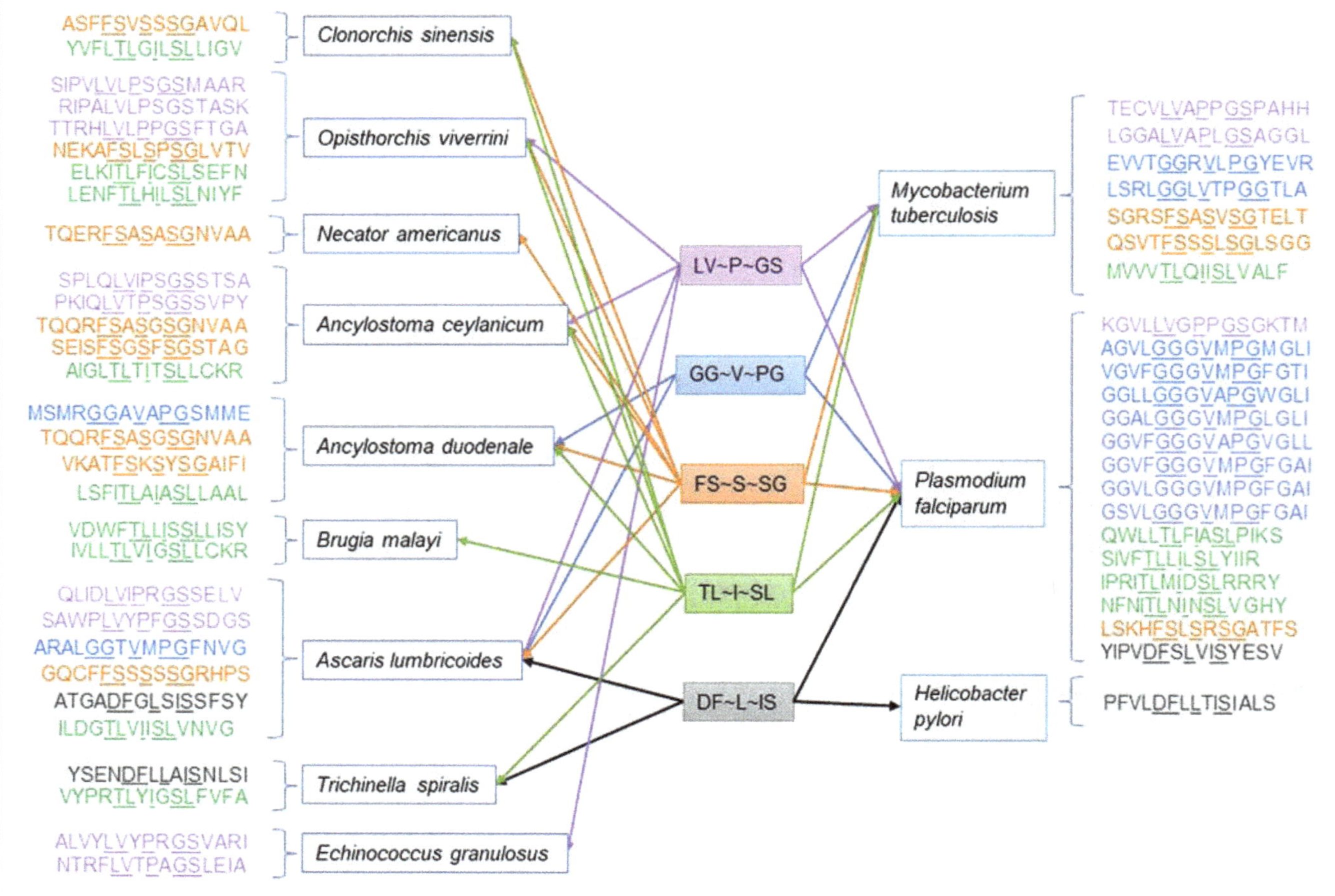

FIGURE 4 | Illustration of networking among high suppressive index T-cell-exposed motifs in helminths and selected co-infections.

a conceptual model, which may shed new light on the immunomodulation phenomenon. The goal of this study was not to identify a definitive set of peptides that are solely responsible for immunomodulation, but rather to highlight potential interplay of T-cell epitopes in an ecosystem in which helminths are present, and also to know how such networking may contribute to immunomodulation of the host.

Our study has several important limitations. Both annotation of helminth proteomes and transcriptomic studies of helminths infecting their hosts are incomplete and challenging (102, 103). Indeed, we do not know in which life stage of the parasite, many proteins are expressed or in which host microenvironment they may have an effect. Thus, we cannot anticipate the quantitative or temporal impact of each protein. In a highly expressed protein, a suppressive motif may be multiplied many times or a moderately suppressive peptide motif may carry more weight if that protein is highly upregulated. Each parasite proteome is large, and to facilitate analysis, we selected certain subsets (surface and secreted proteins) for more detailed evaluation. For most of the helminths studied, only a single proteome is available. We only studied one isolate or reference proteome for each organism, both helminth and the three selected co-infecting pathogens. Polymorphisms of proteins between isolates based on single amino acid changes are sufficient to change MHC binding of peptides and the TCEM presented (104). Furthermore, single amino acid changes impact T-cell interactions across up to 46 potential binding peptides, by changing any of cathepsin processing, MHC binding, or the TCEMs presented (65). Hence, different isolates will have somewhat different networking patterns, but the overall conceptual model will apply.

The starting point for such a networking model is the premise that a T-cell receptor is agnostic as to the source of the amino acid motif of a bound peptide, which the TCR engages in the context of the MHC histotope. A cognate TCR engages a particular pentameric motif whether that occurs in a host protein, a microbiome protein, a helminth, or a co-infecting pathogen. While the flanking and intercalated amino acids in the groove or pocket positions determine MHC binding affinity (and thus the peptide dwell time), they are hidden from the TCR. Only three variables determine the signaling directed to the TCR: whether the TCR engages the pentameric motif or not; how frequently that motif is encountered and hence the population of cognate T cells stimulated to engage it; and the dwell time of the peptide bound in the MHC groove. A precondition is that the peptide is efficiently processed by peptidases in the APC to allow excision of a peptide of appropriate length to bind in the MHC.

The second, and rather obvious, key point is that the repertoire of pentameric amino acid motifs in each recognition pattern is limited to 20^5 or 3.2 million permutations. These may be distributed in at least three different patterns: two recognition patterns based on binding in MHC II and one pattern based on binding in MHC I (58, 60). This limits the maximal repertoire of T-cell differentiation to 9.6 million. This is entirely consistent with estimates of a human's total T-cell count and the essential role of polyspecificity (62, 105). Given this relatively small number, it is not surprising that the large helminth proteomes we examined embodied a large percentage of the total pentameric possibilities, including the common motifs, and showed a high degree of overlap with the other proteomes and organisms examined. This mirrors findings of motif sharing among bacteria, both pathogens and commensal microbiome (57).

A further layer of variables, not addressed in this analysis, lies in the fact that multiple different clones of T cells may have TCR that bind the same TCEM peptide motif but with different affinities, and hence different dwell times, and that may trigger different cytokine outcomes (106). Higher binding affinity, consistent with higher suppressive indices, is reportedly more prone to generate IL-10 upregulation (106, 107). Binding based on less than five amino acid residues, or so-called "near neighbor" binding, further expands the possibilities for lesser binding affinities (108). The multiplicity of T-cell clones, which respond to any specific TCEM with differing binding affinities, do not change the importance of the TCEM cross-reactivity patterns but do expand the degrees of modulation possible.

The examples in **Figures 3** and **4** show, for a small number of TCEM IIA motifs, that shared motifs may be embedded within many different peptides. The differing MHC GEMs, those amino acids that are directed into the MHC pockets (i.e. the non-TCEM amino acids), each determine the affinity of binding to a different set of HLA. We have focused here only on those peptides, which generate the most extreme high suppressive indices. To achieve such a score, a peptide has to be able to bind to almost all HLA alleles with high affinity. Peptides that bind with high affinity to only two or three alleles would not achieve such a high score but would have a potentially suppressive effect in individuals carrying those alleles. This reinforces two points. First, the data shown are illustrations based on the most extreme cases of epitope sharing leading to potential shared immunosuppression, when in fact a much greater span of complexity of epitope networking patterns exists across lesser degrees of binding affinity. Second, regional/ethnic population adaptation to parasites – and by the parasites to their local hosts – may be a selection function of those alleles carried by the native subpopulation binding potentially suppressive peptides with greater affinity, while those of foreign hosts do not. In addition, peptide binding to mouse, or other animal, alleles may differ from human alleles, in some cases limiting the relevance of animal models.

The analyses, even with the limitations noted, suggest that a systems approach in which the immune response is seen as a network of shared T-cell engagement may be needed to fully understand the immunomodulatory functions of helminthiasis. What is extraordinary among the helminths, which initially drew our attention, is the presence of many extremely high suppressive indices, indicative of common TCEM combined with high binding by most or many HLA alleles. In this regard, the helminths, on an individual peptide basis, far outstrip viruses and bacteria we have previously examined, where any suppressive index over 100,000 would be considered very high and where we have only in extremely rare instances observed an index of >1,000,000. Overall, this is likely due to the large helminth proteomes that increase the probability of common TCEM motifs and, when these also bind to MHC, and potentially beneficial modulatory peptides will be selected over evolutionary time.

Where shared TCEM motifs occur between helminth species, it implies that the cognate T-cell population responsive to the first helminth TCEM would also be responsive, or cross-reactive, to the same TCEM where it occurs in a second helminth. If the MHC binding of the first motif is such that it has a long dwell time and is likely to elicit a Treg response (67–70); when that same motif occurs in a second helminth and is bound by the same T-cell clones, the effect of the Treg phenotype would carry over to the response to the second helminth. Induction of relatively few Treg cells may impact the effector cells within the local microenvironment through bystander suppression (109, 110). The lengthy association of the parasite with the host, and the motif sharing among multiple parasites, would ensure a chronic presence of motifs, which have high suppressive indices, thereby fulfilling another requirement for Treg induction, repeated stimulation (111). Whereas protozoal parasites employ antigenic variation as a defensive mechanism to maintain infection (73), helminths employ the continuity of antigenic signaling to modulate the host T cell as a defense, while the surface proteins retain their invasive and other functions. It appears that relatively few Treg responders are needed to overcome a stimulatory response (67).

Mycobacterium tuberculosis, *P. falciparum*, and *H. pylori* were selected as examples of co-infections for analysis based on literature reports of interaction with helminths (7, 13, 14, 18). The widespread sharing of TCEMs among helminths, host, and the three co-infections indicates that there is potential for T-cell repertoires conditioned by exposure to a co-infecting pathogen proteome to be cross-reactive with helminths and vice versa. TCEMs provide the minimal prerequisite for T-cell polyspecificity or cross-reactivity. The shared motif counts in **Table 2** are the maximum possible count of cross-reactions. This count must be further conditioned by MHC binding and peptidase processing and contemporaneous transcription. The degree of sharing is in part a function of the size of the proteome of each organism; the larger the proteome the more chance that rare motifs will be present and also that there will be more shared common motifs. However, such shared motifs can lead to mutual immunomodulatory consequences. Among the motifs that helminths share with the selected co-infections are potentially highly suppressive peptides, indicating, for example, that a Treg response elicited by *M. tuberculosis* may be shared with helminths, or vice versa. Notably, in *M. tuberculosis*, TCEM IIA matches resulting in high suppressive indices were found in 27 proteins of the PE and PE PGRS families, which have been reported to be associated with Treg induction (112, 113). In *P. falciparum*, shared high suppressive index motifs were most frequently found in rifins and in proteins annotated as conserved plasmodium proteins. Rifins are a family of proteins expressed on *P. falciparum*-infected erythrocytes, which have been implicated in immune evasion through binding to immune inhibitory receptors and the development of severe malaria (114, 115). Less sharing was seen in *H. pylori*, which has a smaller proteome and where the interaction with helminths may not be dependent on immune mechanisms (18).

A networking model in which a helminth infection creates a Treg cell-rich microenvironment and simultaneously causes chronic tissue damage, and thus a high rate of host cell division prone to mutations, may also create an environment tolerant to the progression of neoplasia. Treg cells have been demonstrated to be increased in *Opisthorchis* infections (40) and may lead to impaired response to neoepitopes. While multiple mechanisms may trigger carcinogenesis, such a model could explain the emergence of cholangiocarcinoma following prolonged infection with *Clonorchis* or *Opisthorchis* (15, 18). Conversely, the increase in autoimmune, inflammatory, and allergic disease observed in the absence of helminths, or following anthelminthic application, would be consistent with removal of the peptides driving an immunosuppressive Treg-dominated network.

Helminth proteins contain a large number of homopolymers of amino acids along with repetitious simple amino acid motifs. Only a few homopolymers (glycines, leucines, serines, threonines, and tyrosines) contribute to the counts of higher frequency TCEMs; of these, only leucines and tyrosines result in fairly high binding affinity for multiple alleles. While such repeats are a more common feature of eukaryotes than prokaryotes (116) and may offer some selective advantages (117), they do not emerge as a driver of very high suppressive indices in the helminths examined. However, their presence does raise the question of whether multiple occurrences, especially of leucine or tyrosine observed in *L. loa*, might have an additive suppressive effect.

We omitted from consideration proteins under 50 amino acids in length. Some helminth proteomes included a large number of small open reading frames (sORFs). Whether sORFs which generate peptides large enough to bind MHCs may also contribute to the overall epitope landscape is unknown (118, 119). Given species differences in the curation of proteins for inclusion, a comparative analysis is not possible.

In addressing networking as a factor in immunomodulation, we have focused here on the most common TCEM and those that are shared by many helminths. We also noted that a very small percentage of TCEM motifs are unique to any single helminth among those evaluated; these may or may not be motifs rarely found in the immunoglobulinome but are unlikely to be among the most common motifs. **Figure 1** reflects the sharing patterns of motifs among helminth species. There is a range of less common motifs, which also have sharing patterns among the species (as reflected by the grey and red tiles in **Figure 1**). These are motifs that may elicit immune stimulation and potentially have utility in a vaccine. The challenge in designing a vaccine comprising T-cell epitopes is to identify proteins comprising conserved stimulatory epitopes, appropriately processed by cathepsins for MHC presentation, which are not negated by an immunosuppressive motif (120).

It is likely that many mechanisms are contributing simultaneously to immunomodulation. The proteins previously reported (24, 27, 28, 37) may have a primary or secondary role in immune regulation. The cystatins, which have been reported to play an immunomodulatory role in several parasites (121–123), would likely inhibit cathepsin function and, hence, peptide excision for presentation on the MHC. Others may act through the induction of Treg cells or as a downstream consequence of such regulation. Among the previously reported immunomodulators that we analyzed, only *T. spiralis* p53 was found to have a suppressive index over 300,000. Several others had suppressive indices below this level, indicating that they might have a suppressive effect in individuals of certain alleles, or when present in large amounts; the major egg antigen of *S. mansoni* is one example. However, it is important to keep in mind that several of the proteins previously examined for their immunomodulatory role are from helminths that are not human pathogens and they have been examined in animal models, so our analysis of suppressive index based on human alleles examines those out of the host context in which they were tested.

There has been increasing interest in exploiting the immunomodulatory effects of helminths (23, 26), by administering low level live parasite infections, extracts, or recombinant proteins (24, 25, 31). The TCEM networking model put forth here offers an approach to defining predicted immunomodulatory peptides, which have benefited from selection through an evolutionary filter and which may then be tested in a therapeutic model at less risk than a live parasite.

Given the lack of annotation of many individual proteins in the helminth proteomes, and the recognition that we have only worked with one isolate of each species, we have not focused here on highlighting the particular potential highly suppressive peptides for each parasite. Rather we have addressed this as a conceptual model. For every motif example for which we show an unambiguous predicted outcome for most HLA, there are many more subtle effects based on lower suppres- sive indices or particular host HLAs. The systems approach we have taken suggests that the immune response to a given parasite cannot be considered in isolation but should be seen as a part of an epitope ecosystem, or microenvironment, in which the potentially highly suppressive peptides in the helminths network through their common T-cell receptor recognition signals with T-cell epitopes in self proteins, microbiome, in other helminths and in taxonomically unrelated pathogens. It indicates the complexity of T-cell interactions, which may have allowed helminths to evolve to select for the peptides that drive an immunosuppressive repertoire of T cells. Such a repertoire would favor long-term coexistence with the host, or an immunogenetic subpopulation thereof, and facilitate polyparasitism and co-infections. This approach suggests that a different paradigm, in which epitope networking is considered, can contribute to understanding helminth associ ated immunomodulation. It is a paradigm, which is both very simple in conception and profoundly complex to test through a reductionist approach.

AUTHOR CONTRIBUTIONS

RB designed the algorithms, EH planned the study and performed the analyses, and EH and RB wrote the article.

REFERENCES

1. Hotez PJ, Brindley PJ, Bethony JM, King CH, Pearce EJ, Jacobson J. Helminth infections: the great neglected tropical diseases. *J Clin Invest* (2008) 118(4): 1311–21. doi:10.1172/JCI34261
2. Brooker S, Bethony J, Hotez PJ. Human hookworm infection in the 21st century. *Adv Parasitol* (2004) 58:197–288. doi:10.1016/S0065-308X(04)58004-1
3. Herricks JR, Hotez PJ, Wanga V, Coffeng LE, Haagsma JA, Basanez MG, et al. The global burden of disease study 2013: what does it mean for the NTDs? *PLoS Negl Trop Dis* (2017) 11(8):e0005424. doi:10.1371/journal.pntd.0005424
4. McSorley HJ, Maizels RM. Helminth infections and host immune regulation. *Clin Microbiol Rev* (2012) 25(4):585–608. doi:10.1128/CMR.05040-11
5. Harris AR, Russell RJ, Charters AD. A review of schistosomiasis in immigrants in Western Australia, demonstrating the unusual longevity of *Schistosoma mansoni*. *Trans R Soc Trop Med Hyg* (1984) 78(3):385–8. doi:10.1016/0035-9203(84)90129-9
6. Wright EP, Jain S. Human infestation by *Taenia saginata* lasting over 20 years. *Postgrad Med J* (1984) 60(705):495–6. doi:10.1136/pgmj.60.705.495
7. Wammes LJ, Hamid F, Wiria AE, de Gier B, Sartono E, Maizels RM, et al. Regulatory T cells in human geohelminth infection suppress immune responses to BCG and *Plasmodium falciparum*. *Eur J Immunol* (2010) 40(2):437–42. doi:10.1002/eji.200939699
8. Cooper PJ, Chico M, Sandoval C, Espinel I, Guevara A, Levine MM, et al. Human infection with *Ascaris lumbricoides* is associated with suppression of the interleukin-2 response to recombinant cholera toxin B subunit following vaccination with the live oral cholera vaccine CVD 103-HgR. *Infect Immun* (2001) 69(3):1574–80. doi:10.1128/IAI.69.3.1574-1580.2001
9. Stelekati E, Wherry EJ. Chronic bystander infections and immunity to unrelated antigens. *Cell Host Microbe* (2012) 12(4):458–69. doi:10.1016/j.chom.2012.10.001
10. Supali T, Verweij JJ, Wiria AE, Djuardi Y, Hamid F, Kaisar MM, et al. Polyparasitism and its impact on the immune system. *Int J Parasitol* (2010) 40(10):1171–6. doi:10.1016/j.ijpara.2010.05.003
11. Maizels RM, Yazdanbakhsh M. T-cell regulation in helminth parasite infections: implications for inflammatory diseases. *Chem Immunol Allergy* (2008) 94:112–23. doi:10.1159/000154944
12. Babu S, Bhat SQ, Kumar NP, Jayantasri S, Rukmani S, Kumaran P, et al. Human type 1 and 17 responses in latent tuberculosis are modulated by coincident filarial infection through cytotoxic T lymphocyte antigen-4 and programmed death-1. *J Infect Dis* (2009) 200(2):288–98. doi:10.1086/599797
13. George PJ, Anuradha R, Kumaran PP, Chandrasekaran V, Nutman TB, Babu S. Modulation of mycobacterial-specific Th1 and Th17 cells in latent tuberculosis by coincident hookworm infection. *J Immunol* (2013) 190(10):5161–8. doi:10.4049/jimmunol.1203311
14. Chatterjee S, Nutman TB. Helminth-induced immune regulation: implications for immune responses to tuberculosis. *PLoS Pathog* (2015) 11(1): e1004582. doi:10.1371/journal.ppat.1004582
15. Sripa B, Kaewkes S, Sithithaworn P, Mairiang E, Laha T, Smout M, et al. Liver fluke induces cholangiocarcinoma. *PLoS Med* (2007) 4(7):e201. doi:10.1371/journal.pmed.0040201
16. Mostafa MH, Sheweita SA, O'Connor PJ. Relationship between schistosomiasis and bladder cancer. *Clin Microbiol Rev* (1999) 12(1):97–111.

ACKNOWLEDGMENTS

Systems analysis of this type is not possible without the assembly of genomes and proteomes into accessible databases such as EuPathDB, Patric, Wormbase, Uniprot, and the Human Microbiome Project. We are indebted to the consortia, which maintain such databases. The authors thank Erich Marquard Schwarz for insightful discussion and Alleen Hager for computational and editorial assistance.

17. Whary MT, Sundina N, Bravo LE, Correa P, Quinones F, Caro F, et al. Intestinal helminthiasis in Colombian children promotes a Th2 response to *Helicobacter pylori*: possible implications for gastric carcinogenesis. *Cancer Epidemiol Biomarkers Prev* (2005) 14(6):1464–9. doi:10.1158/1055-9965.EPI-05-0095
18. Brindley PJ, da Costa JM, Sripa B. Why does infection with some helminths cause cancer? *Trends Cancer* (2015) 1(3):174–82. doi:10.1016/j.trecan.2015.08.011
19. Cooper PJ. Intestinal worms and human allergy. *Parasite Immunol* (2004) 26(11–12):455–67. doi:10.1111/j.0141-9838.2004.00728.x
20. Correale J, Farez M. Association between parasite infection and immune responses in multiple sclerosis. *Ann Neurol* (2007) 61(2):97–108. doi:10.1002/ana.21067
21. Libbey JE, Cusick MF, Fujinami RS. Role of pathogens in multiple sclerosis. *Int Rev Immunol* (2014) 33(4):266–83. doi:10.3109/08830185.2013.823422
22. Sanya RE, Nkurunungi G, Andia Biraro I, Mpairwe H, Elliott AM. A life without worms. *Trans R Soc Trop Med Hyg* (2017) 111(1):3–11. doi:10.1093/trstmh/trx010
23. Wammes LJ, Mpairwe H, Elliott AM, Yazdanbakhsh M. Helminth therapy or elimination: epidemiological, immunological, and clinical considerations. *Lancet Infect Dis* (2014) 14(11):1150–62. doi:10.1016/S1473-3099(14)70771-6
24. Nascimento Santos L, Carvalho Pacheco LG, Silva Pinheiro C, Alcantara-Neves NM. Recombinant proteins of helminths with immunoregulatory properties and their possible therapeutic use. *Acta Trop* (2017) 166:202–11. doi:10.1016/j.actatropica.2016.11.016
25. Smallwood TB, Giacomin PR, Loukas A, Mulvenna JP, Clark RJ, Miles JJ. Helminth immunomodulation in autoimmune disease. *Front Immunol* (2017) 8: 453. doi:10.3389/fimmu.2017.00453
26. Harnett MM, Harnett W. Can parasitic worms cure the modern world's ills? *Trends Parasitol* (2017) 33(9):694–705. doi:10.1016/j.pt.2017.05.007
27. Finlay CM, Walsh KP, Mills KH. Induction of regulatory cells by helminth parasites: exploitation for the treatment of inflammatory diseases. *Immunol Rev* (2014) 259(1):206–30. doi:10.1111/imr.12164
28. Maizels RM, McSorley HJ. Regulation of the host immune system by helminth parasites. *J Allergy Clin Immunol* (2016) 138(3):666–75. doi:10.1016/j.jaci.2016.07.007
29. McSorley HJ, Loukas A. The immunology of human hookworm infections. *Parasite Immunol* (2010) 32(8):549–59. doi:10.1111/j.1365-3024.2010.01224.x
30. McSorley HJ, Hewitson JP, Maizels RM. Immunomodulation by helminth parasites: defining mechanisms and mediators. *Int J Parasitol* (2013) 43(3–4): 301–10. doi:10.1016/j.ijpara.2012.11.011
31. Navarro S, Pickering DA, Ferreira IB, Jones L, Ryan S, Troy S, et al. Hookworm recombinant protein promotes regulatory T cell responses that suppress experimental asthma. *Sci Transl Med* (2016) 8(362):362ra143. doi:10.1126/scitranslmed.aaf8807
32. Geiger SM, Fujiwara RT, Freitas PA, Massara CL, Dos Santos Carvalho O, Correa-Oliveira R, et al. Excretory-secretory products from hookworm l(3) and adult worms suppress proinflammatory cytokines in infected individuals. *J Parasitol Res* (2011) 2011:512154. doi:10.1155/2011/512154
33. Maizels RM, Philipp M, Ogilvie BM. Molecules on the surface of parasitic nematodes as probes of the immune response in infection. *Immunol Rev* (1982) 61:109–36. doi:10.1111/j.1600-065X.1982.tb00375.x
34. Ferreira I, Smyth D, Gaze S, Aziz A, Giacomin P, Ruyssers N, et al. Hookworm excretory/secretory products induce interleukin-4 (IL-4)+ IL-10+ CD4+

T cell responses and suppress pathology in a mouse model of colitis. *Infect Immun* (2013) 81(6):2104–11. doi:10.1128/IAI.00563-12
35. Lightowlers MW, Rickard MD. Excretory-secretory products of helminth parasites: effects on host immune responses. *Parasitology* (1988) 96(Suppl):S123–66. doi:10.1017/S0031182000086017
36. Coakley G, Maizels RM, Buck AH. Exosomes and other extracellular vesicles: the new communicators in parasite infections. *Trends Parasitol* (2015) 31(10):477–89. doi:10.1016/j.pt.2015.06.009
37. Morais SB, Figueiredo BC, Assis NRG, Alvarenga DM, de Magalhaes MTQ, Ferreira RS, et al. *Schistosoma mansoni* SmKI-1 serine protease inhibitor binds to elastase and impairs neutrophil function and inflammation. *PLoS Pathog* (2018) 14(2):e1006870. doi:10.1371/journal.ppat.1006870
38. Maizels RM, Smith KA. Regulatory T cells in infection. *Adv Immunol* (2011) 112:73–136. doi:10.1016/B978-0-12-387827-4.00003-6
39. Ricci ND, Fiuza JA, Bueno LL, Cancado GG, Gazzinelli-Guimaraes PH, Martins VG, et al. Induction of CD4(+)CD25(+)FOXP3(+) regulatory T cells during human hookworm infection modulates antigen-mediated lymphocyte proliferation. *PLoS Negl Trop Dis* (2011) 5(11):e1383. doi:10.1371/journal.pntd.0001383
40. Kaewraemruaen C, Sermswan RW, Wongratanacheewin S. Induction of regulatory T cells by *Opisthorchis viverrini*. *Parasite Immunol* (2016) 38(11): 688–97. doi:10.1111/pim.12358
41. Taylor MD, Harris A, Babayan SA, Bain O, Culshaw A, Allen JE, et al. CTLA-4 and CD4+ CD25+ regulatory T cells inhibit protective immunity to filarial parasites in vivo. *J Immunol* (2007) 179(7):4626–34. doi:10.4049/jimmunol.179.7.4626
42. Sawant DV, Gravano DM, Vogel P, Giacomin P, Artis D, Vignali DA. Regulatory T cells limit induction of protective immunity and promote immune pathology following intestinal helminth infection. *J Immunol* (2014) 192(6):2904–12. doi:10.4049/jimmunol.1202502
43. Doetze A, Satoguina J, Burchard G, Rau T, Loliger C, Fleischer B, et al. Antigen-specific cellular hyporesponsiveness in a chronic human helminth infection is mediated by T(h)3/T(r)1-type cytokines IL-10 and transforming growth factor-beta but not by a T(h)1 to T(h)2 shift. *Int Immunol* (2000) 12(5):623–30. doi:10.1093/intimm/12.5.623
44. Metenou S, Dembele B, Konate S, Dolo H, Coulibaly SY, Coulibaly YI, et al. At homeostasis filarial infections have expanded adaptive T regulatory but not classical Th2 cells. *J Immunol* (2010) 184(9):5375–82. doi:10.4049/jimmunol.0904067
45. Khan IA, Hakak R, Eberle K, Sayles P, Weiss LM, Urban JF Jr. Coinfection with *Heligmosomoides polygyrus* fails to establish CD8+ T-cell immunity against *Toxoplasma gondii*. *Infect Immun* (2008) 76(3):1305–13. doi:10.1128/IAI.01236-07
46. Marple A, Wu W, Shah S, Zhao Y, Du P, Gause WC, et al. Cutting Edge: helminth coinfection blocks effector differentiation of CD8 T cells through alternate host Th2- and IL-10-mediated responses. *J Immunol* (2017) 198(2): 634–9. doi:10.4049/jimmunol.1601741
47. Walsh CM, Smith P, Fallon PG. Role for CTLA-4 but not CD25+ T cells during *Schistosoma mansoni* infection of mice. *Parasite Immunol* (2007) 29(6):293–308. doi:10.1111/j.1365-3024.2007.00947.x
48. Sachdev D, Gough KC, Flynn RJ. The chronic stages of bovine *Fasciola hepatica* are dominated by CD4 T-cell exhaustion. *Front Immunol* (2017) 8:1002. doi:10.3389/fimmu.2017.01002
49. Huang Y, Mao K, Chen X, Sun MA, Kawabe T, Li W, et al. S1P-dependent interorgan trafficking of group 2 innate lymphoid cells supports host defense. *Science* (2018) 359(6371):114–9. doi:10.1126/science.aam5809
50. Logan J, Navarro S, Loukas A, Giacomin P. Helminth-induced regulatory T cells and suppression of allergic responses. *Curr Opin Immunol* (2018) 54:1–6. doi:10.1016/j.coi.2018.05.007
51. Loukas A, Bethony J, Brooker S, Hotez P. Hookworm vaccines: past, present, and future. *Lancet Infect Dis* (2006) 6(11):733–41. doi:10.1016/S1473-3099(06)70630-2
52. Noon JB, Aroian RV. Recombinant subunit vaccines for soil-transmitted helminths. *Parasitology* (2017) 144(14):1845–70. doi:10.1017/S003118201700138X
53. Jia TW, Melville S, Utzinger J, King CH, Zhou XN. Soil-transmitted helminth reinfection after drug treatment: a systematic review and meta-analysis. *PLoS Negl Trop Dis* (2012) 6(5):e1621. doi:10.1371/journal.pntd.0001621
54. Albonico M, Smith PG, Ercole E, Hall A, Chwaya HM, Alawi KS, et al. Rate of reinfection with intestinal nematodes after treatment of children with mebendazole or albendazole in a highly endemic area. *Trans R Soc Trop Med Hyg* (1995) 89(5):538–41. doi:10.1016/0035-9203(95)90101-9
55. Ahumada V, Garcia E, Dennis R, Rojas MX, Rondon MA, Perez A, et al. IgE responses to *Ascaris* and mite tropomyosins are risk factors for asthma. *Clin Exp Allergy* (2015) 45(7):1189–200. doi:10.1111/cea.12513
56. Loukas A, Prociv P. Immune responses in hookworm infections. *Clin Microbiol Rev* (2001) 14(4):689–703. doi:10.1128/CMR.14.4.689-703.2001
57. Bremel RD, Homan J. Extensive T-cell epitope repertoire sharing among human proteome, gastrointestinal microbiome, and pathogenic bacteria: implications for the definition of self. *Front Immunol* (2015) 6:538. doi:10.3389/fimmu.2015.00538
58. Birnbaum ME, Mendoza JL, Sethi DK, Dong S, Glanville J, Dobbins J, et al. Deconstructing the peptide-MHC Specificity of T cell recognition. *Cell* (2014) 157(5):1073–87. doi:10.1016/j.cell.2014.03.047
59. Wucherpfennig KW. The structural interactions between T cell receptors and MHC-peptide complexes place physical limits on self-nonself discrimination. *Curr Top Microbiol Immunol* (2005) 296:19–37.
60. Rudolph MG, Stanfield RL, Wilson IA. How TCRs bind MHCs, peptides, and coreceptors. *Annu Rev Immunol* (2006) 24:419–66. doi:10.1146/annurev.immunol.23.021704.115658
61. Bremel RD, Homan EJ. An integrated approach to epitope analysis II: a system for proteomic-scale prediction of immunological characteristics. *Immunome Res* (2010) 6(1):8. doi:10.1186/1745-7580-6-8
62. Wucherpfennig KW, Allen PM, Celada F, Cohen IR, De Boer R, Garcia KC, et al. Polyspecificity of T cell and B cell receptor recognition. *Semin Immunol* (2007) 19(4):216–24. doi:10.1016/j.smim.2007.02.012
63. Bogen B, Weiss S. Processing and presentation of idiotypes to MHC-restricted T cells. *Int Rev Immunol* (1993) 10:337–55. doi:10.3109/08830189309061709
64. Weiss S, Bogen B. B-lymphoma cells process and present their endogenous immunoglobulin to major histocompatibility complex-restricted T cells. *Proc Natl Acad Sci U S A* (1989) 86(1):282–6. doi:10.1073/pnas.86.1.282
65. Bremel RD, Homan EJ. Frequency patterns of T-cell exposed amino acid motifs in immunoglobulin heavy chain peptides presented by MHCs. *Front Immunol* (2014) 5:541. doi:10.3389/fimmu.2014.00541
66. Hoglund RA, Lossius A, Johansen JN, Homan J, Benth JS, Robins H, et al. In silico prediction analysis of idiotope-driven T-B cell collaboration in multiple sclerosis. *Front Immunol* (2017) 8:1255. doi:10.3389/fimmu.2017.01255
67. Li MO, Rudensky AY. T cell receptor signalling in the control of regulatory T cell differentiation and function. *Nat Rev Immunol* (2016) 16(4):220–33. doi:10.1038/nri.2016.26
68. Valitutti S. The serial engagement model 17 years after: from TCR triggering to immunotherapy. *Front Immunol* (2012) 3:272. doi:10.3389/fimmu.2012.00272
69. Faroudi M, Zaru R, Paulet P, Muller S, Valitutti S. Cutting edge: T lymphocyte activation by repeated immunological synapse formation and intermittent signaling. *J Immunol* (2003) 171(3):1128–32. doi:10.4049/jimmunol.171.3.1128
70. Gabrysova L, Wraith DC. Antigenic strength controls the generation of antigen-specific IL-10-secreting T regulatory cells. *Eur J Immunol* (2010) 40(5):1386–95. doi:10.1002/eji.200940151
71. Gett AV, Sallusto F, Lanzavecchia A, Geginat J. T cell fitness determined by signal strength. *Nat Immunol* (2003) 4(4):355–60. doi:10.1038/ni908
72. Feng Y, Brazin KN, Kobayashi E, Mallis RJ, Reinherz EL, Lang MJ. Mechanosensing drives acuity of alphabeta T-cell recognition. *Proc Natl Acad Sci U S A* (2017) 114(39):E8204–13. doi:10.1073/pnas.1703559114
73. Zarowiecki M, Berriman M. What helminth genomes have taught us about parasite evolution. *Parasitology* (2015) 142(Suppl 1):S85–97. doi:10.1017/S0031182014001449
74. Blaxter M, Koutsovoulos G. The evolution of parasitism in Nematoda. *Parasitology* (2015) 142(Suppl 1):S26–39. doi:10.1017/S0031182014000791
75. Schwarz EM, Hu Y, Antoshechkin I, Miller MM, Sternberg PW, Aroian RV. The genome and transcriptome of the zoonotic hookworm *Ancylostoma ceylanicum* identify infection-specific gene families. *Nat Genet* (2015) 47(4): 416–22. doi:10.1038/ng.3237
76. Mulvenna J, Sripa B, Brindley PJ, Gorman J, Jones MK, Colgrave ML, et al. The secreted and surface proteomes of the adult stage of the carcinogenic human liver fluke *Opisthorchis viverrini*. *Proteomics* (2010) 10(5):1063–78. doi:10.1002/pmic.200900393

77. Young ND, Campbell BE, Hall RS, Jex AR, Cantacessi C, Laha T, et al. Unlocking the transcriptomes of two carcinogenic parasites, *Clonorchis sinensis* and *Opisthorchis viverrini*. *PLoS Negl Trop Dis* (2010) 4(6):e719. doi:10.1371/journal.pntd.0000719
78. Almeida CR, Stoco PH, Wagner G, Sincero TC, Rotava G, Bayer-Santos E, et al. Transcriptome analysis of *Taenia solium* cysticerci using open reading frame ESTs (ORESTES). *Parasit Vectors* (2009) 2(1):35. doi:10.1186/1756-3305-2-35
79. Bennuru S, Cotton JA, Ribeiro JM, Grote A, Harsha B, Holroyd N, et al. Stage-specific transcriptome and proteome analyses of the filarial parasite *Onchocerca volvulus* and Its *Wolbachia* endosymbiont. *mBio* (2016) 7(6):e2028-2016. doi:10.1128/mBio.02028-16
80. Harris TW, Lee R, Schwarz E, Bradnam K, Lawson D, Chen W, et al. WormBase: a cross-species database for comparative genomics. *Nucleic Acids Res* (2003) 31(1):133–7. doi:10.1093/nar/gkg053
81. Tang YT, Gao X, Rosa BA, Abubucker S, Hallsworth-Pepin K, Martin J, et al. Genome of the human hookworm *Necator americanus*. *Nat Genet* (2014) 46(3):261–9. doi:10.1038/ng.2875
82. Ghedin E, Wang S, Spiro D, Caler E, Zhao Q, Crabtree J, et al. Draft genome of the filarial nematode parasite *Brugia malayi*. *Science* (2007) 317(5845): 1756–60. doi:10.1126/science.1145406
83. Tallon LJ, Liu X, Bennuru S, Chibucos MC, Godinez A, Ott S, et al. Single molecule sequencing and genome assembly of a clinical specimen of *Loa loa*, the causative agent of loiasis. *BMC Genomics* (2014) 15:788. doi:10.1186/1471-2164-15-788
84. Cotton JA, Bennuru S, Grote A, Harsha B, Tracey A, Beech R, et al. The genome of *Onchocerca volvulus*, agent of river blindness. *Nat Microbiol* (2016) 2:16216. doi:10.1038/nmicrobiol.2016.216
85. Korhonen PK, Pozio E, La Rosa G, Chang BC, Koehler AV, Hoberg EP, et al. Phylogenomic and biogeographic reconstruction of the *Trichinella* complex. *Nat Commun* (2016) 7:10513. doi:10.1038/ncomms10513
86. Foth BJ, Tsai IJ, Reid AJ, Bancroft AJ, Nichol S, Tracey A, et al. Whipworm genome and dual-species transcriptome analyses provide molecular insights into an intimate host-parasite interaction. *Nat Genet* (2014) 46(7):693–700. doi:10.1038/ng.3010
87. Huang Y, Chen W, Wang X, Liu H, Chen Y, Guo L, et al. The carcinogenic liver fluke, *Clonorchis sinensis*: new assembly, reannotation and analysis of the genome and characterization of tissue transcriptomes. *PLoS One* (2013) 8(1):e54732. doi:10.1371/journal.pone.0054732
88. Young ND, Nagarajan N, Lin SJ, Korhonen PK, Jex AR, Hall RS, et al. The *Opisthorchis viverrini* genome provides insights into life in the bile duct. *Nat Commun* (2014) 5:4378. doi:10.1038/ncomms5378
89. Cwiklinski K, Dalton JP, Dufresne PJ, La Course J, Williams DJ, Hodgkinson J, et al. The *Fasciola hepatica* genome: gene duplication and polymorphism reveals adaptation to the host environment and the capacity for rapid evolution. *Genome Biol* (2015) 16:71. doi:10.1186/s13059-015-0632-2
90. Berriman M, Haas BJ, LoVerde PT, Wilson RA, Dillon GP, Cerqueira GC, et al. The genome of the blood fluke *Schistosoma mansoni*. *Nature* (2009) 460(7253):352–8. doi:10.1038/nature08160
91. Protasio AV, Tsai IJ, Babbage A, Nichol S, Hunt M, Aslett MA, et al. A systematically improved high quality genome and transcriptome of the human blood fluke *Schistosoma mansoni*. *PLoS Negl Trop Dis* (2012) 6(1):e1455. doi:10.1371/journal.pntd.0001455
92. Tsai IJ, Zarowiecki M, Holroyd N, Garciarrubio A, Sanchez-Flores A, Brooks KL, et al. The genomes of four tapeworm species reveal adaptations to parasitism. *Nature* (2013) 496(7443):57–63. doi:10.1038/nature12031
93. Bremel RD, Homan EJ. An integrated approach to epitope analysis I: dimensional reduction, visualization and prediction of MHC binding using amino acid principal components and regression approaches. *Immunome Res* (2010) 6:7. doi:10.1186/1745-7580-6-7
94. Wattam AR, Abraham D, Dalay O, Disz TL, Driscoll T, Gabbard JL, et al. PATRIC, the bacterial bioinformatics database and analysis resource. *Nucleic Acids Res* (2014) 42(Database issue):D581–91. doi:10.1093/nar/gkt1099
95. Aurrecoechea C, Barreto A, Basenko EY, Brestelli J, Brunk BP, Cade S, et al. EuPathDB: the eukaryotic pathogen genomics database resource. *Nucleic Acids Res* (2017) 45:D581–91. doi:10.1093/nar/gkw1105
96. Vita R, Overton JA, Greenbaum JA, Ponomarenko J, Clark JD, Cantrell JR, et al. The immune epitope database (IEDB) 3.0. *Nucleic Acids Res* (2015) 43(Database issue):D405–12. doi:10.1093/nar/gku938
97. Johnson NL. Systems of frequency curves generated by methods of translation. *Biometrika* (1949) 36(Pt 1-2):149–76. doi:10.2307/2332539
98. Crow JF. Perspective: here's to fisher, additive genetic variance, and the fundamental theorem of natural selection. *Evolution* (2002) 56(7):1313–6. doi:10.1111/j.0014-3820.2002.tb01445.x
99. Lessard S. Fisher's fundamental theorem of natural selection revisited. *Theor Popul Biol* (1997) 52(2):119–36. doi:10.1006/tpbi.1997.1324
100. Bremel RD, Homan EJ. Recognition of higher order patterns in proteins: immunologic kernels. *PLoS One* (2013) 8(7):e70115. doi:10.1371/journal.pone.0070115
101. Kall L, Krogh A, Sonnhammer EL. A combined transmembrane topology and signal peptide prediction method. *J Mol Biol* (2004) 338(5):1027–36. doi:10.1016/j.jmb.2004.03.016
102. Gilabert A, Curran DM, Harvey SC, Wasmuth JD. Expanding the view on the evolution of the nematode dauer signalling pathways: refinement through gene gain and pathway co-option. *BMC Genomics* (2016) 17:476. doi:10.1186/s12864-016-2770-7
103. Viney M. The genomic basis of nematode parasitism. *Brief Funct Genomics* (2018) 17(1):8–14. doi:10.1093/bfgp/elx010
104. Flanagan KL, Wilson KL, Plebanski M. Polymorphism in liver-stage malaria vaccine candidate proteins: immune evasion and implications for vaccine design. *Expert Rev Vaccines* (2016) 15(3):389–99. doi:10.1586/14760584.2016.1125785
105. Mason D. A very high level of crossreactivity is an essential feature of the T-cell receptor. *Immunol Today* (1998) 19(9):395–404.
106. Sprouse ML, Shevchenko I, Scavuzzo MA, Joseph F, Lee T, Blum S, et al. Cutting edge: low-affinity TCRs support regulatory T cell function in autoimmunity. *J Immunol* (2018) 200(3):909–14. doi:10.4049/jimmunol.1700156
107. Sprouse ML, Scavuzzo MA, Blum S, Shevchenko I, Lee T, Makedonas G, et al. High self-reactivity drives T-bet and potentiates Treg function in tissue-specific autoimmunity. *JCI Insight* (2018) 3(2):97322. doi:10.1172/jci.insight.97322
108. Petrova GV, Gorski J. Cross-reactive responses to modified M1(5)(8)-(6)(6) peptides by CD8(+) T cells that use noncanonical BV genes can describe unknown repertoires. *Eur J Immunol* (2012) 42(11):3001–8. doi:10.1002/eji.201242596
109. Belkaid Y, Tarbell K. Regulatory T cells in the control of host-microorganism interactions. *Annu Rev Immunol* (2009) 27:551–89. doi:10.1146/annurev.immunol.021908.132723
110. Tang Q, Bluestone JA. The Foxp3+ regulatory T cell: a jack of all trades, master of regulation. *Nat Immunol* (2008) 9(3):239–44. doi:10.1038/ni1572
111. Levine AG, Arvey A, Jin W, Rudensky AY. Continuous requirement for the TCR in regulatory T cell function. *Nat Immunol* (2014) 15(11):1070–8. doi:10.1038/ni.3004
112. Delogu G, Brennan MJ. Comparative immune response to PE and PE_PGRS antigens of *Mycobacterium tuberculosis*. *Infect Immun* (2001) 69(9):5606–11. doi:10.1128/IAI.69.9.5606-5611.2001
113. Chatrath S, Gupta VK, Dixit A, Garg LC. PE_PGRS30 of *Mycobacterium tuberculosis* mediates suppression of proinflammatory immune response in macrophages through its PGRS and PE domains. *Microbes Infect* (2016) 18(9):536–42. doi:10.1016/j.micinf.2016.04.004
114. Saito F, Hirayasu K, Satoh T, Wang CW, Lusingu J, Arimori T, et al. Immune evasion of *Plasmodium falciparum* by RIFIN via inhibitory receptors. *Nature* (2017) 552(7683):101–5. doi:10.1038/nature24994
115. Goel S, Palmkvist M, Moll K, Joannin N, Lara P, Akhouri RR, et al. RIFINs are adhesins implicated in severe *Plasmodium falciparum* malaria. *Nat Med* (2015) 21(4):314–7. doi:10.1038/nm.3812
116. Sim KL, Creamer TP. Abundance and distributions of eukaryote protein simple sequences. *Mol Cell Proteomics* (2002) 1(12):983–95. doi:10.1074/mcp.M200032-MCP200
117. Haerty W, Golding GB. Low-complexity sequences and single amino acid repeats: not just "junk" peptide sequences. *Genome* (2010) 53(10):753–62. doi:10.1139/G10-063
118. Plaza S, Menschaert G, Payre F. In search of lost small peptides. *Annu Rev Cell Dev Biol* (2017) 33:391–416. doi:10.1146/annurev-cellbio-100616-060516
119. Couso JP, Patraquim P. Classification and function of small open reading frames. *Nat Rev Mol Cell Biol* (2017) 18(9):575–89. doi:10.1038/nrm.2017.58

120. Morais SB, Figueiredo BC, Assis NRG, Homan J, Mambelli FS, Bicalho RM, et al. Schistosoma mansoni SmKI-1 orIts C-terminal fragment induces partial protection against S. mansoni infection in mice. *Front Immunol* (2018) 9:1762. doi:10.3389/fimmu.2018.01762
121. Jang SW, Cho MK, Park MK, Kang SA, Na BK, Ahn SC, et al. Parasitic helminth cystatin inhibits DSS-induced intestinal inflammation via IL-10(+) F4/80(+) macrophage recruitment. *Korean J Parasitol* (2011) 49(3):245–54. doi:10.3347/kjp.2011.49.3.245
122. Sun Y, Liu G, Li Z, Chen Y, Liu Y, Liu B, et al. Modulation of dendritic cell function and immune response by cysteine protease inhibitor from murine nematode parasite *Heligmosomoides polygyrus*. *Immunology* (2013) 138(4):370–81. doi:10.1111/imm.12049
123. Hartmann S, Kyewski B, Sonnenburg B, Lucius R. A filarial cysteine protease inhibitor down-regulates T cell proliferation and enhances interleukin-10 production. *Eur J Immunol* (1997) 27(9):2253–60. doi:10.1002/eji.1830270920

17

Interactions Between the Gut Microbiota and the Host Innate Immune Response Against Pathogens

Hong-Yu Cheng†, Meng-Xia Ning†, De-Kun Chen and Wen-Tao Ma**

Veterinary Immunology Laboratory, College of Veterinary Medicine, Northwest Agriculture and Forestry University, Yangling, China

***Correspondence:**
De-Kun Chen
cdk@nwafu.edu.cn
Wen-Tao Ma
mawentao@nwafu.edu.cn

†These authors have contributed equally to this work

The mammalian intestine is colonized by over a trillion microbes that comprise the "gut microbiota," a microbial community which has co-evolved with the host to form a mutually beneficial relationship. Accumulating evidence indicates that the gut microbiota participates in immune system maturation and also plays a central role in host defense against pathogens. Here we review some of the mechanisms employed by the gut microbiota to boost the innate immune response against pathogens present on epithelial mucosal surfaces. Antimicrobial peptide secretion, inflammasome activation and induction of host IL-22, IL-17, and IL-10 production are the most commonly observed strategies employed by the gut microbiota for host anti-pathogen defense. Taken together, the body of evidence suggests that the host gut microbiota can elicit innate immunity against pathogens.

Keywords: gut microbiota, host innate immunity, antimicrobial peptides, inflammasome, IL-22, IL-17, IL-10

INTRODUCTION

The mammalian intestine is home to a complex and dynamic population of microorganisms, termed the "gut microbiota" (1, 2). These microorganisms, which co-evolved with the host as part of a mutually beneficial relationship (3), include bacteria, fungi and viruses (4, 5). Accumulating evidence indicates that the gut microbiota can participate in the maturation and function of the innate immune system, while also playing many complex roles in the host defense against pathogens (6). On the one hand, the gut microbiota can help repair intestinal mucosal barrier damage (7, 8); on the other hand, gut microbiota mediates host anti-pathogen defenses (9).

In the past decade, studies of germ-free (GF) mice have provided clues to elucidate the complexity of the intestinal microbiota (10, 11) and its importance to host health (12, 13). Mounting research shows that at least a thousand different gut microbiota species, such as *Firmicutes*, *Bacteroidetes*, *Actinobacteria*, *Proteobacteria*, and others, contribute to host defense against harmful microorganisms (14, 15).

Recently, several studies have begun to elucidate the molecular mechanisms underlying how the gut microbiota regulates host innate immunity against pathogens (16, 17), including a role in helping the host resist pathogen colonization. In this review, we summarize the main mechanisms by which commensal bacteria, including certain probiotic species, actively prevent pathogen colonization of the host.

GUT MICROBIOTA AND ANTIMICROBIAL PEPTIDES

Defensins

The α-defensins, microbicidal peptides mainly produced by Paneth cells, are key components of innate immunity. They control pathogen growth within the intestine (18–20) and their production can be directly elicited by both Gram-negative and Gram-positive bacteria, as well as by bacterial metabolites (e.g., lipopolysaccharide, lipoteichoic acid, lipid A, and muramyl dipeptide) (21–23). By contrast, live fungi and protozoa do not appear to stimulate Paneth cells and thus fail to elicit Paneth cell degranulation (21). Nevertheless, recent research has found that the gut microbiota plays an important role in induction of α-defensins expression against pathogens (24). In one *in vitro* study, live *E. coli* or *S. aureus*, live or dead *S. typhimurium*, lipopolysaccharide (LPS), lipid A, lipoteichoic acid (LTA), or liposomes could stimulate isolated intact intestinal crypts, demonstrating that intestinal Paneth cells may contribute to α-defensins secretion by sensing the presence of exogenous bacteria and bacterial antigens (21). To investigate whether gut microbiota possess the same or similar functions, Shipra Vaishnava and colleagues used a CR2-MyD88 Tg mouse model, whereby Paneth cells were the sole cell lineage expressing MyD88, to demonstrate that Paneth cells may directly sense enteric bacteria to trigger the MyD88-dependent antimicrobial program. Furthermore, increased numbers of *Salmonella* were observed to be internalized by mesenteric lymph node (MLN) cells of MyD88$^{-/-}$ and germ-free mice as compared to corresponding numbers observed for wild-type mice (25). Similarly, transcriptional profiles have shown that α-defensin gene (*Defa*) transcripts were less abundant in intestinal microbiota-free mice and TLRs-deficient or MyD88-deficient mice, but could be recovered after stimulation with toll-like receptor (TLR) agonists, specifically agonists of TLR2 or TLR4 (26). Thus, commensal microbiota appears to protect the host against pathogen invasion by triggering enteric Paneth cell TLR-MyD88 signaling. Notably, this mechanism is distinct from the NOD2-dependent antimicrobial response (25, 27, 28), since the former mechanism entails triggering of expression of multiple antimicrobial factors (25). However, several human-based studies have demonstrated that mutations in the NOD2 peptidoglycan sensor actually did reduce secretion of α-defensins (29–33). Therefore, these contradictory human and mouse study results warrant further research. Notably, another study has demonstrated that Cd1d$^{-/-}$ mice exhibited a defect in Paneth cell granule ultrastructure that specifically resulted in an inability to degranulate after bacterial colonization, with an increased load of segmented filamentous bacteria (SFB) also noted (34). Thus, no clear evidence demonstrates that CD1d mediates regulation of gut microbiota via α-defensins expression.

Meanwhile, more recent research has begun to examine the mechanism of how the gut microbiota influences α-defensins secretion. Studies using the Caco-2 IEC line have demonstrated that lactic acid strongly suppresses transcription of the α-defensin gene, while cecal content may include as yet unidentified factors which enhance concomitant α-defensin 5 expression (35). However, contrary to the aforementioned results, Menendez et al. found that *Defa* expression was partially restored *in vivo* by *lactobacillus* administration to antibiotic-treated mice (26). Notably, an emerging role of vitamin D, a *lactobacillus* metabolite, has been recently discovered that exerts an effect opposite on α-defensins expression to that exerted by lactate (36, 37). To reconcile these results, Su et al. used a mouse model and certain feed formulations to demonstrate that VDD- and HFD ± VDD-fed mice exhibited reduced levels of expression of α-defensin and MMP7 (a metalloproteinase that can proteolytically convert pro-α-defensins to their mature and active forms) within ileal crypts as compared to results for control and HFD groups. Moreover, their results demonstrated a critical role of vitamin D signaling in maintaining steady-state expression of α-defensins and MMP7 under physiological conditions. Subsequently, Su et al. have demonstrated that dietary vitamin D deficiency resulted in loss of Paneth cell-specific α-defensins, which may lead to intestinal dysbiosis and endotoxemia (38). Of note, oral administration of α-defensin suppressed *Helicobacter hepaticus* growth *in vivo* (38). Meanwhile, using complementary mouse models of defensin deficiency (MMP7$^{-/-}$) and surplus (HD5$^{+/+}$), Salzman noted defensin-dependent reciprocal shifts in proportions of dominant bacterial species within the small intestine with no changes in total bacterial numbers observed (**Table 1**). Upon further research, this group observed that mice overexpressing HD5 exhibited a significant loss of segmented filamentous bacteria (SFB), resulting in reduced numbers of Th17 cells within the lamina propria (48). However, direct evidence implicating the involvement of SFB in α-defensin production is still lacking and studies on α-defensin regulation by specific commensal microorganisms are still rare, warranting further research. Nevertheless, in view of existing research results, we believe that the discovery of specific microorganisms through research focusing on specific metabolic pathways may be a more fruitful approach.

With regard to β-defensins, which directly kill or inhibit the growth of microorganisms (49), these agents have been shown to exert antimicrobial activity against some species of enteric pathogenic Gram-positive *S. aureus* and *S. pyogenes*, as well as against Gram-negative *P. aeruginosa*, *E. coli* and the yeast *C. albicans* (50). In fact, accumulating evidence has shown that, similarly to α-defensins, β-defensins secretion is also regulated by the gut microbiota. For example, using *in vitro* studies of HT-29 and Caco-2 human colon epithelial cell lines, human fetal intestinal xenografts have been observed to constitutively express hBD-1 but not hBD-2, with upregulation of only the latter in xenografts intraluminally infected with *Salmonella* (51). Meanwhile, it has been independently shown that preincubation of Caco-2 cells with live *E. faecium* significantly reduced *S. typhimurium* internalization by 45.8%, while heat-killed *E. faecium* pretreatment had no effect on pathogen internalization (49). This result aligns with the latest research, which has shown that only live gut microbiota, as modeled using *Lactobacillus acidophilus* PZ 1129 and PZ 1130, *Lactobacillus paracasei*, *Lactobacillus plantarum*, *E. coli* K-12, and *E. coli Nissle 1917*, can strongly induce expression of hBD-2 in Caco-2 intestinal epithelial cells in a time- and dose-dependent manner (39–42)

TABLE 1 | Gut microbiota protects the host against pathogen infections and the relevant mechanisms.

Pathogens	Gut microbiota	Mechanisms	References
Helicobacter hepaticus	*Lactobacillus*	Inducing α-defensin production from Paneth cells	(38)
S. aureus *S. pyogenes* *P. aeruginosa* *E. coli* *C. albicans*	*Lactobacillus acidophilus PZ 1129* *Lactobacillus acidophilus PZ 1130* *Lactobacillus paracasei* *Lactobacillus plantarum* *E. coli K-12* *E. coli Nissle 1917*	Inducing β-defensin production	(39–42)
Klebsiella pneumoniae *Citrobacter rodentium* *Enterococcus* *Plasmodium chabaudi*	*L. reuteri* *Allobaculum spp* *Clostridium spp* *Bacteroides spp*	Inducing IL-22 production	(43–46)
Salmonella typhimurium	*Bacteroides*	Inducing IL-17 production	(47)

(**Table 1**). Notably, the *E. coli* strain *Nissle 1917*, a non-pathogenic Gram-negative strain isolated in 1917 by Alfred Nissle, elicited the most marked expression of induced β-defensin expression *in vitro* (39–42). Interestingly, Schlee et al. constructed several *E. coli Nissle 1917* deletion mutants and pinpointed flagellin as the major stimulatory factor for triggering of β-defensin secretion in the presence of that strain (40). Meanwhile, Wehkamp et al. and others have found that *E. coli Nissle 1917*-induced β-defensin expression in cell culture was mediated by NF-κB- and MAPK/AP-1-dependent pathways (39–42). Nevertheless, *in vivo* studies are still needed to confirm if gut microbiota can induce β-defensins expression to reduce pathogen colonization and control gut homeostasis (**Table 1**). Recently, to further clarify the relationship between gut microbiota and β-defensin secretion, Miani et al. used a mouse model and antibiotic treatment experiments to study the participation of dysbiotic microbiota and a low-affinity aryl hydrocarbon receptor (AHR) allele in the defective pancreatic expression of mBD14 observed in NOD mice. By utilizing 16S rDNA gene sequencing and AHR ligand activity measurements, they demonstrated that gut microbiota-derived molecules, including AHR ligands and butyrate, promoted IL-22 secretion by pancreatic ILCs that subsequently induced mBD14 expression by endocrine cells. Therefore, dysbiotic microbiota and a low-affinity AHR allele appear to explain defective pancreatic mBD14 expression of mBD14 in NOD mice (24). Because only live gut microbiota can stimulate secretion of β-defensins, we believe that specific gut microbiota that possess special metabolic pathway functionality, including pathways for secretion of AHR ligands, may possess the ability to regulate secretion of β-defensins.

C-Type Lectins

The C-type lectins, also key components of innate immunity that control growth of enteric pathogens (52–54), are expressed by multiple small intestinal epithelial lineages (55, 56). REG3γ and REG3β, two C-type lectins, provide protection against infection by specific bacterial pathogens, including *Enterococcus faecalis* (57–59), *Yersinia pseudotuberculosis* (60, 61), and *Listeria monocytogenes* (57). Notably, additional evidence suggests that C-type lectins actually mediate syncytium endosymbiont defenses through prevention of pathogen colonization. To further demonstrate how these lectins control bacterial colonization of the intestinal epithelial surface, Vil-Myd88^{Tg} mice (mice with IEC-restricted Myd88 expression) were used to determine whether surface Myd88 present on epithelial cells was sufficient to restrain bacterial colonization (55). The results showed that secretion of C-type lectins required both activation of the MyD88 pathway (62) and recognition of syncytium endosymbionts by TLRs (63). Furthermore, Earle et al. used a pipeline method to assess intestinal microbiota localization within immunofluorescence images of fixed gut cross-sections. The results indicated that elimination of dietary microbiota-accessible carbohydrates (MACs) resulted in thinning of mucus within the distal colon that increased microbial proximity to the epithelium and heightened inflammatory marker REG3β expression (64). These results align with those from an earlier study of transcriptional profiles of duodenum, jejunum, ileum and colon samples, which demonstrated that MyD88 was essential for syncytium endosymbiont-induced colonic epithelial expression of antimicrobial genes Reg3β and Reg3γ, with Myd88 deficiency associated with both a shift in bacterial diversity and a greater proportion of SFB in the small intestine (65). In fact, other research found that conventionally raised Myd88$^{-/-}$ mice exhibited increased expression of antiviral genes in the colon, which correlated with norovirus infection of the colonic epithelium (65). Therefore, it can be concluded that both the activation of the MyD88 pathway and recognition of syncytium endosymbionts by TLRs are indispensable for triggering C-type lectins secretion (**Figure 1**). Recently, Ju et al. used antibiotic-treated mice to study differences between metronidazole-treated and control groups, and observed reduced abundance of *Turicibacteraceae*, overgrowth of *E. coli* and higher levels of *Reg3β* and *Reg3γ* mRNA for the metronidazole-treated group (66). These results provide a basis for the study of the effects of specific gut syncytium endosymbiont organisms on C-type lectins secretion.

Other accumulating evidence has shown that the mammalian gut contains a rich fungal community that interacts with the immune system through the C-type lectin receptor Dectin-1. To demonstrate whether symbiotic fungi influence C-type lectins secretion that prevents pathogen colonization, Iliev et al. studied mice lacking Dectin-1 and observed increased susceptibility

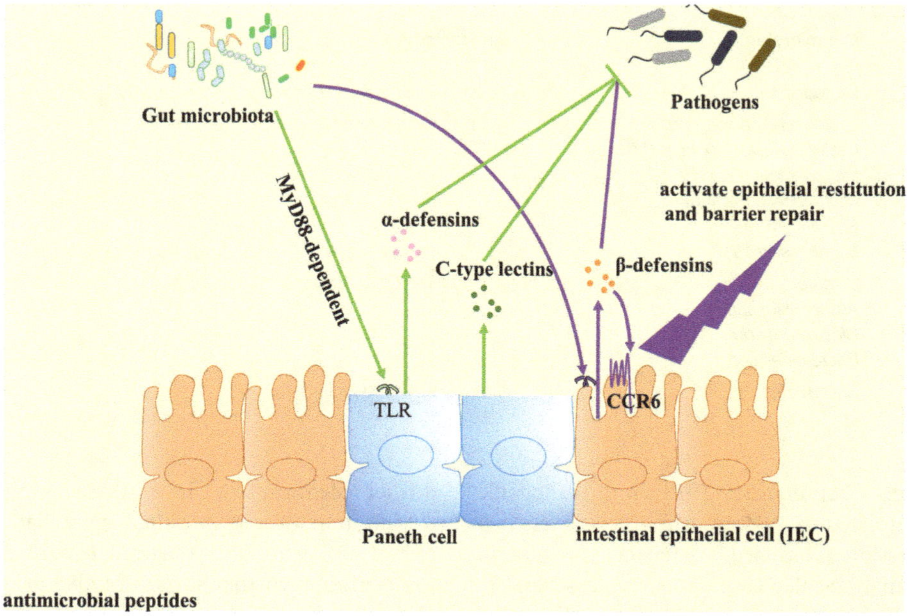

FIGURE 1 | Gut microbiota plays an important role in the induction of antimicrobial peptides expression against pathogens. Antimicrobial peptides are key components of innate immunity to control pathogen growth within the intestine. Accumulated evidence identified that gut microbiota can contribute to the expression of antimicrobial peptides and play a central role in host defense against pathogens. Paneth cells could directly sense gut microbiota through cell-autonomous myeloid differentiation primary response 88 (MyD88)-dependent toll-like receptor (TLR) activation, triggering expression of α-defensins and C-type lectins. With regard to β-defensin, gut microbiota induce β-defensin expression in cell culture mediated by NF-κB- and MAPK/AP-1-dependent pathways *in vitro*. Then β-defensin interacts with intestinal epithelial cell (IEC) through CCR6 to activate epithelial restitution and barrier repair.

to chemically induced colitis due to altered responses to indigenous fungi. Moreover, in humans they identified a gene polymorphism for Dectin-1 (CLEC7A) that is strongly linked to a severe form of ulcerative colitis (67). Independently, Eriksson et al. found that CLR-specific intracellular adhesion molecule-3 grabbing non-integrin homolog-related 3 (SIGNR3) is the closest murine homolog to the human dendritic cell-specific intercellular adhesion molecule-3-grabbing non-integrin (DC-SIGN) receptor. Both receptors recognize similar carbohydrate ligands, such as terminal fucose or high-mannose glycans. Notably, using the dextran sulfate sodium-induced colitis model, IGNR3 has been observed to recognize fungal members of the commensal microbiota, with SIGNR3$^{-/-}$ mice exhibiting a higher level of TNF-α in colon (68). Therefore, symbiotic fungi appear to communicate with the host via the C-type lectin receptor to maintain intestinal homeostasis. However, as yet no direct evidence has been found to determine whether symbiotic fungi can regulate selectin secretion, warranting further research.

GUT MICROBIOTA ELICITS INFLAMMASOME ACTIVATION AGAINST PATHOGENS

Inflammasome activation is an important innate immune pathway that prevents pathogen invasion via secretion of proinflammatory cytokines IL-1β and IL-18, as well as through induction of pyroptosis (69–74). It is well-documented that inflammasomes come from two main sources, namely myeloid- and epithelial-derived inflammasomes. While they share several common features, it should be noted that inflammasomes of distinct origins may exhibit different features and effector functions. For example, from a mechanistic of view, macrophage- and epithelial cell-derived inflammasomes are activated with different intermediate processes. While IL-18 processing is dependent on caspase-11 in IECs, caspase-1 is responsible for the processing of IL-18 in myeloid cells (75). In addition, compared with myeloid cells, IECs constitutively express IL-18, while produce little IL-1β (76–78). Moreover, unlike myeloid inflammasomes, IEC inflammasomes is capable of producing considerable amounts of prostaglandin upon activation (79). Intriguingly, the signaling circuitry between epithelial and myeloid inflammasomes are also different. For example, in homeostasis conditions, both *NLRP3* and *PYCARD* genes have been shown to be highly expressed in murine primary macrophages, while mouse airway epithelial cells can only express a low level of *PYCARD* and cannot express *NLRP3* (80).

Accumulating evidence suggests that gut microbiota can activate NLRC4 and NLRP3 inflammasome pathways against pathogens (81–83). *Enterobacteriaceae* and the pathobiont *Proteus mirabilis*, which are members of the normal flora of the human gastrointestinal tract (84, 85), were shown to induce robust IL-1β production through NLRP3 activation mediated by intestinal Ly6C^{high} monocytes (86, 87). Indeed, recruited Ly6C^{high} monocytes have been shown to express a variety of inflammasome components, such as NAIPs (71, 88, 89), NLRC4

(89), NLRP1 (90, 91), NLRP6 (92, 93), AIM2 (94), caspase-1 (95), caspase-4 (96) (in humans), ASC (93), and IL-18 (87, 97, 98). Meanwhile, Seo et al. have also demonstrated that *Proteus mirabilis* (a Proteobacteria phylum member) induced NLRP3 activation and IL-1β production (86). Interestingly, bacterial components from other *Proteobacteria*, such as LPS produced by *Pseudomonas* spp., have even been shown to induce host mental depression symptoms via NLRP3 inflammasome activation (99). Other interesting lines of research have shown that in addition to gut commensal bacteria, the mammalian gut contains a rich fungal community which also appears to activate the inflammasome pathway. This community includes the human commensal fungus *Candida albicans* (*C. albicans*), which colonizes gastrointestinal and vaginal tract mucosal surfaces and appears to promote inflammasome activation during AOM-DSS-induced colitis (100). In further support of this finding, direct peptide administration experiments had previously demonstrated that candidalysin, a peptide derived from the hypha-specific *ECE1* gene, acted as a fungal trigger for NLRP3 inflammasome-mediated maturation that was sufficient for inducing IL-1β secretion mature macrophages in an NLRP3 inflammasome-dependent manner (101).

In recent studies, numerous other gut microbiota metabolites have also been demonstrated to elicit inflammasome pathways against pathogens. For example, gut microbiota-derived adenosine triphosphate (ATP) has been shown to co-operate with NLRP3 (also known as CIAS1) (102) via the macrophage P2X7 receptor (103) to induce assembly of a cytosolic protein complex containing ASK and caspase-1 (70, 104–106) that eventually leads to inflammasome activation (106). Another important gut microbiota metabolite, short-chain fatty acids (SCFAs), end products of fermentation of dietary fibers by anaerobic intestinal microbiota, have also been implicated in inflammasome activation (107). SCFAs binding to GPR43 on colonic epithelial cells to stimulate K^+ efflux and hyperpolarization has been shown to lead to NLRP3 inflammasome activation, with subsequent acceleration of cell maturation and secretion of IL-1β (108) and IL-18 (77, 109).

GUT MICROBIOTA CAN ENHANCE INTERLEUKIN EXPRESSION TO CLEAR INVADING PATHOGENS

IL-22

IL-22 is important in maintaining mucosal barrier integrity and is produced by many different types of innate immune cells (110–113). This cytokine has been shown to play a host-protective role during infection by a wide range of pathogens, including *Klebsiella pneumoniae* (114), *Citrobacter rodentium* (115, 116), vancomycin-resistant *Enterococcus* (117, 118) and *Plasmodium chabaudi* (119). One IL-22-dependent mechanism involved in pathogen clearance involves the increased presence of antimicrobial proteins within the mucosa (120) that include the following: calprotectin and lipocalin-2, the latter of which binds to the siderophore enterochelin, with both acting to limit iron availability in the gut (120); C-type lectins, which regenerate islet-derivative proteins Reg3β and Reg3γ that control some components of the microbiota (58, 120, 121); and S100A8 and S100A9, two antimicrobial peptides that heterodimerize to form calprotectin, an antimicrobial protein that sequesters zinc and manganese to prevent microbial access to these nutrients (122). Although epithelial antimicrobial defenses also exist, many pathogens can still colonize mucosal surfaces to establish infections (120, 123). Nevertheless, accumulated evidence has shown that IL-22 is rapidly induced in response to pathogen invasion through activation of host AhR via specific gut microbiota-derived molecules (**Figure 2**) (124, 125). For example, *Lactobacillus species* (specifically, *L. reuteri*) can activate IL-22 production by gut type 3 innate lymphoid cells (ILC3) (126–128), while other studies have shown that supplementation with three commensal *Lactobacillus strains* with high tryptophan-metabolizing activities was sufficient to restore intestinal IL-22 production (43, 129). Indeed, additional work has shown that *Lactobacillus species* could utilize tryptophan as an energy source and produce a metabolite, indole-3-aldehyde (IAld), which could then activate AhRs present on ILCs (126, 130). In addition to *Lactobacillus strains*, other recent studies have shown that *Allobaculum* spp. (43), *Escherichia coli* (44), *Clostridium* spp. (45), and *Bacteroides* spp. (46) can also utilize tryptophan to produce IAld and elicit IL-22 production (**Table 1**). Meanwhile, other studies have shown that activated ILCs secrete IL-22 to protect the host against opportunistic pathogens by reducing pathogen colonization (120, 131). In fact, other innate immune cells, such as NKT cells, γδ T cells and macrophages, have very recently been shown to secrete IL-22 under regulation by gut microbiota via the AhR pathway (132). Therefore, gut microbiota may prevent pathogen infection by collectively enhancing IL-22 expression via the AhR pathway.

IL-17

IL-17 is a well-established crucial cytokine that is involved in limiting invasion and dissemination of pathogens, including *Salmonella typhimurium* (133), by both recruitment of neutrophils and by the induction of production of antimicrobial peptides (131, 134). Recent studies have demonstrated that both the abundance and activation status of IL-17-producing intraepithelial lymphocytes (IELs) are modulated by commensal bacteria, with enrichment of the γδT cell population of IELs representing an important source of innate IL-17 production (135, 136). Notably, a comparative study of GF mice and SPF mice has shown that the number of TCRγδ IELs is decreased in GF mice (133). Moreover, in addition to the regulation of IELs numbers, the gut microbiota may also regulate activation of TCRγδ IELs, as reflected by a report showing that production of IL-17 by TCRγδ IELs is decreased in GF mice (137). Meanwhile, antibiotic-treatment and monocolonization of mice have been used to demonstrate that the great majority of γ/δ T cells within peritonea of SPF mice are $CD62L^-$ γδT cells, which are activated γδT cells, with GF mice possessing far fewer $CD62L^-$ γ/δ T cells than SPF mice (47). Notably, additional research suggests that specific commensal bacteria, excluding metronidazole-sensitive anaerobes, such as *Bacteroides* species, are required for maintaining $IL\text{-}1R1^{\pm}$ γδT cells (47), a result

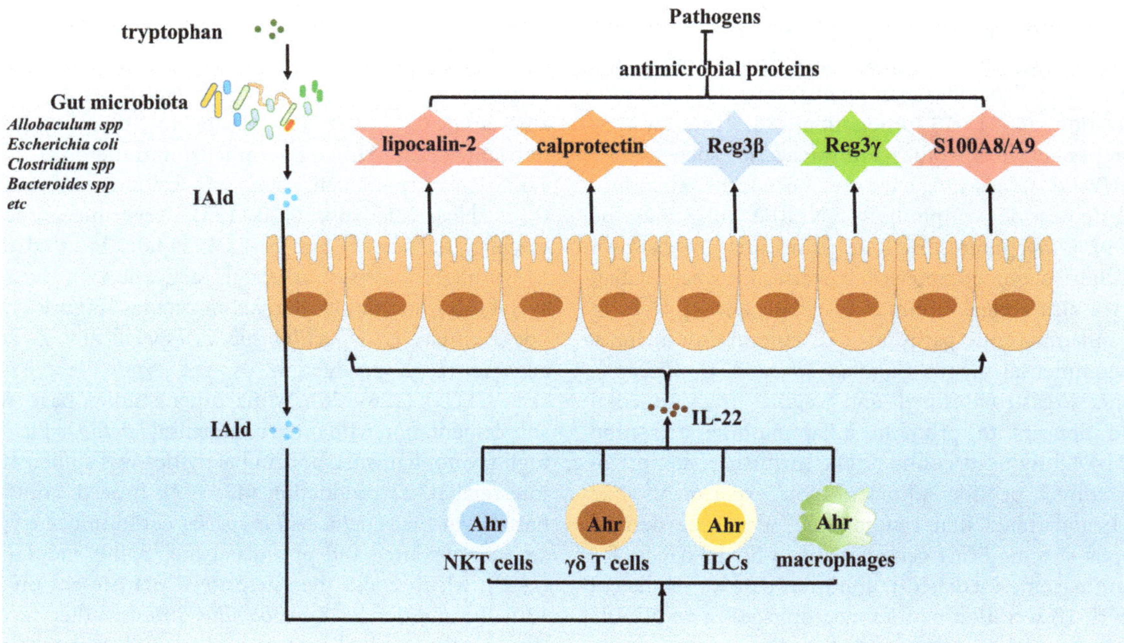

FIGURE 2 | Gut microbiota enhance the expression of IL-22 against invading pathogens. IL-22 is important in maintaining the integrity of mucosal barriers and can be produced by many different types innate immune cells, which induce the expression of various antimicrobial proteins, including lipocalin-2, calprotectin, C-type lectins, S100A8, S100A9, and so on to clear pathogens. Increasing evidence identified that gut microbiota enhances the expression of IL-22 to protect the host against pathogens. The results show that gut microbiota utilize tryptophan as an energy source and produce a metabolite, indole-3-aldehyde (IAld), which in turns activated Ahr on innate immune cells. Once activated, innate immune cells will secrete IL-22, which protects the host against opportunistic pathogens by reducing their colonization.

that aligns with previous research results by another research group (138) (**Table 1**). In conclusion, gut microbiota influences the abundance and activation status of IL-17-producing TCRγδ IELs to protect the host from pathogen infection and to maintain intestinal homeostasis. In addition, lymphoid tissue inducer (LTi) cells and NCR$^-$ ILC3 cells also appear to function as important sources of innate IL-17 production (127). However, few studies have investigated how gut microbiota regulate these cell types, warranting further research in this area.

IL-10

IL-10 is an anti-inflammatory cytokine that plays a central role in regulating the host immune response to pathogens, thereby preventing host damage and maintaining normal tissue homeostasis (139–141). Accumulating evidence suggests that macrophages are an important source of innate IL-10 and that the gut microbiota plays a vital role in mucosal innate IL-10 generation under homeostatic conditions (142–144). For example, studies in GF mice and SPF mice have shown that colonic lamina propria from germ-free mice exhibited lower IL-10 production (142), a reduction later confirmed to be a 50% reduction in steady-state IL-10 levels (142–144). To elucidate the mechanism by which gut microbiota regulate intestinal macrophage IL-10 production, Hayashi et al. used macrophage-specific IL-10-deficient mice to demonstrate that *Clostridium butyricum* (CB), a distinct cluster I *Clostridium* strain, induces IL-10 production to ultimately prevent acute experimental colitis. However, while CB treatment had no effects on IL-10 production by T cells, IL-10-producing F4/80$^{\pm}$CD11b$^{\pm}$CD11c^{int} macrophages accumulated within inflamed mucosa after CB treatment. Subsequently, more rigorous examination demonstrated that CB directly triggered IL-10 production by intestinal macrophages there via the TLR2/MyD88 pathway (144). Meanwhile, Ochi et al. recently found that dietary amino acids directly regulate Il-10 production by small intestine (SI) macrophages. Using mice fed via total parenteral nutrition, a significant decrease of IL-10-producing macrophages in the SI was observed, while IL-10-producing CD4$^{\pm}$ T cells remained intact. Likewise, enteral nutrient deprivation selectively decreased IL-10 production by the monocyte-derived F4/80$^{\pm}$ macrophage population, but had no effect on non-monocytic precursor-derived CD103$^{\pm}$ dendritic cells. Notably, in contrast to regulation of colonic macrophages, replenishment of SI macrophages and their IL-10 production were not regulated by gut microbiota (145). Contrary to results obtained under steady-state conditions, an injury model used to study participation of microbiota to explain observed IL-10 increases post-injury yielded different results. Specifically, comparison of *Il10* mRNA levels in uninjured intact tissue and day-2 post-wound tissue isolated from SPF or GF mice indicated that IL-10 mRNA was induced in post-wound colonic tissue isolated from both SPF and GF mice. Therefore, injury-triggered IL-10 increases appeared to be largely microbiota independent (146), although the reasons remain unclear regarding the differing effects of the gut microbiota observed in different model systems. Nevertheless, we hypothesize that local damage-associated molecular proteins (DAMPs) may regulate immune cells more rapidly and strongly post-intestinal damage, resulting in either a failure of gut microbiota to temporally adjust or a masking of any microbiota-based regulatory effect.

CONCLUDING REMARKS

Gut microbiota resists colonization and growth of invading pathogens through the induction of expression of antimicrobial peptides, IL-22, IL-17, and IL-10 while eliciting inflammasome activation. Because the underlying mechanisms of how the gut microbiota resists pathogenic invasion still remain obscure, future studies are clearly needed to identify gut microbiota functions against various pathogens toward the development of promising strategies to treat infectious diseases. For instance, E. coli Nissle 1917 can induce β-defensin expression mediated by NF-κB- and MAPK/AP-1-dependent pathways (39), while Lactobacillus spp. activate IL-22 production against opportunistic pathogens to reduce colonization (147, 148). Therefore, transplanting suitable specific gut microbiota to compete with specific pathogens could be an effective defense strategy. However, since this strategy poses new disease risks, strategies that restore intestinal homeostasis and promote host immune system may serve to more safely clear pathogens. To this end, identifying specific gut microbiota functions and defining normal gut microbiota populations are necessary first steps toward development of safer strategies for strengthening host defenses against pathogens. Moreover, research on the function and mechanisms of gut microbiota metabolites may facilitate development of novel therapeutic strategies to combat drug-resistant pathogens.

AUTHOR CONTRIBUTIONS

D-KC, W-TM, H-YC, and M-XN designed the structure of the mini-review. H-YC and M-XN wrote the manuscript and drafted the first version of the manuscript. M-XN and W-TM helped revise the manuscript. All authors have reviewed the final version of the manuscript.

FUNDING

This research was supported by the Qinghai province Major R&D and Transformation Project (2018-NK-125), Xianyang Science and Technology Major Project (2017K01-34), Key industrial innovation chains of Shaanxi province (2018ZDCXL-NY-01-06) and PhD research startup fund of Northwest Agriculture and Forestry University (00500/Z109021716).

REFERENCES

1. Jandhyala SM, Talukdar R, Subramanyam C, Vuyyuru H, Sasikala M, Nageshwar Reddy D. Role of the normal gut microbiota. *World J Gastroenterol.* (2015) 21:8787–803. doi: 10.3748/wjg.v21.i29.8787
2. Luthold RV, Fernandes GR, Franco-de-Moraes AC, Folchetti LG, Ferreira SR. Gut microbiota interactions with the immunomodulatory role of vitamin D in normal individuals. *Metabolism.* (2017) 69:76–86. doi: 10.1016/j.metabol.2017.01.007
3. Ayres JS. Cooperative microbial tolerance behaviors in host-microbiota mutualism. *Cell.* (2016) 165:1323–31. doi: 10.1016/j.cell.2016.05.049
4. Foca A, Liberto MC, Quirino A, Marascio N, Zicca E, Pavia G. Gut inflammation and immunity: what is the role of the human gut virome? *Mediators Inflamm.* (2015) 2015:326032. doi: 10.1155/2015/326032
5. Chen B, Chen H, Shu X, Yin Y, Li J, Qin J, et al. Presence of segmented filamentous bacteria in human children and its potential role in the modulation of human gut immunity. *Front Microbiol.* (2018) 9:1403. doi: 10.3389/fmicb.2018.01403
6. Belkaid Y, Hand TW. Role of the microbiota in immunity and inflammation. *Cell.* (2014) 157:121–41. doi: 10.1016/j.cell.2014.03.011
7. Okumura R, Takeda K. Roles of intestinal epithelial cells in the maintenance of gut homeostasis. *Exp Mol Med.* (2017) 49:e338. doi: 10.1038/emm.2017.20
8. Okumura R, Takeda K. Maintenance of intestinal homeostasis by mucosal barriers. *Inflamm Regen.* (2018) 38:5. doi: 10.1186/s41232-018-0063-z
9. Ubeda C, Djukovic A, Isaac S. Roles of the intestinal microbiota in pathogen protection. *Clin Transl Immunol.* (2017) 6:e128. doi: 10.1038/cti.2017.2
10. Biedermann L, Rogler G. The intestinal microbiota: its role in health and disease. *Eur J Pediatr.* (2015) 174:151–67. doi: 10.1007/s00431-014-2476-2
11. Goulet O. Potential role of the intestinal microbiota in programming health and disease. *Nutr Rev.* (2015) 73 Suppl. 1:32–40. doi: 10.1093/nutrit/nuv039
12. Tojo R, Suarez A, Clemente MG, de los Reyes-Gavilan CG, Margolles A, Gueimonde M, et al. Intestinal microbiota in health and disease: role of bifidobacteria in gut homeostasis. *World J Gastroenterol.* (2014) 20:15163–76. doi: 10.3748/wjg.v20.i41.15163
13. Kataoka K. The intestinal microbiota and its role in human health and disease. *J Med Invest.* (2016) 63:27–37. doi: 10.2152/jmi.63.27
14. Gevers D, Knight R, Petrosino JF, Huang K, McGuire AL, Birren BW, et al. The human microbiome project: a community resource for the healthy human microbiome. *PLoS Biol.* (2012) 10:e1001377. doi: 10.1371/journal.pbio.1001377
15. Lloyd-Price J, Abu-Ali G, Huttenhower C. The healthy human microbiome. *Genome Med.* (2016) 8:51. doi: 10.1186/s13073-016-0307-y
16. Lim MY, You HJ, Yoon HS, Kwon B, Lee JY, Lee S, et al. The effect of heritability and host genetics on the gut microbiota and metabolic syndrome. *Gut.* (2017) 66:1031–8. doi: 10.1136/gutjnl-2015-311326
17. Monedero V, Buesa J, Rodriguez-Diaz J. The interactions between host glycobiology, bacterial microbiota, and viruses in the gut. *Viruses.* (2018) 10:96. doi: 10.3390/v10020096
18. Diamond G, Beckloff N, Weinberg A, Kisich KO. The roles of antimicrobial peptides in innate host defense. *Curr Pharm Des.* (2009) 15:2377–92. doi: 10.2174/138161209788682325
19. Hooper LV, Littman DR, Macpherson AJ. Interactions between the microbiota and the immune system. *Science.* (2012) 336:1268–73. doi: 10.1126/science.1223490
20. Kim D, Zeng MY, Nunez G. The interplay between host immune cells and gut microbiota in chronic inflammatory diseases. *Exp Mol Med.* (2017) 49:e339. doi: 10.1038/emm.2017.24
21. Ayabe T, Satchell DP, Wilson CL, Parks WC, Selsted ME, Ouellette AJ. Secretion of microbicidal alpha-defensins by intestinal Paneth cells in response to bacteria. *Nat Immunol.* (2000) 1:113–8. doi: 10.1038/77783
22. Elphick DA, Mahida YR. Paneth cells: their role in innate immunity and inflammatory disease. *Gut.* (2005) 54:1802–9. doi: 10.1136/gut.2005.068601
23. Tanabe H, Ayabe T, Bainbridge B, Guina T, Ernst RK, Darveau RP, et al. Mouse paneth cell secretory responses to cell surface glycolipids of virulent

and attenuated pathogenic bacteria. *Infect Immun.* (2005) 73:2312–20. doi: 10.1128/IAI.73.4.2312-2320.2005

24. Miani M, Le Naour J, Waeckel-Enee E, Verma SC, Straube M, Emond P, et al. Gut microbiota-stimulated innate lymphoid cells support beta-defensin 14 expression in pancreatic endocrine cells, preventing autoimmune diabetes. *Cell Metab.* (2018) 28:557–72.e6. doi: 10.1016/j.cmet.2018.06.012
25. Vaishnava S, Behrendt CL, Ismail AS, Eckmann L, Hooper LV. Paneth cells directly sense gut commensals and maintain homeostasis at the intestinal host-microbial interface. *Proc Natl Acad Sci USA.* (2008) 105:20858–63. doi: 10.1073/pnas.0808723105
26. Menendez A, Willing BP, Montero M, Wlodarska M, So CC, Bhinder G, et al. Bacterial stimulation of the TLR-MyD88 pathway modulates the homeostatic expression of ileal Paneth cell alpha-defensins. *J Innate Immun.* (2013) 5:39–49. doi: 10.1159/000341630
27. MacDonald TT, Monteleone I, Fantini MC, Monteleone G. Regulation of homeostasis and inflammation in the intestine. *Gastroenterology.* (2011) 140:1768–75. doi: 10.1053/j.gastro.2011.02.047
28. Kong S, Zhang YH, Zhang W. Regulation of intestinal epithelial cells properties and functions by amino acids. *Biomed Res Int.* (2018) 2018:2819154. doi: 10.1155/2018/2819154
29. Petnicki-Ocwieja T, Hrncir T, Liu YJ, Biswas A, Hudcovic T, Tlaskalova-Hogenova H, et al. Nod2 is required for the regulation of commensal microbiota in the intestine. *Proc Natl Acad Sci USA.* (2009) 106:15813–8. doi: 10.1073/pnas.0907722106
30. Ramanan D, Tang MS, Bowcutt R, Loke P, Cadwell K. Bacterial sensor Nod2 prevents inflammation of the small intestine by restricting the expansion of the commensal *Bacteroides vulgatus*. *Immunity.* (2014) 41:311–24. doi: 10.1016/j.immuni.2014.06.015
31. Shanahan MT, Carroll IM, Grossniklaus E, White A, von Furstenberg RJ, Barner R, et al. Mouse Paneth cell antimicrobial function is independent of Nod2. *Gut.* (2014) 63:903–10. doi: 10.1136/gutjnl-2012-304190
32. Tan G, Zeng B, Zhi FC. Regulation of human enteric alpha-defensins by NOD2 in the Paneth cell lineage. *Eur J Cell Biol.* (2015) 94:60–6. doi: 10.1016/j.ejcb.2014.10.007
33. Keestra-Gounder AM, Byndloss MX, Seyffert N, Young BM, Chavez-Arroyo A, Tsai AY, et al. NOD1 and NOD2 signalling links ER stress with inflammation. *Nature.* (2016) 532:394–7. doi: 10.1038/nature17631
34. Nieuwenhuis EE, Matsumoto T, Lindenbergh D, Willemsen R, Kaser A, Simons-Oosterhuis Y, et al. Cd1d-dependent regulation of bacterial colonization in the intestine of mice. *J Clin Invest.* (2009) 119:1241–50. doi: 10.1172/JCI36509
35. Sugi Y, Takahashi K, Kurihara K, Nakano K, Kobayakawa T, Nakata K, et al. a-Defensin 5 gene expression is regulated by gut microbial metabolites. *Biosci Biotechnol Biochem.* (2017) 81:242–8. doi: 10.1080/09168451.2016.1246175
36. Jerzynska J, Stelmach W, Balcerak J, Woicka-Kolejwa K, Rychlik B, Blauz A, et al. Effect of *Lactobacillus rhamnosus* GG and vitamin D supplementation on the immunologic effectiveness of grass-specific sublingual immunotherapy in children with allergy. *Allergy Asthma Proc.* (2016) 37:324–34. doi: 10.2500/aap.2016.37.3958
37. Shang M, Sun J. Vitamin D/VDR, probiotics, and gastrointestinal diseases. *Curr Med Chem.* (2017) 24:876–87. doi: 10.2174/0929867323666161202150008
38. Su D, Nie Y, Zhu A, Chen Z, Wu P, Zhang L, et al. Vitamin D signaling through Induction of Paneth cell defensins maintains gut microbiota and improves metabolic disorders and hepatic steatosis in animal models. *Front Physiol.* (2016) 7:498. doi: 10.3389/fphys.2016.00498
39. Wehkamp J, Harder J, Wehkamp K, Wehkamp-von Meissner B, Schlee M, Enders C, et al. NF-kappaB- and AP-1-mediated induction of human beta defensin-2 in intestinal epithelial cells by *Escherichia coli* Nissle 1917: a novel effect of a probiotic bacterium. *Infect Immun.* (2004) 72:5750–8. doi: 10.1128/IAI.72.10.5750-5758.2004
40. Schlee M, Wehkamp J, Altenhoefer A, Oelschlaeger TA, Stange EF, Fellermann K. Induction of human beta-defensin 2 by the probiotic *Escherichia coli* Nissle 1917 is mediated through flagellin. *Infect Immun.* (2007) 75:2399–407. doi: 10.1128/IAI.01563-06
41. Steubesand N, Kiehne K, Brunke G, Pahl R, Reiss K, Herzig KH, et al. The expression of the beta-defensins hBD-2 and hBD-3 is differentially regulated by NF-kappaB and MAPK/AP-1 pathways in an *in vitro* model of Candida esophagitis. *BMC Immunol.* (2009) 10:36. doi: 10.1186/1471-2172-10-36
42. Seo EJ, Weibel S, Wehkamp J, Oelschlaeger TA. Construction of recombinant *E. coli* Nissle 1917 (EcN) strains for the expression and secretion of defensins. *Int J Med Microbiol.* (2012) 302:276–87. doi: 10.1016/j.ijmm.2012.05.002
43. Etienne-Mesmin L, Chassaing B, Gewirtz AT. Tryptophan: A gut microbiota-derived metabolites regulating inflammation. *World J Gastrointest Pharmacol Ther.* (2017) 8:7–9. doi: 10.4292/wjgpt.v8.i1.7
44. Devlin AS, Marcobal A, Dodd D, Nayfach S, Plummer N, Meyer T, et al. Modulation of a circulating uremic solute via rational genetic manipulation of the gut microbiota. *Cell Host Microbe.* (2016) 20:709–15. doi: 10.1016/j.chom.2016.10.021
45. Roager HM, Licht TR. Microbial tryptophan catabolites in health and disease. *Nat Commun.* (2018) 9:3294. doi: 10.1038/s41467-018-05470-4
46. Lee JS, Cella M, McDonald KG, Garlanda C, Kennedy GD, Nukaya M, et al. AHR drives the development of gut ILC22 cells and postnatal lymphoid tissues via pathways dependent on and independent of Notch. *Nat Immunol.* (2011) 13:144–51. doi: 10.1038/ni.2187
47. Duan J, Chung H, Troy E, Kasper DL. Microbial colonization drives expansion of IL-1 receptor 1-expressing and IL-17-producing gamma/delta T cells. *Cell Host Microbe.* (2010) 7:140–50. doi: 10.1016/j.chom.2010.01.005
48. Salzman NH. Paneth cell defensins and the regulation of the microbiome: detente at mucosal surfaces. *Gut Microbes.* (2010) 1:401–6. doi: 10.4161/gmic.1.6.14076
49. Fusco A, Savio V, Cammarota M, Alfano A, Schiraldi C, Donnarumma G. Beta-Defensin-2 and Beta-Defensin-3 reduce intestinal damage caused by *Salmonella typhimurium* modulating the expression of cytokines and enhancing the probiotic activity of *Enterococcus faecium*. *J Immunol Res.* (2017) 2017:6976935. doi: 10.1155/2017/6976935
50. Harder J, Bartels J, Christophers E, Schroder JM. Isolation and characterization of human beta -defensin-3, a novel human inducible peptide antibiotic. *J Biol Chem.* (2001) 276:5707–13. doi: 10.1074/jbc.M008557200
51. O'Neil DA, Porter EM, Elewaut D, Anderson GM, Eckmann L, Ganz T, et al. Expression and regulation of the human beta-defensins hBD-1 and hBD-2 in intestinal epithelium. *J Immunol.* (1999) 163:6718–24.
52. Sotolongo J, Ruiz J, Fukata M. The role of innate immunity in the host defense against intestinal bacterial pathogens. *Curr Infect Dis Rep.* (2012) 14:15–23. doi: 10.1007/s11908-011-0234-4
53. Katakura K, Watanabe H, Ohira H. Innate immunity and inflammatory bowel disease: a review of clinical evidence and future application. *Clin J Gastroenterol.* (2013) 6:415–9. doi: 10.1007/s12328-013-0436-4
54. Thaiss CA, Levy M, Suez J, Elinav E. The interplay between the innate immune system and the microbiota. *Curr Opin Immunol.* (2014) 26:41–8. doi: 10.1016/j.coi.2013.10.016
55. Vaishnava S, Yamamoto M, Severson KM, Ruhn KA, Yu X, Koren O, et al. The antibacterial lectin RegIIIgamma promotes the spatial segregation of microbiota and host in the intestine. *Science.* (2011) 334:255–8. doi: 10.1126/science.1209791
56. Thomas M, Pierson M, Uprety T, Zhu L, Ran Z, Sreenivasan CC, et al. Comparison of porcine airway and intestinal epithelial cell lines for the susceptibility and expression of pattern recognition receptors upon influenza virus infection. *Viruses.* (2018) 10:312. doi: 10.3390/v10060312
57. Abreu MT. Toll-like receptor signalling in the intestinal epithelium: how bacterial recognition shapes intestinal function. *Nat Rev Immunol.* (2010) 10:131–44. doi: 10.1038/nri2707
58. Gallo RL, Hooper LV. Epithelial antimicrobial defence of the skin and intestine. *Nat Rev Immunol.* (2012) 12:503–16. doi: 10.1038/nri3228
59. Mukherjee S, Hooper LV. Antimicrobial defense of the intestine. *Immunity.* (2015) 42:28–39. doi: 10.1016/j.immuni.2014.12.028
60. Dessein R, Gironella M, Vignal C, Peyrin-Biroulet L, Sokol H, Secher T, et al. Toll-like receptor 2 is critical for induction of Reg3 beta expression and intestinal clearance of *Yersinia pseudotuberculosis*. *Gut.* (2009) 58:771–6. doi: 10.1136/gut.2008.168443
61. Burger-van Paassen N, Loonen LM, Witte-Bouma J, Korteland-van Male AM, de Bruijn AC, van der Sluis M, et al. Mucin Muc2 deficiency and weaning influences the expression of the innate defense genes

Reg3beta, Reg3gamma and angiogenin-4. *PLoS ONE.* (2012) 7:e38798. doi: 10.1371/journal.pone.0038798
62. Bel S, Pendse M, Wang Y, Li Y, Ruhn KA, Hassell B, et al. Paneth cells secrete lysozyme via secretory autophagy during bacterial infection of the intestine. *Science.* (2017) 357:1047–52. doi: 10.1126/science.aal4677
63. Valentini M, Piermattei A, Di Sante G, Migliara G, Delogu G, Ria F. Immunomodulation by gut microbiota: role of Toll-like receptor expressed by T cells. *J Immunol Res.* (2014) 2014:586939. doi: 10.1155/2014/586939
64. Earle KA, Billings G, Sigal M, Lichtman JS, Hansson GC, Elias JE, et al. Quantitative imaging of gut microbiota spatial organization. *Cell Host Microbe.* (2015) 18:478–88. doi: 10.1016/j.chom.2015.09.002
65. Larsson E, Tremaroli V, Lee YS, Koren O, Nookaew I, Fricker A, et al. Analysis of gut microbial regulation of host gene expression along the length of the gut and regulation of gut microbial ecology through MyD88. *Gut.* (2012) 61:1124–31. doi: 10.1136/gutjnl-2011-301104
66. Ju T, Shoblak Y, Gao Y, Yang K, Fouhse J, Finlay BB, et al. Initial gut microbial composition as a key factor driving host response to antibiotic treatment, as exemplified by the presence or absence of commensal *Escherichia coli. Appl Environ Microbiol.* (2017) 83:e01107-17. doi: 10.1128/AEM.01107-17
67. Iliev ID, Funari VA, Taylor KD, Nguyen Q, Reyes CN, Strom SP, et al. Interactions between commensal fungi and the C-type lectin receptor Dectin-1 influence colitis. *Science.* (2012) 336:1314–7. doi: 10.1126/science.1221789
68. Eriksson M, Johannssen T, von Smolinski D, Gruber AD, Seeberger PH, Lepenies B. The C-type lectin receptor SIGNR3 binds to fungi present in commensal microbiota and influences immune regulation in experimental colitis. *Front Immunol.* (2013) 4:196. doi: 10.3389/fimmu.2013.00196
69. Franchi L, Eigenbrod T, Munoz-Planillo R, Nunez G. The inflammasome: a caspase-1-activation platform that regulates immune responses and disease pathogenesis. *Nat Immunol.* (2009) 10:241–7. doi: 10.1038/ni.1703
70. Lopez-Castejon G, Brough D. Understanding the mechanism of IL-1beta secretion. *Cytokine Growth Factor Rev.* (2011) 22:189–95. doi: 10.1016/j.cytogfr.2011.10.001
71. Sahoo M, Ceballos-Olvera I, del Barrio L, Re F. Role of the inflammasome, IL-1beta, and IL-18 in bacterial infections. *ScientificWorldJournal.* (2011) 11:2037–50. doi: 10.1100/2011/212680
72. Schmidt RL, Lenz LL. Distinct licensing of IL-18 and IL-1beta secretion in response to NLRP3 inflammasome activation. *PLoS ONE.* (2012) 7:e45186. doi: 10.1371/journal.pone.0045186
73. Kanneganti TD. The inflammasome: firing up innate immunity. *Immunol Rev.* (2015) 265:1–5. doi: 10.1111/imr.12297
74. He Y, Hara H, Nunez G. Mechanism and regulation of NLRP3 inflammasome activation. *Trends Biochem Sci.* (2016) 41:1012–21. doi: 10.1016/j.tibs.2016.09.002
75. Crowley SM, Vallance BA, Knodler LA. Noncanonical inflammasomes: antimicrobial defense that does not play by the rules. *Cell Microbiol.* (2017) 19. doi: 10.1111/cmi.12730
76. Knodler LA, Crowley SM, Sham HP, Yang H, Wrande M, Ma C, et al. Noncanonical inflammasome activation of caspase-4/caspase-11 mediates epithelial defenses against enteric bacterial pathogens. *Cell Host Microbe.* (2014) 16:249–56. doi: 10.1016/j.chom.2014.07.002
77. Thinwa J, Segovia JA, Bose S, Dube PH. Integrin-mediated first signal for inflammasome activation in intestinal epithelial cells. *J Immunol.* (2014) 193:1373–82. doi: 10.4049/jimmunol.1400145
78. Harrison OJ, Srinivasan N, Pott J, Schiering C, Krausgruber T, Ilott NE, et al. Epithelial-derived IL-18 regulates Th17 cell differentiation and Foxp3(+) Treg cell function in the intestine. *Mucosal Immunol.* (2015) 8:1226–36. doi: 10.1038/mi.2015.13
79. Rauch I, Deets KA, Ji DX, von Moltke J, Tenthorey JL, Lee AY, et al. NAIP-NLRC4 inflammasomes coordinate intestinal epithelial cell expulsion with eicosanoid and IL-18 release via activation of caspase-1 and−8. *Immunity.* (2017) 46:649–59. doi: 10.1016/j.immuni.2017.03.016
80. Allen IC, Scull MA, Moore CB, Holl EK, McElvania-TeKippe E, Taxman DJ, et al. The NLRP3 inflammasome mediates *in vivo* innate immunity to influenza A virus through recognition of viral RNA. *Immunity.* (2009) 30:556–65. doi: 10.1016/j.immuni.2009.02.005
81. Franchi L, Kamada N, Nakamura Y, Burberry A, Kuffa P, Suzuki S, et al. NLRC4-driven production of IL-1beta discriminates between pathogenic and commensal bacteria and promotes host intestinal defense. *Nat Immunol.* (2012) 13:449–56. doi: 10.1038/ni.2263
82. Nordlander S, Pott J, Maloy KJ. NLRC4 expression in intestinal epithelial cells mediates protection against an enteric pathogen. *Mucosal Immunol.* (2014) 7:775–85. doi: 10.1038/mi.2013.95
83. Levy M, Thaiss CA, Katz MN, Suez J, Elinav E. Inflammasomes and the microbiota–partners in the preservation of mucosal homeostasis. *Semin Immunopathol.* (2015) 37:39–46. doi: 10.1007/s00281-014-0451-7
84. Endimiani A, Luzzaro F, Brigante G, Perilli M, Lombardi G, Amicosante G, et al. Proteus mirabilis bloodstream infections: risk factors and treatment outcome related to the expression of extended-spectrum beta-lactamases. *Antimicrob Agents Chemother.* (2005) 49:2598–605. doi: 10.1128/AAC.49.7.2598-2605.2005
85. Hardt WD. Journal club. An infection biologist points out an outstanding issue in mucosal immunology. *Nature.* (2009) 459:893. doi: 10.1038/459893e
86. Seo SU, Kamada N, Munoz-Planillo R, Kim YG, Kim D, Koizumi Y, et al. Distinct commensals induce interleukin-1beta via NLRP3 inflammasome in inflammatory monocytes to promote intestinal inflammation in response to injury. *Immunity.* (2015) 42:744–55. doi: 10.1016/j.immuni.2015.03.004
87. Ignacio A, Morales CI, Camara NO, Almeida RR. Innate sensing of the gut microbiota: modulation of inflammatory and autoimmune diseases. *Front Immunol.* (2016) 7:54. doi: 10.3389/fimmu.2016.00054
88. Chen KW, Gross CJ, Sotomayor FV, Stacey KJ, Tschopp J, Sweet MJ, et al. The neutrophil NLRC4 inflammasome selectively promotes IL-1beta maturation without pyroptosis during acute Salmonella challenge. *Cell Rep.* (2014) 8:570–82. doi: 10.1016/j.celrep.2014.06.028
89. Karki R, Lee E, Place D, Samir P, Mavuluri J, Sharma BR, et al. IRF8 regulates transcription of naips for NLRC4 inflammasome activation. *Cell.* (2018) 173:920–33.e13. doi: 10.1016/j.cell.2018.02.055
90. Chi W, Li F, Chen H, Wang Y, Zhu Y, Yang X, et al. Caspase-8 promotes NLRP1/NLRP3 inflammasome activation and IL-1beta production in acute glaucoma. *Proc Natl Acad Sci USA.* (2014) 111:11181–6. doi: 10.1073/pnas.1402819111
91. Kaushal V, Dye R, Pakavathkumar P, Foveau B, Flores J, Hyman B, et al. Neuronal NLRP1 inflammasome activation of Caspase-1 coordinately regulates inflammatory interleukin-1-beta production and axonal degeneration-associated Caspase-6 activation. *Cell Death Differ.* (2015) 22:1676–86. doi: 10.1038/cdd.2015.16
92. Chen GY, Liu M, Wang F, Bertin J, Nunez G. A functional role for Nlrp6 in intestinal inflammation and tumorigenesis. *J Immunol.* (2011) 186:7187–94. doi: 10.4049/jimmunol.1100412
93. Levy M, Thaiss CA, Zeevi D, Dohnalova L, Zilberman-Schapira G, Mahdi JA, et al. Microbiota-modulated metabolites shape the intestinal microenvironment by regulating NLRP6 inflammasome signaling. *Cell.* (2015) 163:1428–43. doi: 10.1016/j.cell.2015.10.048
94. Micaroni M, Stanley AC, Khromykh T, Venturato J, Wong CX, Lim JP, et al. Rab6a/a′ are important Golgi regulators of pro-inflammatory TNF secretion in macrophages. *PLoS ONE.* (2013) 8:e57034. doi: 10.1371/journal.pone.0057034
95. Brough D, Rothwell NJ. Caspase-1-dependent processing of pro-interleukin-1beta is cytosolic and precedes cell death. *J Cell Sci.* (2007) 120(Pt 5):772–81. doi: 10.1242/jcs.03377
96. Pallett MA, Crepin VF, Serafini N, Habibzay M, Kotik O, Sanchez-Garrido J, et al. Bacterial virulence factor inhibits caspase-4/11 activation in intestinal epithelial cells. *Mucosal Immunol.* (2017) 10:602–12. doi: 10.1038/mi.2016.77
97. Guo H, Callaway JB, Ting JP. Inflammasomes: mechanism of action, role in disease, and therapeutics. *Nat Med.* (2015) 21:677–87. doi: 10.1038/nm.3893
98. Thi HTH, Hong S. Inflammasome as a therapeutic target for cancer prevention and treatment. *J Cancer Prev.* (2017) 22:62–73. doi: 10.15430/JCP.2017.22.2.62
99. Maes M, Kubera M, Leunis JC. The gut-brain barrier in major depression: intestinal mucosal dysfunction with an increased translocation of LPS from gram negative enterobacteria (leaky gut) plays a role in the inflammatory pathophysiology of depression. *Neuro Endocrinol Lett.* (2008) 29:117–24. doi: 10.1016/j.jad.2012.02.023

100. Roselletti E, Perito S, Gabrielli E, Mencacci A, Pericolini E, Sabbatini S, et al. NLRP3 inflammasome is a key player in human vulvovaginal disease caused by *Candida albicans*. *Sci Rep.* (2017) 7:17877. doi: 10.1038/s41598-017-17649-8
101. Joly S, Ma N, Sadler JJ, Soll DR, Cassel SL, Sutterwala FS. Cutting edge: *Candida albicans* hyphae formation triggers activation of the Nlrp3 inflammasome. *J Immunol.* (2009) 183:3578–81. doi: 10.4049/jimmunol.0901323
102. Gombault A, Baron L, Couillin I. ATP release and purinergic signaling in NLRP3 inflammasome activation. *Front Immunol.* (2012) 3:414. doi: 10.3389/fimmu.2012.00414
103. Amores-Iniesta J, Barbera-Cremades M, Martinez CM, Pons JA, Revilla-Nuin B, Martinez-Alarcon L, et al. Extracellular ATP activates the NLRP3 inflammasome and is an early danger signal of skin allograft rejection. *Cell Rep.* (2017) 21:3414–26. doi: 10.1016/j.celrep.2017.11.079
104. Franchi L, Kanneganti TD, Dubyak GR, Nunez G. Differential requirement of P2X7 receptor and intracellular K+ for caspase-1 activation induced by intracellular and extracellular bacteria. *J Biol Chem.* (2007) 282:18810–8. doi: 10.1074/jbc.M610762200
105. Dubyak GR. P2X7 receptor regulation of non-classical secretion from immune effector cells. *Cell Microbiol.* (2012) 14:1697–706. doi: 10.1111/cmi.12001
106. Franceschini A, Capece M, Chiozzi P, Falzoni S, Sanz JM, Sarti AC, et al. The P2X7 receptor directly interacts with the NLRP3 inflammasome scaffold protein. *FASEB J.* (2015) 29:2450–61. doi: 10.1096/fj.14-268714
107. den Besten G, van Eunen K, Groen AK, Venema K, Reijngoud DJ, Bakker BM. The role of short-chain fatty acids in the interplay between diet, gut microbiota, and host energy metabolism. *J Lipid Res.* (2013) 54:2325–40. doi: 10.1194/jlr.R036012
108. Grebe A, Hoss F, Latz E. NLRP3 inflammasome and the IL-1 pathway in atherosclerosis. *Circ Res.* (2018) 122:1722–40. doi: 10.1161/CIRCRESAHA.118.311362
109. Munoz-Planillo R, Kuffa P, Martinez-Colon G, Smith BL, Rajendiran TM, Nunez G. K(+) efflux is the common trigger of NLRP3 inflammasome activation by bacterial toxins and particulate matter. *Immunity.* (2013) 38:1142–53. doi: 10.1016/j.immuni.2013.05.016
110. Mabuchi T, Takekoshi T, Hwang ST. Epidermal CCR6^{+} gammadelta T cells are major producers of IL-22 and IL-17 in a murine model of psoriasiform dermatitis. *J Immunol.* (2011) 187:5026–31. doi: 10.4049/jimmunol.1101817
111. Malhotra N, Yoon J, Leyva-Castillo JM, Galand C, Archer N, Miller LS, et al. IL-22 derived from gammadelta T cells restricts *Staphylococcus aureus* infection of mechanically injured skin. *J Allergy Clin Immunol.* (2016) 138:1098–107.e93. doi: 10.1016/j.jaci.2016.07.001
112. Steinbach S, Vordermeier HM, Jones GJ. CD4^{+} and gammadelta T cells are the main producers of IL-22 and IL-17A in lymphocytes from *Mycobacterium bovis*-infected cattle. *Sci Rep.* (2016) 6:29990. doi: 10.1038/srep29990
113. Tyler CJ, McCarthy NE, Lindsay JO, Stagg AJ, Moser B, Eberl M. Antigen-presenting human gammadelta T cells promote intestinal CD4(+) T cell expression of IL-22 and mucosal release of calprotectin. *J Immunol.* (2017) 198:3417–25. doi: 10.4049/jimmunol.1700003
114. Xu X, Weiss ID, Zhang HH, Singh SP, Wynn TA, Wilson MS, et al. Conventional NK cells can produce IL-22 and promote host defense in *Klebsiella pneumoniae* pneumonia. *J Immunol.* (2014) 192:1778–86. doi: 10.4049/jimmunol.1300039
115. Zheng Y, Valdez PA, Danilenko DM, Hu Y, Sa SM, Gong Q, et al. Interleukin-22 mediates early host defense against attaching and effacing bacterial pathogens. *Nat Med.* (2008) 14:282–9. doi: 10.1038/nm1720
116. Ota N, Wong K, Valdez PA, Zheng Y, Crellin NK, Diehl L, et al. IL-22 bridges the lymphotoxin pathway with the maintenance of colonic lymphoid structures during infection with *Citrobacter rodentium*. *Nat Immunol.* (2011) 12:941–8. doi: 10.1038/ni.2089
117. Kinnebrew MA, Ubeda C, Zenewicz LA, Smith N, Flavell RA, Pamer EG. Bacterial flagellin stimulates Toll-like receptor 5-dependent defense against vancomycin-resistant Enterococcus infection. *J Infect Dis.* (2010) 201:534–43. doi: 10.1086/650203
118. Abt MC, Buffie CG, Susac B, Becattini S, Carter RA, Leiner I, et al. TLR-7 activation enhances IL-22-mediated colonization resistance against vancomycin-resistant enterococcus. *Sci Transl Med.* (2016) 8:327ra325. doi: 10.1126/scitranslmed.aad6663
119. Sellau J, Alvarado CF, Hoenow S, Mackroth MS, Kleinschmidt D, Huber S, et al. IL-22 dampens the T cell response in experimental malaria. *Sci Rep.* (2016) 6:28058. doi: 10.1038/srep28058
120. Behnsen J, Jellbauer S, Wong CP, Edwards RA, George MD, Ouyang W, et al. The cytokine IL-22 promotes pathogen colonization by suppressing related commensal bacteria. *Immunity.* (2014) 40:262–73. doi: 10.1016/j.immuni.2014.01.003
121. Stelter C, Kappeli R, Konig C, Krah A, Hardt WD, Stecher B, et al. Salmonella-induced mucosal lectin RegIIIbeta kills competing gut microbiota. *PLoS ONE.* (2011) 6:e20749. doi: 10.1371/journal.pone.0020749
122. Hayden JA, Brophy MB, Cunden LS, Nolan EM. High-affinity manganese coordination by human calprotectin is calcium-dependent and requires the histidine-rich site formed at the dimer interface. *J Am Chem Soc.* (2013) 135:775–87. doi: 10.1021/ja3096416
123. Feinen B, Russell MW. Contrasting roles of IL-22 and IL-17 in murine genital tract infection by *Neisseria gonorrhoeae*. *Front Immunol.* (2012) 3:11. doi: 10.3389/fimmu.2012.00011
124. Quintana FJ. The aryl hydrocarbon receptor: a molecular pathway for the environmental control of the immune response. *Immunology.* (2013) 138:183–9. doi: 10.1111/imm.12046
125. Murray IA, Perdew GH. Ligand activation of the Ah receptor contributes to gastrointestinal homeostasis. *Curr Opin Toxicol.* (2017) 2:15–23. doi: 10.1016/j.cotox.2017.01.003
126. Gao J, Xu K, Liu H, Liu G, Bai M, Peng C, et al. Impact of the gut microbiota on intestinal immunity mediated by tryptophan metabolism. *Front Cell Infect Microbiol.* (2018) 8:13. doi: 10.3389/fcimb.2018.00013
127. Million M, Tomas J, Wagner C, Lelouard H, Raoult D, Gorvel J-P. New insights in gut microbiota and mucosal immunity of the small intestine. *Hum Microbiome J.* (2018) 7–8:23–32. doi: 10.1016/j.humic.2018.01.004
128. Yitbarek A, Taha-Abdelaziz K, Hodgins DC, Read L, Nagy E, Weese JS, et al. Gut microbiota-mediated protection against influenza virus subtype H9N2 in chickens is associated with modulation of the innate responses. *Sci Rep.* (2018) 8:13189. doi: 10.1038/s41598-018-31613-0
129. Natividad JM, Agus A, Planchais J, Lamas B, Jarry AC, Martin R, et al. Impaired aryl hydrocarbon receptor ligand production by the gut microbiota is a key factor in metabolic syndrome. *Cell Metab.* (2018) 28:737–49.e4. doi: 10.1016/j.cmet.2018.07.001
130. Zelante T, Iannitti RG, Cunha C, De Luca A, Giovannini G, Pieraccini G, et al. Tryptophan catabolites from microbiota engage aryl hydrocarbon receptor and balance mucosal reactivity via interleukin-22. *Immunity.* (2013) 39:372–85. doi: 10.1016/j.immuni.2013.08.003
131. Valeri M, Raffatellu M. Cytokines IL-17 and IL-22 in the host response to infection. *Pathog Dis.* (2016) 74:ftw111. doi: 10.1093/femspd/ftw111
132. Krishnan S, Ding Y, Saedi N, Choi M, Sridharan GV, Sherr DH, et al. Gut microbiota-derived tryptophan metabolites modulate inflammatory response in hepatocytes and macrophages. *Cell Rep.* (2018) 23:1099–111. doi: 10.1016/j.celrep.2018.03.109
133. Ismail AS, Severson KM, Vaishnava S, Behrendt CL, Yu X, Benjamin JL, et al. Gammadelta intraepithelial lymphocytes are essential mediators of host-microbial homeostasis at the intestinal mucosal surface. *Proc Natl Acad Sci USA.* (2011) 108:8743–8. doi: 10.1073/pnas.1019574108
134. Witter AR, Okunnu BM, Berg RE. The essential role of neutrophils during infection with the intracellular bacterial pathogen listeria monocytogenes. *J Immunol.* (2016) 197:1557–65. doi: 10.4049/jimmunol.1600599
135. Nielsen MM, Witherden DA, Havran WL. gammadelta T cells in homeostasis and host defence of epithelial barrier tissues. *Nat Rev Immunol.* (2017) 17:733–45. doi: 10.1038/nri.2017.101
136. Krishnan S, Prise IE, Wemyss K, Schenck LP, Bridgeman HM, McClure FA, et al. Amphiregulin-producing gammadelta T cells are vital for safeguarding oral barrier immune homeostasis. *Proc Natl Acad Sci USA.* (2018) 115:10738–43. doi: 10.1073/pnas.1802320115
137. Heiss CN, Olofsson LE. The role of the gut microbiota in development, function and disorders of the central nervous system and the enteric nervous system. *J Neuroendocrinol.* (2019) e12684. doi: 10.1111/jne.12684

138. Mazmanian SK, Liu CH, Tzianabos AO, Kasper DL. An immunomodulatory molecule of symbiotic bacteria directs maturation of the host immune system. *Cell.* (2005) 122:107–18. doi: 10.1016/j.cell.2005.05.007
139. Couper KN, Blount DG, Riley EM. IL-10: the master regulator of immunity to infection. *J Immunol.* (2008) 180:5771–7. doi: 10.4049/jimmunol.180.9.5771
140. Cyktor JC, Turner J. Interleukin-10 and immunity against prokaryotic and eukaryotic intracellular pathogens. *Infect Immun.* (2011) 79:2964–73. doi: 10.1128/IAI.00047-11
141. Iyer SS, Cheng G. Role of interleukin 10 transcriptional regulation in inflammation and autoimmune disease. *Crit Rev Immunol.* (2012) 32:23–63. doi: 10.1615/CritRevImmunol.v32.i1.30
142. Ueda Y, Kayama H, Jeon SG, Kusu T, Isaka Y, Rakugi H, et al. Commensal microbiota induce LPS hyporesponsiveness in colonic macrophages via the production of IL-10. *Int Immunol.* (2010) 22:953–62. doi: 10.1093/intimm/dxq449
143. Rivollier A, He J, Kole A, Valatas V, Kelsall BL. Inflammation switches the differentiation program of Ly6Chi monocytes from antiinflammatory macrophages to inflammatory dendritic cells in the colon. *J Exp Med.* (2012) 209:139–55. doi: 10.1084/jem.20101387
144. Hayashi A, Sato T, Kamada N, Mikami Y, Matsuoka K, Hisamatsu T, et al. A single strain of *Clostridium butyricum* induces intestinal IL-10-producing macrophages to suppress acute experimental colitis in mice. *Cell Host Microbe.* (2013) 13:711–22. doi: 10.1016/j.chom.2013.05.013
145. Ochi T, Feng Y, Kitamoto S, Nagao-Kitamoto H, Kuffa P, Atarashi K, et al. Diet-dependent, microbiota-independent regulation of IL-10-producing lamina propria macrophages in the small intestine. *Sci Rep.* (2016) 6:27634. doi: 10.1038/srep27634
146. Quiros M, Nishio H, Neumann PA, Siuda D, Brazil JC, Azcutia V, et al. Macrophage-derived IL-10 mediates mucosal repair by epithelial WISP-1 signaling. *J Clin Invest.* (2017) 127:3510–20. doi: 10.1172/JCI90229
147. Sassone-Corsi M, Raffatellu M. No vacancy: how beneficial microbes cooperate with immunity to provide colonization resistance to pathogens. *J Immunol.* (2015) 194:4081–7. doi: 10.4049/jimmunol.1403169
148. Crouzet L, Derrien M, Cherbuy C, Plancade S, Foulon M, Chalin B, et al. *Lactobacillus paracasei* CNCM I-3689 reduces vancomycin-resistant *Enterococcus persistence* and promotes *Bacteroidetes resilience* in the gut following antibiotic challenge. *Sci Rep.* (2018) 8:5098. doi: 10.1038/s41598-018-23437-9

18

Commensal Bacteria: An Emerging Player in Defense Against Respiratory Pathogens

Rabia Khan, Fernanda Cristina Petersen and Sudhanshu Shekhar**

Faculty of Dentistry, Institute of Oral Biology, University of Oslo, Oslo, Norway

***Correspondence:**
Rabia Khan
rabia_naeemkhan@hotmail.com
Sudhanshu Shekhar
sudhanshu.shekhar@odont.uio.no

A diverse community of trillions of commensal bacteria inhabits mucosal and epidermal surfaces in humans and plays an important role in defense against pathogens, including respiratory pathogens. Commensal bacteria act on the host's immune system to induce protective responses that prevent colonization and invasion by pathogens. On the other hand, these bacteria can directly inhibit the growth of respiratory pathogens by producing antimicrobial products/signals and competing for nutrients and adhesion sites. Such mechanisms preserve the niche for commensal bacteria and support the host in containing respiratory infections. Herein, we discuss current evidence on the role of commensal bacteria in conferring protection against respiratory pathogens and the underlying mechanisms by which these bacteria do so. A deeper knowledge of how commensal bacteria interact with the host and pathogens might provide new insights that are poised to aid in the development of vaccines and therapeutics that target infectious diseases.

Keywords: host, commensal, pathogen, lungs, vaccine

INTRODUCTION

Since the inception of the Human Microbiome Project in 2007, a plethora of knowledge has accumulated that throws light on diverse and crucial roles played by commensal bacteria in homeostasis and disease (1, 2). With the help of advances in omic and systems biology technologies, our knowledge of the composition, genetics, and functional capacity of commensal bacteria is growing at a fast pace. It is becoming clear that commensal bacteria, which reside in various parts of the human body, such as the gut and airways, correspond approximately to the total number of human cells (about 1:1 ratio), and exert a profound impact on regulation of immunophysiological functions, including but not limited to, metabolism, ontogeny, and pathogen defense (3, 4). Several recent studies have shown that commensals promote resistance to gut pathogens that is mutually beneficial to the host and the commensal microbiota (5–7). However, imbalances in the microbial communities can occur, and are linked to many diseases, such as inflammatory bowel disease, allergies, asthma, diabetes, and obesity (8). It remains scantily understood how these bacteria execute their functional activities against respiratory pathogens. Respiratory infections are of utmost importance, as they inflict substantial social and economic burden on people across the world in general and in low and lower-middle income countries in particular (9–11). Additionally, current therapeutic and prophylactic interventions against respiratory diseases have major constraints, such as rapid emergence of anti-microbial resistance and disruption of the normal microbiota by use of antibiotics. Unraveling the interactions between commensals and pathogens may allow the exploitation of inhibitory properties of commensals to combat pathogens causing respiratory diseases. In this review article, we provide an overview of the current state of knowledge about the role of commensal bacteria in protective immunity to respiratory pathogens and the mechanisms involved in commensal bacteria mediated defenses. Understanding the relationship between commensal bacteria, host, and pathogen is a way forward to develop safe and effective prophylactics and therapeutics against pathogens.

COMMENSAL BACTERIA MEDIATED PROTECTION

Protection in Mouse Models

Much of what is known about the direct role of commensal bacteria in protection against respiratory pathogens stems from studies using various mouse models, including germ-free and antibiotic-treated mice (12–23). Following lung infection with *Streptococcus pneumoniae*, numerous studies have shown that antibiotic-treated mice display significantly higher pathogen loads and increased pathologies in the lungs compared with sham-treated mice (15, 21). Likewise, germ-free mice showed enhanced levels of bacterial burden when subjected to *S. pneumoniae* and *Klebsiella pneumoniae* lung infections (15). Similar to the protection conferred by fecal microbiota transplant (FMT) against intestinal pathogens, FMT in gut microbiota-depleted mice restored pulmonary bacterial clearance early after *S. pneumoniae* infection (21). In case of mouse models of *Mycobacterium tuberculosis* infection, gut microbiota disruption after pre- and post-antibiotic treatment showed decreased resistance to infection in the lungs, which was associated with severe histopathological changes, such as pulmonary granulomas (24). Furthermore, antibiotic-induced dysbiosis changed the microbiota diversity in the gut and promoted lung colonization by *M. tuberculosis* (25). Similar protective effect was conferred after mice having antibiotic-induced disrupted microbiota received an intranasal infectious dose of influenza A virus (12). In a different study, FMT into germ-free mice led to reconstitution of the gut microbiota that facilitated increased survival against lethal influenza A virus infection (26). Overall, these studies employing multiple experimental approaches provide *in vivo* evidence that underscores a profound contribution of commensal bacteria in defense against diverse respiratory pathogens.

Even though antibiotic-treated and germ-free mice have proven to be a crucial tool in understanding the role of the microbiota in pathogen defense, there are potential pitfalls that need consideration while interpreting results from studies involving these animals. Germ-free animals lack all detectable microbes in different organs and have an impaired immune system, whereas antibiotics are used to deplete specific microbiota (27). Although these two approaches provide crucial information on the function of the microbiota in general, the specific contribution of the microbiota found in different body compartments, such as the lung microbiota, in immunity to respiratory infections is unclear. This is important because the lung microbiota, which in healthy adults seems to mainly consist of a small number of bacteria originating from the oral cavity, plays a significant role in respiratory health, and disease (28–30). Additionally, there is a need for models that can answer a more direct question about protection in the presence of a fully developed immune system. To address this issue, researchers have attempted to deplete the lung microbiota in mice by a combination of aerosolized vancomycin and neomycin via nasal route, which resulted in a significant reduction in the lung commensal microbiota, with the advantage of minimally affecting the gut microbiota (31, 32). But the possibility of antibiotic spread to the nearby tissues/organs harboring different microbiota remains, requiring future studies to focus on developing better models to fill in this pitfall.

The microbiota consists of a large number of bacterial species, and therefore, it is of great interest to specifically identify commensal species that protect from respiratory pathogens. Recent studies have evaluated the protective efficacy of commensal bacterial species in respiratory infections. Oral administration of *Bifidobacterium longum* (BB536), but not saline, in mice significantly reduced viral loads, pulmonary pathology, and body weight loss following intranasal challenge with influenza virus, suggesting a protective role for this commensal bacterium in influenza infection (33). Similarly, oral or nasal inoculation of mice with different strains of *Lactobacillus*, e.g., *L. gasseri* (TMC0356), *L. rhamnosus* (CRL 1505), and *L. brevis* (KB290), conferred protective immunity to influenza virus infections (34–36). Furthermore, *L. rhamnosus* (CRL 1505) exerted a protective effect in mice subjected to an intranasal challenge with respiratory syncytial virus infection (37, 38). These data indicate a prophylactic role for commensal bacteria against viral pathogens. In order to assess therapeutic significance, *B. longum* (MM2) was orally administered in mice infected with influenza virus. Mice that received *B. longum* (MM2) ameliorated infection, as determined by decreased body weight loss, viral titers, and inflammation, compared with control mice (39). Protective effect induced by these probiotic bacteria is not confined to respiratory infections with viruses, but can be applicable to bacterial pathogens (37–40). Intake of *B. longum* (5^{1A}) in mice not only demonstrated protective effect against infection with *K. pneumoniae*, but also suppressed inflammatory changes in the lung (40). Very recently, we have demonstrated that intranasal immunization of mice with the commensal *Streptococcus mitis* conferred protection against lung infection with *S. pneumoniae* strains D39 (serotype 2) and TIGR4 (serotype 4), which illuminates the unique ability of *S. mitis* to offer resistance to different pneumococcal serotypes (41). Two recent studies performed by independent groups further show that the gut colonizer bacterium *Helicobacter hepaticus* influences the composition of the gut microbiota and the outcome of *M. tuberculosis* infection in mouse models (42, 43). Mice subjected to intestinal colonization with *H. hepaticus*, when challenged by intranasal route with *M. tuberculosis*, reflected higher mycobacterial burden in the lungs compared with the controls (42). This increased mycobacterial burden in the *H. hepaticus*-colonized mice coincided with severe *M. tuberculosis*-mediated pulmonary pathologies, mainly characterized by granulomas and tissue damage, and accumulation/production of inflammatory leukocytes/cytokines (42). Similar to these results, mice colonized with *H. hepaticus* eliminated subunit-vaccine-induced protective immunity to lung infection with *M. tuberculosis* (43). Taken together, these findings indicate that commensal bacteria can be harnessed for prophylactic and therapeutic purposes, provided utmost precaution on the possible negative effects of enriching for specific colonizers of the microbiota.

Protection in Humans

Relatively little information is available on whether commensal bacteria can prevent respiratory infections in humans. Oral commensals, such as *Streptococcus oralis* and *Streptococcus salivarius*, can induce protection against middle ear inflammation, referred to as otitis media, which is primarily caused by respiratory pathogens, such as *S. pneumoniae* and *Haemophilus influenzae* (44–46). Upon intranasal administration of *S. salivarius* and *S. oralis*, children susceptible to acute otitis media displayed reduced recurrences of disease with no side effects (44). Contrarily, a nasal spray containing oral commensals, e.g., *S. mitis* and *S. oralis*, in susceptible children under 4 years of age showed no significant effect regarding the number of episodes of recurrent otitis media compared to the placebo group (46). The discrepancy in these studies might be due to differences in bacterial doses, inoculation regimens, and combinations, which need to be analyzed in light of new technologies (e.g., metagenomics and next generation sequencing) and concepts like dysbiosis. The fact that antibiotics were used together with the streptococcal nasal spray in the first study, but not in the second, is also an important factor to consider. In controlled infection studies in humans, nasopharyngeal colonization by the commensal *Neisseria lactamica* provided protection against the respiratory pathogen *Neisseria meningitidis* (47, 48). Furthermore, in a block-randomized challenge trial, 310 healthy individuals (18–25 years) were intranasally inoculated with live *N. lactamica* or sham and the bacterial carriage was monitored for 26 weeks (48). All those who developed nasopharyngeal colonization by *N. lactamica* revealed a significant reduction in the *N. meningitidis* carriage compared with sham-treated ones (48). These studies show that commensal bacteria not only show inhibitory/displacing effects on the carriage of respiratory pathogens but also highlight the ease and safety with which these bacteria can be used to contain infections in humans. It is however notable that most bacteria with high pathogenic potential, such as those in the above examples, are also part of the healthy microbiome (49). The reason as to why these pathogens cause diseases is attributed to various host and microbial factors, including viral infections (49). Dysbiosis in particular, such as a result of antibiotic use has been associated with a reduction in the prevalence of respiratory commensal bacteria like *Corynebacterium* spp. and *Dolosigranulum* spp. in the nasopharynx of healthy infants. These are considered to reduce the colonization by *S. pneumoniae*, *H. influenzae*, and *S. aureus* in the respiratory tract (50). It is further shown that respiratory syncytial virus infection in children below 2 years of age was positively correlated with nasopharyngeal *H. influenzae* and *Streptococcus* microbiota clusters and inversely correlated with *Staphylococcus aureus* (51). Transcriptomic analysis of the children infected with *H. influenzae* and *Streptococcus* clusters presented greater expression of immune components, suggesting that nasopharyngeal microbiota can influence host immunity (51). In line with this, prolonged antibiotic treatment in early life has also been annexed with an increased risk for respiratory infections in infants (52, 53). Thus, these studies shine light on the effect of the microbiota perturbations caused by antibiotics on host susceptibility to respiratory infections, particularly during the critical life period of immune maturation.

MECHANISMS OF COMMENSAL BACTERIA MEDIATED PROTECTION

A pertinent question however remains as to what are the underlying mechanisms by which commensal bacteria perform their protective function against respiratory pathogens. Emerging data thus far indicate that commensal bacteria confer protection in two ways: host-mediated immunity (acting on the host's immune system) and direct action (directly inhibiting/killing pathogens and competing for colonization).

Host-Mediated Immunity

A wealth of emerging evidence indicates that both the lung and gut microbiota are involved in the regulation of immune responses during lung infections (28, 54). However, it is difficult to assess the specific contributions of the lung and gut microbiota to protective immunity to respiratory pathogens, mainly due to three reasons: (1) the gut microbiota is the largest and most diverse community of commensals that significantly influences the outcome of immunity in the lungs as well as gut; (2) the gut is the largest lymphoid organ in the body because of which it occupies a central position in host-microbiota studies; and (3) we do not have optimal models to ascertain their specific roles in immunity. Despite an important role for these commensal bacteria in promoting resistance against respiratory pathogens, the mechanistic basis for this resistance remains unclear. Several studies have shown a potential defect in innate immunity and subsequent adaptive immunity in the lung, when signals from commensal bacteria are abrogated (12, 14, 25, 55). Key innate immune cells that are recruited to the lungs and are involved in protective immunity include macrophages, natural killer (NK) cells, and mucosal-associated invariant T (MAIT) cells (12, 14, 25, 55). The pulmonary macrophages in mice depleted of the microbiota by antibiotics reflected reduced expression of the macrophage-associated antiviral genes, such as Irf 7, Ifnb, Mx1, Tnfa, Il6, and Il1b following influenza virus infection (14). This corresponded with reduced response to IFN-γ, IFN-α, or influenza infection in macrophages from the mice treated with antibiotics. *In vivo* experiments in mice also indicated that the alveolar macrophage response was impaired during viral infection, which was characterized by down-regulation of most of the antiviral genes activated *ex vivo* (14). Wang et al. demonstrated a new mechanism in mice colonized with *S. aureus* where $CD11b^{+}$ M2 alveolar macrophages, stimulated with Toll-like receptor (TLR) 2, play a protective role in influenza infection (56). Another innate immune cell type is MAIT cell that is shown to play an important role in microbiota mediated mycobacterial immunity (25). Flow cytometric analysis reflected that mice depleted of the microbiota had reduced number of lung MAIT cells, characterized by MR1-5-OP-RU tetramer^{+}TCRβ^{+} phenotype, which expressed significantly lower IL-17A compared with control mice, suggesting that lung MAIT cells may function to contain early pulmonary *M. tuberculosis* infection (25). Furthermore, NK cells from germ-free mice did not induce anti-influenza immunity because macrophages and dendritic cells failed to produce type 1 IFN in response to infection (55). Cumulatively, these data suggest that microbiota-derived signals provide a stimulus that maintains the potency of the lung innate immune system needed for invoking effective immunity (**Figure 1**).

Adaptive immunity follows innate immunity and is crucial for specific immunity against respiratory pathogens (57–59). Rabbit antisera raised against *S. mitis* show cross-reactivity with *S. pneumoniae* (59). Similar to IgG mediated cross-reactivity, IgA antibodies from the sera, nasal wash, and bronchoalveolar lavage of mice vaccinated with *S. mitis* cross-reacted with *S. pneumoniae* serotypes 2 and 4 (41). On the other hand, human CD4^{+} T cells expressing IL-17A, which are reactive to *S. mitis*, show cross-reactivity toward *S. pneumoniae* in an *in vitro* culture system (60). Intranasal vaccination of mice with *S. mitis* led to an increased production of IL-17A by CD4^{+} T cells in the lungs compared to PBS-treated control mice (41). These results are in line with the evidence that the gut commensal segmented filamentous bacteria (SFB) regulate pulmonary Th17 immunity to the fungal pathogen *Aspergillus fumigatus* (19). In a mouse model of influenza viral infection, it is shown that commensal bacteria regulate virus-specific CD4^{+} and CD8^{+} T cells and antibodies following lung infection with virus (12). Overall, commensal bacteria mediated adaptive immunity to respiratory pathogens include both humoral (IgG and IgA) and T cell-mediated responses.

Involvement of the gut microbiota in protective immunity to pulmonary pathogens illustrates a pathogenic nexus between the microbiota and the "gut-lung axis," underscoring a profound protective influence of the gut commensals over several pathogens residing at distant anatomical compartments of the body (61). The gut microbiota mediated control of the lung immunopathology is also evident from studies demonstrating the susceptibility of animals with the altered gut microbiota to allergic lung diseases (20). On the other hand, dysbiosis in the lung microbiota can change the composition of the gut microbiota. For example, mice subjected to lung infection with influenza virus infection or intranasal instillation of lipopolysaccharide disturbed the gut microbiota homeostasis, which supports the fact that the gut and lungs are closely linked in a way that they affect each other's microbiology and physiology (62, 63). Moreover, how the gut microbiota controls the lung immunity has recently been explored by few key studies in mouse models of pulmonary bacterial infections. Brown *et al.* performed a well-designed and comprehensive study that sheds light on a major innate immune mechanism used by the microbiota to clear lung infections in mouse models (15). In antibiotic-treated mice, there was an increased growth of *S. pneumoniae* and *K. pneumoniae* in the lungs after bacterial inoculation compared to sham-treated mice, which was associated with reduced production of innate immune factors, such granulocyte–macrophage colony-stimulating factor (GM-CSF) (15). *In vivo* neutralization of GM-CSF into antibiotic-treated mice, which received the microbiota from the sham-treated mice and had restored pulmonary bacterial clearance, resulted in making these mice prone to infections (15). These findings suggest that GM-CSF is essential for the microbiota to execute their functional activities against both Gram-positive (*S. pneumoniae*) and Gram-negative (*K. pneumoniae*) pathogens. It was further demonstrated that GM-CSF programs alveolar macrophage function via an extracellular signal-regulated kinase (ERK)-specific signaling pathway leading to increased pathogen killing via reactive oxygen species (ROS) (15). Several studies have implicated pattern recognition receptor (PRR) ligands produced by the gut microbiota in controlling immune responses outside the intestinal tract (16, 64). Following antibiotic-mediated depletion of the microbiota in mice, early clearance of *K. pneumoniae* was impaired and this could be rescued by injection of bacterial Nod-like receptor (NLR) ligands (the NOD1 ligand MurNAcTri(DAP) and NOD2 ligand muramyl dipeptide [MDP]), but not bacterial TLR ligands (16). Defects in early innate immunity were found to be due to reduced ROS-mediated killing of bacteria by alveolar macrophages (16). Interestingly, upon treatment of mice with antibiotics and NLR ligands orally prior to *S. pneumoniae* lung infection, neutralization of GM-CSF abrogated the rescue of respiratory clearance (15). Taking account of all these data, it is clear that the microbiota and NLR ligands regulate lung innate immunity to respiratory pathogens via GM-CSF, highlighting crucial mechanisms of the gut-lung axis of communication. In addition, the gut commensal SFB has been reported to provide protection in immunocompromised (Rag$^{-/-}$) mice by partially enhancing neutrophil resolution during pneumococcal lung infection, which corresponded with reduced expression of the anti-phagocytic molecule CD47 (65). Like NK cells, another lymphoid cell population referred to as group 3 lymphoid cells that produce IL-22 (IL-22^{+}ILC3), a cytokine involved in pathogen defense, has been implicated in gut commensal bacteria-induced protection against *S. pneumoniae* (66). Disruption of commensal bacteria by antibiotics decreased the influx of IL-22^{+}ILC3 cells into the lungs of new born mice, which made them more prone to pneumococcal infection compared with control mice. This effect was reversed when ILC3 cells were adoptively transferred or exogenous IL-22 administered in mice (66). Thus, these immune mechanisms furnish crucial information on how the gut microbiota controls protective immunity to lung infections (**Figure 1**).

Direct Action

Commensal bacteria resist colonization of pathogens by using wide range of direct mechanisms for niche competition, such as secretion of inhibitory substances and nutrient competition, enlisting the exploitative, and interference modes of competition (67). Recent studies dissected novel mechanisms used by resident commensals to inhibit and contain respiratory pathogens, such as

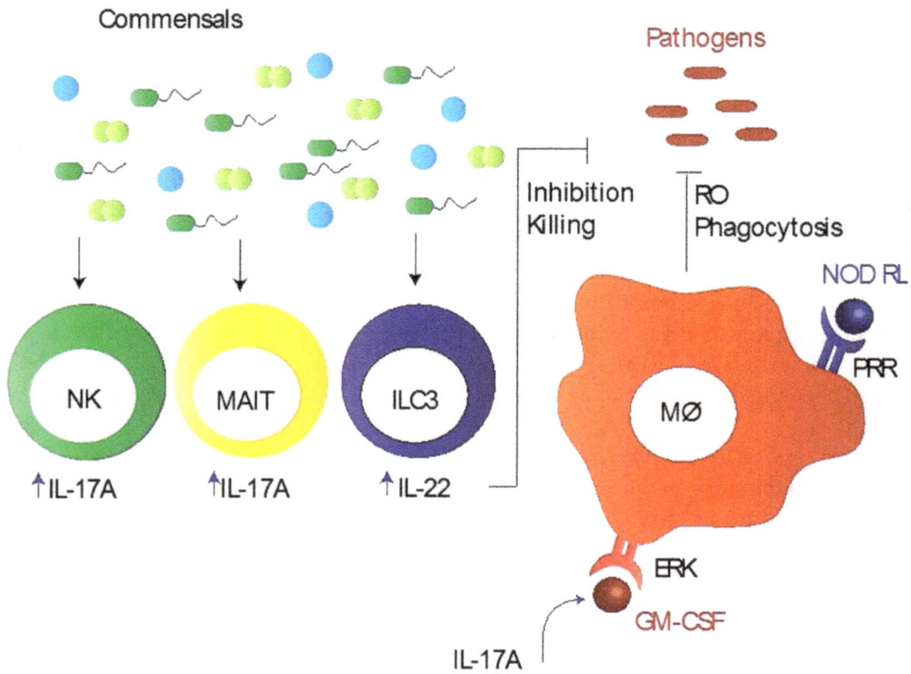

FIGURE 1 | Commensal bacteria mediated innate immunity to respiratory pathogens. Commensal bacteria stimulate various innate immune cells, particularly alveolar macrophages (Mϕ), mucosa-associated invariant T (MAIT) cells, group 3 innate lymphoid cells (ILC3), and natural killer (NK) cells, to induce early protection. These bacteria promote pathogen killing via granulocyte–macrophage colony-stimulating factor (GM-CSF), which stimulates pathogen killing and clearance by alveolar macrophages (Mϕ) through phagocytosis, reduced reactive oxygen species (RO), and extracellular signal regulated kinase (ERK) signaling. Intrapulmonary GM-CSF production in response to infection is regulated by the microbiota via interleukin-17A (IL-17A). Pattern recognition receptor (PRR) expressed by Mϕ recognizes PRR ligands, such as nod-like receptor ligands (NOD RL), leading to the activation of Mϕ. NK and MAIT cells when activated by commensal bacteria produce large quantities of IL-17A, whereas ILC3 cells secrete IL-22, aiding in inhibition/killing of various respiratory pathogens.

disruption of biofilms, exploitation of host resources to generate antimicrobial products, and down-regulation of virulence genes. This highlights the complexity and diversity of mechanisms involved in direct inhibition (68–70). The well-documented mechanism by which commensal bacteria can directly inhibit the pathogen growth and compete with them is the production of ribosomally produced antimicrobials called bacteriocins (71, 72). For example, *S. salivarius* produces a wide range of bacteriocins, which is a major mechanism that antagonizes *S. pneumoniae* (71, 73–75). More recently, it is also demonstrated that *S. salivarius* reduces the *S. pneumoniae* colonization by blocking the adhesion sites, suggesting multiple mechanisms used by this commensal to inhibit pathogens (76). Apart from ribosomally encoded bacteriocins, commensal bacteria encode non-ribosomally produced bioactive antimicrobials to compete with pathogens (77). Zipperer et al. showed that the nasal commensal *Staphylococcus lugdunensis* directly inhibits the growth of *S. aureus* through a novel cyclic antimicrobial peptide named "Lugdunin." Lugdunin possessed bactericidal activity against all tested strains of *S. aureus in vitro*. Moreover, in animal model, the co-colonization of *S. lugdunensis* and *S. aureus* resulted in competitive exclusion of *S. aureus* (77). The use of purified antimicrobials or bacterial strains encoding antimicrobials may serve as a source of new generation of antibiotics to deal with multidrug resistant strains, such as methicillin resistant *S. aureus*. One mechanism, which contributes to competitive advantage for colonization of commensal bacteria to preserve their niche and to suppress the growth of pathogens, includes the production of hydrogen peroxide. Epidemiological data show a negative correlation between *S. pneumoniae* and *S. aureus* and presumably, the reason for increased *S. aureus* related otitis media after use of pneumococcal vaccine (78, 79). One possible mechanism implicated to define this negative association is hydrogen peroxide mediated inhibition of *S. aureus* by pneumococcal hydrogen peroxide (80).

Nutrient competition is also a strategy used by commensal bacteria to reduce the fitness of pathogens by competing for the same pool of resources (81). Stubbendieck et al. recently showed that isolates of *Corynebacterium* spp. inhibited *Staphylococcus* spp. *in vitro*. This inhibition was due to reduced iron bioavailability, mediated by siderophore-induced sequestration of iron by *Corynebacterium* spp. (82). Another novel mechanism of commensal mediated inhibition is through the production of secreted enzymes. Iwase et al. first demonstrated the negative correlation between the commensal *Staphylococcus epidermidis* and pathogenic *S. aureus* in human nasal samples. To gain further insight to explain this negative association, they identified the inhibitory factor produced by *S. epidermidis* as serine protease, which inhibits the biofilm formation and

TABLE 1 | Examples of direct mechanisms of colonization resistance used by commensal bacteria against respiratory pathogens.

Commensal bacteria	Anatomical location	Mechanism of inhibition	Respiratory pathogens	References
Streptococcus salivarius	Oral cavity	Ribosomally synthesized antimicrobials (Bacteriocins)	*Streptococcus pneumoniae* *Streptococcus pyogenes*	(71)
Staphylococcus lugdunensis	Skin, and nasal cavity	Non-ribosomally synthesized antimicrobials (Lugdunin)	*Staphylococcus aureus*	(77)
Corynebacterium accolens	Skin, and nasal cavity	Metabolic products with antimicrobial properties (Free fatty acids)	*Streptococcus pneumoniae*	(69)
Staphylococcus epidermidis	Skin and nasal cavity	Secreted enzymes (Serine protease)	*Staphylococcus aureus*	(68)
Streptococcus pneumoniae	Nasopharynx, and oral cavity	Hydrogen peroxide (H_2O_2) mediated killing	*Staphylococcus aureus*	(80)
Corynebacterium spp.	Skin and nasal cavity	Nutrient competition (Iron limitation by siderophore production)	*Staphylococcus* spp.	(82)

human nasal colonization by *S. aureus* (68). Follow-up study from the same group showed that intranasal colonization of mice with serine protease producing *S. epidermidis* inhibited colonization with methicillin resistant *S. aureus* (83). Commensal bacteria also exploit the host resources to generate metabolic compounds with antimicrobial properties to suppress the growth of respiratory pathogens. An elegant study by Bomar et al. investigated the mechanistic explanation for correlation between increased abundance of *Corynebacterium* species and reduced *S. pneumoniae* colonization (69). Interestingly, they found that *Corynebacterium accolens* encodes lipase, which catalyzes the hydrolysis of host triacylglycerolsto to produce free fatty acids with antibacterial properties that suppress the growth of *S. pneumoniae* (69). Taken together, the above examples evidently suggest that antagonistic interactions exist in the polymicrobial community utilizing wide range of mechanisms by which commensal bacteria inhibit respiratory pathogens. Advanced understanding of existing mechanisms using both *in vitro* and *in vivo* models and further elucidation of novel mechanisms may enable us to exploit commensals to inhibit respiratory pathogens. Mechanisms used by commensal bacteria to directly inhibit/kill respiratory pathogens are exemplified in **Table 1**.

CONCLUSIONS AND FUTURE INSIGHTS

Advanced research technologies have been applied to evaluate the contribution of commensal bacteria to respiratory infections. Accumulating evidence indicates an important role for commensal bacteria in defense against respiratory pathogens, which paves the way to target these bacteria for the development of vaccines and therapeutics that provide optimal protection with safety and low cost. Moreover, the use of modern experimental tools to decipher the novel mechanisms used by commensals to inhibit pathogens may assist in designing novel therapeutics with targeted approach focusing exclusively on the pathogen inhibition without disrupting the homeostatic microbial community. Future studies are required to address the following questions: (1) What are the underlying mechanisms by which the trio of commensals, pathogens, and host interact with each other? (2) What could be the long-term consequences of using commensal bacteria-based vaccines/therapeutics on the host, pathogens, and the microbiota? (3) What are the effects of medical manipulations, such as antibiotics and probiotics, on the biology of commensal bacteria? (4) How can we use commensal bacteria-expressed bacteriocins for protection against respiratory pathogens? (5) Which specific commensal bacterial species of the microbiota are directly involved in protection immunity to different pathogens? (6) How can we use commensal microbiota/bacteria to correct dysbiosis? A sincere exploration of these questions may have implications for the clinical use of commensal bacteria with inhibitory properties against pathogens. This may be important to bypass the drawbacks associated with currently available options, such as antimicrobial resistance.

AUTHOR CONTRIBUTIONS

RK, FP, and SS wrote and revised the manuscript. All authors assisted in the conception of this review and acquisition of relevant literature. All authors gave approval of the last version to be published.

FUNDING

This work was supported by a grant from the Norwegian Research Council (Grant number - 241011).

REFERENCES

1. Turnbaugh PJ, Ley RE, Hamady M, Fraser-Liggett CM, Knight R, Gordon JI. The human microbiome project. *Nature.* (2007) 449:804–10. doi: 10.1038/nature 06244
2. Gevers D, Knight R, Petrosino JF, Huang K, McGuire AL, Birren BW, et al. The human microbiome project: a community resource for the healthy human microbiome. *PLoS Biol.* (2012) 10:e1001377. doi: 10.1371/journal.pbio.1001377
3. Sender R, Fuchs S, Milo R. Revised estimates for the number of human and bacteria cells in the body. *PLoS*

Biol. (2016) 14:e1002533. doi: 10.1371/journal.pbio.1002533

4. Wang BH, Yao MF, Lv LX, Ling ZX, Li LJ. The human microbiota in health and disease. *Eng Prc.* (2017) 3:71–82. doi: 10.1016/J.ENG.2017.01.008
5. Kamada N, Seo SU, Chen GY, Nunez G. Role of the gut microbiota in immunity and inflammatory disease. *Nat Rev Immunol.* (2013) 13:321–35. doi: 10.1038/nri3430
6. Abt MC, Pamer EG. Commensal bacteria mediated defenses against pathogens. *Curr Opin Immunol.* (2014) 29:16–22. doi: 10.1016/j.coi.2014.03.003
7. Buffie CG, Pamer EG. Microbiota-mediated colonization resistance against intestinal pathogens. *Nat Rev Immunol.* (2013) 13:790–801. doi: 10.1038/nri3535
8. Carding S, Verbeke K, Vipond DT, Corfe BM, Owen LJ. Dysbiosis of the gut microbiota in disease. *Microb Ecol Health Dis.* (2015) 26:26191. doi: 10.3402/mehd.v26.26191
9. Epaud R. An update on paediatric respiratory diseases. *Eur Respir Rev.* (2018) 27:180013. doi: 10.1183/16000617.0013-2018
10. Alimi Y, Lim WS, Lansbury L, Leonardi-Bee J, Nguyen-Van-Tam JS. Systematic review of respiratory viral pathogens identified in adults with community-acquired pneumonia in Europe. *J Clin Virol.* (2017) 95:26–35. doi: 10.1016/j.jcv.2017.07.019
11. Fogel N, Tuberculosis: A disease without boundaries. *Tuberculosis.* (2015) 95:527–531. doi: 10.1016/j.tube.2015.05.017
12. Ichinohe T, Pang IK, Kumamoto Y, Peaper DR, Ho JH, Murray TS. Microbiota regulates immune defense against respiratory tract influenza A virus infection. *Proc Natl Acad Sci USA.* (2011) 108:5354–9. doi: 10.1073/pnas.1019378108
13. Fagundes CT, Amaral FA, Vieira AT, Soares AC, Pinho V, Nicoli JR, et al. Transient TLR activation restores inflammatory response and ability to control pulmonary bacterial infection in germfree mice. *J Immunol.* (2012) 188:1411–20. doi: 10.4049/jimmunol.1101682
14. Abt MC, Osborne LC, Monticelli LA, Doering TA, Alenghat T, Sonnenberg GF, et al. Commensal bacteria calibrate the activation threshold of innate antiviral immunity. *Immunity.* (2012) 37:158–70. doi: 10.1016/j.immuni.2012.04.011
15. Brown RL, Sequeira RP, Clarke TB. The microbiota protects against respiratory infection via GM-CSF signaling. *Nat Commun.* (2017) 8:1512. doi: 10.1038/s41467-017-01803-x
16. Clarke TB, Early innate immunity to bacterial infection in the lung is regulated systemically by the commensal microbiota via nod-like receptor ligands. *Infect Immun.* (2014) 82:4596–606. doi: 10.1128/IAI.02212-14
17. Gauguet S, D'Ortona S, Ahnger-Pier K, Duan B, Surana NK, Lu R, et al. Intestinal microbiota of mice influences resistance to Staphylococcus *aureus* pneumonia. *Infect Immun.* (2015) 83:4003–14. doi: 10.1128/IAI.00037-15
18. Lankelma JM, Birnie E, Weehuizen AF, Scicluna BP, Belzer C, Houtkooper RH, et al. The gut microbiota as a modulator of innate immunity during melioidosis. *PLoS Neglect Trop D.* (2017) 11:e0005548. doi: 10.1371/journal.pntd.0005548
19. McAleer JP, Nguyen LH, Chen K, Kumar P, Ricks DM, Binnie M, et al. Pulmonary Th17 antifungal immunity is regulated by the gut microbiome. *J Immunol.* (2016) 197:97–107. doi: 10.4049/jimmunol.1502566
20. Samuelson DR, Welsh DA, Shellito JE. Regulation of lung immunity and host defense by the intestinal microbiota. *Front Microbiol.* (2015) 6:1085. doi: 10.3389/fmicb.2015.01085
21. Schuijt TJ, Lankelma JM, Scicluna BP, de Sousa e Melo F, Roelofs JJ, de Boer JD, et al. The gut microbiota plays a protective role in the host defence against pneumococcal pneumonia. *Gut.* (2016) 65:575–83. doi: 10.1136/gutjnl-2015-309728
22. Wu S, Jiang ZY, Sun YF, Yu B, Chen J, Dai CQ, et al. Microbiota regulates the TLR7 signaling pathway against respiratory tract influenza A virus infection. *Curr Microbiol.* (2013) 67:414–22. doi: 10.1007/s00284-013-0380-z
23. Chen LW, Chen PH, Hsu CM. Commensal microflora contribute to host defense against escherichia coli pneumonia through Toll-Like Receptors. *Shock.* (2011) 36:67–75. doi: 10.1097/SHK.0b013e3182184ee7
24. Khan N, Vidyarthi A, Nadeem S, Negi S, Nair G, Agrewala JN. Alteration in the gut microbiota provokes susceptibility to tuberculosis. *Front Immunol.* (2016) 7:529. doi: 10.3389/fimmu.2016.00529
25. Dumas A, Corral D, Colom A, Levillain F, Peixoto A, Hudrisier D, et al., The host microbiota contributes to early protection against lung colonization by *Mycobacterium tuberculosis*. *Front Immunol.* (2018) 9:2656. doi: 10.3389/fimmu.2018.02656
26. Rosshart SP, Vassallo BG, Angeletti D, Hutchinson DS, Morgan AP, Takeda K, et al. Wild mouse gut microbiota promotes host fitness and improves disease resistance. *Cell.* (2017) 171:1015–28.e13. doi: 10.1016/j.cell.2017.09.016
27. Kennedy EA, King KY, Baldridge MT. Mouse microbiota models: comparing germ-free mice and antibiotics treatment as tools for modifying gut bacteria. *Front Physiol.* (2018) 9:1534. doi: 10.3389/fphys.2018.01534
28. Mathieu E, Escribano-Vazquez U, Descamps D, Cherbuy C, Langella P, Riffault S, et al. Paradigms of lung microbiota functions in health and disease, particularly, in asthma. *Front Physiol.* (2018) 9:1168. doi: 10.3389/fphys.2018.01168
29. Hilty M, Burke C, Pedro H, Cardenas P, Bush A, Bossley C, et al. Disordered microbial communities in asthmatic airways. *PLoS ONE.* (2010) 5:e8578. doi: 10.1371/journal.pone.0008578
30. Venkataraman A, Bassis CM, Beck JM, Young VB, Curtis JL, Huffnagle GB, et al. Application of a neutral community model to assess structuring of the human lung microbiome. *MBio.* (2015) 6:e02284-14. doi: 10.1128/mBio.02284-14
31. Le Noci V, Guglielmetti S, Arioli S, Camisaschi C, Bianchi F, Sommariva M, et al. Modulation of pulmonary microbiota by antibiotic or probiotic aerosol therapy: a strategy to promote immunosurveillance against lung metastases. *Cell Rep.* (2018) 24:3528–38. doi: 10.1016/j.celrep.2018.08.090
32. Zarogoulidis P, Kioumis I, Porpodis K, Spyratos D, Tsakiridis K, Huang H, et al. Clinical experimentation with aerosol antibiotics: current and future methods of administration. *Drug Des Devel Ther.* (2013) 7:1115–34. doi: 10.2147/DDDT.S51303
33. Iwabuchi N, Xiao JZ, Yaeshima T, Iwatsuki K. Oral administration of bifidobacterium longum ameliorates influenza virus infection in mice. *Biol Pharm Bull.* (2011) 34:1352–5. doi: 10.1248/bpb.34.1352
34. Kawase M, He F, Kubota A, Yoda K, Miyazawa K, Hiramatsu M. Heat-killed *Lactobacillus gasseri* TMC0356 protects mice against influenza virus infection by stimulating gut and respiratory immune responses. *FEMS Immunol Med Microbiol.* (2012) 64:280–8. doi: 10.1111/j.1574-695X.2011.00903.x
35. Zelaya H, Tada A, Vizoso-Pinto MG, Salva S, Kanmani P, Aguero G, et al. Nasal priming with immunobiotic Lactobacillus rhamnosus modulates inflammation-coagulation interactions and reduces influenza virus-associated pulmonary damage. *Inflamm Res.* (2015) 64:589–602. doi: 10.1007/s00011-015-0837-6
36. Waki N, Yajima N, Suganuma H, Buddle BM, Luo D, Heiser A, et al. Oral administration of Lactobacillus brevis KB290 to mice alleviates clinical symptoms following influenza virus infection. *Lett Appl Microbiol.* (2014) 58:87–93. doi: 10.1111/lam.12160
37. Chiba E, Tomosada Y, Vizoso-Pinto MG, Salva S, Takahashi T, Tsukida K, et al. Immunobiotic *Lactobacillus rhamnosus* improves resistance of infant mice against respiratory syncytial virus infection. *Int Immunopharmacol.* (2013) 17:373–82. doi: 10.1016/j.intimp.2013.06.024
38. Tomosada Y, Chiba E, Zelaya H, Takahashi T, Tsukida K, Kitazawa H, et al. Nasally administered *Lactobacillus rhamnosus* strains differentially modulate respiratory antiviral immune responses and induce protection against respiratory syncytial virus infection. *BMC Immunol.* (2013) 14:40. doi: 10.1186/1471-2172-14-40
39. Kawahara T, Takahashi T, Oishi K, Tanaka H, Masuda M, Takahashi S, et al. Consecutive oral administration of Bifidobacterium longum MM-2 improves the defense system against influenza virus infection by enhancing natural killer cell activity in a murine model. *Microbiol Immunol.* (2015) 59:1–12. doi: 10.1111/1348-0421.12210
40. Vieira AT, Rocha VM, Tavares L, Garcia CC, Teixeira MM, Oliveira SC, et al. Control of Klebsiella pneumoniae pulmonary infection and immunomodulation by oral treatment with the commensal probiotic Bifidobacterium longum 5(1A). *Microbes Infect.* (2016) 18:180–9. doi: 10.1016/j.micinf.2015.10.008
41. Shekhar S, Khan R, Schenck K, Petersen FC. Intranasal immunization with the commensal Streptococcus mitis confers protective immunity against pneumococcal lung infection. *Appl Environ Microbiol.* (2019). 85:e02235-18. doi: 10.1128/AEM.02235-18

42. Majlessi L, Sayes F, Bureau JF, Pawlik A, Michel V, Jouvion G, et al. Colonization with Helicobacter is concomitant with modified gut microbiota and drastic failure of the immune control of *Mycobacterium tuberculosis*. *Mucosal Immunol.* (2017) 10:1178–89. doi: 10.1038/mi.2016.140
43. Arnold IC, Hutchings C, Kondova I, Hey A, Powrie F, Beverley P, et al. Helicobacter hepaticus infection in BALB/c mice abolishes subunit-vaccine-induced protection against *M. tuberculosis*. *Vaccine.* (2015) 33:1808–14. doi: 10.1016/j.vaccine.2015.02.041
44. La Mantia I, Varricchio A, Ciprandi G. Bacteriotherapy with *Streptococcus salivarius* 24SMB and Streptococcus oralis 89a nasal spray for preventing recurrent acute otitis media in children: a real-life clinical experience. *Int J Gen Med.* (2017) 10:171–5. doi: 10.2147/IJGM.S137614
45. Marchisio P, Santagati M, Scillato M, Baggi E, Fattizzo M, Rosazza C, et al. *Streptococcus salivarius* 24SMB administered by nasal spray for the prevention of acute otitis media in otitis-prone children. *Eur J Clin Microbiol Infect Dis.* (2015) 34:2377–83. doi: 10.1007/s10096-015-2491-x
46. Tano K, Hakansson EG, Holm SE, Hellstrom S. A nasal spray with alpha-haemolytic streptococci as long term prophylaxis against recurrent otitis media. *Int J Pediatr Otorhi.* (2002) 62:17–23. doi: 10.1016/S0165-5876(01)00581-X
47. Evans CM, Pratt CB, Matheson M, Vaughan TE, Findlow J, Borrow R, et al. Nasopharyngeal colonization by *Neisseria lactamica* and induction of protective immunity against *Neisseria meningitidis*. *Clin Infect Dis.* (2011) 52:70–7. doi: 10.1093/cid/ciq065
48. Deasy AM, Guccione E, Dale AP, Andrews N, Evans CM, Bennett JS, et al. Nasal inoculation of the commensal neisseria lactamica inhibits carriage of neisseria meningitidis by young adults: a controlled human infection study. *Clin Infect Dis.* (2015) 60:1512–20. doi: 10.1093/cid/civ098
49. Henriques-Normark B, Normark S. Commensal pathogens, with a focus on Streptococcus pneumoniae, and interactions with the human host. *Exp Cell Res.* (2010) 316:1408–14. doi: 10.1016/j.yexcr.2010.03.003
50. Teo SM, Mok D, Pham K, Kusel M, Serralha M, Troy N, et al. The infant nasopharyngeal microbiome impacts severity of lower respiratory infection and risk of asthma development. *Cell Host Microbe.* (2015) 17:704–15. doi: 10.1016/j.chom.2015.03.008
51. de Steenhuijsen Piters WA, Heinonen S, Hasrat R, Bunsow E, Smith B, Suarez-Arrabal MC, et al. Nasopharyngeal microbiota, host transcriptome, and disease severity in children with respiratory syncytial virus infection. *Am J Respir Crit Care Med.* (2016) 194:1104–15. doi: 10.1164/rccm.201602-0220OC
52. Arboleya S, Sanchez B, Milani C, Duranti S, Solis G, Fernandez N, et al. Intestinal microbiota development in preterm neonates and effect of perinatal antibiotics. *J Pediatr.* (2015) 166:538–44. doi: 10.1016/j.jpeds.2014.09.041
53. Kuppala VS, Meinzen-Derr J, Morrow AL, Schibler KR. Prolonged initial empirical antibiotic treatment is associated with adverse outcomes in premature infants. *J Pediatr.* (2011) 159:720–5. doi: 10.1016/j.jpeds.2011.05.033
54. Man WH, de Steenhuijsen Piters WA, Bogaert D, The microbiota of the respiratory tract: gatekeeper to respiratory health. *Nat Rev Microbiol.* (2017) 15:259–70. doi: 10.1038/nrmicro.2017.14
55. Ganal SC, Sanos SL, Kallfass C, Oberle K, Johner C, Kirschning C, et al. Priming of natural killer cells by nonmucosal mononuclear phagocytes requires instructive signals from commensal microbiota. *Immunity.* (2012) 37:171–86. doi: 10.1016/j.immuni.2012.05.020
56. Wang J, Li F, Sun R, Gao X, Wei H, Li LJ, et al. Bacterial colonization dampens influenza-mediated acute lung injury via induction of M2 alveolar macrophages. *Nat Commun.* (2013) 4:2106. doi: 10.1038/ncomms3106
57. Shekhar S, Khan R, Ferreira DM, Mitsi E, German E, Rorvik GH, et al. Antibodies reactive to commensal *Streptococcus mitis* show cross-reactivity with virulent *Streptococcus pneumoniae* serotypes. *Front Immunol.* (2018) 9:747. doi: 10.3389/fimmu.2018.00747
58. Shekhar S, Schenck K, Petersen FC. Exploring host-commensal interactions in the respiratory tract. *Front Immunol.* (2017) 8:1971. doi: 10.3389/fimmu.2017.01971
59. Skov Sorensen UB, Yao K, Yang Y, Tettelin H, Kilian M. Capsular polysaccharide expression in commensal streptococcus species: genetic and antigenic similarities to *Streptococcus pneumoniae*. *MBio.* (2016) 7: e01844-16. doi: 10.1128/mBio.01844-16
60. Engen SA, Rukke HV, Becattini S, Jarrossay D, Blix IJ, Petersen FC, et al. The oral commensal streptococcus mitis shows a mixed memory Th cell signature that is similar to and cross-reactive with *Streptococcus pneumoniae*. *PLoS ONE.* (2014) 9:e104306. doi: 10.1371/journal.pone.0104306
61. Dumas A, Bernard L, Poquet Y, Lugo-Villarino G, Neyrolles O. The role of the lung microbiota and the gut-lung axis in respiratory infectious diseases. *Cell Microbiol.* (2018) 20:e12966. doi: 10.1111/cmi.12966
62. Looft T, Allen HK. Collateral effects of antibiotics on mammalian gut microbiomes. *Gut Microbes.* (2012) 3:463–7. doi: 10.4161/gmic.21288
63. Sze MA, Tsuruta M, Yang SW, Oh Y, Man SF, Hogg JC, et al. Changes in the bacterial microbiota in gut, blood, and lungs following acute LPS instillation into mice lungs. *PLoS ONE.* (2014) 9:e111228. doi: 10.1371/journal.pone.0111228
64. Chu H, Mazmanian SK. Innate immune recognition of the microbiota promotes host-microbial symbiosis. *Nat Immunol.* (2013) 14:668–75. doi: 10.1038/ni.2635
65. Felix KM, Jaimez IA, Nguyen TV, Ma H, Raslan WA, Klinger CN, et al. Gut microbiota contributes to resistance against pneumococcal pneumonia in immunodeficient Rag(-/-) mice. *Front Cell Infect Microbiol.* (2018) 8:118. doi: 10.3389/fcimb.2018.00118
66. Gray J, Oehrle K, Worthen G, Alenghat T, Whitsett J, Deshmukh H. Intestinal commensal bacteria mediate lung mucosal immunity and promote resistance of newborn mice to infection. *Sci Transl Med.* (2017) 9:eaaf9412. doi: 10.1126/scitranslmed.aaf9412
67. Stubbendieck RM, Straight PD. Multifaceted interfaces of bacterial competition. *J Bacteriol.* (2016) 198:2145–55. doi: 10.1128/JB.00275-16
68. Iwase T, Uehara Y, Shinji H, Tajima A, Seo H, Takada K, et al. Staphylococcus epidermidis Esp inhibits Staphylococcus aureus biofilm formation and nasal colonization. *Nature.* (2010) 465:346-U100. doi: 10.1038/nature09074
69. Bomar L, Brugger SD, Yost BH, Davies SS, Lemon KP. *Corynebacterium accolens* releases antipneumococcal free fatty acids from human nostril and skin surface triacylglycerols. *Mbio.* (2016) 7:e01725-15. doi: 10.1128/mBio.01725-15
70. Ramsey MM, Freire MO, Gabrilska RA, Rumbaugh KP, Lemon KP. *Staphylococcus aureus* shifts toward commensalism in response to corynebacterium species. *Front Microbiol.* (2016) 7:1230. doi: 10.3389/fmicb.2016.01230
71. Santagati M, Scillato M, Patane F, Aiello C, Stefani S. Bacteriocin-producing oral streptococci and inhibition of respiratory pathogens. *FEMS Immunol Med Microbiol.* (2012) 65:23–31. doi: 10.1111/j.1574-695X.2012.00928.x
72. Janek D, Zipperer A, Kulik A, Krismer B, Peschel A. High frequency and diversity of antimicrobial activities produced by nasal staphylococcus strains against bacterial competitors. *PLoS Pathog.* (2016) 12:e1005812. doi: 10.1371/journal.ppat.1005812
73. Tagg JR, Streptococcal bacteriocin-like inhibitory substances: some personal insights into the bacteriocin-like activities produced by streptococci good and bad. *Probiot Antimicro.* (2009) 1:60–6. doi: 10.1007/s12602-008-9002-7
74. Walls T, Power D, Tagg J. Bacteriocin-like inhibitory substance (BLIS) production by the normal flora of the nasopharynx: potential to protect against otitis media? *J Med Microbiol.* (2003) 52:829–33. doi: 10.1099/jmm.0.05259-0
75. Wescombe PA, Heng CK, Burton JP, Chilcott CN, Tagg JR. *Streptococcal bacteriocins* and the case for *Streptococcus salivarius* as model oral probiotics. *Future Microbiol.* (2009) 4:819–35. doi: 10.2217/fmb.09.61
76. Manning J, Dunne EM, Wescombe PA, Hale JD, Mulholland EK, Tagg JR, et al. Investigation of *Streptococcus salivarius*-mediated inhibition of pneumococcal adherence to pharyngeal epithelial cells. *BMC Microbiol.* (2016) 16:225. doi: 10.1186/s12866-016-0843-z
77. Zipperer A, Konnerth MC, Laux C, Berscheid A, Janek D, Weidenmaier C, et al. Human commensals producing a novel antibiotic impair pathogen colonization. *Nature.* (2016) 535:511–6. doi: 10.1038/nature18634
78. Regev-Yochay G, Dagan R, Raz M, Carmeli Y, Shainberg B, Derazne E, et al. Association between carriage of *Streptococcus pneumoniae* and *Staphylococcus aureus* in children. *Jama-J Am Med Assoc.* (2004) 292:716–20. doi: 10.1001/jama.292.6.716
79. Bogaert D, van Belkum A, Sluijter M, Luijendijk A, de Groot R, Rumke HC, et al. Colonisation by *Streptococcus pneumoniae* and

Staphylococcus aureus in healthy children. *Lancet.* (2004) 363:1871–2. doi: 10.1016/S0140-6736(04)16357-5
80. Regev-Yochay G, Trzcinski K, Thompson CM, Malley R, Lipsitch M. Interference between *Streptococcus pneumoniae* and *Staphylococcus aureus: in vitro* hydrogen peroxide-mediated killing by *Streptococcus pneumoniae. J Bacteriol.* (2006) 188:4996–5001. doi: 10.1128/JB.00317-06
81. Kamada N, Chen GY, Inohara N, Nunez G. Control of pathogens and pathobionts by the gut microbiota. *Nat Immunol.* (2013) 14:685–90. doi: 10.1038/ni.2608
82. Stubbendieck RM, May DS, Chevrette MG, Temkin MI, Wendt-Pienkowski E, Cagnazzo J, et al. Competition among nasal bacteria suggests a role for siderophore-mediated interactions in shaping the human nasal microbiota. *Appl Environ Microbiol.* (2018) AEM.02406–18. doi: 10.1128/AEM.02406-18
83. Park B, Iwase T, Liu GY. Intranasal application of S. epidermidis prevents colonization by methicillin-resistant *Staphylococcus aureus* in mice. *PLoS ONE.* (2011) 6:e25880. doi: 10.1371/journal.pone.0025880

Permissions

All chapters in this book were first published by Frontiers; hereby published with permission under the Creative Commons Attribution License or equivalent. Every chapter published in this book has been scrutinized by our experts. Their significance has been extensively debated. The topics covered herein carry significant findings which will fuel the growth of the discipline. They may even be implemented as practical applications or may be referred to as a beginning point for another development.

The contributors of this book come from diverse backgrounds, making this book a truly international effort. This book will bring forth new frontiers with its revolutionizing research information and detailed analysis of the nascent developments around the world.

We would like to thank all the contributing authors for lending their expertise to make the book truly unique. They have played a crucial role in the development of this book. Without their invaluable contributions this book wouldn't have been possible. They have made vital efforts to compile up to date information on the varied aspects of this subject to make this book a valuable addition to the collection of many professionals and students.

This book was conceptualized with the vision of imparting up-to-date information and advanced data in this field. To ensure the same, a matchless editorial board was set up. Every individual on the board went through rigorous rounds of assessment to prove their worth. After which they invested a large part of their time researching and compiling the most relevant data for our readers.

The editorial board has been involved in producing this book since its inception. They have spent rigorous hours researching and exploring the diverse topics which have resulted in the successful publishing of this book. They have passed on their knowledge of decades through this book. To expedite this challenging task, the publisher supported the team at every step. A small team of assistant editors was also appointed to further simplify the editing procedure and attain best results for the readers.

Apart from the editorial board, the designing team has also invested a significant amount of their time in understanding the subject and creating the most relevant covers. They scrutinized every image to scout for the most suitable representation of the subject and create an appropriate cover for the book.

The publishing team has been an ardent support to the editorial, designing and production team. Their endless efforts to recruit the best for this project, has resulted in the accomplishment of this book. They are a veteran in the field of academics and their pool of knowledge is as vast as their experience in printing. Their expertise and guidance has proved useful at every step. Their uncompromising quality standards have made this book an exceptional effort. Their encouragement from time to time has been an inspiration for everyone.

The publisher and the editorial board hope that this book will prove to be a valuable piece of knowledge for researchers, students, practitioners and scholars across the globe.

List of Contributors

Nian-Zhang Zhang, Meng Wang, Jun-Ling Hou, Jin-Lei Wang and Fu-Kai Zhang
State Key Laboratory of Veterinary Etiological Biology, Key Laboratory of Veterinary Parasitology of Gansu Province, Lanzhou Veterinary Research Institute, Chinese Academy of Agricultural Sciences, Lanzhou, China

Qi Gao
State Key Laboratory of Veterinary Etiological Biology, Key Laboratory of Veterinary Parasitology of Gansu Province, Lanzhou Veterinary Research Institute, Chinese Academy of Agricultural Sciences, Lanzhou, China
Hunan Entry-Exit Inspection and Quarantine Bureau, Changsha, China

Ling-Ying Hu
Fujian Yongcheng Agricultural and Animal Husbandry Sci-Tech Group, Fuzhou, China

Xing-Quan Zhu
State Key Laboratory of Veterinary Etiological Biology, Key Laboratory of Veterinary Parasitology of Gansu Province, Lanzhou Veterinary Research Institute, Chinese Academy of Agricultural Sciences, Lanzhou, China
Jiangsu Co-innovation Center for the Prevention and Control of Important Animal Infectious Diseases and Zoonoses, College of Veterinary Medicine, Yangzhou University, Yangzhou, China

Hany M. Elsheikha
Faculty of Medicine and Health Sciences, School of Veterinary Medicine and Science, University of Nottingham, Loughborough, United Kingdom

Bo Wang
Department of Mathematics, University of Leicester, Leicester, United Kingdom

Jinfeng Liu and Fangli Lu
Department of Parasitology, Zhongshan School of Medicine, Sun Yat-sen University, Guangzhou, China
Key Laboratory of Tropical Disease Control of Ministry of Education, Sun Yat-sen University, Guangzhou, China

Shiguang Huang
School of Stomatology, Jinan University, Guangzhou, China

Young Sang Hwang, Ji-Hun Shin and Jung-Pyo Yang
Department of Parasitology and Tropical Medicine, Seoul National University College of Medicine, and Institute of Endemic Diseases, Seoul National University, Seoul, South Korea

Bong-Kwang Jung
Department of Parasitology and Tropical Medicine, Seoul National University College of Medicine, and Institute of Endemic Diseases, Seoul National University, Seoul, South Korea
Institute of Parasitic Diseases, Korea Association of Health Promotion, Seoul, South Korea

Sang Hyung Lee
Department of Neurosurgery, Seoul National University College of Medicine, SMG-SNU Boramae Medical Center, Seoul, South Korea

Eun-Hee Shin
Department of Parasitology and Tropical Medicine, Seoul National University College of Medicine, and Institute of Endemic Diseases, Seoul National University, Seoul, South Korea
Seoul National University Bundang Hospital, Seongnam, South Korea

Yuli Cheng, Xing Zhu, Xiaohuan Wang, Qinghui Zhuang, Xu Huyan, Ximeng Sun, Jingjing Huang and Xinping Zhu
Department of Medical Microbiology and Parasitology, School of Basic Medical Sciences, Capital Medical University, Beijing, China

Bin Zhan
Department of Pediatrics, National School of Tropical Medicine, Baylor College of Medicine, Houston, TX, United States

Hironori Bando, Youngae Lee, Ji Su Ma, Shun Tanaka, Miwa Sasai and Masahiro Yamamoto
Department of Immunoparasitology, Research Institute for Microbial Diseases, Osaka University, Osaka, Japan
Laboratory of Immunoparasitology, WPI Immunology Frontier Research Center, Osaka University, Osaka, Japan

Naoya Sakaguchi and Ariel Pradipta
Department of Immunoparasitology, Research Institute for Microbial Diseases, Osaka University, Osaka, Japan

De-Hua Lai and Zhao-Rong Lun
State Key Laboratory of Biocontrol, Center for Parasitic Organisms, School of Life Sciences, Guangzhou, China

Jianfa Liu
Department of Pathology and Pathogenic Biology, Medical College of Ningbo University, Ningbo, China

Yoshifumi Nishikawa
National Research Center for Protozoan Diseases, Obihiro University of Agriculture and Veterinary Medicine, Obihiro, Japan

Ximena Volpini, Laura F. Ambrosio, Laura Fozzatti, Constanza Insfran, Cinthia C. Stempin, Laura Cervi and Claudia Cristina Motran
Departamento de Bioquímica Clínica, Facultad de Ciencias Químicas, Universidad Nacional de Córdoba, Córdoba, Argentina
Centro de Investigaciones en Bioquímica Clínica e Inmunología (CIBICI), CONICET, Haya de la Torre y Medina Allende, Ciudad Universitaria, Córdoba, Argentina

Juliana Barreto de Albuquerque and Jens V. Stein
Theodor Kocher Institute, University of Bern, Bern, Switzerland

Danielle Silva dos Santos
Laboratory on Thymus Research, Oswaldo Cruz Institute, Oswaldo Cruz Foundation, Rio de Janeiro, Brazil

Juliana de Meis
Laboratory on Thymus Research, Oswaldo Cruz Institute, Oswaldo Cruz Foundation, Rio de Janeiro, Brazil
National Institute of Science and Technology on Neuroimmunomodulation (INCT-NIM), Rio de Janeiro, Brazil

Friederike Ebner, Ankur Midha and Susanne Hartmann
Department of Veterinary Medicine, Institute of Immunology, Freie Universität Berlin, Berlin, Germany

Mathias Kuhring
Bioinformatics Unit (MF1), Department for Methods Development and Research Infrastructure, Robert Koch Institute, Berlin, Germany
Core Unit Bioinformatics, Berlin Institute of Health (BIH), Berlin, Germany
Berlin Institute of Health Metabolomics Platform, Berlin Institute of Health (BIH), Berlin, Germany
Max Delbrück Center (MDC) for Molecular Medicine, Berlin, Germany

Aleksandar Radonić
Center for Biological Threats and Special Pathogens: Highly Pathogenic Viruses (ZBS 1), Robert Koch Institute, Berlin, Germany

Bernhard Y. Renard
Bioinformatics Unit (MF1), Department for Methods Development and Research Infrastructure, Robert Koch Institute, Berlin, Germany

Muhammad Ehsan, WenJuan Wang, Javaid Ali Gadahi, Muhammad Waqqas Hasan, MingMin Lu, YuJian Wang, XinChao Liu, Muhammad Haseeb, RuoFeng Yan, LiXin Xu, XiaoKai Song and XiangRui Li
Department of Preventive Veterinary Medicine, College of Veterinary Medicine, Nanjing Agricultural University, Nanjing, China

Ningbo Xia, Taifang Zhou, Xiaohan Liang, Shu Ye, Pengfei Zhao, Jichao Yang and Yanqin Zhou
State Key Laboratory of Agricultural Microbiology, Huazhong Agricultural University, Wuhan, China

Junlong Zhao
State Key Laboratory of Agricultural Microbiology, Huazhong Agricultural University, Wuhan, China
Hubei Cooperative Innovation Center for Sustainable Pig Production, Wuhan, China
Key Laboratory of Preventive Medicine in Hubei Province, Wuhan, China

Bang Shen
State Key Laboratory of Agricultural Microbiology, Huazhong Agricultural University, Wuhan, China
Key Laboratory of Preventive Medicine in Hubei Province, Wuhan, China

Fana Alem Kidane, Taniya Mitra, Patricia Wernsdorf and Dieter Liebhart
Clinic for Poultry and Fish Medicine, Department for Farm Animals and Veterinary Public Health, University of Veterinary Medicine Vienna, Vienna, Austria

Michael Hess
Clinic for Poultry and Fish Medicine, Department for Farm Animals and Veterinary Public Health, University of Veterinary Medicine Vienna, Vienna, Austria
Christian Doppler Laboratory for Innovative Poultry Vaccines, University of Veterinary Medicine Vienna, Vienna, Austria

Cong Wang, Qian Yu, Tian Xing, Shoubin Chen, Lei Liu, Li Yu, Jian Du and Qingli Luo
Department of Pathogen Biology, Provincial Laboratories of Pathogen Biology and Zoonoses, School of Basic Medicine, Anhui Medical University, Hefei, China

Weisheng Cheng
Department of Medical Genetics, Zhongshan School of Medicine, Sun Yat-sen University, The Key Laboratory of Tropical Disease Control, Ministry of Education, Guangzhou, China

Jilong Shen and Yuanhong Xu
Department of Pathogen Biology, Provincial Laboratories of Pathogen Biology and Zoonoses, School of Basic Medicine, Anhui Medical University, Hefei, China
Department of Clinical Laboratory, The First Affiliated Hospital of Anhui Medical University, Hefei, China

Radheshyam Maurya
Department of Animal Biology, School of Life Science, University of Hyderabad, Hyderabad, India

Parna Bhattacharya, Ranadhir Dey and Hira L. Nakhasi
Division of Emerging and Transfusion Transmitted Diseases, Center for Biologics Evaluation and Research, Food and Drug Administration, Silver Spring, MD, United States

Anuradha Rajamanickam, Saravanan Munisankar and Yukthi Bhootra
National Institutes of Health - National Institute of Research in Tuberculosis (ICMR) - International Center for Excellence in Research, Chennai, India

Chandra Kumar Dolla
National Institute of Research in Tuberculosis (ICMR), Chennai, India

Thomas B. Nutman
Laboratory of Parasitic Diseases, National Institute of Allergy and Infectious Diseases, National Institutes of Health, Bethesda, MD, United States

Subash Babu
National Institutes of Health - National Institute of Research in Tuberculosis (ICMR) - International Center for Excellence in Research, Chennai, India
Laboratory of Parasitic Diseases, National Institute of Allergy and Infectious Diseases, National Institutes of Health, Bethesda, MD, United States

E. Jane Homan and Robert D. Bremel
EigenBio LLC, Madison, WI, United States

Hong-Yu Cheng, Meng-Xia Ning, De-Kun Chen and Wen-Tao Ma

Veterinary Immunology Laboratory, College of Veterinary Medicine, Northwest Agriculture and Forestry University, Yangling, China

Rabia Khan, Fernanda Cristina Petersen and Sudhanshu Shekhar

Faculty of Dentistry, Institute of Oral Biology, University of Oslo, Oslo, Norway

Index

www.ingramcontent.com/pod-product-compliance
Lightning Source LLC
LaVergne TN
LVHW082157200926
848484LV00008B/2175